Temporary Anchorage Devices
in ORTHODONTICS

Temporary Anchorage Devices in ORTHODONTICS

Ravindra Nanda, BDS, MDS, PhD
UConn Orthodontic Alumni Endowed Chair
Professor and Head
Department of Craniofacial Sciences
Chair, Division of Orthodontics
School of Dental Medicine
University of Connecticut Health Center
Farmington, Connecticut

Flavio Andres Uribe, DDS
Assistant Professor
Division of Orthodontics
Department of Craniofacial Sciences
School of Dental Medicine
University of Connecticut Health Center
Farmington, Connecticut

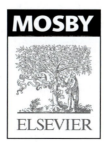

11830 Westline Industrial Drive
St. Louis, Missouri 63146

TEMPORARY ANCHORAGE DEVICES IN ORTHODONTICS   ISBN: 978-0-323-04807-1

Copyright © 2009 by Mosby, Inc., an affiliate of Elsevier Inc.

All rights reserved. No part of this publication may be reproduced or transmitted in any form or by any means, electronic or mechanical, including photocopy, recording, or any information storage and retrieval system, without permission in writing from the publisher. Permissions may be sought directly from Elsevier's Rights Department: phone: (+1) 215 239 3804 (US) or (+44) 1865 843830 (UK); fax: (+44) 1865 853333; e-mail: healthpermissions@elsevier.com. You may also complete your request on-line via the Elsevier website at http://www.elsevier.com/permissions.

Notice

Neither the Publisher nor the Authors assume any responsibility for any loss or injury and/or damage to persons or property arising out of or related to any use of the material contained in this book. It is the responsibility of the treating practitioner, relying on independent expertise and knowledge of the patient, to determine the best treatment and method of application for the patient.

The Publisher

Library of Congress Control Number 2008920327

ISBN: 978-0-323-04807-1

Vice President and Publisher: Linda Duncan
Senior Editor: John J. Dolan
Developmental Editor: Courtney Sprehe
Publishing Services Manager: Patricia Tannian
Senior Project Manager: Anne Altepeter
Text Designer: Paula Catalano
Cover Design Direction: Paula Catalano

Printed in China

Last digit is the print number: 9 8 7 6 5 4 3 2

Working together to grow libraries in developing countries

www.elsevier.com | www.bookaid.org | www.sabre.org

ELSEVIER   BOOK AID International   Sabre Foundation

To Catherine, for all of the love and support you have given me

To Renu, Seema, Anjuli, and my grandchildren; you make every day of my life a pleasure

Contributors

Ahu Acar, DDS, PhD
Associate Professor
Department of Orthodontics
Faculty of Dentistry
Marmara University
Istanbul, Turkey

George Anka, DDS, MS
Associate Professor
Department of Orthodontics
Nihon University Dental College
Tokyo, Japan
Head Orthodontist
Sekido Orthodontic Office
Tama-shi, Tokyo, Japan

Peter R. Diedrich, Prof Dr Dr
Department of Orthodontics
University of Aachen
Aachen, Germany

Nejat Erverdi, DDS, PhD
Professor
Department of Orthodontics
Faculty of Dentistry
Marmara University
Istanbul, Turkey

Ulrike B. Fritz, Prof Dr
Department of Orthodontics
University of Aachen
Aachen, Germany

Peter Göellner, Dr med dent
Department of Orthodontics
University of Berne
Berne, Switzerland
Private Orthodontic Practice
Berne, Switzerland

Britta A. Jung, Dr med dent
Department of Orthodontics
Johannes Gutenberg-University Mainz
Mainz, Germany

Ryuzo Kanomi, DDS, PhD
Private Practice, Orthodontics
Himeji, Japan

Hiroshi Kawamura, DDS, DDSc
Professor and Chair
Department of Maxillofacial Surgery
Tohoku University
Sendai, Miyagi, Japan

Martin Kunkel, Prof Dr med, Dr med dent
Senior Consultant
Department of Oral and Maxillofacial Surgery
Johannes Gutenberg-University Mainz
Mainz, Germany

Morten Godtfredsen Laursen, DDS
Clinical Assistant Professor
Department of Orthodontics
University of Aarhus
Aarhus, Denmark
Certified Specialist in Orthodontics
Private and Community Orthodontic Practice
Aarhus, Denmark

Kee-Joon Lee, DDS, PhD
Assistant Professor
Department of Orthodontics
College of Dentistry
Yonsei University
Seoul, Korea

James Cheng-Yi Lin, DDS
Clinical Assistant Professor
Department of Orthodontics and Pediatric Dentistry
School of Dentistry
National Defense Medical University
Taipei, Taiwan
Attending Orthodontist
Department of Orthodontics and Craniofacial
Dentistry
Chang Gung Memorial Hospital
Taipei, Taiwan
Dr. James Lin and Associates' Orthodontic and
Implant Center (private practice)
Taipei, Taiwan

Eric Jein-Wein Liou, DDS, MS
Associate Professor
Department of Orthodontics
Graduate School of Craniofacial Medicine
Chang Gung University
Taoyung, Taiwan
Associate Professor and Director
Department of Orthodontics and Craniofacial
Dentistry
Chang Gung Memorial Hospital
Taipei, Taiwan

Birte Melsen, Dr Odont, DDS
Professor
Department of Orthodontics
University of Aarhus
School of Dentistry
Aarhus, Denmark

Kuniaki Miyajima, DDS, MS, PhD
Adjunct Professor
Department of Orthodontics
St. Louis University Center for Advanced Dental Education
St. Louis, Missouri

Hiroshi Nagasaka, DDS, DDSc
Clinical Professor
Department of Maxillofacial Surgery
Tohoku University
Sendai, Miyagi, Japan
Director
Department of Oral Surgery
Miyagi Children's Hospital
Sendai, Miyagi, Japan

Ravindra Nanda, BDS, MDS, PhD
UConn Orthodontic Alumni Endowed Chair
Professor and Head
Department of Craniofacial Sciences
Chair, Division of Orthodontics
School of Dental Medicine
University of Connecticut Health Center
Farmington, Connecticut

Makoto Nishimura, DDS, DDSc
Part-Time Lecturer
Division of Oral Dysfunction Science
Department of Oral Health and Development Sciences
Graduate School of Dentisty
Tohoku University
Sendai, Japan
Orthodontic Faculty
SAS Orthodontic Centre
Ichiban-cho Dental Office
Sendai, Miyagi, Japan

Hyo-Sang Park, DDS, MS, PhD
Associate Professor
Department of Orthodontics
Kyungpook National University
School of Dentistry
Daegu, Korea
Clinical Director in the Student Clinic
Department of Orthodontics
Kyungpook University Hospital
Daegu, Korea

Young-Chel Park, DDS, PhD
Professor and Dean
Department of Orthodontics
College of Dentistry
Yonsei University
Seoul, Korea

A. Korrodi Ritto, DDS, PhD
Private Practice
Leiria, Portugal

Jeffery A. Roberts, DDS, MSD
Private Practice
Roberts Orthodontics
Indianapolis, Indiana

W. Eugene Roberts, DDS, PhD, DHC(Med)
Jarabak Professor and Head
Section of Orthodontics
Indiana University School of Dentistry
Indianapolis, Indiana
Associate Professor
Department of Oral and Maxillofacial Implantology
University of Lille II
Faculty of Medicine
Lille, France

Junji Sugawara, DDS, DDSc
Visiting Clinical Professor
Division of Orthodontics
Department of Craniofacial Science
School of Dental Medicine
University of Connecticut
Farmington, Connecticut
Director
SAS Orthodontic Centre
Ichiban-cho Dental Office
Sendai, Miyagi, Japan

Flavio Andres Uribe, DDS
Assistant Professor
Division of Orthodontics
Department of Craniofacial Sciences
School of Dental Medicine
University of Connecticut Health Center
Farmington, Connecticut

Serdar Üşümez, DDS, PhD
Associate Professor and Chair
Department of Orthodontics
Gaziantep University
Faculty of Dentistry
Gaziantep, Turkey

Sunil Wadhwa, DDS
Assistant Professor
Department of Craniofacial Sciences
University of Connecticut
School of Dental Medicine
Farmington, Connecticut

Heiner Wehrbein, Prof Dr med, Dr med dent
Professor and Head
Department of Orthodontics
Johannes Gutenberg-University Mainz
Mainz, Germany

Preface

Patient compliance, anchorage preservation, and lack of anchor units often present a perplexing problem for orthodontists, mainly because of a lack of effective devices. Headgear, which is used to control anchorage and requires patient cooperation, is a device that has been used in orthodontics for at least 100 years. Despite longevity in the field, however, the use of headgear has enjoyed only moderate success. In recent years, with the introduction of temporary anchorage devices (TADs), a paradigm shift has occurred in the overall perspective toward patient compliance, preservation of anchorage, and facilitation of treatment for various difficult malocclusions. As happens with every innovation, the learning curve is steep as a result of lack of evidence-based prospective studies related to stability, applications, and long-term results.

No one person can claim to be an expert in the application of TADs, since the technique is young and results are still short term. For this reason, I invited clinicians who have been instrumental in pioneering this technique to participate in the creation of this book. They have helped me to compile a book that is clear and concise in describing some of the basic principles involved in the application of TADs for different types of malocclusions. The book is not designed to be an exhaustive compendium of every application of TADs that has been reported. Instead, the primary emphasis is on the detailed description of methods that have been shown to be successful and have the potential to become mainstream in clinical orthodontics. The text will appeal to both academics and clinicians, since equal importance has been given to both theoretical and practical aspects. Each chapter covers its topics in great detail and is accompanied by extensive illustrations and references.

ORGANIZATION

Part I, Biological Perspective, addresses the use of endosseous miniscrews and the biological response to TADs. Chapter 1 reviews the historical perspective of implant development relative to the current concepts of bone physiology, surgery, healing, and integration. It is written to help clinicians develop a scientific perspective for the effective use of miniscrews. Chapter 2 looks at bone biology and the factors that predict stability behind mechanically retained and osseous-integrated orthodontic TADs.

Part II, Diagnosis and Treatment Planning, looks at these aspects for orthodontic cases that require skeletal anchorage. Chapter 3 reviews ideal sites for the placement of mini-implants and how to apply orthodontic force using three-dimensional finite element models (3D FEM). Chapter 4 provides a unique perspective of the K-1 system, since the chapter author designed the K-1 System. Chapter 5 details what factors should be addressed when deciding to use skeletal anchorage, including the indications for when skeletal anchorage should be used and the possible failures and adverse effects.

Part III, Biomechanics Considerations, offers pragmatic discussions regarding the application of sound biomechanical principles involved in moving teeth with the help of skeletal anchorage. Chapter 6 addresses the fundamental biomechanical principles of miniscrew-driven orthodontics and explains the practical application of these principles. Chapter 7 reviews different clinical scenarios in which skeletal anchorage may provide an advantage to conventional treatment mechanics.

Part IV, Anchorage Device Systems and Clinical Applications, explores the different types of anchorage device systems and the "clinical applications" of these systems, with an emphasis on practical applications and avoidance of common mistakes and pitfalls. Chapter 8 addresses the appliances, mechanics, and treatment strategies for orthognathic-like orthodontics in Class I and II dentoalveolar protrusion, Class III dentoalveolar protrusion, anterior open bite, and Class II mandibular retrognathism. Chapter 9 details the management of the occlusal plane using TADs and looks at the dimensions of occlusal plane in space and force application and devices. Chapter 10 reviews the treatment limitations that come with missing teeth, tooth movement using TADs, and congenital missing teeth. Chapter 11 addresses various methods for bone anchorage, including microimplants, resorbable screws, bracket head–type microimplants, and noninvasive miniplates. Chapter 12 provides information on mini- or micro-screw implants. Chapter 13 details the advantages and disadvantage of using titanium microscrews, as well as screw design, implant insertion, typical implant sites, complications, and failure rates. Chapter 14 looks at the use of conventional dental implants versus TADs for orthodontic anchorage.

Part V, Skeletal Anchorage, concludes the book by looking specifically at the different aspects of skeletal anchorage. Chapter 15 addresses the features of orthodontic miniplates and screws, indications for skeletal anchorage systems (SAS) treatment, timing of treatment, positioning of miniplates, orthodontic mechanics of SAS, and surgical procedures for implantation and removal of miniplates. Chapter 16 details the clinical use of different orthodontic implants to correct different malocclusions. The treatment methods presented in this chapter are compared with the conventional method and the benefits of the implant method are clarified.

Chapter 17 reviews the anatomical considerations in palatal implant placement, radiographic evaluation of bone height at the implant site, preparation of the surgical template for positioning the implant, the surgical method, evaluation of the implant placement method, and various orthodontic mechanics used with palatal implants. Chapter 18 looks at commonly used skeletal orthodontic anchorage devices and discusses their clinical use and potential benefits. Specifically, the chapter focuses on the use of palatal implants for orthodontic treatment tasks.

CONTRIBUTORS

The authors who have contributed to this book are clinically active; many of them are engaged in clinical and laboratory research in bone biology, tooth movement, clinical orthodontics, and biomechanics. Therefore, most of the arguments put forward in this textbook are based on current research findings. However, when conclusive evidence was not available, we presented a consensus founded on a significant depth of experience and available scientific data.

NOTE FROM THE EDITOR

I was fortunate to work with a group of authors who are among the most prominent in the field of orthodontics. We hope that our efforts will serve as a stimulus for further research in this increasingly important area of clinical orthodontics and also provide the much-needed impetus toward general acceptability of TADs in day-to-day orthodontics.

Ravindra Nanda

Acknowledgments

I owe a heartfelt thanks to my contributors. Without their cooperation, this effort could not have come to fruition. They are innovators, scientists, and super clinicians in the truest sense, and they have helped to pioneer a new way to address the correction of malocclusions. I hope they will appreciate the final result and will forget about my constant pleas to meet deadlines.

Flavio Uribe deserves special recognition for helping me prepare this book during every stage of its development. I am very fortunate to have a colleague like him, who in his own right is a thoughtful clinician and a prolific writer. A special thanks to Sunil Wadhwa for his advice and comments, which were easy to incorporate in development of the book.

I also express my gratitude both to Gaby Hricko, who during her residency did exhaustive literature research that was instrumental in helping me decide on potential contributors, and Madhur Upadhyay, who helped me in the final stages of preparing the manuscript, especially with proofreading of various chapters.

A book like this is not possible without the encouragement of the publisher. I express my sincere thanks to Senior Editor John Dolan for taking up this project and helping me at every step, and my deep gratitude to Courtney Sprehe, my developmental editor, for being the driving force for this book from day one.

Ravindra Nanda

Contents

Part I   **BIOLOGICAL PERSPECTIVE**

Chapter 1   Endosseous Miniscrews: Historical, Vascular, and Integration Perspectives, 3
W. Eugene Roberts and Jeffery A. Roberts

Chapter 2   Biological Response to Orthodontic Temporary Anchorage Devices, 14
Sunil Wadhwa and Ravindra Nanda

Part II   **DIAGNOSIS AND TREATMENT PLANNING**

Chapter 3   Radiographic Evaluation of Bone Sites for Mini-Implant Placement, 25
Kuniaki Miyajima

Chapter 4   Miniature Osseointegrated Implants for Orthodontics Anchorage, 49
Ryuzo Kanomi and W. Eugene Roberts

Chapter 5   Factors in the Decision to Use Skeletal Anchorage, 73
Birte Melsen and Morten Godtfredsen Laursen

Part III   **BIOMECHANICS CONSIDERATIONS**

Chapter 6   Biomechanical Principles in Miniscrew-Driven Orthodontics, 93
Young-Chel Park and Kee-Joon Lee

Chapter 7   Skeletal Anchorage Based on Biomechanics, 145
Flavio Andres Uribe and Ravindra Nanda

Part IV   **ANCHORAGE DEVICE SYSTEMS AND CLINICAL APPLICATIONS**

Chapter 8   Appliances, Mechanics, and Treatment Strategies Toward Orthognathic-Like Treatment Results, 167
Eric Jein-Wein Liou and James Cheng-Yi Lin

Chapter 9   Controlled Occlusal Plane Changes Using Temporary Anchorage Devices, 198
George Anka

Chapter 10   Management of Missing Teeth Using Temporary Anchorage Devices, 223
George Anka

Chapter 11   Skeletal Anchorage: Different Approaches, 238
A. Korrodi Ritto

Chapter 12   Clinical Application of Microimplants, 260
Hyo-Sang Park

Chapter 13   Clinical Suitability of Titanium Microscrews for Orthodontic Anchorage, 287
Ulrike B. Fritz and Peter R. Diedrich

Chapter 14   Treatment Planning with Endosseous Implants for Orthodontic Anchorage and Prosthodontic Restorations, 295
Flavio Andres Uribe and Ravindra Nanda

Part V   **SKELETAL ANCHORAGE**

Chapter 15   Skeletal Anchorage System Using Orthodontic Miniplates, 317
Junji Sugawara, Makoto Nishimura, Hiroshi Nagasaka, and Hiroshi Kawamura

Chapter 16   Bone Anchorage: a New Concept in Orthodontics, 342
Nejat Erverdi and Serdar Üşümez

Chapter 17   Palatal Anchorage, 374
Nejat Erverdi and Ahu Acar

Chapter 18   Skeletal Anchorage in Orthodontics Using Palatal Implants, 392
Heiner Wehrbein, Britta A. Jung, Martin Kunkel, and Peter Göellner

PART I
BIOLOGICAL PERSPECTIVE

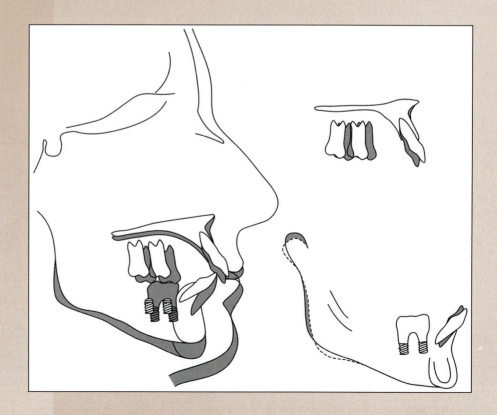

CHAPTER 1

Endosseous Miniscrews: Historical, Vascular, and Integration Perspectives

W. Eugene Roberts and Jeffery A. Roberts

The explosive development of temporary anchorage devices (TADs) presents a professional dilemma for orthodontists. Although a large body of evidence supports *osseointegrated* anchorage, most miniscrew and microscrew systems currently are not designed for osseous integration (osseointegration) and were marketed with little or no fundamental scientific verification. Clinical applications have superseded the scientific rationale for their effective use. In the absence of adequate (evidence-based) research, clinicians must rely on a limited number of basic science studies, supplemented by scientific interpolation of fundamental data derived from investigations of other types of endosseous implants. Historically, the current surge in miniscrews resembles the initial development of dental implants. At present, the only reliable means for discriminating among miniscrew systems is using the fundamental principles of bone biology, osseointegration, and biocompatibility. The "state of the art" is "clinician, beware."

This chapter reviews the historical perspective of implant development relative to current concepts of bone physiology, surgery, healing, and integration. The purpose is to help clinicians develop a scientific perspective for effective use of miniscrews. Bone physiological principles are important in selecting a device and developing a realistic perspective for using it effectively to treat specific malocclusions. No single system is optimal for all clinical applications. The anchorage needs of each patient are unique because of the nature of the malocclusion, the host response to the invasive device(s), and the biomechanical approaches favored by the clinician.

DEFINITION AND DESIGN

The TADs compose a broad array of implants used to support orthodontic treatment. As presently defined, all TADs are invasive devices and are best reserved for problems that cannot be effectively managed with conventional mechanics (Figure 1-1, *A*). The anchorage component may be a biocompatible wire attached to the endosseous base of an implant designed for prosthetic use. Furthermore, a nonfunctional osseointegrated implant may serve as an abutment for surgically assisted, rapid palatal expansion (Figure 1-1, *B*). The products with the longest clinical history of efficacy are osseointegrated fixtures originally designed for prosthetic purposes.[1-3]

Most current miniscrews are titanium (Ti) or titanium alloy and are manufactured with a smooth, machined surface that is not designed to osseointegrate. By definition, TADs are temporary devices; no long-term functional or esthetic role is planned. Thus, most TADs are removed after orthodontic treatment. However, some osseointegrated TADs may be covered with soft tissue ("put to sleep") or retained for sustained prosthetic function (see Figure 1-1, *B*). At present, the most common TADs include miniscrews, microscrews, miniature implants (mini-implants), palatal implants, modified bone plates, and retromolar implants, as well as functionally loaded prosthetic implants. In addition, a TAD may be a temporary prosthetic component (e.g., bracket attached to gold crown) that is removed after treatment (Figure 1-2). Therefore, TADs can range from nonintegrated miniscrews to implant-supported prostheses (ISPs) with temporary orthodontic attachments.

BACKGROUND

At the Bone Research Laboratory at the University of Pacific in San Francisco, the authors performed a series of experiments to develop orthodontic anchorage devices.[1,4-8] Titanium miniscrews, 2 mm in diameter with an acid-etched surface, were tested in rabbits, dogs, and monkeys from 1980 to 1988. The devices were very predictable when placed in extraoral sites such as rabbit femur and nasal bones,[5,7,9,10] but the intraoral use of the miniscrews in dogs and monkeys was less successful (failure rate, ~25%-50%). Failure was defined as

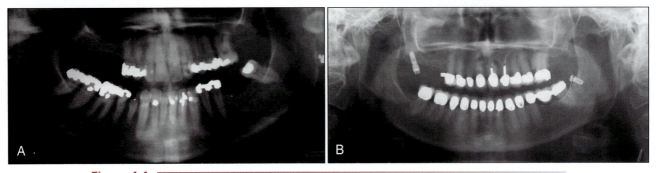

Figure 1-1
A, Severe, Class III, partially edentulous malocclusion in 41-year-old woman complicated by insulin-dependent diabetes mellitus and end-stage renal disease. **B,** Left retromolar implant (TAD) was used to align and move the third molar mesially to serve as an abutment for a fixed prosthesis; it will be removed. Because of the patient's health problems, orthognathic surgery was not a viable option. The compromise treatment in the maxillary arch was pre-prosthetic alignment to open space between the teeth and move the left segment mesially. The right maxillary implant in the tuberosity region was originally a temporary anchorage device (TAD), but it was retained to serve as a posterior abutment for a removable partial denture.

mobility or exfoliation of the anchorage fixture. Similar to current reports,[11-13] there were significant anatomical limitations relative to where miniscrews could be placed. Furthermore, soft tissue irritation of cheek, tongue, and alveolar mucosa was a significant problem. The biomechanical possibilities were compromised because of a lack of torsional resistance, particularly when immediately loaded. Unless miniscrews are osseointegrated, the most reliable mechanics are for the line of force to pass through the implant, not ideal for treatment of most malocclusions. The use of lever arms to improve the line of force may result in unfavorable moments on the implant.

It is important to note that the limitations of the miniscrews tested more than 20 years ago in the authors' laboratory are similar to the current predictability for these devices.[14-17] Thus, it is apparent that the biological efficacy of miniscrews is lagging the rapid increase in their clinical use. This scenario is similar to the initial development of dental implants before the well-documented introduction of "osseointegration" in the early 1980s.[18]

The 2-mm, acid-etched Ti miniscrews developed in the authors' laboratory were never used in patients because the intraoral animal data were considered inadequate to secure institutional review board (IRB) approval for a clinical trial. Because of the long history of clinical success without any serious complications (e.g., osteomyelitis, neoplasms), standard Branemark (Swedish) prosthetic fixtures were adapted for orthodontic anchorage. These relatively large implants (3.75 × 7 mm) could not be placed in the alveolar ridge if space closure and arch consolidation were the objectives of treatment (see Fig. 1-1). For mandibular anchorage, the retromolar area was selected as the optimal site. Indirect anchorage evolved as the most effective mechanism for most applications.[1] To a lesser extent, the tuberosity region of the maxilla has served as an osseous site for anchorage implants (see Fig. 1-1, B) A prospective clinical trial of implant anchorage demonstrated that osseointegrated anchorage is a highly reliable clinical procedure.[19]

The machine tools and methods for manufacturing Ti and Ti alloy screws have improved dramatically in the past 20 years, as illustrated by the functional designs of supramucosal heads for many miniscrew systems. At present, the major problem with TADs is the inability to achieve osseointegration routinely with most current devices. To our knowledge, the osseointegrated K-1 System (see Chapter 4) developed by Dr. Ryuzo Kanomi is the only osseointegrated miniscrew for orthodontic application.[9,20] As miniscrew technology matures, other osseointegrated systems will likely evolve.

PERSPECTIVES

Dental implant anchorage has progressed from nonintegrated screws (1940s)[7] to osseointegrated devices (1972 to present). The first documented use of osseointegrated orthodontic anchorage apparently was in a patient treated from 1972 to 1975 by Dr. Tom Horton (Columbus, Georgia) and Dr. Hilt Tatum (Opelika, Alabama). Dr. Horton corrected a buccal crossbite (scissors-bite) with a bite plate and cross-elastics anchored by an osseointegrated Ti blade implant, custom-made and placed by Dr. Hilt Tatum, a pioneer in the field of implant dentistry. In addition to placing the first osseointegrated implant for orthodontic

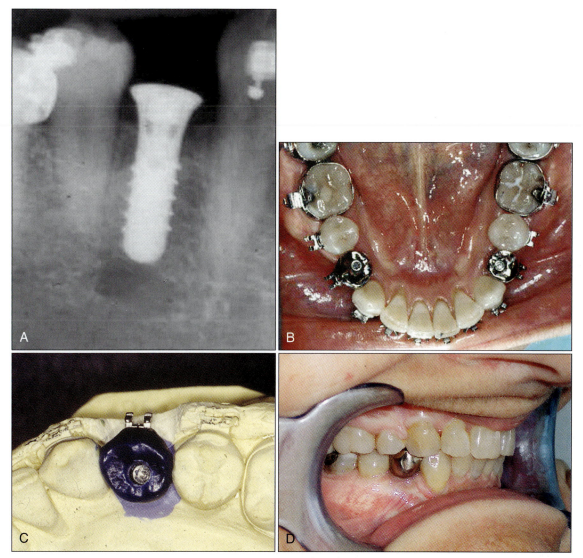

Figure 1-2

Severe relapse of Class II, Division 1 malocclusion in 47-year-old brachycephalic woman. A deep-bite malocclusion was treated 35 years earlier with extraction of four first premolars. **A,** Treatment required opening spaces to replace the mandibular premolars with implants. **B,** Orthodontic brackets were attached to the wax pattern for the crowns before investing and casting in gold. **C,** The crowns with attached brackets served as TADs for leveling and finishing the mandibular arch. **D,** After treatment the gold crowns were recovered and the brackets removed with a stone. The crowns were polished and retained as the permanent prostheses.

anchorage, Dr. Tatum was the developer of the maxillary sinus bone graft procedure[21] and numerous other dental implant innovations.[22-27]

The field of dental implantology originally embraced what was actually an osseointegration "failure" (fibrous implant interface) with the semiphysiological term "pseudoperiodontium."[28-30] However, subsequent research demonstrated that the fibrous interface was actually avascular scar tissue; furthermore, mobile implants with a "pseudoperiodontium" had a high failure rate. Titanium blade or cobalt-chromium alloy (Vitallium) blade dental implants have had many years of functional service. Most favorable reports involve blades that achieved osseointegration despite being immediately loaded.[31-33] The most reliable dental implant devices currently in use are osseointegrated systems, based directly or indirectly on the biological concept introduced by Brånemark and his collegues.[18,34] This developmental progression likely will repeat itself with respect to miniscrews because osseointegration is a mature technology with high reliability. Extension of the biotechnology of osseointegration to miniscrews would be an important advance for TAD anchorage.

COMMON QUESTIONS

To frame the current development of miniscrews in a clinical context, it is helpful to address questions frequently asked by clinicians.

Are Miniscrews a New Concept in Bone Biology?

No; there is a long history of similar devices in bone biology and osseous surgery. Miniscrews have long been used for attaching bone plates in orthopedic,[35] plastic,[36] orthognathic,[37] and neurosurgical[38] procedures. The principal use of miniscrews in orthognathic surgery is for attaching bone fixation plates to stabilize fractures and osteotomy segments. One of the first reports of clinical orthodontics using miniscrew anchorage employed the screws typically used to attach bone plates.[39]

Is Osseointegration an Important Goal for Miniscrew Anchorage?

Yes; for optimal reliability and stability, osseointegration has been a proven scientific concept in medicine and dentistry for more than three decades. Osseointegrated miniscrews have also served as anchorage for orthopedic devices if the therapeutic load is less than 3 newtons (N).[40] To date, the only mini-implant (miniscrew) that attempts to achieve osseointegration routinely is the K-1 System of Kanomi.[9,20]

Are Nonintegrated Miniscrews an Important Step in the Progression to User-Friendly Osseointegrated Devices?

Yes; the wide interest in miniscrews has focused the orthodontic profession on the importance of "rigid osseous" anchorage. Much literature from outside the United States has failed to document the serious health risk associated with the clinical use of miniscrew TADs. This safety data will assist North American investigators in securing ethical approval for future developmental studies at the clinical level. Continuing research and development will provide improved products to serve a large, newly created market.

DENTAL IMPLANTS FOR ORTHODONTIC ANCHORAGE

In 1984, Roberts et al.[7] reviewed the literature on the use of endosseous devices for orthodontic anchorage. The first clinical report of implant anchorage was in 1969 by Dr. Leonard Linkow.[41-43] (The senior author has interacted with Dr. Linkow as a fellow faculty member at the Maxillofacial Implantology Program, University of Lille, Faculty of Medicine, for more than 20 years.) Although not well known to orthodontists, Dr. Linkow pioneered many aspects of dental implants with respect to prosthetic dentistry and has remained active in the field for more than 50 years. The blade implants originally used by Linkow and his orthodontic colleagues were limited in effectiveness because they were not osseointegrated. Mobility caused by the "pseudoperiodontium" at the interface (scar tissue) probably limited the life expectancy of most blade implants used for orthodontic anchorage. Thus, it can be argued that the blade-anchored "implantodontics" of Linkow and his colleagues were indeed the first orthodontic TADs that had the potential for long-term masticatory function. Importantly, blade-supported prostheses were the first devices to serve the critical function of restoring and maintaining the *vertical dimension of occlusion* (VDO). To correct and maintain the VDO in a patient with a partially edentulous acquired malocclusion, a TAD must resist masticatory loading and maintain the VDO at least during active orthodontic treatment (Figure 1-3). Most current miniscrews and other TADs do not have the capability for restoring the VDO.

The first report of a surgical fixation screw for orthodontic anchorage was in 1983 by Creekmore and Eklund.[44] In 1990, Roberts et al.[1] published the first documented case report with posttreatment follow-up of an osseointegrated screw used for retromolar anchorage. Use of a nonintegrated miniscrew for orthodontic anchorage was first reported by Kanomi in 1997.[39] Much TAD literature has been published in the past decade and is reviewed throughout this text.

BONE VASCULAR CONSIDERATIONS

A schematic series of drawings based on histological studies[4,5,7,10] is helpful for understanding the bone response to insertion of a Ti screw. A drawing of cortical bone with an internal trabecular network shows the fundamental osseous features: periosteum, cortical bone, trabecular bone, and marrow (Figure 1-4). The blood supply of trabecular bone and marrow is derived from transcortical vessels that traverse the cortex in haversian and Volkmann canals.

In the mandible the vascular supply of the marrow and endosteal trabecular bone is primarily through the inferior alveolar artery. Internal vascularity of the maxilla is provided primarily by transcortical branches of the greater palatine and posterior superior maxillary arteries. Thus, the buccal and lingual cortices of the alveolar processes have a radial arterial system, meaning the arterial supply is through transcortical arteries that enter the endosteal space and supply capillaries that permeate the peripheral cortex. The venous return for cortical bone is provided by the subperiosteal venous plexus (Figure 1-5).[45]

It is important to remember that any disruption of the periosteum, such as reflecting a mucoperiosteal flap, will compromise the venous return of the operated site, increase the size of the postoperative blood clot (potentially a hematoma), and decrease the localized healing potential. When placing a TAD, it is best to minimize the disruption of the mucoperiosteum by opening the operative site with a soft tissue punch rather than

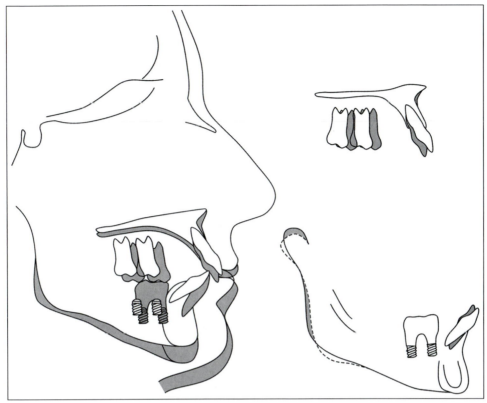

Figure 1-3
Prosthodontist referred this 65-year-old female because her partially edentulous malocclusion was "unrestorable." The vertical dimension of occlusion (VDO) was opened about 1 cm with four osseointegrated TADs (3.75 × 4–mm Nobel Biocare Craniofacial Fixtures) supporting a bilateral temporary fixed prostheses that was removed after treatment. The patient's occlusion was restored with bilateral fixed prostheses in the maxillary arch and a removable partial denture in the mandibular arch. Note that the restoration of the VDO and maxillary space closure was associated with more inferior repositioning of the maxilla and mandible. In addition, the mandible increased about 4 mm in length over the 36-month course of treatment.

making an incision and raising a mucoperiosteal flap. To avoid mucosal trauma, the punch should be of a slightly larger diameter than the surgical instruments used to prepare the miniscrew site (Figure 1-6). The trend to limit periosteal disruption when placing miniscrews parallels the current emphasis on flapless implant placement.[46-48] Three-dimensional (3D) imaging of the implant site is particularly important for flapless implant placement.[49]

PRESURGICAL ASSESSMENT OF MINISCREW SITE

A critical presurgical consideration is selection of a site with adequate bone to support a miniscrew.[11-13] Schnelle et al.[50] digitally assessed pretreatment and posttreatment panoramic radiographs and found that the most favorable sites for miniscrew placement were at the midroot level mesial to the maxillary first molars and mesial or distal to mandibular first molars. Other studies have shown that panoramic radiographs are unreliable for demonstrating osseous structure[51] or axial inclination of teeth[52] because they are two-dimensional (2D) compressions of distorted 3D projections.[49,53] Panoramic imaging has been used for determining relative bone thickness[50] but is notoriously inaccurate for demonstrating 3D anatomical features critical to miniscrew placement.[54] Periapical radiographs provide a more reliable 2D view, but the only practical methods for accurately determining anatomical details of mineralized tissues are 3D imaging (cone-beam or spiral CT).

Recently, Deguchi et al.[13] used computed tomography (CT) to demonstrate that subperiosteal cortical bone thickness was greatest near first molars in both arches. Selection of a miniscrew site in partially edentulous patients may be more problematic because of alveolar ridge atrophy and expansion of the maxillary

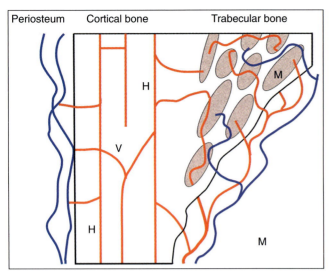

Figure 1-4
Section of a long bone shows the periosteum, cortical bone, and trabecular bone. Note that the arterial supply *(red)* originates from the internal nutrient artery *(left)* in the marrow *(M)*. Arterioles and capillaries provide surface circulation for trabeculae but serve as an internal blood supply for cortical bone via the haversian *(H)* and Volkmann *(V)* canals. The venous circulation *(blue)* for trabecular bone is through the internal nutrient vein in the marrow *(left)*, but venous return of the cortical bone is provided by periosteal veins.

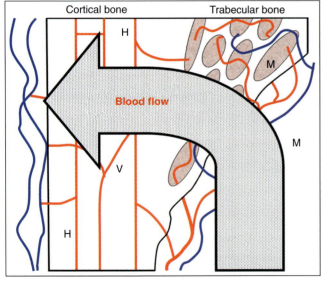

Figure 1-5
Blood flow through cortical bone is from the marrow to the periosteum. It is important for surgeons to realize that raising a mucoperiosteal flap during implant placement compromises the blood supply and destroys the cambium (inner osteogenic) layer of the periosteum. *H,* Haversian canal; *V,* Volkmann canal; *M,* marrow.

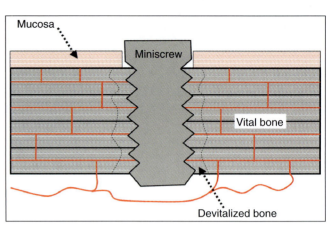

Figure 1-6
A minimal surgical procedure is recommended for placing miniscrews in cortical bone. The least disruptive approach for removing mucosa is a tissue punch; then a hole is drilled in the bone and the self-tapping TAD screwed into place. Even with the most atraumatic technique, the internal collateral blood supply is disrupted, resulting in a layer of devitalized bone within about 1 mm of the implant surface.

sinus. Using skulls and radiographic studies of other patients[11,13,50] to predict the mass and quality of alveolar bone for a specific patient is unreliable. In Figure 1-7, for example, a partially edentulous woman has an enlarged sinus mesial to the maxillary right second molar but appears to have adequate mass of cortical and trabecular bone in the tuberosity area (see Figure 1-7, *A*). Presurgical cone-beam CT is essential for reliably assessing the thickness of cortical bone, the trabecular density, and the position of surgical hazards such as the maxillary sinus, greater palatal neurovascular bundle, mental foramen, and inferior alveolar canal (see Figure 1-7, *B*). The need for precise placement of miniscrews in this patient cannot be reliably predicted from a panoramic radiograph.

POSTOPERATIVE HEALING AND INTEGRATION

When installed, a self-tapping endosseous implant (with miniscrew) is retained by a layer of nonvital bone about

Figure 1-7
A, Conventional panoramic radiograph shows an enlarged maxillary sinus on the mesial side of the right second molar *(dotted circle)*. Because of the distortions inherent in panoramic radiographs, it is unclear if there is adequate bone mesial to the molar for placement of a miniscrew. *B,* An i-CAT cone-beam CT scan of the same patient demonstrates that the area mesial to the right maxillary molar is a high risk site for a miniscrew because the bone beneath the sinus is only about 2 mm thick, as shown in sections 79 to 81.

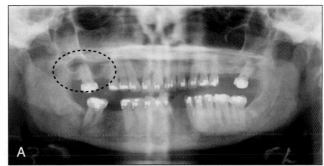
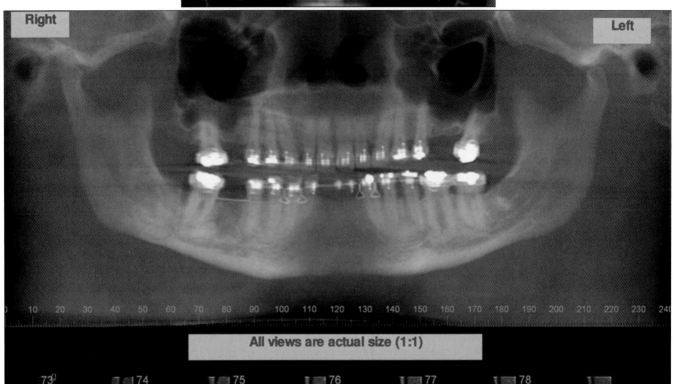

1 mm in thickness.[4,5,7] The devitalization is caused by surgical trauma, inflammation, and disruption of the complex collateral (haversian) blood supply of cortical bone. The layer of devitalized bone is increased by more traumatic surgery and overheating of the osseous tissue with burs, taps, and insertion of the implant.

Self-drilling screws have been used for osseous surgery for more than half a century.[55] The interface devitalization and postoperative healing response for self-drilling miniscrews are less clear than for tapped preparations and self-tapping screws. After 6 weeks in situ, more bone formation is noted near miniscrews in the mandible than in the maxilla.[16] However, the bone-labeling pattern of both sites is consistent with a *regional acceleratory phenomenon* (RAP), meaning the rate of bone turnover progressively decreases when moving away from the implant surface.

The crushing of bone to create an intraosseous site for a self-drilling miniscrew is an important variable in TAD compatibility that should be studied in detail. The crushing may significantly disrupt the vascular supply of supporting bone, creating a denser layer of nonvital bone that is more resistant to bone resorption. This may be an advantage for short-term retention of a nonintegrated miniscrew. On the contrary, bone crushing may increase intraosseous inflammation, enhancing the postoperative restorative response. It is difficult to predict whether a crushed interface will be an advantage or a disadvantage for miniscrew retention.

Tapered screws, along with self-tapping and self-drilling designs, are currently in use. Each design is advantageous for different types of bone.[56] Tapered screws are the preferred design for retention in cancellous bone; cylindrical self-tapping screws are advantageous for relatively thick cortical bone; and the self-drilling design is optimal for thin cortical bone. When cortical bone is thicker, self-drilling screws can produce substantial bone damage because the compression of a rigid structural material (mineralized bone) may produce a blowout defect at the endosteal surface of cortical bone.[57] If screws with an endosteal blowout defect are immediately loaded, there is likely to be less intact osseous interface to resist displacement. All osseous wounds (e.g., fractures, osteotomies, bone screws) produce a postoperative healing reaction, which Frost[58] defined as an RAP. With miniscrews, the RAP manifests as intense bone remodeling within 1 mm of the screw interface; the prevalence of remodeling foci progressively decreases as the distance increases from the implant surface.[16]

The failure of miniscrews is usually noted during the postoperative healing period. Six weeks after inserting 102 miniscrews (6-8 mm in length) in multiple intraoral sites in dogs, 20 failed (were loose or lost).[16] All these screws were unloaded. There was no significant difference in pull-out strength at 6 weeks compared with the immediate postoperative period for miniscrews that were retained and had not become loose. For these successful screws, bone contact at the interface ranged from 79% to 95%. This study demonstrates that miniscrews have about a 20% failure rate for the first 6 weeks, even in the absence of therapeutic loading. Immediate loading may increase the failure rate, but there are no specific, well-controlled studies of miniscrew failure caused by immediate loading.

OSSEOINTEGRATION

Metallic screws are manufactured by turning a rod-shaped blank on a lathe. The usual machining process results in a smooth, polished surface that is contaminated with residue from the tools. Osseointegration of the titanium surface is inhibited by both the smooth surface and the manufacturing contaminants (e.g., iron, nickel) that permeate the surface.[34] Acid etching of Ti miniscrews removes contaminants and increases the roughness (microtexture) of the surface. Acid-etched Ti screws routinely achieve osseointegration.[7]

Postoperative healing and the response to therapeutic loads have been described for Ti miniscrews with an acid-etched surface that are installed as self-tapping fixtures. Healing of cortical bone devitalized or otherwise compromised by endosseous surgery occurs through a bone-remodeling mechanism (Figure 1-8). After a 6-week healing phase, these TADs routinely osseointegrate in rabbit bone.[7] A comparable healing period in humans is 4 months.[5] The nonvital interface and supporting bone remodel through an RAP,[59,60] which lasts about 1 year for most bone screws in human cortical

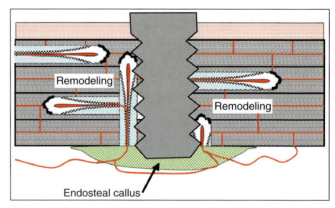

Figure 1-8

Postoperative healing of the cortical bone supporting a miniscrew involves the formation of an endosteal callus and an intense remodeling response, deemed a regional acceleratory phenomenon (RAP). Note that cutting/filling cones, remodeling interfacial bone in a vertical direction, emanate from the endosseous surface. If the interface is biocompatible and micromotion is controlled, titanium implants usually osseointegrate because of progressive remodeling to replace the nonvital bone interface.

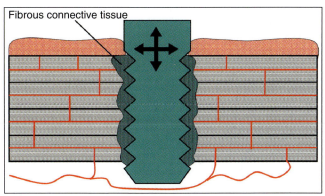

Figure 1-9
In the presence of micromotion *(arrows)* the postoperative bone-remodeling response may fail to osseointegrate the implant, and the interface reverts to fibrous connective tissue. The fibrous interface of nonintegrated miniscrews is responsible for mobility and movement of the loaded TADs within bone.

bone. The postoperative stability of a miniscrew depends on the thickness of the cortex and timing of the remodeling response to replace devitalized bone. Stability at any point in time is difficult to predict for miniscrews because most current devices have a smooth, machined surface that is unlikely to osseointegrate. Furthermore, the micromotion associated with functional and therapeutic loading is conducive to forming a layer of fibrous connective tissue at the interface (Figure 1-9). This layer of scar tissue is the functional equivalent of a nonunion in orthopedics.[4,18]

The postoperative implant RAP has been demonstrated with bone scintillation (scintigraphy) scans in humans.[61] High bone turnover activity is noted for 12 weeks in the mandible and 20 weeks in the maxilla. When endosseous implants fail to integrate, the amount of bone remodeling near the interface decreases.[62]

STABILITY AND FAILURE

The failure of Ti miniscrews to osseointegrate contributes to instability and a relatively high failure rate. Miniscrews are usually loaded immediately and have a "success rate" of 50% to 89%.[15,17] Conversely, up to 11% to 50% of current miniscrews fail to serve as adequate TADs during orthodontic treatment. Although nonintegration renders miniscrews easier to remove at the end of active treatment, this advantage is not sufficient to offset the high failure rate.

Because of the fibrous connective tissue interface, miniscrews used for orthodontic anchorage move relative to supporting bone.[63] The bone-modeling mechanism for movement of nonintegrated Ti implants has been described.[1] Orthodontic anchorage is often critical when miniscrews are the preferred treatment option.

Even a 1-mm to 2-mm lack of stability for a TAD may significantly compromise treatment outcome. Similar to prosthetic implants, osseointegration would probably improve the stability and success rate of miniscrews. Developing an osseointegrated miniscrew that could be easily removed at the end of treatment would be a significant advance in the field.

SUMMARY

- Most current miniscrew and microscrew systems have been marketed with little or no fundamental scientific verification of their osseous compatibility under unloaded and loaded conditions.
- The most popular temporary anchorage devices (TADs) are miniscrews made of commercially pure titanium (Ti) or titanium alloy.
- Most current miniscrews have a smooth, machined surface that is not conducive to osseointegration.
- The bone supporting self-tapping miniscrews is subject to an intense postoperative remodeling response known as rapid acceleratory phenomenon (RAP).
- Most miniscrews fail to integrate, so the bone-implant interface tends to evolve into a layer of fibrous connective tissue.
- During clinical use, miniscrews are expected to display varying degrees of mobility relative to supporting bone.
- The current 25% to 50% failure rate is unlikely to improve for nonintegrated miniscrews.
- Osseointegration would considerably improve miniscrew reliability.
- The profession should demand more scientific rigor in the development of skeletal anchorage devices.
- The current approach is "clinician, beware."

REFERENCES

1. Roberts WE, Marshall KJ, Mozsary PG: Rigid endosseous implant utilized as anchorage to protract molars and close an atrophic extraction site, *Angle Orthod* 60(2):135-152, 1990.
2. Wehrbein H et al: The use of palatal implants for orthodontic anchorage: design and clinical application of the orthosystem, *Clin Oral Implants Res* 7(4):410-416, 1996.
3. Kokich VG: Managing complex orthodontic problems: the use of implants for anchorage, *Semin Orthod* 2(2):153-160, 1996.
4. Roberts WE et al: Rigid endosseous implants for orthodontic and orthopedic anchorage, *Angle Orthod* 59(4):247-256, 1989.
5. Roberts WE: Bone tissue interface, *J Dent Educ* 52(12):804-809, 1988.
6. Roberts WE: Bone tissue interface, *Int J Oral Implantol* 5(1):71-74, 1988.
7. Roberts WE et al: Osseous adaptation to continuous loading of rigid endosseous implants, *Am J Orthod* 86(2):95-111, 1984.
8. Roberts WE: Rigid endosseous anchorage and tricalcium phosphate (TCP)–coated implants, *Calif Dent Assoc J* 12(12):158-161, 1984.
9. Roberts WE: Bone physiology, metabolism, and biomechanics in orthodontic practice. In Graber TM, Vanarsdall RL Jr, Vig KWL, editors: *Orthodontics: current principles and techniques*, St Louis, 2005, Mosby-Elsevier, pp 221-292.

10. Roberts WE et al: Implants: bone physiology and metabolism, *Calif Dent Assoc J* 15(10):54-61, 1987.
11. Poggio PM et al: "Safe zones": a guide for miniscrew positioning in the maxillary and mandibular arch, *Angle Orthod* 76(2):191-197, 2006.
12. Kim HJ et al: Soft-tissue and cortical-bone thickness at orthodontic implant sites. *Am J Orthod Dentofacial Orthop* 130(2):177-182, 2006.
13. Deguchi T et al: Quantitative evaluation of cortical bone thickness with computed tomographic scanning for orthodontic implants, *Am J Orthod Dentofacial Orthop* 129(6):721, e7-12, 2006.
14. Fritz U, Ehmer A, Diedrich P: Clinical suitability of titanium microscrews for orthodontic anchorage: preliminary experiences, *J Orofac Orthop* 65(5):410-418, 2004.
15. Cheng SJ et al: A prospective study of the risk factors associated with failure of mini-implants used for orthodontic anchorage, *Int J Oral Maxillofac Implants* 19(1):100-106, 2004.
16. Huja SS et al: Biomechanical and histomorphometric analyses of monocortical screws at placement and 6 weeks postinsertion, *J Oral Implantol* 32(3):110-116, 2006.
17. Miyawaki S et al: Factors associated with the stability of titanium screws placed in the posterior region for orthodontic anchorage, *Am J Orthod Dentofacial Orthop* 124(4):373-378, 2003.
18. Albrektsson T et al: Osseointegrated titanium implants: requirements for ensuring a long-lasting, direct bone-to-implant anchorage in man, *Acta Orthop Scand* 52(2):155-170, 1981.
19. Roberts WE et al: Implant-anchored orthodontics for partially edentulous malocclusions in children and adults, *Am J Orthod Dentofacial Orthop* 126(3):302-304, 2004.
20. Roberts WE, Kanomi R, Hohlt WF: Miniature implants and retromolar fixtures for orthodontic anchorage. In Bell WH, editor: *Advances in oral and maxillofacial surgery*, St Louis, 2006, Mosby-Elsevier, pp 205-214.
21. Tatum H Jr: Maxillary and sinus implant reconstructions, *Dent Clin North Am* 30(2):207-229, 1986.
22. Tatum OH Jr: Osseous grafts in intra-oral sites, *J Oral Implantol* 22(1):51-52, 1996.
23. Tatum H Jr, Lebowitz M, Borgner R: Restoration of the atrophic, edentulous mandible, *J Oral Implantol* 20(2):124-134, 1994.
24. Tatum OH Jr et al: Sinus augmentation: rationale, development, long-term results, *N Y State Dent J* 59(5):43-48, 1993.
25. Smiler DG et al: Sinus lift grafts and endosseous implants: treatment of the atrophic posterior maxilla, *Dent Clin North Am* 36(1):151-186 (discussion, 187-188), 1992.
26. Tatum OH Jr: Maxillary implants, *Fla Dent J* 60(2):23-27, 1989.
27. Tatum H Jr: Endosteal implants, *CDA J* 16(2):71-76, 1988.
28. Babbush CA: Endosseous blade-vent implants: a research review, *J Oral Surg* 30(3):168-175, 1972.
29. Cranin AN, Dennison TA: Construction techniques for blade and anchor implants, *J Am Dent Assoc* 83(4):833-839, 1971.
30. Linkow LI: Endosseous blade-vent implants: a two-year report, *J Prosthet Dent* 23(4):441-448, 1970.
31. Di Stefano D et al: Immediately loaded blade implant retrieved from a after a 20-year loading period: a histologic and histomorphometric case report, *J Oral Implantol* 32(4):171-176, 2006.
32. Cappuccilli M, Conte M, Praiss ST: Placement and post-mortem retrieval of a 28-year-old implant: a clinical and histologic report, *J Am Dent Assoc* 135(3):324-329, 2004.
33. Proussaefs P, Lozada J: Evaluation of two Vitallium blade-form implants retrieved after 13 to 21 years of function: a clinical report, *J Prosthet Dent* 87(4):412-415, 2002.
34. Albrektsson T, Jacobsson M: Bone-metal interface in osseointegration, *J Prosthet Dent* 57(5):597-607, 1987.
35. Seitz WH Jr et al: External fixator pin insertion techniques: biomechanical analysis and clinical relevance, *J Hand Surg [Am]* 16(3):560-563, 1991.
36. Goldman ND et al: Malar augmentation with self-drilling single-screw fixation, *Arch Facial Plast Surg* 2(3):222-225, 2000.
37. Steinhauser EW: Bone screws and plates in orthognathic surgery, *Int J Oral Surg* 11(4):209-216, 1982.
38. Caton WL 3rd et al: A new self-drilling skull traction device with flexion-extension modification: technical note, *J Neurosurg* 50(4):528-530, 1979.
39. Kanomi R: Mini-implant for orthodontic anchorage, *J Clin Orthod* 31(11):763-737, 1997.
40. Parr JA et al: Sutural expansion using rigidly integrated endosseous implants: an experimental study in rabbits, *Angle Orthod* 67(4):283-290, 1997.
41. Linkow LI, Chercheve R: *Theories and techniques of oral implantology*, St Louis, 1970, Mosby.
42. Linkow LI: Implanto-orthodontics, *J Clin Orthod* 4:685-705, 1970.
43. Linkow LI: The endosseous blade implant and its use in orthodontics, *Int J Orthod* 18:149-154, 1969.
44. Creekmore TD, Eklund MK: Possibility of skeletal anchorage, *J Clin Orthod* 17:266-267, 1983.
45. Chanavaz M: Anatomy and histophysiology of the periosteum: quantification of the periosteal blood supply to the adjacent bone with ^{85}Sr and gamma spectrometry, *J Oral Implantol* 21(3):214-219, 1995.
46. Fortin T et al: Effect of flapless surgery on pain experienced in implant placement using an image-guided system, *Int J Oral Maxillofac Implants* 21(2):298-304, 2006.
47. Oh TJ, Shotwell JL, Billy EJ, Wang HL: Effect of flapless implant surgery on soft tissue profile: a randomized controlled clinical trial, *J Periodontol* 77(5):874-882, 2006.
48. Wittwer G et al: Computer-guided flapless transmucosal implant placement in the mandible: a new combination of two innovative techniques, *Oral Surg Oral Med Oral Pathol Oral Radiol Endod* 101(6):718-723, 2006.
49. Hatcher DC, Dial C, Mayorga C: Cone beam CT for pre-surgical assessment of implant sites, *J Calif Dent Assoc* 31(11):825-833, 2003.
50. Schnelle MA et al: A radiographic evaluation of the availability of bone for placement of miniscrews, *Angle Orthod* 74(6):832-837, 2004.
51. Laster WS et al: Accuracy of measurements of mandibular anatomy and prediction of asymmetry in panoramic radiographic images, *Dentomaxillofac Radiol* 34(6):343-349, 2005.
52. Yeo DK, Freer TJ, Brockhurst PJ: Distortions in panoramic radiographs, *Aust Orthod J* 18(2):92-98, 2002.
53. Reuter I, Ritter W, Kaeppler G: Triple images on panoramic radiographs, *Dentomaxillofac Radiol* 28(5):316-319, 1999.
54. Schulze R, Schalldach F, d'Hoedt B: [Effect of positioning errors on magnification factors in the mandible in digital panorama imaging], *Mund Kiefer Gesichtschir* 4(3):164-170, 2000.
55. Lehv SP: A headless self-drilling screw, *Am J Surg* 80(5):608-609, 1950.
56. Lohr J et al: [Comparative in vitro studies of self-boring and self-tapping screws: histomorphological and physical-technical studies of bone layers], *Mund Kiefer Gesichtschir* 4(3):159-163, 2000.
57. Sowden D, Schmitz JP: AO self-drilling and self-tapping screws in rat calvarial bone: an ultrastructural study of the implant interface, *J Oral Maxillofac Surg* 60(3):294-299 (discussion, 300), 2002.
58. Frost HM: The biology of fracture healing: an overview for clinicians. Part II, *Clin Orthop* (248):294-309, 1989.
59. Frost HM: The regional acceleratory phenomenon: a review, *Henry Ford Hosp Med J* 31(1):3-9, 1983.

60. Mueller M et al: A systemic acceleratory phenomenon (SAP) accompanies the regional acceleratory phenomenon (RAP) during healing of a bone defect in the rat, *J Bone Miner Res* 6(4):401-410, 1991.
61. Meidan Z et al: Technetium 99m–MDP scintigraphy of patients undergoing implant prosthetic procedures: a follow-up study, *J Periodontol* 65(4):330-335, 1994.
62. Schliephake H, Berding G: Evaluation of bone healing in patients with bone grafts and endosseous implants using single photon emission tomography (SPECT), *Clin Oral Implants Res* 9(1):34-42, 1998.
63. Liou EJ, Pai BC, Lin JC: Do miniscrews remain stationary under orthodontic forces? *Am J Orthod Dentofacial Orthop* 126(1):42-47, 2004.

CHAPTER 2

Biological Response to Orthodontic Temporary Anchorage Devices

Sunil Wadhwa and Ravindra Nanda

In the past decade, use of implantable devices for anchorage control during orthodontic treatment has increased dramatically. These implantable devices include conventional titanium (Ti) endosseous dental implants, palatal implants, Ti miniscrews, and mini–bone plates.[1] To be successful, these implantable devices must be stable in the bone for the duration of orthodontic treatment. Retention of orthodontic implantable devices is obtained either by allowing for osseointegration of the device or by the intrinsic design of the device (screw threads), which renders immediate retention within the bone.

This chapter reviews the bone biology and factors predicting stability for mechanically retained and osseointegrated orthodontic temporary anchorage devices (TADs). Frequently prescribed drugs that may affect orthodontic TADs are also reviewed.

HISTORY OF ORTHODONTIC IMPLANTABLE DEVICES

Almost 60 years ago, the first orthodontic TAD was placed in the mandibles of dogs. Gainsforth et al.[2] placed cobalt-chromium alloy (Vitallium) screws in the mandibles of dogs as anchors for the application of orthodontic forces. Despite some success, the resultant tooth movement was limited because implants loosened within 1 month after application of orthodontic forces. Over the next 40 years, few studies were published on orthodontic TADs. Linkow et al.[3] reported on blade implants to retract teeth using rubber bands, and Sherman[4] recommended that implants be stabilized by a nonloading bone-healing period before application of orthodontic forces.

In the 1980s, animal studies laid the framework for analyzing the effectiveness of orthodontic TADs. Gray et al.[5] examined the movement of Bioglass-coated and Vitallium endosseous implants loaded with constant orthodontic forces in the femurs of rabbits. After 28 days of healing, no statistically significant movement occurred at any of the force levels (60, 120, and 180 grams [g]) for either type of implant. In addition, histological evaluation revealed a connective tissue encapsulation with the Vitallium implant and an implant-bone bond with the Bioglass implant. Roberts et al.[6] reported similar results with Ti implants in the femurs of rabbits (6-12 weeks of healing) loaded with 100 g for 4 to 8 weeks. During the healing period, 3 days after implant placement, there was extensive bone formation, particularly at the endosteal margin of the surgical defect. In addition, by the end of 6 weeks, a rigid bone-implant interface was achieved. During the loading period, 19 of 20 loaded implants remained rigid. The authors concluded that "6 weeks is an adequate healing period, prior to loading, to attain rigid stability and avoid spontaneous fracture and that titanium endosseous implants have potential as a source of firm osseous anchorage for orthodontics and dentofacial orthopedics."[6]

Human case reports on the use of orthodontic TADs were also published in the early 1980s. For example, Creekmore and Eklund[7] inserted a Vitallium screw just below the anterior nasal spine in a patient with maxillary incisor elongation. After 10 days, they attached an elastic thread from the archwire to the head of the screw. In 1 year the upper incisors had intruded 6 mm, and the Vitallium bone screw had remained stable throughout the treatment. Roberts et al.[8] used a traditional two-stage endosseous implant for orthodontic anchorage to translate two mandibular molars mesially 10 to 12 mm into an atrophic edentulous ridge. After the 3 years of treatment, the endosseous implant remained rigid. Polarized light analyses revealed that about 80% of the endosseous portion of the implant was in direct contact with mature lamellar bone.

Other orthodontic TADs besides traditional dental implants were developed in the early 1990s. Block and Hoffman[9] used a textured disk with a hydroxyapatite coating on one side and an internal thread on the other side to provide palatal orthodontic anchorage. They found that placement of palatal implants in dogs and monkeys provided absolute anchorage to move teeth orthodontically without moving the implant. Kanomi[10] described the use of small Ti bone screws for orthodontic anchorage. Mini–bone screws (1.2 mm in diameter, 6 mm in length) were placed in the alveolar bone between the root apices of the mandibular central incisors. After healing and the uncovering of the mini-implant, an elastic chain was tied to mandibular central incisor brackets and the implant. After 4 months the mandibular incisors had been intruded 6 mm without any patient discomfort, root resorption, or periodontal pathology. Sugawara and his team in Japan reported a new skeletal anchorage system consisting of a Ti miniplate temporarily fixed in the maxilla or mandible. The miniplates were used for intrusion of lower molars in open-bite malocclusions; the open bite improved significantly with little extrusion of the lower incisors.[11-13]

Freudenthaler et al.[14] described one of the first reports on immediately loaded, mechanically retained orthodontic TADs. Eight patients received 12 bicortical Ti screws as anchorage units for orthodontic molar protraction. After insertion of the screws, orthodontic forces were applied immediately. Of the 12 screws, three were prematurely removed. The remaining nine screws remained stationary throughout the duration of treatment. The authors concluded that "the total treatment time is reduced as the screws can be loaded immediately."[14]

In 2005, Kim et al.[15] described the use of drill-free screws; 32 (16 self-tapping, 16 drill-free) screws were inserted into the jaws of two beagles. A pilot-drilling bur was used before inserting the traditional self-tapping screws. Forces of 200 to 300 g were applied using nickel-titanium (Ni-Ti) coil springs 1 week after insertion. At 12 weeks, mobility was tested, and the screws with the surrounding bone were prepared for histomorphometric evaluation. The screws in the drill-free group showed less mobility and more bone-to-metal contact compared with the self-tapping group, although osseointegration was generally found in both groups. Huja et al.[16,17] found similar results with drill-free Ti screws.

BIOLOGICAL PROCESSES

Dr. J.B. Cope proposed classifying orthodontic TADs into two groups: (1) those that are osseointegrated and (2) those that have mechanical retention (Figure 2-1). The biological processes are quite different between the two groups (Table 2-1).

OSSEOINTEGRATED DEVICES

The insertion of an orthodontic TAD into bone initiates a series of biological processes, including formation of a blood clot, alteration in nuclear morphology of the osteocytes surrounding the site of implantation, and formation of new bone.

After placement of an orthodontic TAD, the surface comes in contact with blood and is covered by a biofilm.

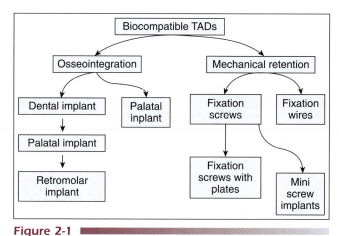

Figure 2-1
Biocompatible Temporary Anchorage Devices *(TADs)*. *(Redrawn from Cope JB: Classification of temporary anchorage devices, 2005. www.orthoTADS.com.)*

TABLE 2-1	Biological Response to Osseointegrated and Mechanically Retained Temporary Anchorage Devices (TADs)	
Postimplant Period	Osseointegrated	Mechanically Retained
Immediate	Biofilm, formation of blood clot	—
1 day	Red blood cells and inflammatory cells	Attachment of osteoblasts to titanium surfaces
3-5 days	Appearance of osteoblasts Decrease in inflammatory cells	—
1-4 weeks	Bone remodeling	Bone remodeling

The biofilm contains fibrinogen and serine proteases of the complement and coagulation system.[18] Red blood cells (RBCs) and platelets then attach to the biofilm, resulting in a fibrin-containing blood clot that forms at the bone-TAD interface.[18,19] The blood clot also may contain polygonal bone chips, apparently resulting from the surgical preparation or TAD insertion.[20]

After 1 day, RBCs and inflammatory cells (mainly neutrophils) are present between the bone and TAD. Within the bone adjacent to the device, appearance of the osteocytes is altered, with empty osteocytic lacunae and pyknotic osteocytic nuclei extending up to 100 μm in the bone adjacent to the TAD.[21,22]

From 3 to 7 days after implantation, inflammatory cell infiltration gradually disappears, and spindle-shaped or flattened cells start to appear in the interface between preexisting bone and orthodontic TADS.[21]

From 2 to 4 weeks after TAD placement, cuboidal osteoblasts are clearly visible at the bone-TAD interface. Interestingly, new collagen fibers run circumferentially around the TAD cavity, whereas the course of the fibers of existing bone corresponds to the long axis of the bone. Numerous bone-modeling units containing multinucleated osteoclasts and blood vessels[22] also appear in the cortical bone surrounding the device.

Six weeks after TAD placement, active bone remodeling appears to decrease, and a region of empty osteocytic lacunae is still seen adjacent to the newly deposited bone.[23]

After the nonloading healing period and osseous integration, application of orthodontic loading to the TAD causes increased bone tissue turnover and increased density of the adjacent alveolar bone compared with the unloaded control. Despite increased bone tissue turnover, however, the TAD maintains osseointegration even after 32 weeks of orthodontic loading.[24,25] In addition, no significant differences in bone remodeling are seen around the bone-TAD interface within areas of compression, tension, or shear.[26,27] (See Table 2-1.)

MECHANICALLY RETAINED DEVICES

In screw-shaped, mechanically retained orthodontic TADs, areas of the screw in direct contact with the bone are responsible for primary mechanical stability of the device; other areas show gaps hundreds of microns in size between the device surface and the bone. In the areas where small gaps exist between the screw surface and bone, the biological process is similar to that previously described. In direct-contact areas, however, the biological response is different. In areas of direct contact with the screw, no invasion of inflammatory cells occurs in the first week. Instead, 1 day after insertion, not only are mineralized bone tissue contacts present between the surface of the implant and bone, but the osteoblasts are also attached firmly to the Ti implant surface.[28] After 1 to 2 weeks, in the areas in direct contact with the bone, the bone is resorbed and replaced with newly formed, viable bone. Despite this temporary loss of hard-bone contact, the implants remain clinically stable.[29] This process does not seem to be affected if the screw is immediately loaded or if there is a healing period before external loading begins.[28] (See Table 2-1.)

STABILITY OF ANCHORAGE DEVICES

As with the biological processes, the factors that predict stability also differ between osseointegrated and mechanically retained TADs.

MECHANICALLY RETAINED DEVICES

Stability of TADs immediately after insertion, called *primary stability*, is critical in determining success in the early loading phase, particularly in TADs immediately loaded. Primary stability depends on the geometric design of the implant, bone quality, insertion technique, and tip moment.[30]

Many studies have examined the geometric design and stability of orthodontic TADs. Geometric designs of screws that seem to have a positive effect on primary stability include conical shape, greater outer diameter,[30] increased length,[31-33] and use of abutments (attachments to screw for placing orthodontic force).[34]

Placement of TADs in areas of higher bone mineral density (BMD) increases the primary stability.[16,30,33] How TADs are placed also influences the primary stability. Initially, placement of screw-type TADs either requires or does not require the drilling of a pilot hole. A recent study indicated that drill-free screws have increased bone-metal contact, greater bone area, and less mobility than screws that require the drilling of a pilot hole.[15] In addition, for screws that require a pilot hole, the smaller predrilling diameters increase the insertion and removal torques.[30]

Excessive loading of mechanically retained TADs has been associated with increased failure rates. Butcher et al.[35] recently found that increased *tip moments* (magnitude of orthodontic force × length of lever arm) at the bone rim caused decreased stability mechanically retained TADs. Tip moments greater than 900 centinewtons (cN) mm were found to cause decreased stability of mechanically retained TADs after 22 and 70 days of loading.

To increase primary stability of mechanically retained TADs, particularly in areas of decreased BMD (maxilla), these studies suggest using a longer, wider, drill-free screw with a short abutment.

OSSEOINTEGRATED DEVICES

Two major factors affecting osseointegration are primary stability and a no-loading healing period. Primary stability is critical to the processes of osseointegration of the TAD. In one study, when Ti implants were placed in the mandible of rats so that they did not make contact with the mandibular bone, no bone-implant contact was observed, even after 9 months of a no-load healing period.[36]

Roberts et al.[6] and Sherman[4] both advocated a no-load healing before the application of orthodontic forces to the osseointegrated TADs. Immediate or early loading of these TADs caused decreased stability[4] and spontaneous fracture of the bone[6] in animal models.

OVERLAP BETWEEN OSSEOINTEGRATED AND MECHANICALLY RETAINED ANCHORAGE DEVICES

Mechanically retained orthodontic TADs are associated with early or immediate loading, a lack of osseointegration, and the ability to withstand lesser orthodontic forces. In contrast, osseointegrated TADs are associated

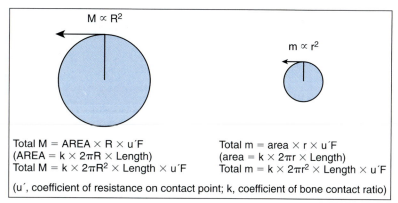

Figure 2-2
Difference in Removal Torque for Screws with Different Radii. Removal torque is proportional to the screw radius and bone contact area, which is proportional to the screw radius under the same bone contact ratio. Therefore, removal torque is proportional to the square of the screw radius. If the radius is reduced to one third or one fourth, removal torque will decrease to one ninth or one sixteenth, respectively. *(From Kim JW, Ahn SJ, Chang YI: Am J Orthod Dentofacial Orthop 128(2):190-194, 2005.)*

with delayed loading, osseointegration, and the ability to withstand greater orthodontic forces. However, recent research and the development of new types of TADs have made the distinction between the two types less clear.

EARLY LOADING ON OSSEOINTEGRATED DEVICES

Waiting for osseointegration before applying orthodontic forces may not be important in predicting TAD failure. Chen et al.[37] used finite element analysis to compare the stress and failure of osseointegrated and nonosseointegrated palatal implants caused by the application of a 5-newton (N) orthodontic force. They found that nonosseointegrated implants had greater stresses on the surface than osseointegrated implants. However, the stresses did not result in loss of anchorage or failure of the implant. The authors concluded that "waiting for osseointegration might be unnecessary for an orthodontic implant."[37]

OSSEOINTEGRATION OF MECHANICALLY RETAINED DEVICES

For all miniscrew TADs, waiting for osseointegration before applying orthodontic loads is unnecessary. However, whether the miniscrews become osseointegrated during orthodontic treatment depends on the type and surface properties of the miniscrew. Studies using the Aarhus Anchorage System screw suggested that a fibrous interface between the screw and bone allows easy removal of the orthodontic miniscrew.[38,39] Another study showed that miniscrews 2 mm in diameter and 17 mm in length (Leibinger, Tuttlingen, Germany) do not remain absolutely stationary throughout orthodontic loading; the miniscrews tipped forward significantly, by an average of 0.4 mm at the screw head.[40] The authors hypothesized that the miniscrews moved because they were not osseointegrated and because a layer of fibrous tissue was interposed between the miniscrews and the surrounding bone. Histologically, however, osseointegration has been documented in miniscrews (Osas; Epoch Medical, Seoul, South Korea), measuring 1.6 mm in diameter, after waiting 1 week before applying an orthodontic force of 200 to 300 g for 11 weeks.[15] Deguchi et al.[41] reported similar results. Miniscrews may be easy to remove because of the decreased width of the screw, not the lack of osseointegration (Figure 2-2).

ORTHODONTIC FORCES APPLIED TO ANCHORAGE DEVICES

A recent review compared loading protocols for osseointegrated and mechanically retained orthodontic TADs[42]; 11 articles met selection criteria.* In the five studies with osseointegrated TADs, the no-load healing period was 2 to 12 months, and the range of applied orthodontic forces was 80 to 550 g. In the six studies with mechanically retained TADs, four applied orthodontic forces immediately after TAD insertion two applied force after 2 weeks. The orthodontic forces in the studies ranged from 150 to 500 g. Therefore, a similar magnitude of orthodontic forces is used for both osseointegrated and mechanically retained TADs (Table 2-2).

---

*References 14, 24, 33, 39, 40, 43-48.

TABLE 2-2 Comparison Review of TAD Loading Protocols

Study	Sample*/Age	Number/Type of Appliance	Time Before Loading	Force Applied (grams)	Anchorage Time (months)	Failure
Bernhart et al.[43]	21: 15 F, 6 M 25.8 ± 9.9 (12.7-48.1) yr	21 mini-implants	4.2 mo	—	11.6	3
Cheng et al.[44]	44: 38 F, 6 M 29 ± 8.9 (13-55) yr	92 miniscrews	2-4 wk	100-200	—	15
Costa et al.[39]	14	16 miniscrews	Immediately loaded	—	—	—
Freudenthaler et al.[14]	8: 4 F, 4 M 22.1 (13-46) yr	15 screws	Immediately loaded	150	11.3	1
Gelgör et al.[45]	25: 18 F, 7 M 13.9 (11.3-16.5) yr	25 screws	Immediately loaded	500	3-6.2 (4.6)	—
Higuchi and Slack[46]	7: 5 F, 2 M 33.1 (22-41) yr	14 implants	4-6 mo	Initially, 150-200 Later, 400	36	0
Liou et al.[40]	16 22-29 yr	32 miniscrews	2 wk	400	9	—
Miyawaki et al.[33]	51: 42 F, 9 M 21.8 ± 7.8 yr	134 screws	Immediately loaded	<200	12	10
Ödman et al.[47]	9: 6 F, 3 M 47 (17-64) yr	23 implants	3-9 mo	—	4-33 (17)	0
Trisi and Rebaudi[48]	41 patients	Orthoimplants	2-12 mo	80-120	2-15	0
Wehrbein et al.[24]	4: 2 F, 2 M 18-27 yr	6 orthoimplants	1 (0), others (12 wk)	200-600	8-20	0

From Ohashi E et al: *Angle Orthod* 76(4):721-727, 2006.
*Total: F, females; M, males.

COMMON DRUGS THAT MAY AFFECT ANCHORAGE DEVICES

CYCLOOXYGENASE-2 INHIBITORS

Cyclooxygenase (COX) is the rate-limiting enzyme responsible for the conversion of arachidonic acid into prostaglandins. There are two isoforms of the enzyme: COX-1, which is constitutively expressed, and COX-2, which is inducible. In bone cells, the increase in prostaglandin levels caused by various stimuli depends on the induction of COX-2. In animal models, inhibitors of COX-2 cause a delay in fracture healing.[49] However, there are no reports of COX-2 inhibitors affecting the osseointegration of dental implants, possibly because of a lack of studies, or because osseointegration and bone healing occur by separate biological processes. A recent report showed that genes are expressed differently during osseointegration of Ti implants than in normal bone osteotomy healing.[50]

BISPHOSPHONATES

Bisphosphonates are a class of drugs that inhibits the resorption of bone. Administered orally or intravenously, the two classes of bisphosphonates are nonnitrogenous and nitrogenous, each with different mechanisms of action. The *nonnitrogenous* bisphosphonates are metabolized in the cell to compounds that compete with adenosine triphosphate (ATP); the *nitrogenous* bisphosphonates block the enzyme farnesyl diphosphate synthase. Bisphosphonates are used in a variety of conditions that cause bone fragility, including osteoporosis, osteitis deformans, osteogenesis imperfecta, and in cancer patients, bone metastasis.

Bisphosphonates do not seem to interfere with osseointegration of Ti implants in animal models[51] and may even increase bone-implant contact and removal torque in animal models with reduced bone mass.[52,53] However, an increase in the incidence of osteonecrosis of the jaws has recently become evident in cancer patients taking nitrogenous bisphosphonates intravenously.

Clinical diagnosis of osteonecrosis of the jaws is usually made by the presence of exposed bone in the oral cavity for an extended time (Figure 2-3). Although some patients may be asymptomatic, more frequently they have symptoms when the site becomes secondarily infected or the soft tissues are traumatized by the sharp edges of the exposed bone. Typical signs and symptoms include pain, soft tissue swelling, and tooth

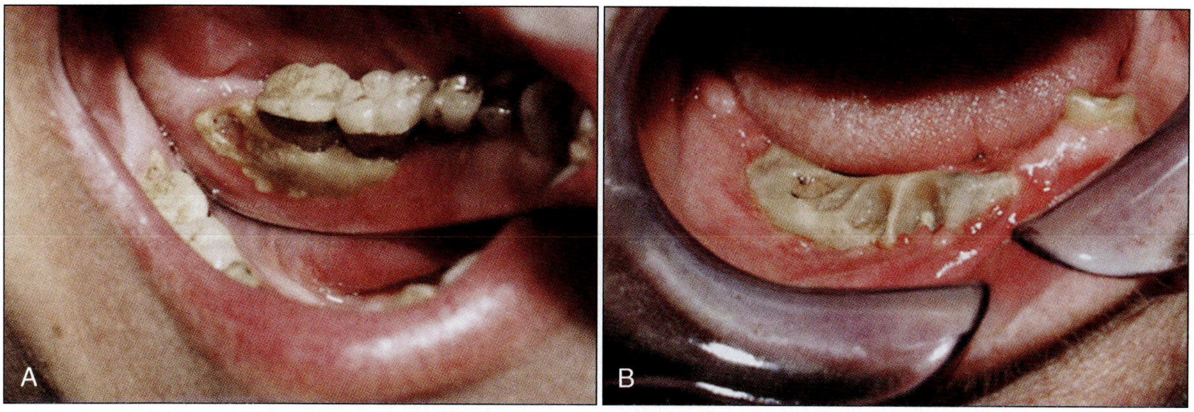

Figure 2-3

A, Spontaneous bone exposure of the posterior mandible, lingual aspect. **B,** Nonhealing extraction sites with exposed alveolar bone. *(From Ruggiero SL, Fantasia J, Carlson E: Oral Surg Oral Med Oral Pathol Oral Radiol Endod 102(4):433-441, 2006.)*

loosening. Histopathological analysis of biopsy specimens from osteonecrotic bone demonstrates tissue with lacunae devoid of bone cells. If the site is secondarily infected, the presence of bacteria and inflammatory cells consistent with osteomyelitis may also be noted.[54,55]

Of patients who develop bisphosphonate-related osteonecrosis of the jaw, 94% are cancer patients receiving intravenous nitrogenous bisphosphonate therapy. The mandible is more likely to be affected than the maxilla, and 60% of these cancer patients recently had dental surgical procedures.[56] Expert panels recommend that elective dental procedures should not be performed in cancer patients taking bisphosphonates.[57-59] Therefore, clinicians should not perform orthodontics, let alone place TADs, in these patients.

In other recent case reports, osteoporosis patients taking nitrogenous bisphosphonate have developed osteonecrosis of the jaw. The estimated incidence of nitrogenous bisphosphonate–related osteonecrosis of the jaw in patients taking oral bisphosphonate for osteoporosis is 1 : 140,000.[60] (To put this risk in perspective, the National Weather Service estimates that the chance of being struck by lightning is 1 : 400,000.) However, some experts believe that many new cases of bisphosphonate-related osteonecrosis of the jaw are emerging, and that the incidence will be much greater. Nevertheless, the American Dental Association now recommends the following:

> Treatment plans for patients taking oral bisphosphonates should be considered carefully, since implant placement requires the preparation of the osteotomy site . . . Before implant placement, the dentist and the patient should discuss the risks, benefits and treatment alternatives, which may include but are not limited to periodontal, endodontic or nonimplant prosthetic treatments . . . [T]his discussion should be documented and the patient's written acknowledgment of that discussion and consent for the chosen course of treatment should be obtained.[60]

In addition, the American Society of Bone and Mineral Research recommends that in osteoporosis patients taking bisphosphonates, "Dental surgery should be limited to that required for good dental health and undertaken only when more conservative non-surgical therapies are either not appropriate or ineffective."[61]

Therefore, placement of TADs in patients taking nitrogenous bisphosphonates for osteoporosis is inadvisable.

CONCLUSION

The biological response and the factors that predict stability differ between mechanically retained and osseous integrated TADs. However, recent research and the development of new types of TADs have made the distinction less clear. Despite the relative ease in placing these devices, careful attention should be paid to the medical history of these patients.

REFERENCES

1. Heymann GC, Tulloch JF: Implantable devices as orthodontic anchorage: a review of current treatment modalities, *J Esthet Restor Dent* 18(2):68-79 (discussion, 80), 2006.
2. Gainsforth BL et al: A study of orthodontic anchorage possibilities in basal bone, *Am J Orthod Oral Surg* 31:406-417, 1945.
3. Linkow LI: The endosseous blade implant and its use in orthodontics, *Int J Orthod* 7(4):149-154, 1969.
4. Sherman AJ: Bone reaction to orthodontic forces on vitreous carbon dental implants, *Am J Orthod* 74(1):79-87, 1978.
5. Gray JB et al: Studies on the efficacy of implants as orthodontic anchorage, *Am J Orthod* 83(4):311-317, 1983.
6. Roberts WE et al: Osseous adaptation to continuous loading of rigid endosseous implants, *Am J Orthod* 86(2):95-111, 1984.
7. Creekmore TD, Eklund MK: Possibility of skeletal anchorage, *J Clin Orthod* 17:266-267, 1983.

8. Roberts WE, Marshall KJ, Mozsary PG: Rigid endosseous implant utilized as anchorage to protract molars and close an atrophic extraction site, *Angle Orthod* 60(2):135-152, 1990.
9. Block MS, Hoffman DR: A new device for absolute anchorage for orthodontics, *Am J Orthod Dentofacial Orthop* 107(3):251-258, 1995.
10. Kanomi R: Mini-implant for orthodontic anchorage, *J Clin Orthod* 31(11):763-767, 1997.
11. Umemori M et al: Skeletal anchorage system for open-bite correction, *Am J Orthod Dentofacial Orthop* 115(2):166-174, 1999.
12. Sugawara J: Orthodontic reduction of lower facial height in open bite patients with skeletal anchorage system: beyond traditional orthodontics, *World J Orthod* 6(suppl):24-26, 2005.
13. Sugawara J et al: Distal movement of maxillary molars in non-growing patients with the skeletal anchorage system, *Am J Orthod Dentofacial Orthop* 129(6):723-733, 2006.
14. Freudenthaler JW, Haas R, Bantleon HP: Bicortical titanium screws for critical orthodontic anchorage in the mandible: a preliminary report on clinical applications, *Clin Oral Implants Res* 12(4):358-363, 2001.
15. Kim JW, Ahn SJ, Chang YI: Histomorphometric and mechanical analyses of the drill-free screw as orthodontic anchorage, *Am J Orthod Dentofacial Orthop* 128(2):190-194, 2005.
16. Huja SS et al: Pull-out strength of monocortical screws placed in the maxillae and mandibles of dogs, *Am J Orthod Dentofacial Orthop* 127(3):307-313, 2005.
17. Huja SS et al: Biomechanical and histomorphometric analyses of monocortical screws at placement and 6 weeks postinsertion, *J Oral Implantol* 32(3):110-116, 2006.
18. Nygren H, Tengvall P, Lundstrom I: The initial reactions of TiO_2 with blood, *J Biomed Mater Res* 34(4):487-492, 1997.
19. Park JY, Davies JE: Red blood cell and platelet interactions with titanium implant surfaces, *Clin Oral Implants Res* 11(6):530-539, 2000.
20. Franchi M et al: Biological fixation of endosseous implants, *Micron* 36(7-8):665-671, 2005.
21. Futami T et al: Tissue response to titanium implants in the rat maxilla: ultrastructural and histochemical observations of the bone-titanium interface, *J Periodontol* 71(2):287-298, 2000.
22. Traini T et al: Bone microvascular pattern around loaded dental implants in a canine model, *Clin Oral Invest* 10(2):151-156, 2006.
23. Slaets E et al: Early cellular responses in cortical bone healing around unloaded titanium implants: an animal study, *J Periodontol* 77(6):1015-1024, 2006.
24. Wehrbein H et al: Bone-to-implant contact of orthodontic implants in humans subjected to horizontal loading, *Clin Oral Implants Res* 9(5):348-353, 1998.
25. Saito S et al: Endosseous titanium implants as anchors for mesiodistal tooth movement in the beagle dog, *Am J Orthod Dentofacial Orthop* 118(6):601-607, 2000.
26. Wehrbein H, Yildirim M, Diedrich P: Osteodynamics around orthodontically loaded short maxillary implants: an experimental pilot study, *J Orofac Orthop* 60(6):409-415, 1999.
27. Melsen B, Lang NP: Biological reactions of alveolar bone to orthodontic loading of oral implants, *Clin Oral Implants Res* 12(2):144-152, 2001.
28. Meyer U et al: Ultrastructural characterization of the implant/bone interface of immediately loaded dental implants, *Biomaterials* 25(10):1959-1967, 2004.
29. Berglundh T et al: De novo alveolar bone formation adjacent to endosseous implants, *Clin Oral Implants Res* 14(3):251-262, 2003.
30. Wilmes B et al: Parameters affecting primary stability of orthodontic mini-implants, *J Orofac Orthop* 67(3):162-174, 2006.
31. Gedrange T et al: An evaluation of resonance frequency analysis for the determination of the primary stability of orthodontic palatal implants: a study in human cadavers, *Clin Oral Implants Res* 16(4):425-431, 2005.
32. Chen CH et al: The use of microimplants in orthodontic anchorage, *J Oral Maxillofac Surg* 64(8):1209-1213, 2006.
33. Miyawaki S et al: Factors associated with the stability of titanium screws placed in the posterior region for orthodontic anchorage, *Am J Orthod Dentofacial Orthop* 124(4):373-378, 2003.
34. Motoyoshi M et al: Biomechanical effect of abutment on stability of orthodontic mini-implant: a finite element analysis, *Clin Oral Implants Res* 16(4):480-485, 2005.
35. Buchter A et al: Load-related implant reaction of mini-implants used for orthodontic anchorage, *Clin Oral Implants Res* 16(4):473-479, 2005.
36. Lioubavina-Hack N, Lang NP, Karring T: Significance of primary stability for osseointegration of dental implants, *Clin Oral Implants Res* 17(3):244-250, 2006.
37. Chen F et al: Anchorage effect of osseointegrated vs nonosseointegrated palatal implants, *Angle Orthod* 76(4):660-665, 2006.
38. Melsen BV et al: Miniscrew implants: the Aarhus Anchorage System, *Semin Orthod* 11(1):24-31, 2005.
39. Costa A, Raffainl M, Melsen B: Miniscrews as orthodontic anchorage: a preliminary report, *Int J Adult Orthod Orthognath Surg* 13(3):201-209, 1998..
40. Liou EJ, Pai BC, Lin JC: Do miniscrews remain stationary under orthodontic forces? *Am J Orthod Dentofacial Orthop* 126(1):42-47, 2004.
41. Deguchi T et al: The use of small titanium screws for orthodontic anchorage, *J Dent Res* 82(5):377-381, 2003.
42. Ohashi E et al: Implant vs screw loading protocols in orthodontics, *Angle Orthod* 76(4):721-727, 2006.
43. Bernhart T et al: Short epithetic implants for orthodontic anchorage in the paramedian region of the palate: a clinical study, *Clin Oral Implants Res* 12:624-631, 2001.
44. Cheng SJ, Tsong IY, Lee JJ, Kok SH: A prospective study of the risk factors associated with failure of mini-implants used for orthodontic anchorage, *Int Oral Maxillofac Implants* 19:100-106, 2004.
45. Gelgör IE et al: Intraosseous screw-supported uppermolar distalization, *Angle Orthod* 74:838-850, 2004.
46. Higuchi KW, Slack JM: The use of titanium fixtures for intraoral anchorage to facilitate orthodontic tooth movement, *Int J Oral Maxillofac Implants* 6:338-344, 1991.
47. Ödman J, Lekholm U, Jemt T, Thilander B: Osseointegrated implants as orthodontic anchorage in the treatment of partially edentulous adult patients, *Eur J Orthod* 16:187-201, 1994.
48. Trisi P, Rebaudi A: Progressive bone adaptation of titanium implants during and after orthodontic load in human, *Int J Periodont Restor Dent* 22:31-43, 2002.
49. Radi ZA, Khan NK: Effects of cyclooxygenase inhibition on bone, tendon, and ligament healing, *Inflamm Res* 54(9):358-366, 2005.
50. Ogawa T, Nishimura I: Genes differentially expressed in titanium implant healing, *J Dent Res* 85(6):566-570, 2006.
51. Chacon GE et al: Effect of alendronate on endosseous implant integration: an in vivo study in rabbits, *J Oral Maxillofac Surg* 64(7):1005-1009, 2006.
52. Duarte PM et al: Alendronate therapy may be effective in the prevention of bone loss around titanium implants inserted in estrogen-deficient rats, *J Periodontol* 76(1):107-114, 2005.
53. Narai S, Nagahata S: Effects of alendronate on the removal torque of implants in rats with induced osteoporosis, *Int J Oral Maxillofac Implants* 18(2):218-223, 2003.
54. Ruggiero SL, Fantasia J, Carlson E: Bisphosphonate-related osteonecrosis of the jaw: background and guidelines for diagnosis, staging and management, *Oral Surg Oral Med Oral Pathol Oral Radiol Endod* 102(4):433-441, 2006.
55. Nase JB, Suzuki JB: Osteonecrosis of the jaw and oral bisphosphonate treatment, *J Am Dent Assoc* 137(8):1115-1119 (quiz, 1169-1170), 2006.

56. Woo SB, Hellstein JW, Kalmar JR: Narrative [corrected] review: bisphosphonates and osteonecrosis of the jaws, *Ann Intern Med* 144(10):753-761, 2006.
57. Van Poznak C, Estilo C: Osteonecrosis of the jaw in cancer patients receiving IV bisphosphonates, *Oncology (Huntingt)* 20(9):1053-1062 (discussion, 1065-1066), 2006.
58. Tanvetyanon T, Stiff PJ: Management of the adverse effects associated with intravenous bisphosphonates, *Ann Oncol* 17(6):897-907, 2006.
59. Migliorati CA et al: Managing the care of patients with bisphosphonate-associated osteonecrosis: an American Academy of Oral Medicine position paper, *J Am Dent Assoc* 136(12):1658-1668, 2005.
60. American Dental Association: Dental management of patients receiving oral bisphosphonate therapy: expert panel recommendations, *J Am Dent Assoc* 137(8):1144-1150, 2006.
61. Shane E, Goldring S, Christakos S: Osteonecrosis of the jaw: more research needed, *J Bone Miner Res* 21(10):1503-1505, 2006.

PART II

DIAGNOSIS AND TREATMENT PLANNING

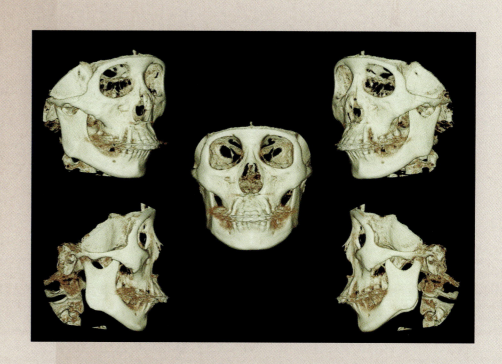

CHAPTER 3

Radiographic Evaluation of Bone Sites for Mini-Implant Placement

Kuniaki Miyajima

Temporary anchorage devices (TADs) such as the mini-implant have proven efficacy in providing "absolute anchorage" in orthodontics. However, some failures have been reported at insertion and during tooth movement. The most serious adverse outcome is injury to the root, which may occur not only at insertion, but also with tooth movement if the screw and root are in close contact. A less serious complication is loosening of the mini-implant, resulting from inflammation or excessive orthodontic force, regardless of primary stability obtained during surgery.

RADIOGRAPHY AND COMPUTED TOMOGRAPHY

To avoid TAD failures, clinicians must consider the ideal sites for mini-implant placement and understand how forces need to be applied. Radiographic information is a prerequisite in determining the ideal site for mini-implant placement. A two-dimensional (2D) panoramic radiograph usually suffices to determine the implant placement area, although there are inherent limitations. In Figure 3-1, for example, the panoramic radiograph *(A)* shows a mini-implant placed through what appears to be the root of a tooth, whereas the posteroanterior (PA) cephalometric radiograph *(B)* shows that the mini-implant was actually far from the teeth, in the external oblique ridge.

Three-dimensional computed tomography (3D CT) is sometimes required to obtain more detailed information of the potential implant sites, such as bone depth, bone density, and distance between adjacent roots. Software applications are useful in devising a precise plan, especially when the mini-implant is to be placed between roots or near the sinus.

The CT scanner, first described for medical use by Hounsfield[1] in 1973, has since been applied to analyze bone depth, width, and density of teeth, as well as the distance between roots, and to map precisely other anatomical structures, such as the maxillary sinus.[2] With this information, clinicians can find the most suitable site for TAD placement.

Many CT scanners use cone beams, resulting in less irradiation to the rest of the body while providing sharper and realistic images. The cone-beam (CB) CT scanners currently available for craniofacial applications are NewTom 3G (Aperio Services, Sarasota, Florida), i-CAT (Imaging Sciences International, Hatfield, Pennsylvania), CB MercuRay (Hitachi Medical, Tokyo, Japan), and the 3DX multiimage micro CT scanner (Morita, Tokyo).

Radiographic analysis software has also been developed, including SimPlant (Materialise, Belgium), i-VIEW (Morita), i-dent (IGS, Israel), i-cat (i-cat Corp, Osaka, Japan).[3] Most of these programs were developed originally for use with dental implants in edentulous areas. However, such software allows visual and quantitative assessment of the site, as well as calculation of the distances between any two points on the 3D models, making it also useful in orthodontic treatment planning.

The radiographic data provided by the CT scan can then be used for the fabrication of the surgical stent. During surgery, a surgical guide is a safe and reliable tool that allows precise insertion of the mini-implant at the designated site.

STUDY MODELS

The mini-implant is one of several TADs widely accepted and used by clinicians. I and my colleagues have performed 3D finite element model (FEM) analysis[4] and animal studies[5] using miniscrews for orthodontic anchorage.

FINITE ELEMENT MODEL ANALYSIS

Using the software program COSMOS/M (version 1.75), alveolar bone was modeled to a width of 10 mm,

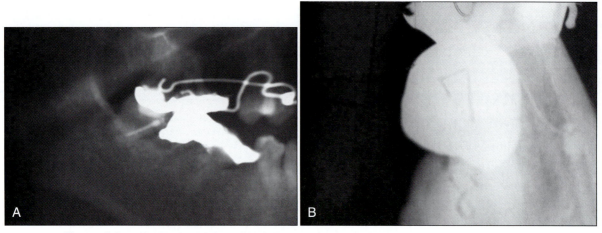

Figure 3-1
Mini-Implant Placed on External Oblique Ridge. **A,** In the two-dimensional (2D) panoramic radiograph, the mini-implant appears to be placed into the tooth root. This is an example of the limitation of 2D radiography. **B,** In the periapical x-ray study, taken from the axial direction, the same mini-implant is seen to be far from the teeth.

depth of 10 mm, and height of 30 mm (comprising 2.0 mm of cortical bone covering 28 mm of spongy bone). A linear static model for the 3D FEM analysis was applied.[4] This model consisted of 6293 elements and 18,879 degrees of freedom. To test this 3D FEM, all the experiments were performed based on the assumption that the implants and the surrounding alveolar bone were osseointegrated. The proposed miniscrew implant for model 1 was 1.0 mm in diameter and 5 mm in length (Figure 3-2), whereas that of model 2 was 2.0 mm in diameter and 15 mm in length. The following load combinations were applied on these two models:

1. Amount: 100 grams (g) of tractional load.
2. Three different angles of direction: loads at 0, 45, and 90 degrees perpendicular to the bone surface were applied individually on the implant head and 4 mm away from the neck (Figure 3-3).

To determine the effect of varying the height of the tractional point above the alveolar surface, 1-, 2-, and 4-mm distances above the cortical bone surface were tested using model 1 (Figure 3-4).

Table 3-1 shows the mechanical properties of different components of current 3D FEM models. The stress distributions and deflections in the implants and surrounding alveolar bone were calculated using the COSMOS/M linear static module.

Results

The 3D FEM analysis revealed the same "pattern" of stress distributions and deflections in both model 1 and model 2, although the values were much larger in model 1 than in model 2. The findings are summarized as follows[4]:

1. The greatest stress on the surrounding alveolar bone was distributed at the cervical area (Figure 3-5).
2. The greatest stress on the implant was distributed at the cervical area (Figure 3-6).
3. Stress increased with the angle, from 0 degrees to 45 and to 90 degrees (Table 3-2).
4. Values of stress distribution in model 1 were almost six times larger with a directional angle of 0 and 45 degrees, and 3.4 times larger with an angle of 90 degrees, compared with those of model 2 (see Table 3-2).
5. Stress created at a point 4 mm above the bone surface was about 3.2 times greater than that at 1 mm above the surface when tractional force was applied horizontally (Table 3-3).

Conclusions

Stress was distributed on the neck areas of both the implant and the alveolar bone, where most inflammation is seen after mini-implant insertion. One significant issue is the diameter of the mini-implant. A mini-implant 1 mm in diameter created almost six times more stress at the neck of the alveolar bone area than one with a 2-mm diameter.

In addition to the magnitude of force applied, the direction of the force application should also be considered to prevent failure of the mini-implant. Even when the amount of force is the same, the point of force application on the mini-implant is critical. Therefore, gingival depth should be considered in addition to cortical bone depth.

ANIMAL STUDY

The purpose of the animal study was to prove the applicability of the FEM study to live subjects.[5] The actual intraoral situation may be different from that premised by a computer as a result of factors such as bacterial plaque and the chewing function in animals.

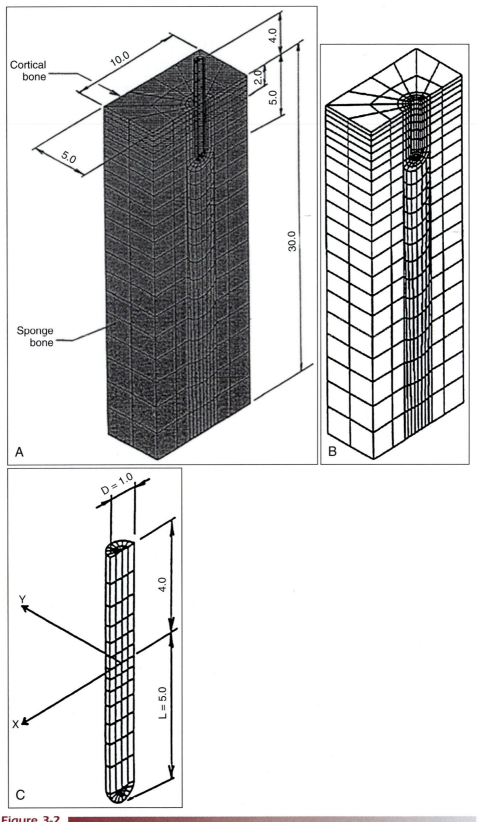

Figure 3-2
Finite Element Model (FEM) Analysis: Model 1. The alveolar bone was modeled with 10 mm of width, 10 mm of height, and 30 mm of depth. The mini-implant in model 1 was 1.0 mm in diameter with a length of 5 mm. **A,** Overall view. **B,** Alveolar bone. **C,** Implant.

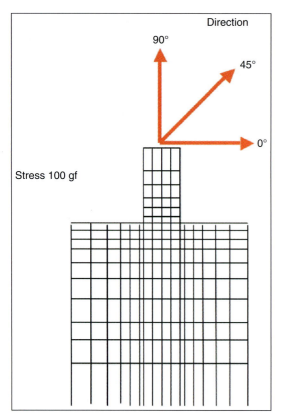

Figure 3-3
Tractional loads of 100 g (*gf,* grams of force) are individually applied on the implant head, 4 mm away from the neck in three directions (0, 45, and 90 degrees perpendicular to the bone surface).

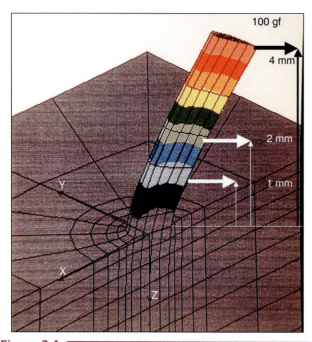

Figure 3-4
Using model 1, assumed heights of 1, 2, and 4 mm were used to determine the effect of varying the placement of the tractional point (height) from the alveolar surface.

TABLE 3-1	Mechanical Properties of Three-Dimensional (3D) Finite Element Model (FEM)		
Component	**Elasticity Coefficient**		**Poisson's Ratio**
Cortical bone	1.4×10^4 MPa (1.43×10^6 gf/mm^2)		0.30
Spongy bone	7.9×10^3 MPa (8.06×10^5 gf/mm^2)		0.30
Implant	1.1×10^4 MPa (1.085×10^7 gf/mm^2)		0.34

MPa, megapascals; *gf,* grams of force.

Four adult beagle dogs were used to study maxillary canine intrusion. On one side, the labial alveolar bone mesial to the canine received a miniscrew implant 6 mm long, while the labial alveolar bone mesial to the other canine received an implant 3 mm long. Both had the same screw diameter of 1.0 mm. A lingual button with a band was placed on the canine. The mucoperiosteal flap was opened and the alveolar bone denuded. Denuded cortical bone was drilled to the length of each mini-implant (3 mm and 6 mm) with a 0.9-mm water-cooled pilot drill. The mini-implants were inserted with a miniature screwdriver. Soon after implant placement, 100-g nickel-titanium (Ni-Ti) closed-coil springs were placed between the implant head and the canine lingual button on both sides (Figure 3-7).

Data were collected soon after the placement of the implant and 3 months later, at the end of the experiments, using photographs of the oral cavity and periapical radiographs. At the end of the orthodontic intrusion, the animals were anesthetized, and the periimplant alveolar bone with the implants was dissected and soft x-ray studies performed (SRO-M50, Sofron, Tokyo). The mini-implants and the surrounding bone were prepared for histologic calcified tissue sections using conventional laboratory techniques.

Results

No implant failure was found during the 3-month experimental period in either the short-screw or long-screw implants. Clinical measurements indicated that the canines on both sides were intruded and tipped mesially by an average of 3.5 mm over the 3-month period. There was no difference between the long and the short screw lengths in the amount of canine movement. Radiographic findings also indicated no significant difference in the periodontal condition on both sides (Figure 3-8) or any observable signs of root resorption.

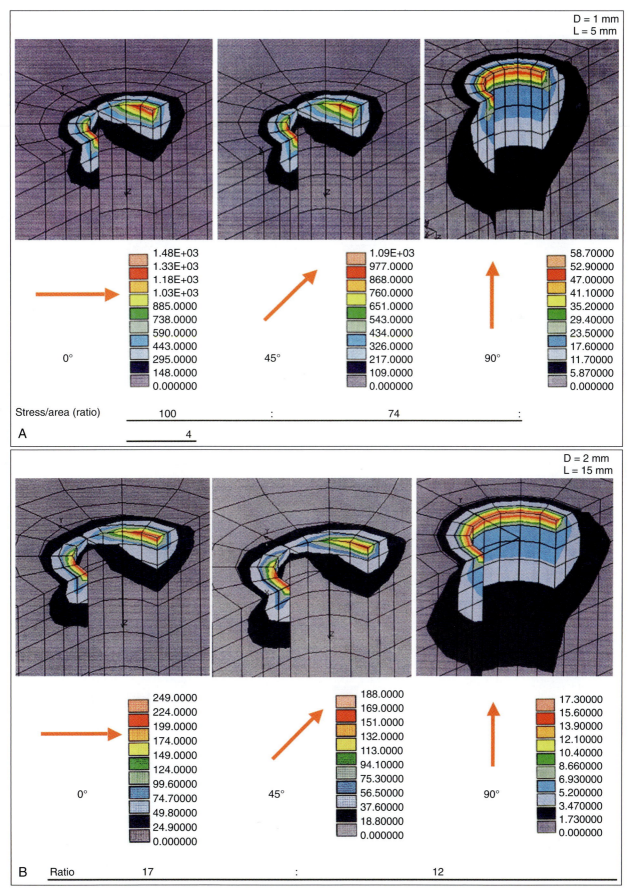

Figure 3-5

Results of FEM Study: Bone Stress. Maximum stress on the surrounding alveolar bone was distributed on the cervical area. **A**, Model 1. **B**, Model 2.

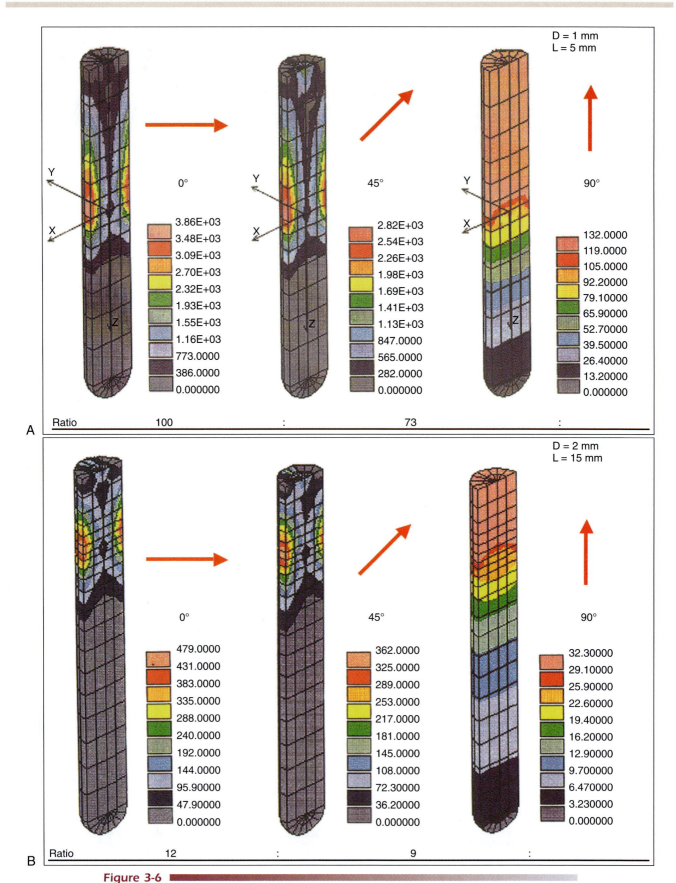

Figure 3-6

Results of FEM Study: Implant Stress. Maximum stress of the implant body was distributed on the cervical area. **A,** Model 1. **B,** Model 2.

TABLE 3-2	Stress Distribution on Alveolar Bone and Implant in 3D FEM Analysis*		
Model (dimensions)	Force Direction (degrees)	Alveolar Bone (gf/mm^2)	Implant (gf/mm^2)
Model 1	0	1480	3860
D: 1 mm	45	1090	2820
L: 5 mm	90	59	132
Model 2	0	249	479
D: 2 mm	45	188	362
L: 15 mm	90	17	32

*FEM analysis revealed that vertical traction causes about 25 times more stress on the alveolar bone in model 1 and 14 times more in model 2 than horizontal traction. Model 1 received six times more stress on the alveolar bone than model 2.
D, Diameter; gf, grams of force; L, length.

TABLE 3-3	Amount of Stress Produced at Different Heights of Applied Force	
Height of Tractional Point above Bone	Alveolar Bone (cN/mm^2)	Implant (Model 1) (cN/mm^2)
1 mm	459	925
2 mm	796	1860
4 mm	1480	3860

cN, centinewtons.

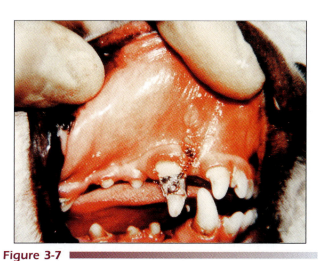

Figure 3-7
The 100-g Ni-Ti closed-coil springs were placed between the implant head and the canine lingual button on both sides.

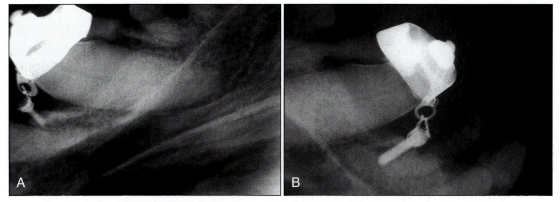

Figure 3-8
Periapical x-ray (**A**) and soft x-ray (**B**) studies show no significant difference in the periodontal conditions on both sides.

Histological study revealed that the surrounding bone did not osseointegrate to most of the implant surface of either short-screw or long-screw implants. Nevertheless, the teeth moved, and no implant failure was seen. Therefore, complete osseointegration may not be needed for orthodontic anchorage purposes.

Conclusions

The FEM study proved that screw length does not affect results as long as the screw diameter is the same. Mini-implants with a 1-mm diameter were stable with 100 g of tractional force.

CASE STUDIES

Based on FEM and animal studies, mini-implants of 1-mm diameter and 6-mm length were fabricated for clinical use. However, most mini-implants of this size were not stable, presumably because of the difference in bone density between beagle dogs and humans. Therefore, larger miniscrews were selected, ISA (Biodent, Tokyo), with a 1.4-mm diameter and a 6-mm length, which were found to be stable.

The following two case reports describe patients with dolicofacial and brachyfacial features.

CASE REPORT 3-1: DOLICOFACIAL PATIENT

Figure 3-9 shows a 3D reconstruction of the skull of this dolicofacial patient, initially planned to undergo orthognathic surgery. However, orthodontic treatment using TADs was considered when the patient rejected orthognathic surgery. Upper and lower anterior, premolar, and molar alveolar bone areas were used to plan the placement of the mini-implants. A medical CT scan was obtained for this purpose.

Nine sliced images on a panoramic view were selected in the upper anterior area, after determining the approximate area where a mini-implant would be placed (Figure 3-10, *A*). One of the views was selected for a close-up and used to measure bone depth between the labial and palatal cortical layers. Because this patient had a long face, there was sufficient alveolar bone space vertically (Figure 3-10, *B*). The alveolar bone width measured 7.39 mm.

Bone density for the upper anterior area was also measured; the red bar on the left in Figure 3-11 indicates the mini-implant. The bone density both inside and outside the implant area was evaluated. The mean density value inside the implant area was 603.91 Hounsfield units (HU), whereas the bone density outside the implant area was 691.03 HU. Both the labial and the palatal cortical bone had high density values, and the bone farther from the implant was denser than the bone surrounding the implant.

Another nine sliced views are shown on Figure 3-12, *A*, depicting the alveolar area selected for mini-implant placement distal to the canine. Figure 3-12, *B*, shows a close-up view of this area. The upper-right figure shows a cross-sectional view of this bone and the mini-implant (red bar). The horizontal distance between the buccal and the palatal cortical bone was 8.54 mm. The bone density of this area appeared deficient, as seen in Figure 3-13, which suggested that immediate loading was contraindicated.

For the molar area, a site distal to the first molar was chosen to receive the implant (Figure 3-14, *A*). The vertical distance from the selected implant site to the maxillary sinus (Figure 3-14, *B*) was measured at 10.23 mm. This distance was large enough to accommodate a monocortical implant.

The anatomical characteristics of the lower incisor area were different from those of the upper incisor area. Indeed, morphologically the alveolar bone width between the labial and the lingual cortical bone is generally smaller in the lower incisor region, especially in patients with long-face patterns (Figure 3-15, *A*). The cross-sectional view of the lower incisor area revealed a very thin alveolar bone width, only 4.78 mm (Figure 3-15, *B*). Careful selection of the implant length was required. Fortunately, the bone density for the implant site under consideration was sufficiently high for good primary stability on insertion of the mini-implant (Figure 3-16).

In the lower premolar area, the mini-implant was designed to be placed between the canine and the first

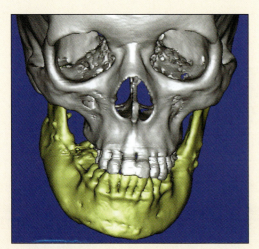

Figure 3-9 Three-dimensional (3D) reconstruction using 3D CT and associated software shows skull of the patient with dolicofacial features.

CASE REPORT 3-1: DOLICOFACIAL PATIENT—cont'd

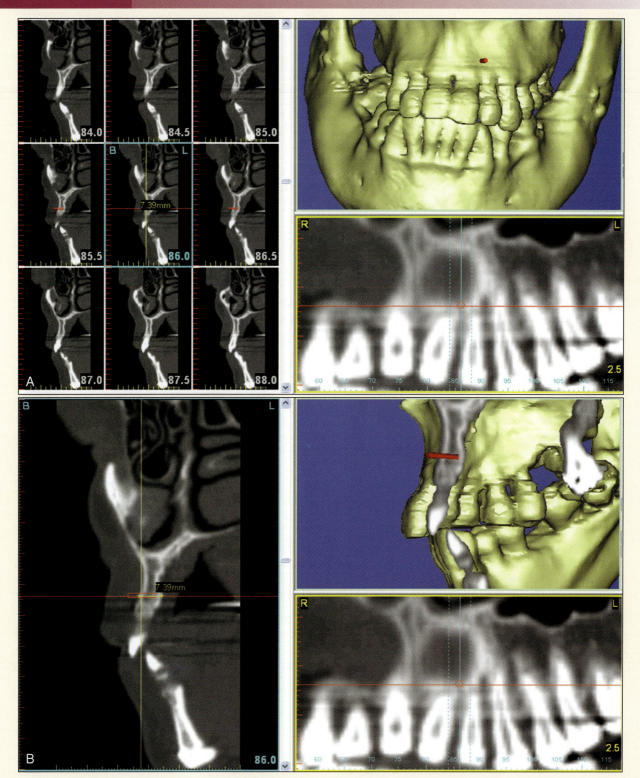

Figure 3-10 **A**, Nine sliced images of the upper anterior area. Panoramic view was used to estimate where the mini-implant should be placed. **B**, Close-up view was used to measure bone depth between the labial and palatal cortical layers. This patient demonstrated a long facial vertical pattern. There was enough vertical space, but the horizontal distance was short. Actual measurement is 7.39 mm.

Continued

CASE REPORT 3-1: DOLICOFACIAL PATIENT—cont'd

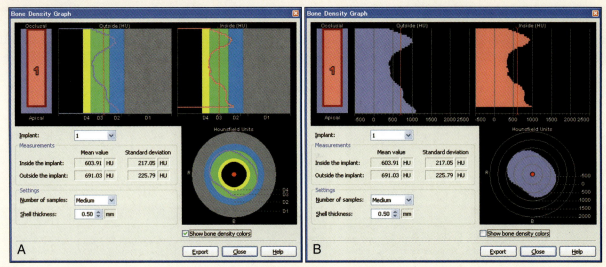

Figure 3-11 **A,** Bone density graphs of the upper anterior area based on bone quality classification system (D1, compact bone to D4, low-density trabecular bone) where the labial and palatal cortical bones showed high-density values. The bone outside the implant was denser than the bone inside the implant. **B,** Same bone density graph in Hounsefield units.

premolar (Figure 3-17, *A*). The cross-sectional view of this area reveals that bone depth along the mini-implant from the buccal surface to the lingual surface was 11.20 mm (Figure 3-17, *B*). In cases where the bone density might not be sufficient, a long screw that can reach the lingual cortical layer and provide bicortical anchorage is required. In this case, however, the bone density around the mini-implant site appeared adequate, although the buccal surface had less bone density (Figure 3-18).

The lower premolar area was deemed appropriate to retain the mini-implant. In the lower molar area, a site mesial to the first molar area was designated to receive the mini-implant as temporary anchorage (Figure 3-19, *A*).

In this dolicofacial patient, the distance along the planned mini-implant site from the buccal to the lingual bone surface was 15.94 mm. The vertical distance from the tip of the planned mini-implant to the mandibular canal was 14.54 mm. There was no defined external oblique ridge in this high-angle patient. Thus, the mini-implant could not be placed perpendicular to the tooth axis, as seen by the cross-sectional view on Figure 3-19, *B*. The bone density graph showed that the buccal surface had compact bone; however, the trabecular bone in the mandibular body was significantly less dense (Figure 3-20). Bone density analysis for this patient revealed that reliable bone did not exist in the molar area, so a wider mini-implant was selected.

Text continued on p. 43

CASE REPORT 3-1: DOLICOFACIAL PATIENT—cont'd

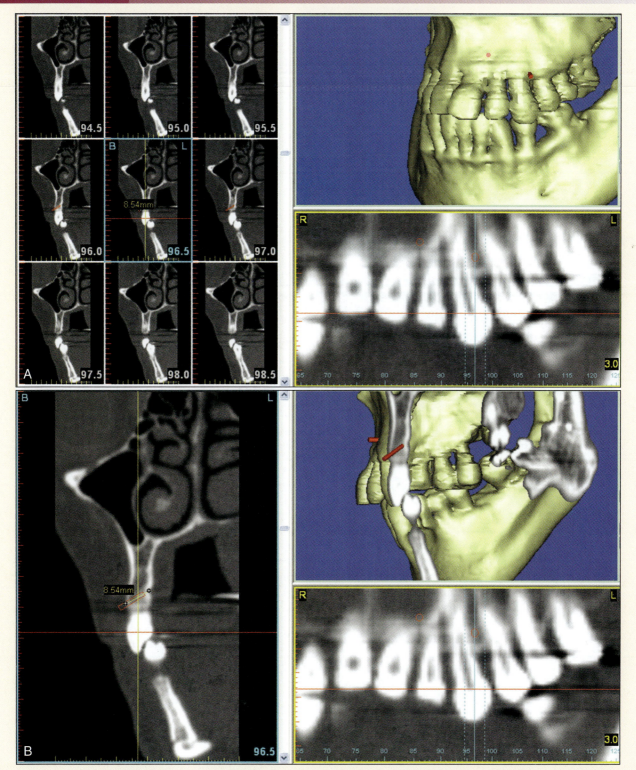

Figure 3-12 **A,** Nine sliced images of the premolar area. **B,** Close-up view of the premolar area. *Upper right,* Cross-sectional view of the bone and the mini-implant *(red bar)*. The horizontal distance between the buccal and palatal cortical bone was 8.54 mm.

Continued

PART II Diagnosis and Treatment Planning

CASE REPORT 3-1: DOLICOFACIAL PATIENT—cont'd

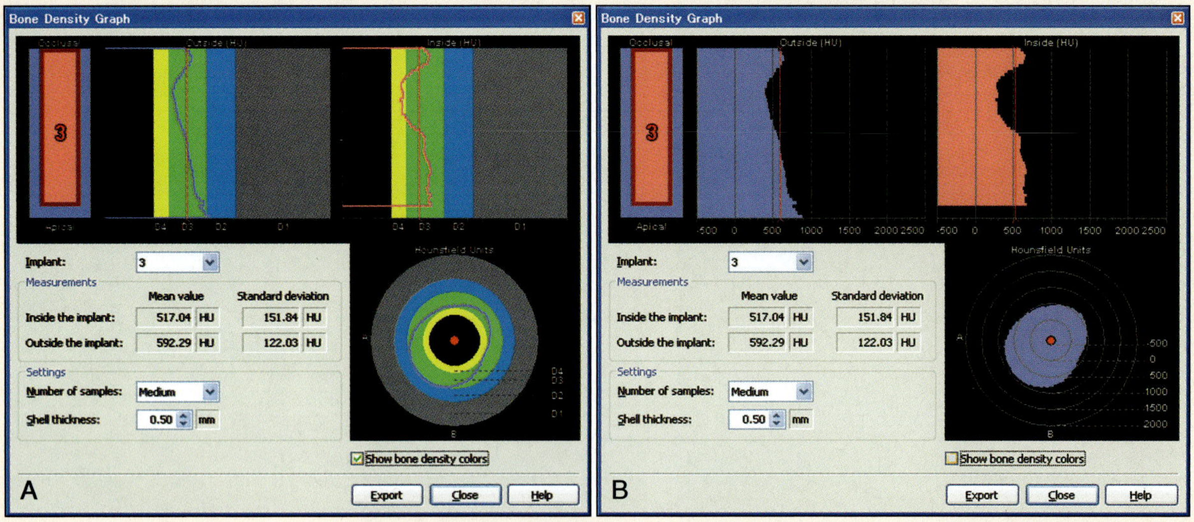

Figure 3-13 **A,** Bone density graphs of the premolar area based on bone quality classification system (D1, compact bone to D4, low-density trabecular bone). The bone density of this area appeared decreased, and immediate loading was contraindicated. **B,** Same bone density graph in Hounsfield units.

CASE REPORT 3-1: DOLICOFACIAL PATIENT—cont'd

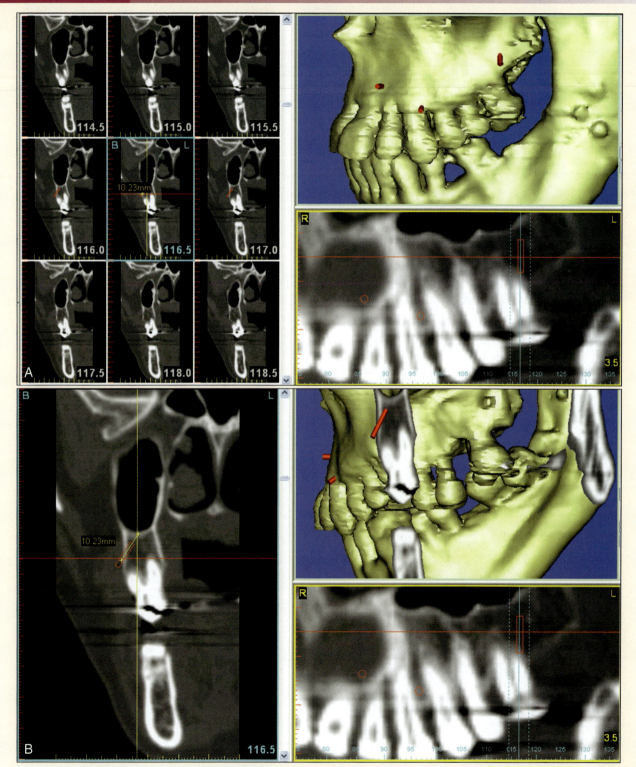

Figure 3-14 **A,** Nine sliced images of the molar area. A site distal to the first molar was chosen to receive the implant. **B,** The bone depth of the infrazygomatic area was 10.23 mm if measured from the implant tip to the maxillary sinus.

Continued

CASE REPORT 3-1: DOLICOFACIAL PATIENT—cont'd

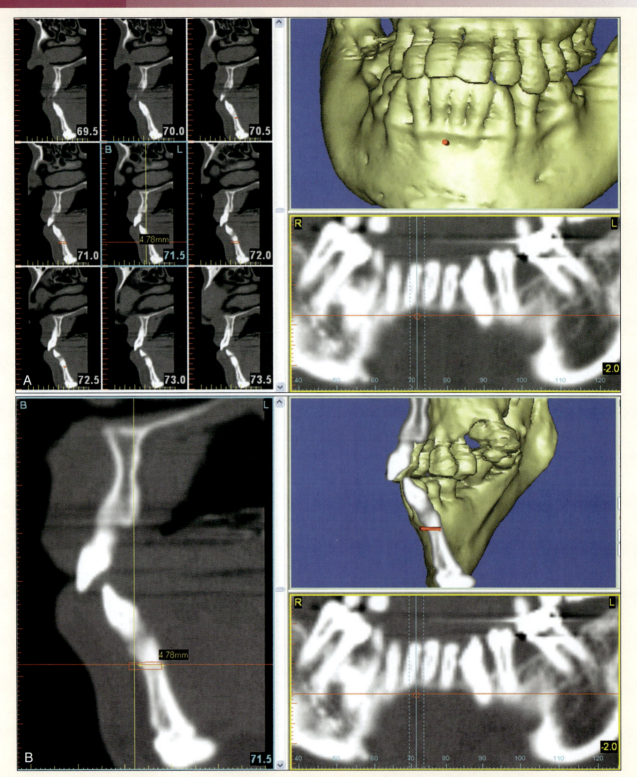

Figure 3-15 A, Lower incisor area showing a lingual cortical bone layer. The long-faced patient has a short distance between the labial and the lingual cortical bone width. B, Cross-sectional view of the lower incisor area revealed a very thin alveolar bone.

3 Radiographic Evaluation of Bone Sites for Mini-Implant Placement   39

CASE REPORT 3-1: DOLICOFACIAL PATIENT—cont'd

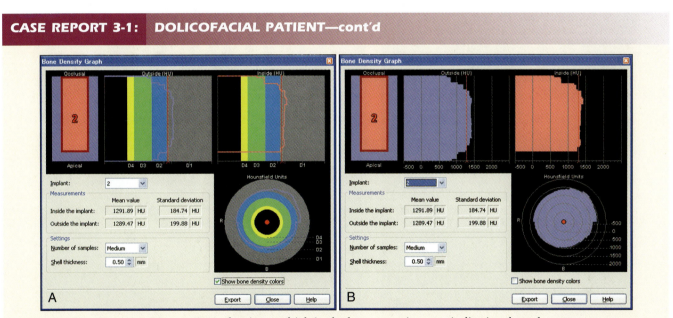

Figure 3-16 **A,** Bone density was high in the lower anterior area, indicating that adequate primary stability could be expected. **B,** Bone density in the lower anterior area. In the upper graph the bone density was almost the same from the labial surface to the lingual surface.

Continued

CASE REPORT 3-1: DOLICOFACIAL PATIENT—cont'd

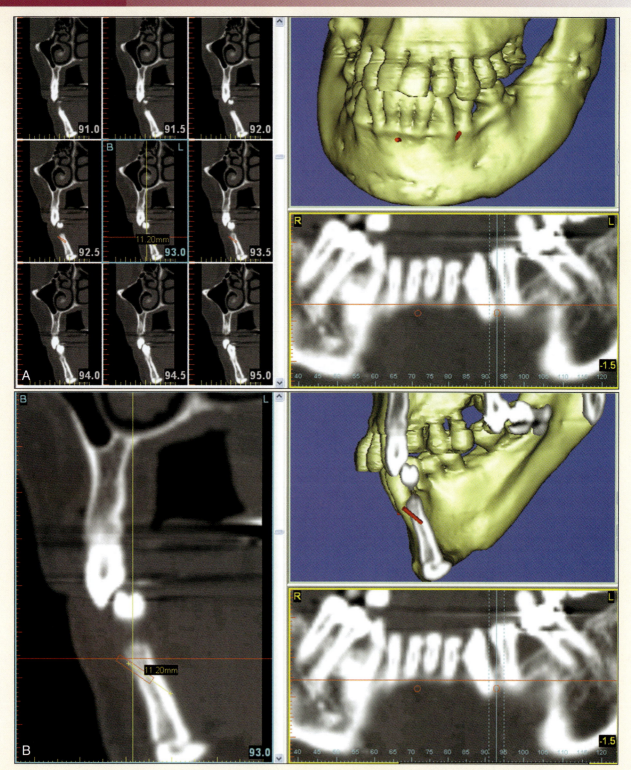

Figure 3-17 **A,** Placement of a mini-implant was planned between the canine and the first premolar in the lower premolar area. **B,** Cross-sectional view of the lower premolar area showed that bone depth along the mini-implant from the buccal surface to the lingual surface was 11.2 mm.

3 Radiographic Evaluation of Bone Sites for Mini-Implant Placement 41

CASE REPORT 3-1: DOLICOFACIAL PATIENT—cont'd

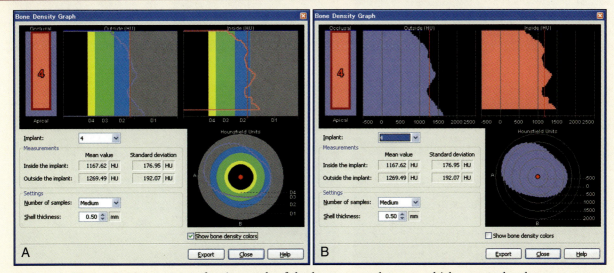

Figure 3-18 **A,** Bone density graph of the lower premolar area, which appeared to have adequate bone quality for retention of the mini-implant. **B,** If bone density had been reduced, a longer screw (bicortical anchorage) would have been required. However, the bone density in this area, both inside and outside the mini-implant site, appeared to be adequate (although slightly reduced in the buccal surface).

Continued

CASE REPORT 3-1: DOLICOFACIAL PATIENT—cont'd

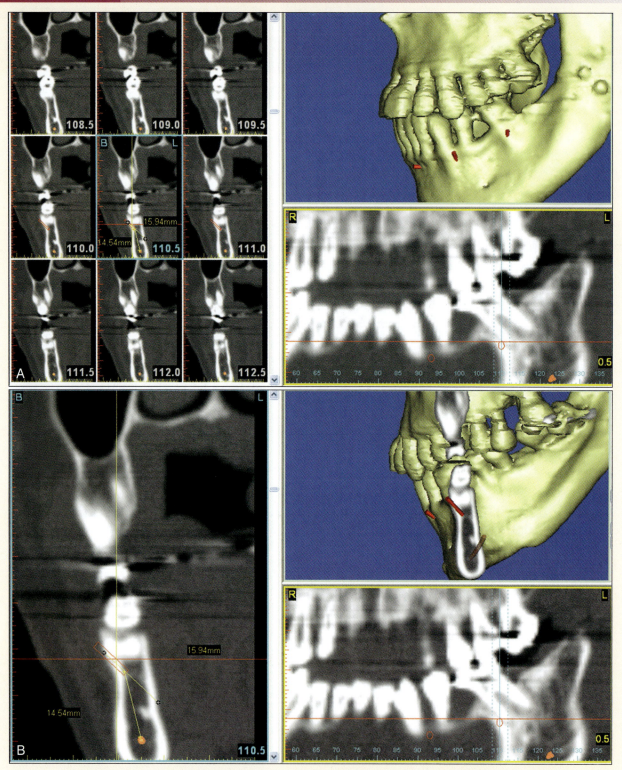

Figure 3-19 **A,** Three-dimensional CT image of the lower molar area. A site mesial to the first molar area was planned to receive a mini-implant as a temporary anchorage. The distance along the planned mini-implant to the lingual bone surface was 15.94 mm, and the distance from the tip of the planned mini-implant to the mandibular canal was 14.54 mm. There was no external oblique ridge (as seen in this area for this high-angle patient), and the bone shape was almost the same as that of the premolar area. **B,** Cross-sectional view shows that the mini-implant could not be placed perpendicular to the tooth axis.

CASE REPORT 3-1: DOLICOFACIAL PATIENT—cont'd

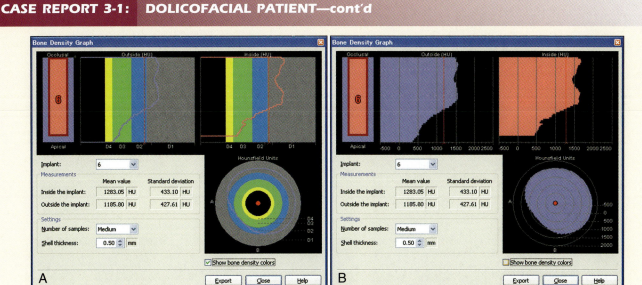

Figure 3-20 **A,** Bone density graph of the lower molar area. **B,** Bone density graph shows that the buccal surface had compact bone, but only weak trabecular bone existed inside the mandibular body.

CASE REPORT 3-2: BRACHYFACIAL PATIENT

In contrast to the previous patient with a dolicofacial pattern, this patient had a brachyfacial pattern. A 3DX (CB CT) scan was taken to evaluate the 3D bone structure and determine proper mini-implant placement. Brachyfacial patients usually have denser bone than dolicofacial patients but have less vertical space in the alveolar bone for placement of a mini-implant. Figure 3-21, *A,* shows 3D CT images of the upper anterior area. A panoramic view revealed a maxillary sinus enlarged in a downward direction making the placement of the mini-implant difficult. Additionally, the 3D CT images revealed limited alveolar bone width, especially if the mini-implant was to be placed horizontally. The distance along the designated mini-implant site from the labial to the palatal surface was 10.19 mm.

In the lower anterior area, the CT scan indicated that across the designated mini-implant site, there was only 6.65 mm between the cortical surfaces (Figure 3-21, *B*). Such CT data must be carefully considered when determining the length and placement direction of the mini-implant.

In the premolar area, the maxillary sinus showed downward enlargement, and the buccal area looked small (Figure 3-22, *A*). One of the nine sliced views was selected to determine the appropriate mini-implant length and position (Figure 3-22, *B*). In contrast to the dolicofacial patient, this brachyfacial patient had a reduced vertical height; only 8.08 mm from the labial surface to the lower portion of the maxillary sinus. The cross-sectional view reveals the positions of the planned upper and lower mini-implants. The lower anatomical width was 12.02 mm to the lingual bone surface.

In the molar area (Figure 3-23, *A*), the maxillary sinus showed downward enlargement, and there was only a small space around the roots of the upper first molar. Only 5.69 mm was observed from the buccal surface to the lateral surface of the maxillary sinus (Figure 3-23, *B*). In contrast, the lower molar area had sufficient space because of a prominent buccal extension of the oblique ridge; therefore the mini-implant could be placed almost vertically (Figure 3-24). The distance from the tip of the mini-implant to the mandibular canal was 9.84 mm. The anatomical characteristics of this area permitted easy insertion of the mini-implant.

Continued

CASE REPORT 3-2: BRACHYFACIAL PATIENT—cont'd

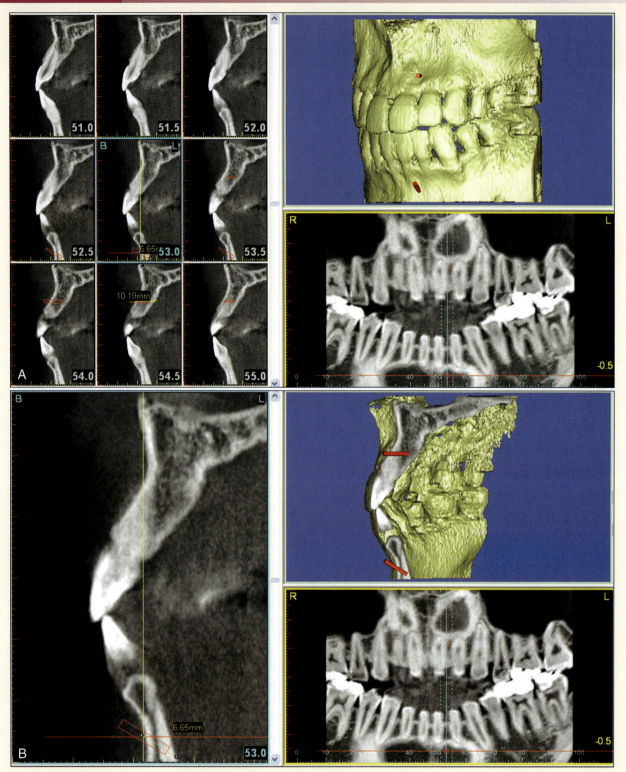

Figure 3-21 **A,** Three-dimensional CT images of the upper anterior area. The panoramic view shows that the maxillary sinus has enlarged in a downward direction, making placement of the mini-implant difficult. The 3D CT image showed there was sufficient space, especially if the mini-implant were placed horizontally. **B,** Three-dimensional CT images of the lower anterior area show a distance of only 6.65 mm between the cortical surfaces along the selected mini-implant site.

CASE REPORT 3-2: BRACHYFACIAL PATIENT—cont'd

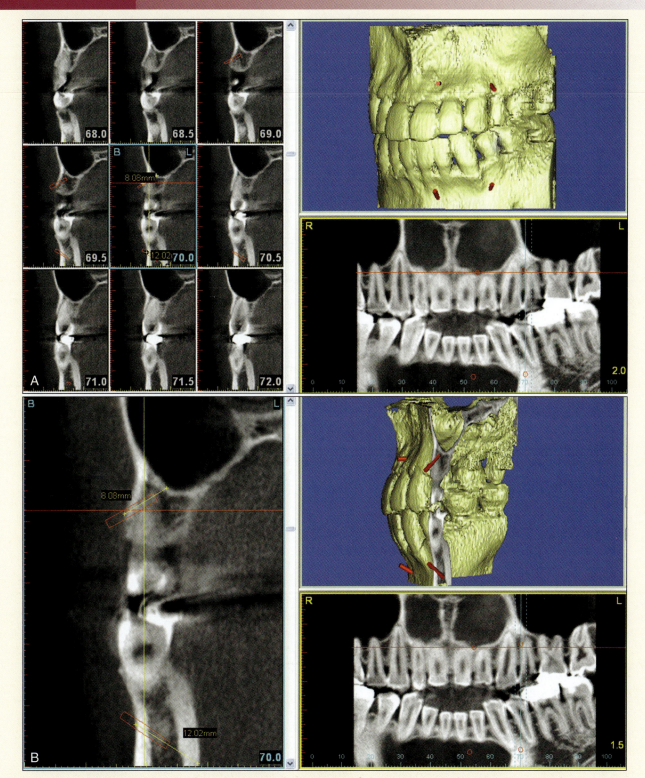

Figure 3-22 **A,** Three-dimensional CT image of the upper premolar area. Downward enlargement was seen in the maxillary sinus, and the buccal area showed a small space for mini-implant placement. **B,** View of one of the nine sliced images, used to select the mini-implant site.

Continued

CASE REPORT 3-2: BRACHYFACIAL PATIENT—cont'd

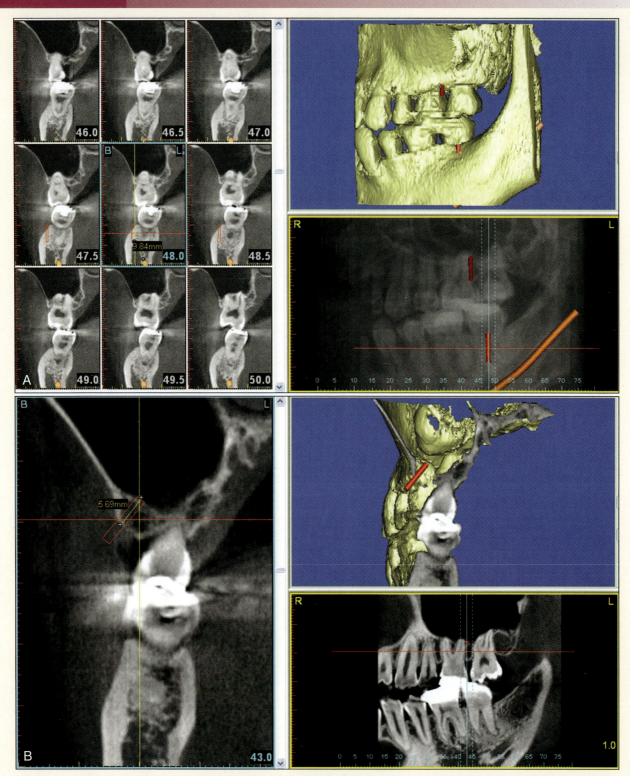

Figure 3-23 **A,** In the molar area the maxillary sinus showed downward enlargement, with only minimal space around the roots of the upper first molar for mini-implant placement. **B,** Measurement showed a depth of 5.69 mm from the buccal surface to the lateral border of the maxillary sinus.

CASE REPORT 3-2: BRACHYFACIAL PATIENT—cont'd

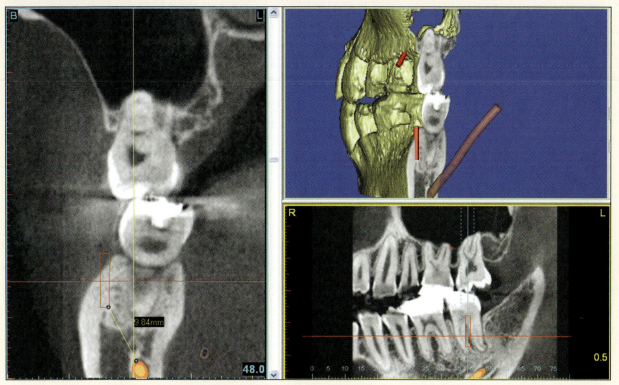

Figure 3-24 Prominent external oblique ridge in relation to the lower molar area, allowing for a mini-implant to be positioned almost vertically.

CONCLUSION

Computed tomography can provide a fully reconstructed 3D model of the maxilla and the mandible, as well as additional diagnostic information on dental root positioning, morphology of sites for TAD placement, and location of critical anatomical structures. CT scanning and its associated software provide the most effective radiographic modality in the diagnostic evaluation of patients for TADs in orthodontics and permits the immediate formulation of a treatment plan.

REFERENCES

1. Hounsfield GN: Computerized transverse axial scanning (tomography). 1. Description of system, *Br J Radiol* 46:1016-1022, 1973.
2. Macchi A, Carrafiello G, Cacciafesta V, et al: Three-dimensional digital modeling and setup, *Am J Orthod Dentofacial Orthop* 129:605-610, 2006.
3. Gerig G, Jomier M, Chakos M, et al: A new validation tool for assessing and improving 3-D object segmentation. In Niessen W, Viergever M, editors: *Medical image computing and computer-assisted intervention* (MICCAI: 4th International Conference, Utrecht, The Netherlands), Berlin, 2001, Springer-Verlag.
4. Miyajima K, Sana M: FEM analysis of mini-implants as orthodontic anchorage. In Davidovitch Z, Mah J, editors: *Biological mechanisms of tooth eruption, resorption and replacement by implants*, Boston, 1998, Harvard Society for the Advancement of Orthodontics.
5. Miyajima K, Saito S, Sana M, et al: Three-dimensional finite element models and animal studies of the use of mini-screws for orthodontic anchorage: In McNamara JA, editor: *Craniofacial growth series*, vol 42. *Implants, microimplants, onplants, and transplants*, Ann Arbor, Mich, 2005, Needham Press.

ADDITIONAL READING

Block MS, Hoffman DR: A new device for absolute anchorage for orthodontics, *Am J Orthod Dentofacial Orthop* 107:251-258, 1990.

Cope BC: Temporary anchorage devices in orthodontics: a paradigm shift, *Semin Orthod* 11:3-9, 2005.

Costa A, Pasta G, Bergamaschi G: Intraoral hard and soft tissue depths for temporary anchorage devices, *Semin Orthod* 11:10-15, 2005.

Creekmore TD, Eklund MK: The possibility of skeletal anchorage, *J Clin Orthod* 17:266-269, 1983.

Duyck J, Ronald HJ, Van Oosterwyck H, et al: The influence of static and dynamic loading on marginal bone reactions around osseointegrated implants: an animal experimental study, *Clin Oral Implant Res* 12:207-218, 2001.

Frost HM: The regional accelerated phenomenon: a review, *Henry Ford Hosp Med J* 31:3-9, 1985.

Hoblt WF: Using the palatal onplant for absolute anchorage. In McNamara JA, editor: *Craniofacial growth series*, vol 42. *Implants, microimplants, onplants, and transplants*, Ann Arbor, Mich, 2005, Needham Press.

Kanomi R: Mini-implant for orthodontic anchorage, *J Clin Orthod* 31:763-767, 1997.

Lagravere MO, Hansen L, Harzer W, et al: Plane orientation for standardization in 3-dimensional cephalometric analysis with computerized tomography imaging, *Am J Orthod Dentofacial Orthop* 129:601-604, 2006.

Lum LB, Beirne R, Curtis DA: Histological evaluation of hydroxylapatite-coated versus uncoated titanium blade implants in delayed and immediately loaded applications, *Int J Oral Maxillofac Implants* 6:456-462, 1991.

Melsen B, Verna C: Miniscrew implants: the Aarhus Anchorage System, *Semin Orthod* 11:24-31, 2005.

Melsen B: Mini-implants: where are we? *J Clin Orthod* 34(9):539-547, 2005.

Mitani H, Brodie AG: Three plane analysis of tooth movement, growth and angular changes with cervical traction, *Angle Orthod* 40:80-94, 1970.

Miyajima K: Diagnosis and treatment planning of mini-implant orthodontics, Las Vegas, 2006, American Association of Orthodontists.

Piva LM, Brito HHA, Leite HR, et al: Effects of cervical headgear and fixed appliances on the space available for maxillary second molars, *Am J Orthod Dentofacial Orthop* 128:366-371, 2005.

Ricketts RM: The influence of orthodontic treatment on facial growth and development, *Angle Orthod* 30:103-133, 1960.

Roberts WE, Marshall KJ, Mozsary PG: Rigid endosseous implant utilized as anchorage to protract molars and close an atrophic extraction site, *Angle Orthod* 60:135-152, 1990.

Roberts WE, Smith RK, Zilberman Y, et al: Osseous adaptation to continuous loading of rigid endosseous implants, *Am J Orthod Dentofacial Orthop* 86:95-111, 1984.

Saito S, Sugimoto N, Morohashi T, et al: Endosseous titanium implants can function as anchors for mesiodistal tooth movement in the beagle dog, *Am J Orthod Dentofacial Orthop* 118:601-607, 2000.

Sugawara J, Baik UB, Umemori M, et al: Treatment and post treatment dentoalveolar changes following intrusion of mandibular molars with application of a skeletal anchorage system (SAS) for open bite correction, *Int J Adult Orthod Orthognath Surg* 17:243-253, 2002.

Sugawara J: New surgical orthodontics for Class III correction in combination with a skeletal anchorage system (SAS), Las Vegas, 2006, American Association of Orthodontists.

Umemori M, Sugawara J, Nagasaka H, et al: Skeletal anchorage system for open-bite correction, *Am J Orthop* 115:166-174, 1999.

CHAPTER 4

Miniature Osseointegrated Implants for Orthodontics Anchorage

Ryuzo Kanomi and W. Eugene Roberts

Temporary anchorage devices (TADs) have developed into important orthodontic adjuncts for expanding the scope of biomechanical therapy and enhancing clinical outcomes.[1-3] However, most of the devices currently available have significant limitations because they are not designed to osseointegrate.[4,5] The development of miniscrews is similar to the evolution of endosseous implants to support dental prostheses more than 20 years ago.[6]

The initial prostheses, as well as the first report of endosseous implant anchorage for orthodontics, relied on biocompatible metallic devices not designed to osseointegrate.[7] Immediate loading was advocated to develop persistent implant mobility, thought to be a desirable physiological characteristic and deemed "fibro-osseous integration" or a "pseudoperiodontium." Histological studies subsequently demonstrated that fibro-osseous integration was actually an encapsulation of the implant by relatively acellular fibrous connective tissue.[6] A pseudoperiodontium was distinct from the highly vascular and cellular principal elements of the periodontium: periodontal ligament and epithelial attachment. Thus, fibro-osseous integration was the physiological equivalent of the scar tissue that characterizes an orthopedic nonunion. Considering this biological reality, it was not surprising that dental implants designed to achieve fibro-osseous integration had a poor success rate in most patients. The persistent micromotion produces inflammation and progressive resorption,[8] resulting in a vicious cycle of inflammation that eventually manifests as pain, infection, and exfoliation of the implant.

The modern era of highly successful dental implants began with the well-documented efforts of Branemark and colleagues in routinely achieving rigid osseous fixation of endosseous titanium fixtures.[6] Although the obvious initial market for osseointegrated implants was prosthetics, the similarity of the rigid fixtures to ankylosed teeth led to osseous anchorage for orthodontics. Osseointegrated anchorage was one of the most important developments in orthodontics in the twentieth century. Rigid osseous anchorage has had a high rate of success in orthodontics for more than 20 years.[1,2,9-11]

EVOLUTION OF MINISCREWS

Placement of miniscrews or microscrews in the alveolar process is an increasingly popular intraalveolar procedure. In general, the anchorage achieved with this type of TAD is less reliable than osseointegrated devices,[12,13] although the surgical procedure is relatively simple. The most popular locations are on the labial surface of the alveolar process in both arches, superior to the roots of the maxillary incisors, or in the palate. The sites selected are usually between the roots of teeth or apical to them. The original miniscrews used for orthodontic anchorage were the anchor screws supplied with surgical fixation plates.[14,15] In general, these screws engaged the cortical plate of the alveolus as a thread-retained device. The minscrews were immediately loaded, with no attempt to achieve osseointegration. The efficacy of miniscrews as bone anchorage devices has been documented in animal studies.[16]

After extensive experience with nonintegrated miniscrews, the senior author designed a one-stage, miniature intraalveolar implant that routinely achieves osseointegration (K-1 System). Clinical trial of the K-1 System has been promising. Two case reports are presented to demonstrate the utility of the K-1 System for intruding and retracting maxillary incisors.

THE K-1 SYSTEM

The K-1 System features osseointegrated mini-implants specifically designed for orthodontic anchorage to facilitate tooth movement that cannot be accomplished with conventional anchorage. Minimal bone and interradicular space is required for safe drilling of the 1.2-mm-diameter holes, into which the miniscrews are inserted as self-tapping fixtures. The most frequently used implants are 4 mm and 6 mm in length, but 8-mm implants are also available. Indications for implant anchorage include canine retraction, intrusion of incisors, intrusion of molars, and retraction of buccal segments. To intrude maxillary incisors, K-1 screws are placed a few millimeters below the lower border of the piriform aperture. Intrusive force is delivered to the maxillary incisors through a ligature wire tied from the implants to an eyelet attached to the archwire.

Computed tomography (CT) imaging is used for evaluating potential implant sites. Using the three-dimensional (3D) images, surgical stents are prepared to help ensure accurate placement of the TADs. Because the devices are designed to osseointegrate, they must be placed early in treatment to allow 3 months or more of undisturbed healing to achieve osseointegration before installing the transmucosal abutment and orthodontically loading the devices.

CASE REPORT 4-1: TEMPOROMANDIBULAR DISORDER

A woman age 23 years, 7 months with a history of temporomandibular disorder (TMD) presented for orthodontic consultation with a chief complaint of "jaw pain and crooked front teeth." Clinical examination of the face revealed a hyperdivergent, convex face with a decreased lower facial height (Figure 4-1, A and B). The pretreatment photographic series documented a Class II, Division 1 malocclusion with an 8-mm overjet and 6-mm overbite (~60% overlap of mandibular incisor). About 5 mm of maxillary and 7 mm of mandibular crowding were associated with a deep curve of Spee (Figure 4-1, C-G). The pretreatment panoramic radiograph showed a relatively normal dentition except for endodontic treatment and temporary crowns on the mandibular left and maxillary right first molars. In addition, the mandibular third molars were distally inclined and partially impacted (Figure 4-1, H).

Mounting the casts in the centric relation (Cr) position revealed an asymmetric, 5-mm anterior-posterior shift secondary to a prematurity on the palatal cusp of the maxillary right third molar (Figure 4-1, I-O). From a functional perspective, the malocclusion was a severe full-cusp Class II discrepancy. The patient's habitual, maximal intercuspation relation was defined as the centric occlusion (Co) position. The large Co → Cr shift and prematurity were considered the principal etiological factors in the TMD history reported by the patient.

Cephalometric analysis in the Co position documented relatively normal protrusion of the maxillary apical base (SNA, 80.5 degrees) and a retrusive mandibular apical base (SNB, 73.5 degrees). The ANB of 7 degrees was deceptively low because of the 5-mm Co → Cr shift. From a therapeutic perspective, the ANB was greater than 10 degrees when the mandible was in the Cr position. Figure 4-1, P, provides additional cephalometric values.

It was important for the patient to recognize that this was a severe skeletal malocclusion that usually required orthognathic surgery. The patient was concerned about jaw surgery, preferring a more conservative option. She accepted a treatment plan with mini-implants as anchorage devices. As part of the informed-consent process, she was told that the severity of her malocclusion may exceed what was realistic even with osseointegrated implant anchorage,

and that orthognathic surgery may ultimately be necessary. A relatively long treatment time was anticipated, so good oral hygiene and periodontium maintenance by a periodontist were essential. The patient accepted the treatment plan involving extraction of both mandibular first molars and both maxillary first premolars. She was informed that K-1 implants would be needed apical to the maxillary incisors to intrude and retract the maxillary anterior segment.

The initial phase of treatment was to resolve the TMD symptoms with splint therapy and prepare the surgical stent to place the K-1 implants apical to the maxillary incisors (Figure 4-2). While the implants were healing and osseointegrating, active orthodontic treatment was initiated in the mandibular arch (Figure 4-3). The treatment sequence was to extract the mandibular first molars, retract the canines, resolve mandibular anterior crowding, and achieve space closure with as much mesial movement of the buccal segments as possible. The posterior anchorage units for the alignment of the mandibular arch were the mandibular second molars. The second molars moved mesially, so the supracrestal fibers were expected to tip the third molars mesially, improving their axial inclination and eliminating the soft tissue coverage over the distal aspect of their crowns. After the deep curve of Spee was partially corrected, the maxillary first premolars were extracted, and the maxillary arch was banded, bonded, and leveled.

A cone-beam CT image was used before the second surgical procedure to locate the healed mini-implants (Figure 4-4). The 3D image revealed the extrusion and protrusion of the maxillary incisors after the initial leveling and canine retraction procedures. Figure 4-5 is a panoramic radiograph demonstrating progress in alignment of the mandibular anterior segment and retraction of the maxillary canines. Vertical traction was applied to the maxillary anterior segment with stainless steel ligatures originating from the K-1 mini-implants. Figure 4-6 documents the progression of active treatment to create a full-cusp Class II molar relationship, intrude the maxillary incisors, and reduce the maxillary anterior protrusion. It also illustrates the intermaxillary alignment at the end of space closure and the correction of the interincisal relationship. The Co → Cr discrepancy was eliminated, but it was necessary to

CASE REPORT 4-1: TEMPOROMANDIBULAR DISORDER—cont'd

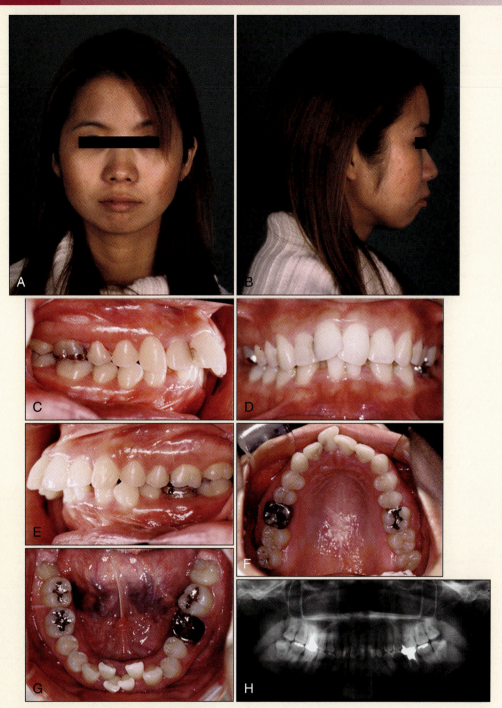

Figure 4-1 Woman with Temporomandibular Disorder (age 23 yr, 7 mo). **A** and **B**, Pretreatment facial photographs. **C** to **G**, Pretreatment intraoral photographs. **H**, Pretreatment panoramic radiograph. **I** to **O**, Photographs of the pretreatment relationship of the casts mounted in the centric relation position document a functional shift associated with a posterior prematurity. **P**, Pretreatment cephalometric analysis. *FMA*, Frankfort mandibular angle; *FMIA*, Frankfort mandibular incisor angle; *IMPA*, incisor mandibular plane angle; *UI*, upper incisor; *LI*, lower incisor; *NA*, nasion to point A; *NB*, nasion to point B.

Continued

52 PART II Diagnosis and Treatment Planning

CASE REPORT 4-1: TEMPOROMANDIBULAR DISORDER—cont'd

80.5
73.5
―――
7.0

FMA 32.0°
FMIA 46.5°
IMPA 101.5°
U1 to NA 27.0°, 11.0 mm
L1 to NB 35.5°, 11.5 mm
Interincisal 110.0°

Figure 4-1, cont'd For legend see p. 51.

CASE REPORT 4-1: TEMPOROMANDIBULAR DISORDER—cont'd

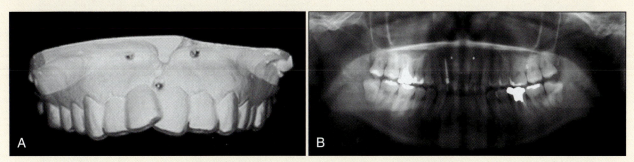

Figure 4-2 Lead makers embedded in a heat-pressure–adapted plastic stent (A) are used to plan the position for K-1 anchorage implants apical to the maxillary incisors (B).

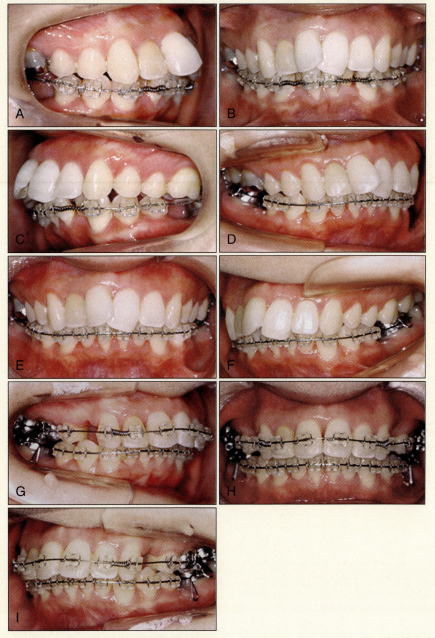

Figure 4-3 Intraoral photographs document treatment progress at 9 months (A-C), 12 months (D-F), and 15 months (G-I).

Continued

CASE REPORT 4-1: TEMPOROMANDIBULAR DISORDER—cont'd

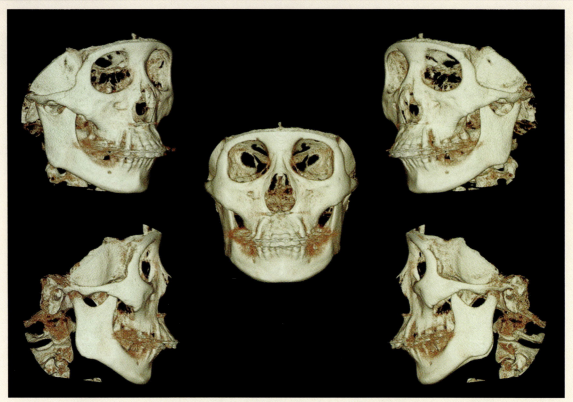

Figure 4-4 Cone-beam CT images before uncovering the K-1 anchorage implants show the flaring of the maxillary incisors before initiating intrusion and retraction.

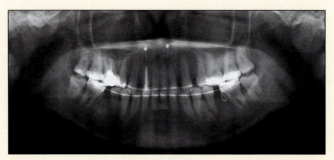

Figure 4-5 Panoramic radiograph showing treatment progress, with alignment of the mandibular anterior segment and retraction of the maxillary canines.

hold the maxillary molars with high-pull headgear and mesially translate the mandibular second molars about 8 mm. Eliminating the Class II molar relationship, complicated by the 5-mm functional shift, required careful management of differential anchorage. This was the major factor in the relatively long duration for space closure, which was not completed until 37 months into treatment.

Posttreatment facial photographs show that a favorable lip profile was achieved despite the severe mandibular retrusion at presentation (Figure 4-7, A and B). The corresponding intraoral photographic series revealed that a near-ideal interdigitation was achieved from first premolar to first premolar, and the posterior buccal occlusion was finished in a full-cusp Class II molar relationship (Figure 4-7, C-F). A posttreatment panoramic radiograph demonstrated ideal second-order correction in the maxillary arch and satisfactory axial inclination of the mandibular dentition (Figure 4-7, H). The severity of the malocclusion required an active

| CASE REPORT 4-1: TEMPOROMANDIBULAR DISORDER—cont'd |

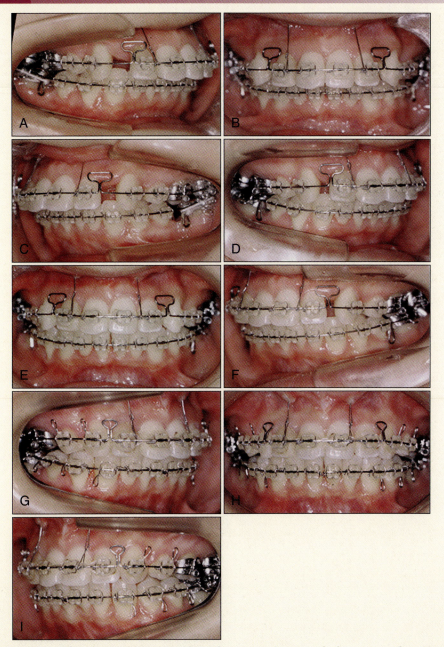

Figure 4-6 After the anchorage implants have osseointegrated, they are used to intrude the maxillary anterior incisors. Intraoral photographs document treatment progress at 20 months **(A-C)**, 24 months **(D-F)**, and 37 months **(G-I)**.

treatment time of about 4 years. Additional treatment to achieve more ideal axial inclination of mandibular premolars was not indicated because of evolving periodontal compromise. Gingival recession and bone loss were noted on the mesial of the mandibular second molars. It was deemed prudent to terminate fixed-appliance treatment to pursue periodontal treatment to stabilize the loss of attachment.

Cephalometric analysis after active treatment demonstrated a primarily dentoalveolar correction of the malocclusion (Figure 4-8, *A*). Although the mandibular plane angle (MPA) closed 1 degree, there was only a 0.5-degree increase in SNB. Furthermore, the cone-beam CT images used to construct the sagittal plane for cephalometric analysis revealed an increase in the superior position of the right

Continued

CASE REPORT 4-1: TEMPOROMANDIBULAR DISORDER—cont'd

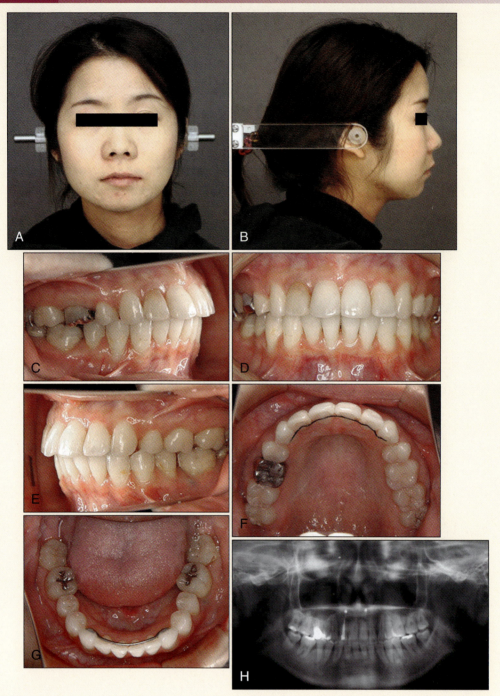

Figure 4-7 A and B, Posttreatment facial photographs (age 27 yr, 7 mo). C to G, Posttreatment intraoral photographs. H, Posttreatment panoramic radiograph.

mandibular condyle. This change in mandibular morphology is consistent with the increase in mandibular length (Ar-Pg) documented in the cephalometric superimposition (Figure 4-8, B), and appears to reflect the morphological mechanism for the correction of the asymmetric 5-mm Co → Cr discrepancy.

Anterior cranial base superimposition of the initial and final cephalometric images shows that the maxillary dentition was intruded and that a forward rotation of the mandible decreased the lower facial height (Figure 4-8, C). The lips were slightly retracted, and the interlabial position moved superiorly. Superimposition on the relatively stable

CASE REPORT 4-1: TEMPOROMANDIBULAR DISORDER—cont'd

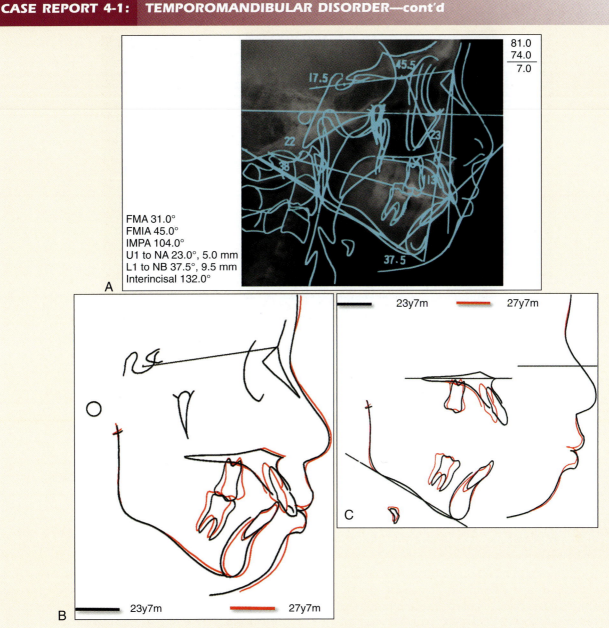

Figure 4-8 A, Posttreatment cephalometric analysis. B, Superimposition of pretreatment and posttreatment cephalometric tracings document intrusion and retraction of maxillary incisors as well as a more anterior position of the mandible. C, Superimpositions on the maxilla, mandible, and upper face profile reveal changes in dental and facial structures.

internal maxillary structures demonstrated the intrusion and retraction of the maxillary incisors. The modest intrusion of the maxillary molars was caused by high-pull headgear wear. Mandibular superimposition on the inferior portion of the symphysis and mandibular plane revealed about 3 mm of incisor intrusion and asymmetric translation of the second molars to close the first molar extraction sites. The mandibular occlusal photograph shows that the right second molar is more anteriorly positioned than the contralateral second molar (see Figure 4-7, C-G). These data demonstrate the differential tooth movement that was necessary to resolve the severe skeletal malocclusion, complicated by an asymmetric Cr → Co shift. The 8 mm of mesial translation of the mandibular right second and third molars to correct the shift was the principal factor associated with the relatively long treatment time of approximately 4 years.

Continued

CASE REPORT 4-1: TEMPOROMANDIBULAR DISORDER—cont'd

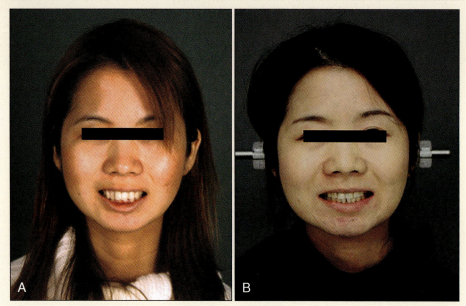

Figure 4-9 Comparison of **A**, pretreatment (age 23 yr, 7 mo), and **B**, posttreatment (age 27 yr, 7 mo), facial photographs shows the improvement of facial form in the frontal plane.

The excellent dental esthetics achieved are complemented by the improved facial form (Figure 4-9, A and B). The patient was particularly pleased with the improvement in her profile, especially because it was achieved without orthognathic surgery. The authors believe that the intrusion and retraction of the maxillary incisors with K-1 anchorage was essential to achieving a good result for this severe, asymmetric malocclusion. Although the periodontal deterioration of the mandibular second molars was a disappointment, the overall result of treatment was gratifying.

CASE REPORT 4-2: DENTOALVEOLAR DYSPLASIA

A woman age 20 years, 11 months presented for orthodontic consultation with a noncontributory medical, dental, and family history. The chief complaint was protrusive lips and crowded lower incisors. Clinical examination revealed that facial balance was near ideal (Figure 4-10, A and B), which suggested that the malocclusion was a dentoalveolar dysplasia. The intraoral photographic series showed Class I buccal segments, overjet of 3 mm, overbite of 4 mm, and about 7 mm of crowding in the mandibular anterior segment (Figure 4-10, C-G). Evaluation of the initial panoramic radiograph documented a relatively healthy dentition compromised by two devitalized teeth with crowns (maxillary left central incisor and mandibular right first molar) (Figure 4-10, H). The mandibular third molars were horizontally impacted. The initial cephalometric analysis showed a bimaxillary retrusion of the apical bases of the jaws (SNA, 78.5 degrees; SNB, 74.5 degrees) with a modest relative retrusion of the mandible (ANB, 4 degrees) (Figure 4-10, I). Mounting the casts on an articulator revealed a 3-mm symmetrical mandibular shift from centric relation (Cr) to centric occlusion (Co) (Figure 4-10, J-N). The patient had no history of TMD and was unaware of the asymptomatic functional shift.

The treatment plan was to extract maxillary first premolars and mandibular second premolars. Bilateral K-1 implants were prescribed to intrude and retract the maxillary incisors. The surgical stent was fabricated to ensure accurate placement of the anchorage implants with respect to the roots of the incisors (Figure 4-11). Before initiation of active treatment, the K-1 implants were inserted according to the surgical sequence illustrated in Figure 4-12. After extraction of both maxillary first premolars and both mandibular second premolars, the arches were leveled. Canine retraction was accomplished by placing open-coil springs between the canines and lateral incisors and cinching back the archwires. Simultaneously, mandibular first molars were moved mesially with open-coil springs placed between the mandibular first and second premolars. A series of intraoral photographs illustrates the progress of canine retraction and mandibular first molar protraction (Figure 4-13). The

CASE REPORT 4-2: DENTOALVEOLAR DYSPLASIA—cont'd

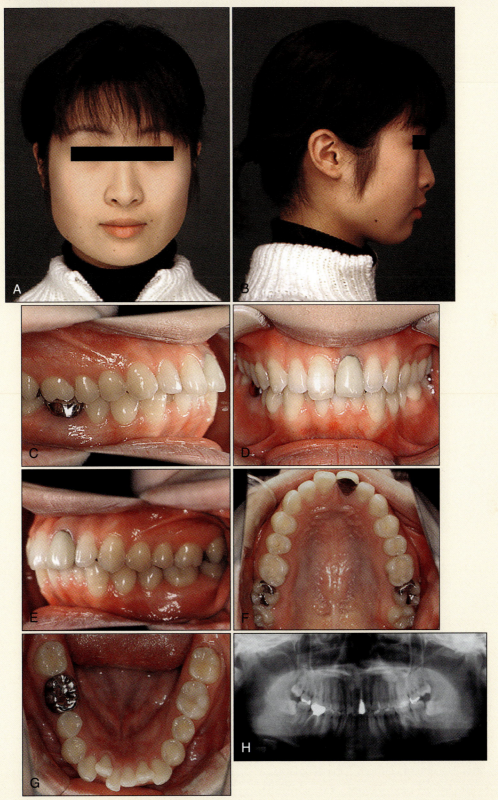

Figure 4-10 Woman with Dentoalveolar Dysplasia (age 20 yr, 11 mo). A and B, Pretreatment facial photographs. C to G, Pretreatment intraoral photographs. H, Pretreatment panoramic radiograph. I, Pretreatment cephalometric analysis. J to N, Photographs of the pretreatment relationship of the casts mounted in the centric relation position document an anterior-posterior functional shift.

Continued

CASE REPORT 4-2: DENTOALVEOLAR DYSPLASIA—cont'd

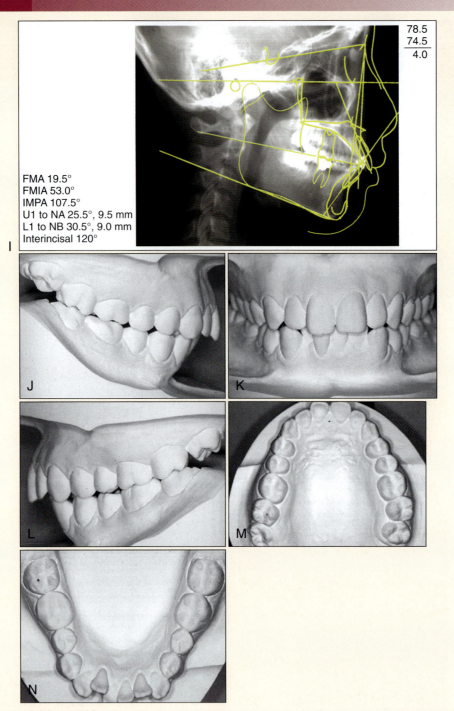

Figure 4-10, cont'd

overbite increased as the mandibular first molars tipped mesially.

Five months after placement of the K-1 mini-implants, a second surgical procedure uncovered the implants. The submerged implants were located with an intraoral metal detector; the overlying mucosa was injected with local anesthetic containing a vasoconstrictor; an incision exposed the implants; and soft tissue was sutured around the head of the TADs (Figure 4-14). After the head of the implant was exposed, a supramucosal slide-on attachment was secured to each implant, and steel ligatures were used for traction between the implants and eyelets soldered to the archwire between the maxillary central and lateral incisors (Figure 4-15). The maxillary incisors were intruded by the traction ligatures attached to the implants, and the mandibular arch was flattened with a stainless steel arch-

CASE REPORT 4-2: DENTOALVEOLAR DYSPLASIA—cont'd

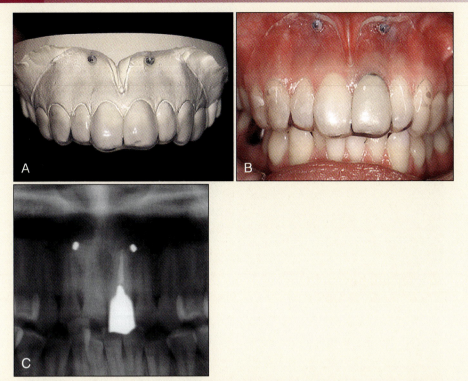

Figure 4-11 Lead makers embedded in a heat-pressure–adapted plastic stent (**A**) are used to plan the position for K-1 anchorage implants apical to the maxillary incisors (**B** and **C**).

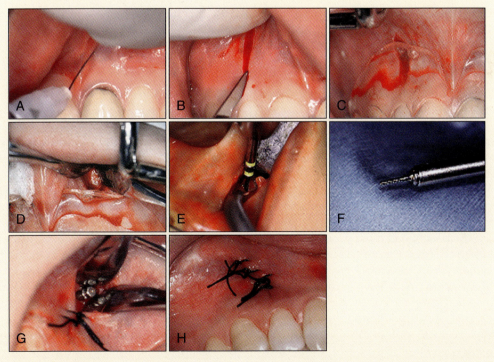

Figure 4-12 First operation, to place K-1 anchorage implants. The sequence of events follows: **A**, anesthesia; **B**, incision; **C**, stent in place; **D**, evacuation; **E**, drilling; **F**, implant in driver; **G**, insertion; **H**, suture.

Continued

CASE REPORT 4-2: DENTOALVEOLAR DYSPLASIA—cont'd

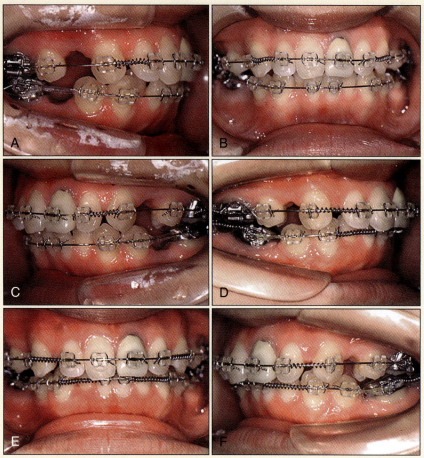

Figure 4-13 Intraoral photographs document progress at 10 weeks (**A-C**) and 28 weeks (**D-F**) after the first operation to place the anchorage implants.

wire. Figure 4-16 shows the progress of the postoperative intrusion and space closure. Space closure was accomplished with sliding-wire mechanics in the mandibular arch and a rectangular steel archwire with bilateral T loops in the maxillary arch. In addition, Class II elastics were used to help protract the mandibular molars. Figure 4-17 provides radiographic and photographic documentation of the K-1 implant mechanism used for intrusion and retraction of the maxillary incisors.

After treatment the patient had a less protrusive profile and was pleased with the result (Figure 4-18, *A* and *B*). The intraoral photographic series depicted a near-ideal Class I occlusion with fixed retainers in the maxillary and mandibular anterior segments (Figure 4-18, *C-G*). A posttreatment panoramic radiograph shows good second-order correction, except for the diverging roots of the mandibular right first molar and second premolar (Figure 4-18, *H*). Because there is no functional occlusion on the maxillary third molars, it was recommended that they be extracted. A maxillary occlusal film reveals slight blunting of the maxillary molar roots (Figure 4-18, *I*).

The immediate posttreatment cephalometric analysis demonstrated that a well-balanced skeletal and dental relationship was achieved (Figure 4-19, *A*). A comparison of pretreatment and posttreatment cephalometric values showed an overall improvement in the dental and skeletal morphology, but no net change in the ANB angle of 4 degrees (Figure 4-19, *B* and *C*). Superimposition of the initial and final cephalometric films on the anterior cranial base documented the retraction of the maxillary and mandibular incisors and lips (Figure 4-19, *D*). The maxillary superimposition reveals a 3-mm to 4-mm intrusion of the maxillary incisors. Mandibular superimposition shows that the mandibular incisors were tipped about 2 mm distally. Superimposition on the profile of the upper face provided further documentation of the reduction in lip protrusion (Figure 4-19, *E*). It should be noted that the reduced lip protrusion in this patient reflects the ideal of Japanese society, which tends to prefer a flatter lip profile than that desired by most Western Caucasians.

After active treatment and removal of the traction ligatures, soft tissue formed over the implants and their supra-

CASE REPORT 4-2: DENTOALVEOLAR DYSPLASIA—cont'd

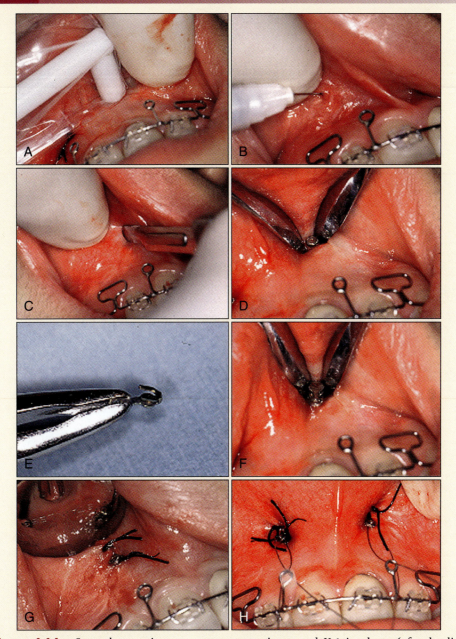

Figure 4-14 Second operation, to uncover osseointegrated K-1 implants (after healing period of 5 months). The sequence of events follows: **A,** detection; **B,** anesthesia; **C,** incision; **D,** evacuation; **E,** abutment; **F,** attachment; **G** and **H,** suture and tying.

mucosal attachments. A third surgical procedure was performed to remove the K-1 implants and attachments. The soft tissue around the implants was anesthetized; an incision exposed the site; the attachments were removed with a utility plier; and the implants were unscrewed with the specially designed driver used to install them. Although the implants were osseointegrated and did not move during treatment, the surface area of the osseointegration did not prevent the screws from being readily removed (Figure 4-20). However, it is important to increase removal torque slowly when removing the implants to avoid shearing them off. This is an important design consideration for osseointegrated TADs. They must have adequate torsional strength, to resist sufficient shear between the implant threads and the bone, in order to disrupt the rigid osseous interface when they are unscrewed. This design objective is impor-

Continued

CASE REPORT 4-2: DENTOALVEOLAR DYSPLASIA—cont'd

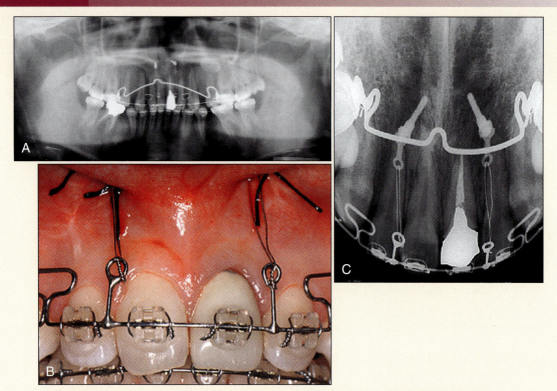

Figure 4-15 After the second operation, traction is shown in the superior direction to intrude the maxillary incisors. **A**, Panoramic radiograph. **B**, Intraoral photograph. **C**, Maxillary occlusal radiograph.

tant for easy removal of the screws after active treatment is completed.

The patient was well satisfied with the treatment results and regularly returned for follow-up visits to evaluate the stability of the correction. Two years after treatment, another set of records was collected. Facial form (Figure 4-21, A and B) and the interdigitation of the right buccal segment (Figure 4-21, C-G) were unchanged. There was a slight relapse (~1 mm) of the left buccal interdigitation to a more Class II relationship. No other changes were noted. A follow-up panoramic film documented the health of the dentition (Figure 4-21, H). Cephalometric evaluation 2 years after treatment showed that the ANB angle had increased 0.5 degree because of a progressive increase in the SNA angle to 79.5 degrees (Figure 4-21, I). In comparison, SNA was 78.5 degrees before treatment and 79.0 degrees at the end of active treatment. These changes were apparently caused by the more anterior position of the maxillary incisor roots as they were intruded and tipped posteriorly. Overall, the final result was deemed to be very good.

Text continued on p. 72

CASE REPORT 4-2: DENTOALVEOLAR DYSPLASIA—cont'd

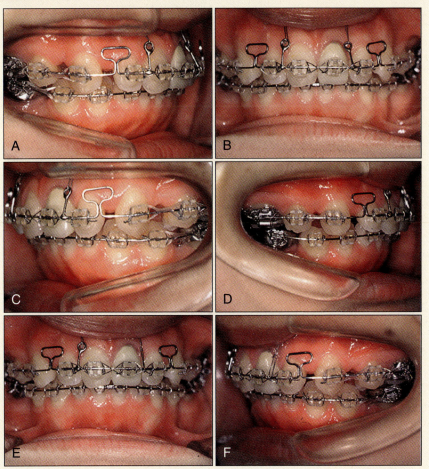

Figure 4-16 Intraoral photographs document progress at 4 weeks **(A-C)** and 9 weeks **(D-F)** after the second operation to load the anchorage implants.

Continued

CASE REPORT 4-2: DENTOALVEOLAR DYSPLASIA—cont'd

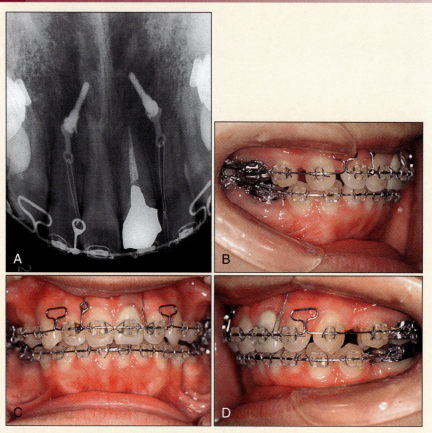

Figure 4-17 Maxillary occlusal radiograph (**A**) and intraoral photographs (**B-D**) reveal progress at 16 weeks after the second operation to load the anchorage implants.

CASE REPORT 4-2: DENTOALVEOLAR DYSPLASIA—cont'd

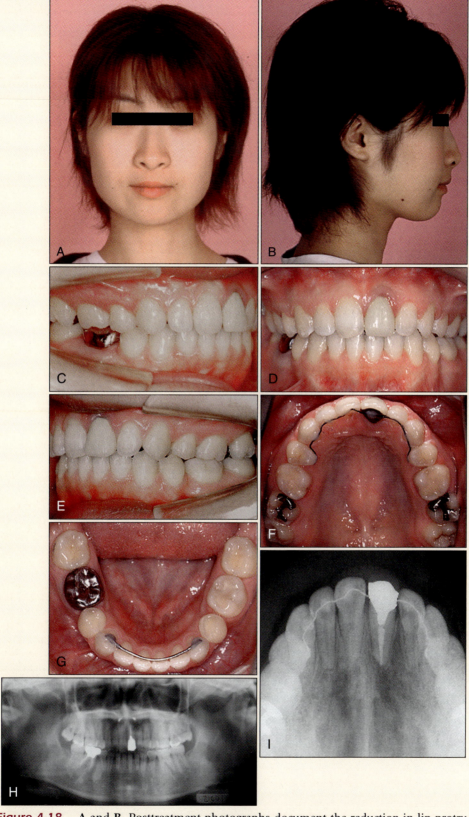

Figure 4-18 **A** and **B,** Posttreatment photographs document the reduction in lip protrusion (patient age: 22 yr, 2 mo). **C** to **G,** Posttreatment intraoral photographs. **H,** Posttreatment panoramic radiograph. **I,** Maxillary occlusal radiograph.

Continued

CASE REPORT 4-2: DENTOALVEOLAR DYSPLASIA—cont'd

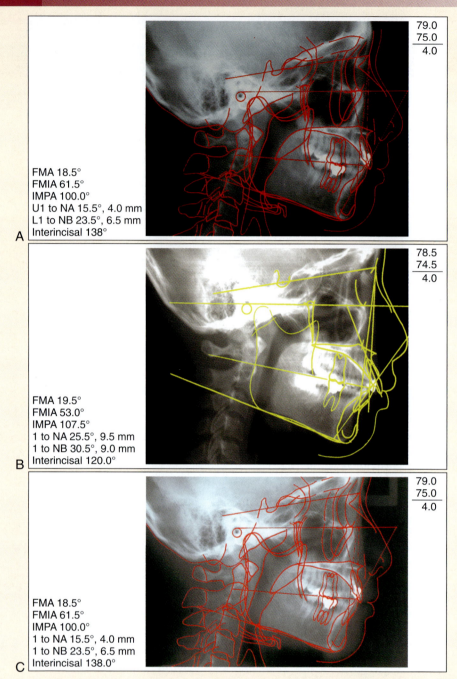

Figure 4-19 A, Posttreatment cephalometric analysis. B and C, Comparison of pretreatment and posttreatment cephalometric analyses.

CASE REPORT 4-2: DENTOALVEOLAR DYSPLASIA—cont'd

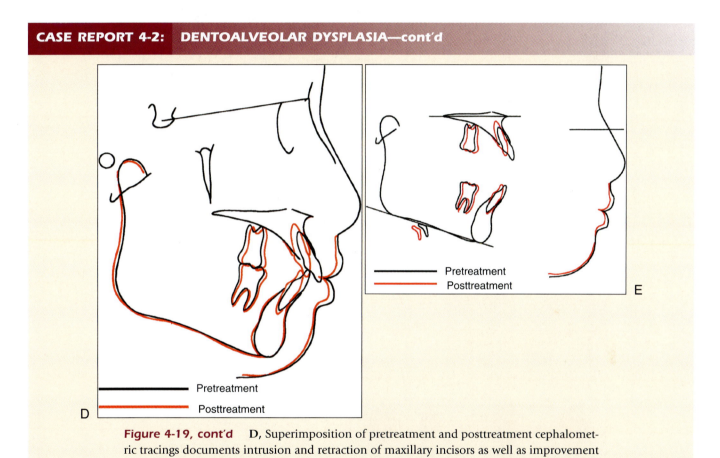

Figure 4-19, cont'd D, Superimposition of pretreatment and posttreatment cephalometric tracings documents intrusion and retraction of maxillary incisors as well as improvement in lip profile. E, Superimpositions on the maxilla, mandible, and upper face profile reveal changes in dental and facial structures.

Continued

CASE REPORT 4-2: DENTOALVEOLAR DYSPLASIA—cont'd

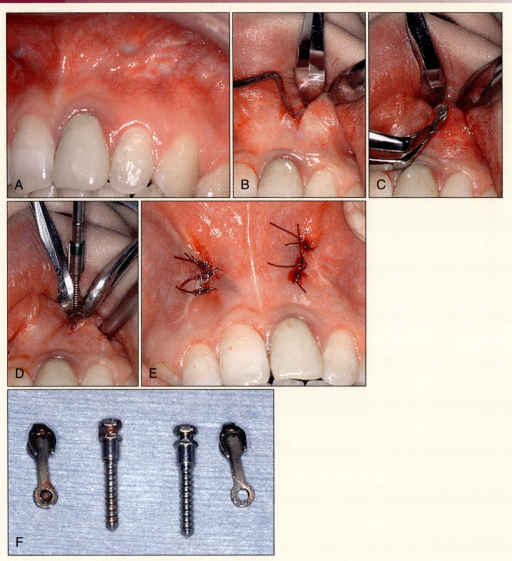

Figure 4-20 Procedure for removing K-1 anchorage implants after the end of active treatment. **A,** K-1 implant and supramucosal attachment submerged under the mucosa covering the interradicular bone between the maxillary central and lateral incisors. **B** and **C,** Exposure and removal of attachments. **D,** Removal of the implant. **E,** Sutures after removal of two K-1 implants, **F,** K-1 implants and attachments immediately after removal.

CASE REPORT 4-2: DENTOALVEOLAR DYSPLASIA—cont'd

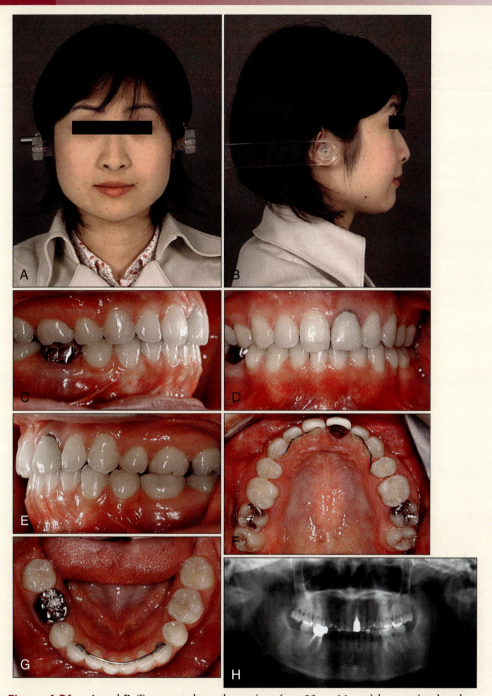

Figure 4-21 **A** and **B,** Two years later the patient (age 23 yr, 11 mo) has retained a pleasing facial form. **C** to **G,** Intraoral photographs 2 years after treatment show that the Class I relationship for the right side was maintained, but the left side slipped into a slight Class II buccal relationship. **H,** Panoramic radiograph 2 years after treatment documents the stability of the radiographic result.

Continued

CASE REPORT 4-2: DENTOALVEOLAR DYSPLASIA—cont'd

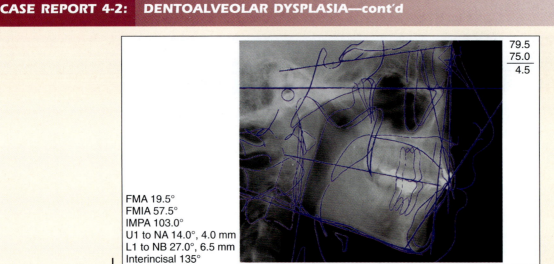

FMA 19.5°
FMIA 57.5°
IMPA 103.0°
U1 to NA 14.0°, 4.0 mm
L1 to NB 27.0°, 6.5 mm
Interincisal 135°

Figure 4-21, cont'd **I,** Cephalometric analysis 2 years after treatment shows a slight increase in the ANB relationship (4.0-4.5 degrees). Otherwise, the treatment result has been stable.

CONCLUSION

The K-1 mini-implant system routinely achieves osseointegration after about 3 months of postoperative healing. To avoid longer treatment time, the TADs should be placed before or at the start of active treatment. By the time initial leveling is accomplished, healing is completed, and the osseointegrated fixtures are available for anchorage. Case reports have documented the use of K-1 implants for intruding and retracting maxillary incisors. These devices are proving to be more reliable than nonintegrated miniscrew TADs, particularly when there is an extrusive load on the implant. The osseointegrated TADs are easily removed after treatment, an important design characteristic of the K-1 System. Both cases reported were young adults, but the incisor intrusion mechanism has been used effectively in growing children and adolescents.

ACKNOWLEDGMENT

We appreciate the assistance of Dr. Jeffery A. Roberts in editing the manuscript.

REFERENCES

1. Roberts WE, Marshall KJ, Mozsary PG: Rigid endosseous implant utilized as anchorage to protract molars and close an atrophic extraction site, *Angle Orthod* 60(2):135-152, 1990.
2. Wehrbein H, Merz BR: Aspects of the use of endosseous palatal implants in orthodontic therapy, *J Esthet Dent* 10(6):315-324, 1998.
3. Janssens F et al: Use of an onplant as orthodontic anchorage, *Am J Orthod Dentofacial Orthop* 122(5):566-570, 2002.
4. Cope JB: Temporary anchorage devices in orthodontics: a paradigm shift, *Semin Orthod* 11(1):3-9, 2005.
5. Mah J, Bergstrand F: Temporary anchorage devices: a status report, *J Clin Orthod* 39(3):132-136 (discussion, 136; quiz, 153), 2005.
6. Albrektsson T et al: Osseointegrated titanium implants: requirements for ensuring a long-lasting, direct bone-to-implant anchorage in man, *Acta Orthop Scand* 52(2):155-170, 1981.
7. Babbush CA: Endosseous blade-vent implants: a research review, *J Oral Surg* 30(3):168-175, 1972.
8. Roberts WE et al: Rigid endosseous implants for orthodontic and orthopedic anchorage, *Angle Orthod* 59(4):247-256, 1989.
9. Odman J et al: Osseointegrated implants as orthodontic anchorage in the treatment of partially edentulous adult patients, *Eur J Orthod* 16(3):187-201, 1994.
10. Drago CJ: Use of osseointegrated implants in adult orthodontic treatment: a clinical report, *J Prosthet Dent* 82(5):504-509, 1999.
11. Keles A, Erverdi N, Sezen S: Bodily distalization of molars with absolute anchorage, *Angle Orthod* 73(4):471-482, 2003.
12. Miyawaki S et al: Factors associated with the stability of titanium screws placed in the posterior region for orthodontic anchorage, *Am J Orthod Dentofacial Orthop* 124(4):373-378, 2003.
13. Cheng SJ et al: A prospective study of the risk factors associated with failure of mini-implants used for orthodontic anchorage, *Int J Oral Maxillofac Implants* 19(1):100-106, 2004.
14. Creekmore TD, Eklund MK: Possibility of skeletal anchorage, *J Clin Orthod* 17:266-267, 1983.
15. Kanomi R: Mini-implant for orthodontic anchorage, *J Clin Orthod* 31(11):763-767, 1997.
16. Deguchi T et al: The use of small titanium screws for orthodontic anchorage, *J Dent Res* 82(5):377-381, 2003.

CHAPTER 5

Factors in the Decision to Use Skeletal Anchorage

Birte Melsen and Morten Godtfredsen Laursen

Two major factors in the increased use of skeletal anchorage devices are (1) difficulty in obtaining satisfactory compliance from patients, which has led orthodontists to focus on appliances that function independently of compliance (compliance-free anchorage), and (2) the growing number of adult and elderly patients in whom reduced dentition rules out the use of conventional appliances.

Conventional anchorage is based on the rule of thumb that more teeth deliver anchorage against the displacement of fewer teeth. Because there is no lower limit for the force that can produce tooth movement,[1,2] none of these appliances can deliver "absolute anchorage." Another compliance-free anchorage approach is the *differential moment* concept, in which the stimulus to the anchorge unit is "translatory movement," whereas the stimulus to the unit of teeth to be moved is "tipping." The differential moment approach is based on tipping being easier to accomplish than translatory movement, and thus anchorage is preserved.[3]

Although some conventional or compliance-free anchorage systems have been able to provide differentiated anchorage, none of the suggested methods has yet been able to deliver the absolute anchorage desired by orthodontists.[4] Only through ankylosed teeth and skeletal anchorage systems has "absolute anchorage" been achieved.[5,6] Many different systems of skeletal anchorage have been introduced over the last decade.[7]

CLASSIFICATION

Skeletal anchorage systems can be classified into two categories according to their origin (Box 5-1). One group has been developed from dental implants and is characterized by an intraosseous part that is surface-treated to enhance the osseointegration. This category includes palatal and retromolar implants.[8,9] These devices are inserted as dental implants with a predrilling procedure, followed by a healing period for osseointegration before loading is accomplished. A special variant in this category is the *onplant* introduced by Block and Hoffman.[10]

The onplant is considered less invasive because it is not placed into bone but rather between the periosteum of the palate and the bone using a tunneling procedure. It consists of a titanium hydroxyapatite coated disk with a threaded hole that is placed toward the mucosa; an abutment can be inserted to serve as anchorage.

The other category of skeletal anchorage originates from surgical screws and is characterized by a polished intraosseous part with a surgical screw attached; it is loaded immediately after insertion.[4,11,12] The two main groups are (1) miniplates with various transmucosal extensions[13-17] and (2) single screws or mini-implants.[4,11,12,18-27]

Depending on the configuration of the head, mini-implants can be used as direct or indirect anchorage. The head of the mini-implant may be formed as a button around which a wire or elastic can be tied. Some of these may also have a hole in the neck through which a wire can be pulled. Both these approaches allow for only one-point contact and application of a force from the tooth or teeth to be displaced to the anchorage screw. Other mini-implants have a bracketlike head into which a wire can be ligated and connected with a bracket on a tooth to make a consolidated unit, which can then be used for anchorage.[27]

INDICATIONS

Skeletal anchorage is most frequently used to replace conventional anchorage, especially headgear, thereby reducing problems with compliance.[12,19,28,29,31-33] Some case reports and clinical studies have also demonstrated that skeletal anchorage can widen the spectrum of orthodontics, allowing treatment previously considered impossible.[8,23,27,34-41]

Table 5-1 summarizes select clinical studies that resulted from a PubMed search using the keywords *skeletal anchorage* and *orthodontics*. Only clinical studies and case reports are included*; the outcome of animal

---

*References 7, 11, 12, 15, 17, 28-31, 33, 39, 40, 42-57.

TABLE 5-1 Select Clinical Trials and Case Reports on Skeletal Anchorage in Orthodontics

Study	Year	Type of Anchorage	Type of Study	Number in Study*	Purpose of Anchorage
Kuroda et al.[69]	2007	Miniscrews, miniplates	Clinical trial	75 P	Not mentioned
Jeon et al.[51]	2006	Miniscrew	Case report	1 P	Molar and premolar intrusion
Chae[52]	2006	Microimplant	Case report	1 P	Vertical control
Kircelli et al.[56]	2006	Miniscrew	Clinical trial	10 P	Molar distalization
De Clerck and Cornelis[53]	2006	Miniplates	Case report	1 P	Class III traction
Sugawara et al.[32]	2006	Miniplates	Clinical trial	25 P	Molar distalization
Tseng et al.[54]	2006	Mini-implants	Clinical trial	45 I	Not mentioned
Kircelli et al.[56]	2006	Miniplates	Case report	1 P	Maxillary protraction
Bengi et al.[30]	2006	Miniplates	Case report	1 P	Canine distalization
Koudstaal et al.[55]	2006	Miniplates	Clinical trial	13 P	Maxillary expansion
Sugawara[40]	2005	Miniplates	Case reports	3 P	Molar intrusion
Gelgör et al.[31]	2004	Miniscrew	Clinical trial	25 P	Molar distalization
Park and Kwon[46]	2004	Miniscrew	Case report	3 P	Anchorage in extraction cases
Kuroda et al.[39]	2004	Miniscrew	Case report	1 P	Molar intrusion
Yao et al.[47]	2004	Miniscrew	Case report	1 P	Upper molar intrusion
Erverdi et al.[17]	2004	Miniplates	Clinical trial	10 P	Upper molar intrusion
Giancotti et al.[48]	2004	Miniscrew	Case report	1 P	Eruption of ectopic molar
Sugawara et al.[49]	2004	Miniplates	Clinical trial	15 P	Mandibular molar distalization
Maino et al.[22]	2003	Miniscrew	Case reports	3 P	Multiple applications
Sugawara et al.[37]	2002	Miniplates	Clinical trial	9 P	Mandibular molar intrusion
Sherwood et al.[15]	2002	Miniplates	Clinical trial	4 P	Maxillary molar intrusion
Chung et al.[44]	2002	Miniplate	Case report	1 P	Canine retraction
Armbruster and Block[29]	2001	Onplant	Case report	1 P	Retraction of anterior teeth
Lee et al.[28]	2001	Mini-implant	Case report	1 P	Anchorage for retraction
Park et al.[12]	2001	Mini-implant	Case report	1 P	Anchorage for retraction
Costa et al.[11]	1998	Mini-implant	Case report	1 P	Front retraction
Jenner and Fitzpatrick[43]	1985	Miniplates	Case report	1 P	Front retraction
Creekmore and Eklund[42]	1983	Miniscrew	Case report	1 P	Incisor intrusion

*P, Patient(s); I, implants.

BOX 5-1 Classification of Extradental Intraoral Anchorage

I. As developed from dental implant
   Treated surface; lag time for loading
   - Palatal implants
   - Onplants
   - Retromolar implants
   - Orthodontic implants
II. As developed from surgical screws
   Smooth surface; immediate loading
   - Miniplates: one-point contact
   - Mini-implants: one-point contact
   - Aarhus mini-implant: three-dimensional control

---

experiments depends on the species. Randomized controlled trials (RCTs), as suggested by Feldmann and Bondenmark,[58] are difficult to perform with skeletal anchorage systems.

One could argue that skeletal anchorage should not be used to replace conventional anchorage just because it is compliance free. Many other compliance-free appliances have been introduced in orthodontics, but because of Newton's third law, no intraoral appliance can deliver "absolute anchorage." Not even satisfactory compliance can provide absolute anchorage, which is sometimes required for the correction of alveolar protrusion.[12,21]

In an essential argument against skeletal anchorage, Kesling[59] claimed that many problems addressed by miniscrews could even be characterized as iatrogenic, resulting from the application of a flawed biomechanical system. He considered that the following problems purported to be "solved" by miniscrews are actually caused by treatment:

1. Deepening of the anterior bite when closing posterior spaces.
2. Difficulties associated with intruding anterior teeth and correcting dental midlines.
3. Need for heavy forces to overcome sliding and active friction and to correct Class II and Class III interarch discrepancies.

Skeletal anchorage should not be used as a shortcut around insufficient biomechanical knowledge. It should be emphasized, however, that skeletal anchorage can help clinicians widen their spectrum of orthodontics by permitting treatment previously not possible. For example, Melsen et al.[60] performed retraction and intrusion of anterior teeth against a surgical wire placed through the infrazygomatic crest in patients with missing molars (Figure 5-1). Roberts et al.[8,34,35] used a retromolar orthodontic implant to displace the second and third molars into the extraction space of a first molar, without displacing any teeth in a posterior direction.

Limiting skeletal anchorage to patients who can truly benefit results in the following indications:

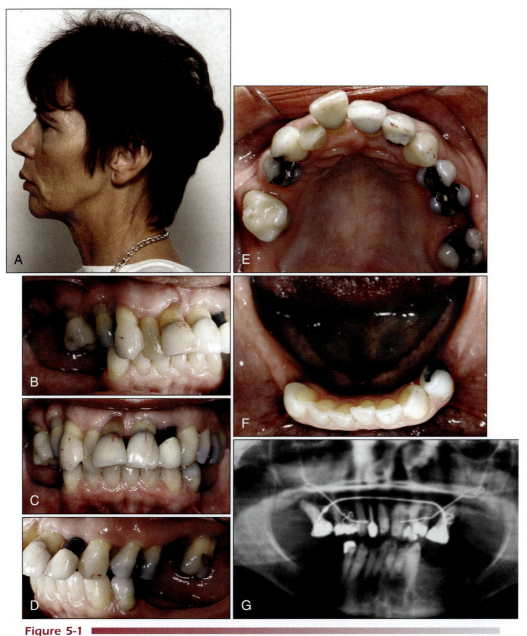

Figure 5-1
A to **F**, Adult woman with pronounced degenerated dentition and no posterior occlusion.
G to **J**, Zygoma ligatures used as anchorage for intrusion and retraction of upper front teeth.
K to **N**, Patient after treatment and reconstruction of anterior teeth.

Continued

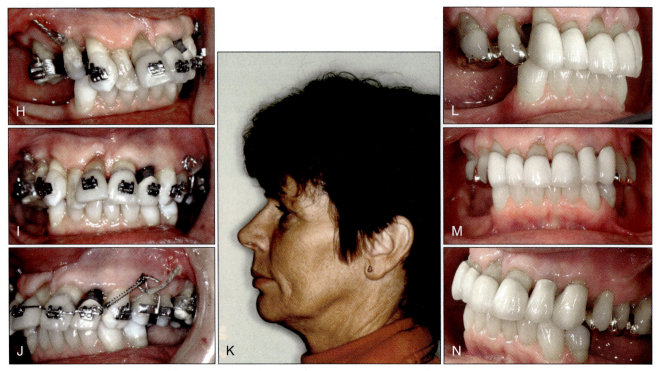

Figure 5-1, cont'd   For legend see p. 75.

- Patients with insufficient teeth for the application of conventional anchorage (Figure 5-2).
- Patients in whom forces to the reactive unit would generate adverse effects (Figures 5-3 and 5-4).
- Patients with a need for asymmetric tooth movements in all planes of space (Figure 5-5).
- In select patients, as an alternative to orthognathic surgery (Figure 5-6).
- As anchorage for tooth movements, to generate bone for a dental implant (Figure 5-7).

FAILURES

Although one aspect of evaluating skeletal anchorage is to define clearly the indications for its use, another is to list the failures and possible adverse effects. Three types of reports have focused on the failures: laboratory tests, animal studies, and clinical cases.

Mechanical strength of skeletal anchorage devices has been analyzed using laboratory tests or stress calculations. Carano et al.[61] tested the resistance of three skeletal anchorage screws (Dentos, Leone, Mini-Screw-Anchorage System [MAS]) of identical length (11 mm) and diameter (1.5 mm) to fracture during bending and torsion. They concluded that the steel screws resisted deformation better than the titanium (Ti) screw. (Surgical steel is recommended only for emergency surgery, and Ti screws are routinely used for maxillofacial surgery.) The torsion in relation to the applied couple did not differ among the three products. Dalstra et al.[62] created mathematical model of the impact of the diameter on the internal stress. They demonstrated that the stress values, and thus the fracture risk, increased dramatically with a reduction in the diameter below 1.5 mm (Figure 5-8).

Primary stability has been studied in animal experiments, with the pig most often used. Büchter et al.[63] inserted mini-implants into the mandibles of pygmy pigs, and the torsion necessary to loosen the implants was evaluated along a range of 0 to 900 centinewtons (cN) They concluded that the implants could be loaded immediately if the force level was controlled. The extrapolation of these results for use in humans should be done with care, as the cortex density and thickness of the minipig is not comparable to that of humans. Wilmes et al.[64] evaluated the insertion torque of five different mini-implants (two designs with different diameter and different lengths) into the pelvic bone of pigs. They concluded that the design, the pilot drilling, and the cortical thickness all had a significant influence on the system's primary stability. The factors identified related to the mini-implant, the handling procedure, and the host. The influence of the magnitude of torque applied to insert the orthodontic mini-implants was evaluated in 41 patients by Motoyoshi et al.,[65] who concluded that the low (<5 newtons per centimeter

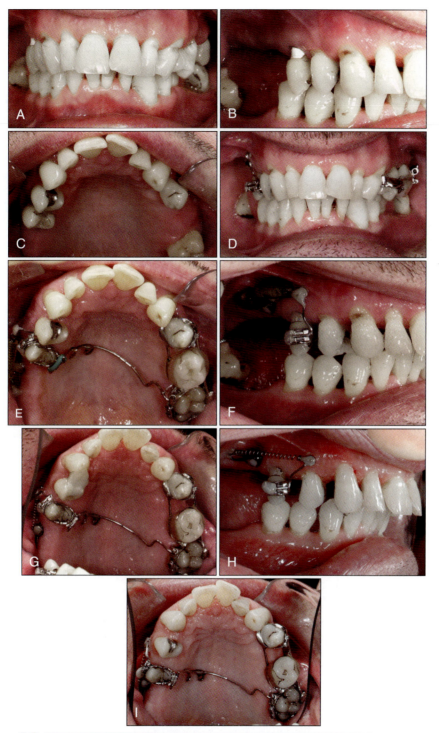

Figure 5-2

A to C, Patient with large overjet and insufficient teeth for conventional anchorage. D to F, Mini-implant in the infrazygomatic crest was used as anchorage for distal displacement of all teeth in the right side of the upper arch, starting with the second premolar. To control the rotation, a transpalatal arch was inserted into a vertical tube on the left side. G, One month of treatment. H and I, Four months of treatment. J and K, Eight months of treatment. The second premolar is now in a Class I relationship and is consolidated to the mini-implant; thus it can serve as anchorage for the distal movement of the first premolar. L to N, Consolidated premolars can indirectly serve as anchorage for retraction of the upper front teeth.

Continued

Figure 5-2, cont'd For legend see p. 77.

[N/cm]) and the high (>10 N/cm) torque values increased the risk of failure. The torque needed for inserting the mini-implants depended on both the cut and diameter of the threaded part and the density and thickness of the bone; both screw and host are important.

Failure rate in the clinical setting is low, although the sample size in all cases has been limited, as seen in the number of parameters evaluated.[66-68] None of the reports defines the failure in detail. The devices evaluated apparently had only moderate influence on the failure rate, but the choice of implant in relation to the clinical problem may be important.

In clinical studies, failures are synonymous with the loss of the mini-implant, and the failure rate varies between 10% and 30%. Factors such as fracture of the mini-implant, infection, and damage to the teeth should also be considered.

PREDICTORS OF CLINICAL FAILURE

Clinical failure is most likely related to the following:
- The design and dimension of the mini-implant.
- The handling at insertion and the timing and level of force applied to the host.
- The quantity and quality of bone at the insertion site.

As yet, however, a distinction has not been made among the different types of failures.

The initial stability is crucial for the maintenance of the anchorage. Failure rates did not differ between mini-plates and freestanding miniscrews.[67] In a prospective study, the following authors found that anatomical location and the periimplant soft tissue were factors of importance for the prognosis. According to Miyawaki et al.,[66] factors such as thin diameter of the screw, high mandibular plane angle, and periimplant inflammation can be considered risks. Kuroda et al.[69] found that the insertion procedure was a major prognostic factor because more anchorage units were lost after flap surgery than with predrilling directly through the mucosa.[69] Tseng et al.[54] found four failures among 45 mini-implants of four different lengths. Because all four failures involved shorter implants and three were in the mandible, the authors concluded that the site was a significant factor related to failure.

AARHUS FAILURE STUDY

To analyze the type of failure and its consequence on the treatment outcome, a prospective study was initiated in the Department of Orthodontics, School of Dentistry, University of Aarhus, Denmark, in 2004. The anchorage devices were inserted by the author, the professors, and postgraduate students who had no previous experience with insertion of implants or skeletal anchor-

Text continued on p. 84

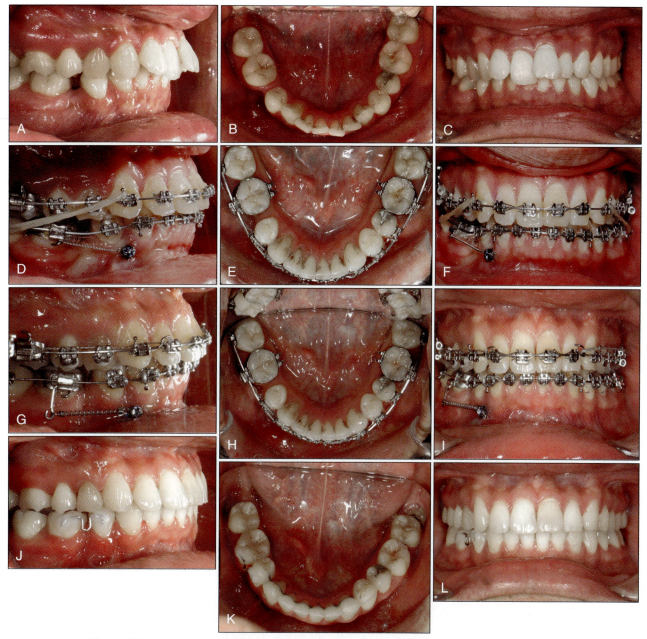

Figure 5-3

A to **C**, Adult patient with agenesis of second premolar in the right side. The space is closed partly through mesial tipping of the first molar and partly through distal tipping of anterior teeth. **D** to **F**, During uprighting of the lower molar, the mini-implant is used to keep the molar crown in place. The leveling will consequently lead to mesial tipping and intrusion of the anterior teeth. **G** to **I**, After leveling the molar is displaced mesially with a Sentalloy coil spring. The displacement is done with sliding mechanics to avoid rotation of the molar. **J** to **L**, Result of treatment. The space of the missing premolar has been closed, and the molar relationship is consequently mesial. An equilibration is needed to improve the occlusion. *(Courtesy Jörg Thorman.)*

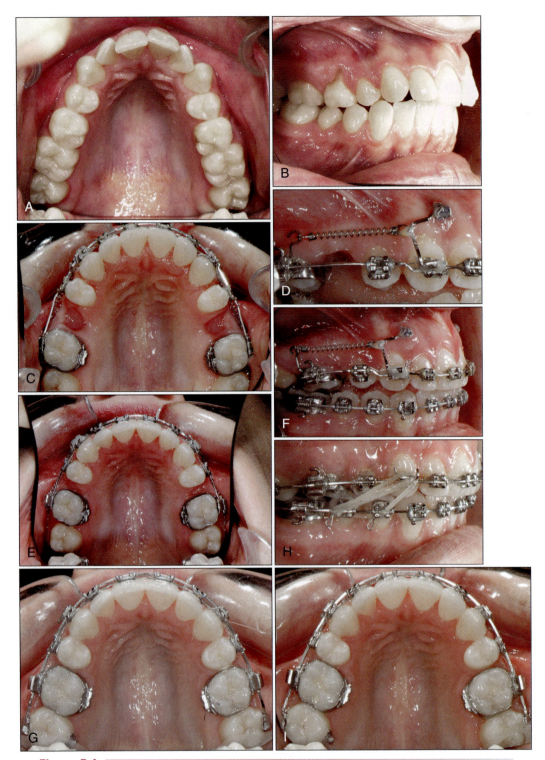

Figure 5-4

A and B, Patient with agenesis of second upper premolars. C and D, Two mini-implants were inserted between the canines and the laterals and used as anchorage for the mesial displacement of the molars. To avoid impingement of the coil spring in the canine region, the spring is extending from the molar to a wire connecting the screw head with the canine bracket. E to G, Height of the point of application and the force direction is controlled by height of the power arms. H and I, Day of screw removal. The occlusion is reinforced by light up-and-down elastics. *(Courtesy Jörg Thorman.)*

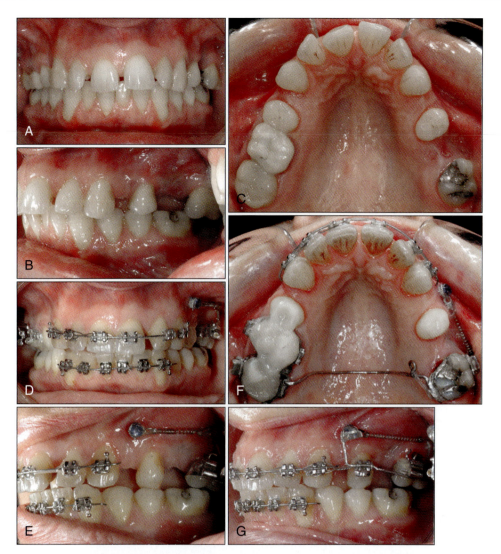

Figure 5-5

A to **C**, Patient in need of asymmetric tooth movement. The plan is to place a single dental implant in the upper first premolar region and achieve a full occlusion on the upper second molar. This is solved by 6-mm mesial displacement of the upper left second molar and slight reciprocal (mesial and distal) movement of the upper left canine and second premolar. **D** to **F**, Mini-implant is inserted between the upper left canine and the second premolar and used as direct anchorage to mesialize the second molar, with a Sentalloy coil attached to a power arm. To guide the second molar into the planned position, a hinge is placed across the palate. The bite is raised with Triad, which serves as anchorage for the hinge and allows movement of the second molar without occlusal interferences. **G**, Mini-implant is used for direct and indirect anchorage. A stainless steel wire passes from the mini-implant through the slot of the premolar bracket and on top of the attachment of the second molar band, to give an intrusive component during mesialization. **H** to **J**, Simultaneous mesialization and uprighting of the second molar. The uprighting spring is attached to the indirect anchorage. Palatally, a Sentalloy coil is applied between power arms of the second molar, and the mini-implant is anchored to the second premolar to control for rotation of the second molar. **K** to **M**, Mini-implant has been removed and a dental implant placed. **N** and **O**, Unintentional amalgam markers in the left maxillary first molar region depict the total mesial displacement of the second molar. *(Case treated and described by Morten Godtfredsen Laursen.)*

Continued

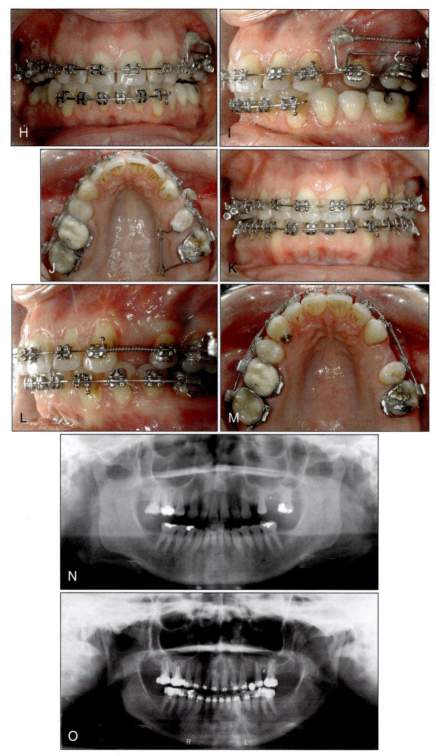

Figure 5-5, cont'd For legend see p. 81.

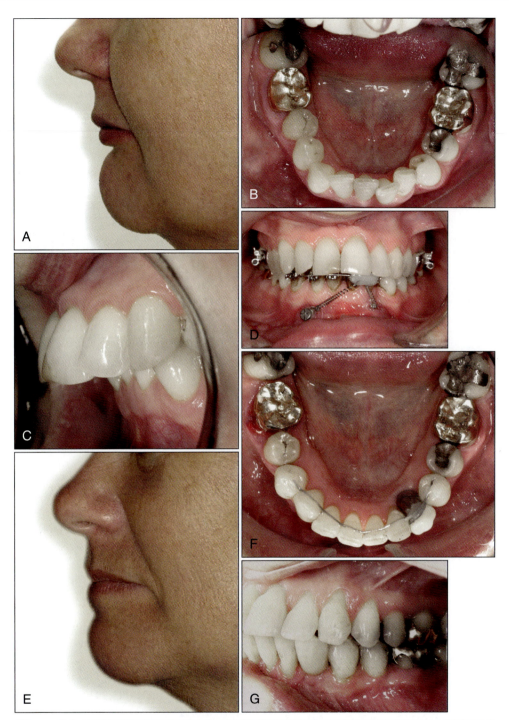

Figure 5-6

A to **C**, Woman age 47 years with pronounced alveolar retrognathism in the mandible leading to an increased overjet. The mandibular arch was asymmetric because an ankylosed canine had been removed in the left side. The patient did not want surgery, which would have involved a sagittal split osteotomy with advancement of the mandible, followed by a reduction of the pronounced symphysis. **D**, Two mini-implants were inserted into the symphysis and used as anchorage for a forward displacement of the lower arch. Hypertrophy of the mucosa occurred as a reaction to the activity of the insertion of the mentalis muscle close to the protruding mini-implants. **E** to **G**, Profile and occlusion after treatment. An implant was used to replace the lost left canine. *(Case treated by Karen Haarbo.)*

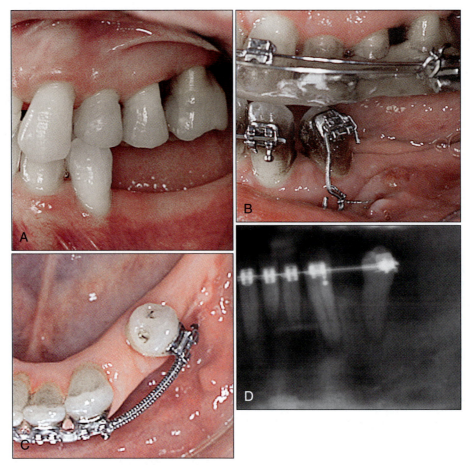

Figure 5-7

A, Patient with missing molars and lower left second premolar. Note the atrophic alveolar process. **B,** The premolar is displaced distally against a submucosal screw to generate bone for a dental implant distal to the canine. **C** and **D,** After treatment. Note the regeneration of the width and height of the alveolar process. *(Case treated by Daniela Garbo.)*

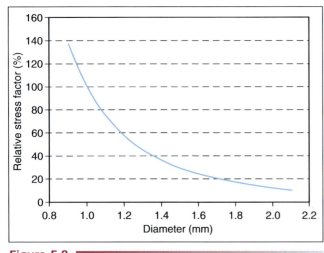

Figure 5-8

Relationship between stress and screw diameter. *(From Dalstra M, Cattaneo PM, Melsen B:* Orthodontics *7:53-62, 2004.)*

age devices. The mini-implants were inserted following instruction by the author. The devices used were the Absoanchor screw, which was preferentially used in the interradicular area of the maxilla, and the Aarhus mini-implant (Figure 5-9). The Absoanchor screws were inserted following the procedure prescribed by Kyung et al.[21]

To insert the Aarhus mini-implant, an orthodontic wire template indicating the approximate insertion site was fixed with light-curing composite, and a periapical radiograph was taken to provide exact information on the insertion site and direction. The mini-implants were self-cutting, and no mucosal incision was necessary (Figure 5-10).

After a thorough washing of the mucosa with 0.2% chlorhexidine, the mini-implants were inserted with a manual screwdriver. The shredded part was inserted into the bone, and screwdriver turning stopped when the neck of the implant touched the periosteum.

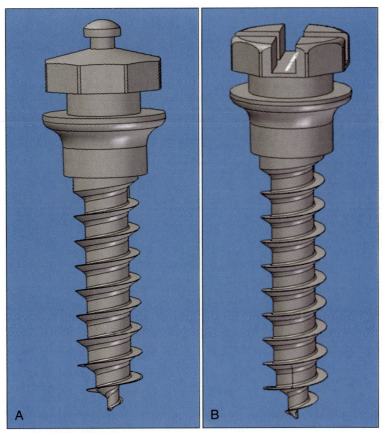

Figure 5-9
A, Aarhus mini-implant with buttonlike head to which a Sentalloy spring can be attached. B, Aarhus mini-implant with bracketlike head into which a wire can be inserted so that the mini-implant can serve as indirect anchorage.

The mini-implants were inserted in the maxilla (in the palate), the alveolar process and the infrazygomatic crest, the mandible in the symphysis, and the alveolar process, as well as in the retromolar area. The mini-implants were used both as direct and indirect anchorage, and the anchorage unit was loaded immediately with 50 cN.

The following tooth movements were performed against the skeletal anchorage:
- Molar uprighting
- Molar uprighting and mesial movement
- Molar mesial movement
- Molar intrusion
- Premolar intrusion
- Premolar distal movement in the case of missing molars
- Midline correction
- Incisor intrusion and proclination
- Incisor retraction

Of the first 180 mini-implants inserted, 19 failed (16 in the first few weeks). The overall failure rate was 10.5%; interestingly, all the failures were related to direct anchorage mechanics. No specific tendency was found regarding the type of tooth movement. The site was a factor, however, in that the implants inserted in the palate had the lowest success rate (2/4 = 50%), and those in the retromolar area in the mandible had the highest success rate (5/5 = 100%). The site played only a minor role in the failures.

Based on the records of each patient, the time and circumstances of the failures were analyzed. Most failures, occurring weeks after insertion, were the first mini-implant inserted by each dentist, indicating a certain learning curve. Success correlated highly with how the screwdriver was held during insertion and whether it was stabilized in the palm, or whether the hand drilling was steady without change in direction. In contrast, failure was associated with holding the screwdriver like a pencil, as often seen in novices inserting the screw. This observation led to the development of a training exercise using a plastic model to explain differences in screwdriver positioning (Figure 5-11).

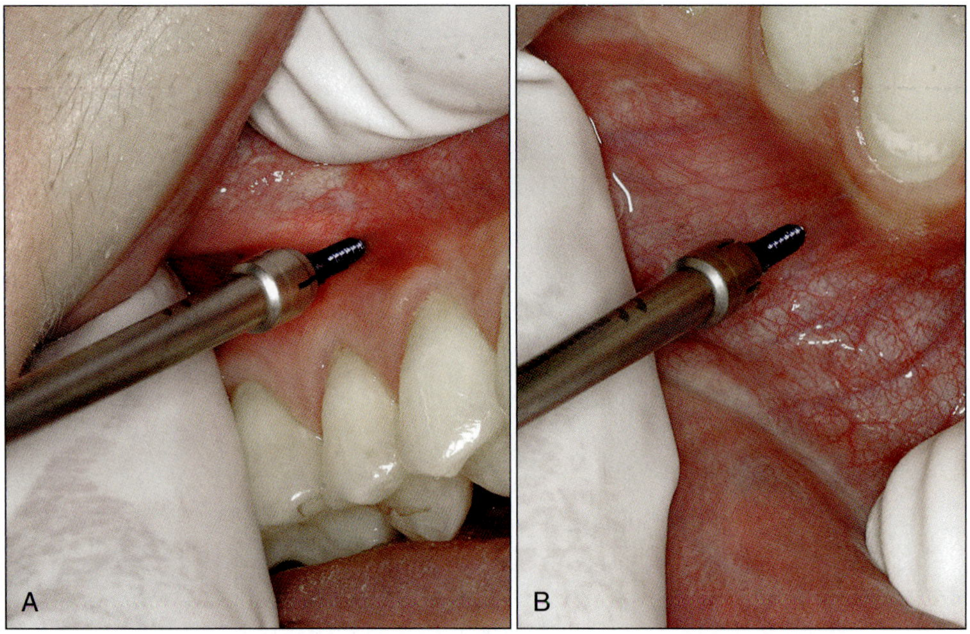

Figure 5-10
A and **B**, Insertion is done through the mucosa directly with a hand-driven screwdriver.

In all the patients who experienced failure within the first weeks, no primary stability was obtained during insertion.

Three of the seven failures observed several months after insertion were related to increased bone turnover in the region of the mini-implants, a result of either ongoing resorption of deciduous teeth (one failure) or remodeling that occurred in front of teeth being displaced toward the mini-implant (two failures). Four of the 19 implants were loosened or removed because of infection. All these had been placed in nonattached gingiva, and the ligature used to fix the coil spring or the wire to the bracketlike head of the implants was placed around the "bracket," similar to a bracket placed on a tooth. The loose end of the ligature can lead to both irritation and plaque accumulation (Figure 5-12).

TYPES OF FAILURE AND SOLUTIONS

Based on reports in the literature and observations from the ongoing study, implant failures can be related to the device, the dentist, or the patient.

FAILURE RELATED TO THE DEVICE
- *Problem:* Fracture occurs, resulting from thin screw diameter or low strength in screw neck area, which will be submitted to greater stress at removal.
  Solution: Choose a slightly conical screw with a solid neck and a diameter compatible with the bone quality.
- *Problem:* Infection around the screw, because not all the transmucosal part has a smooth surface.
  Solution: Choose a screw system with variable neck lengths so that all the transmucosal part is smooth.

FAILURE RELATED TO THE DENTIST
- *Problem:* In the case of self-drilling screws, excessive pressure is used at the start of the insertion, leading to fracture of the cutting tip (see Figure 5-9).
  Solution: Perform the insertion manually using delicate force until the screw "grips."
- *Problem:* The screw is tightened excessively. Once the smooth part (the neck) has reached the periosteum, it is crucial to stop turning the screw; otherwise, it will become loose.
  Solution: Perform the insertion manually, and be aware of changes in the force needed to turn the screwdriver.
- *Problem:* When screws with a bracketlike head are used, turning a ligature around the screw will make it impossible for the patient to keep the screw area free of inflammation.
  Solution: The ligature should be placed on top of the screw in the slot perpendicular to the one in which the wire is resting, and it should be fixed with a composite gel (see Figure 5-12).
- *Problem:* Loosening occurs, resulting from "wiggling" forces during insertion because of faulty handling of the screwdriver or during removal of the screwdriver.
  Solution: During insertion, keep the base of the screwdriver stabilized toward the palm of the hand while turning the screwdriver. It is important that

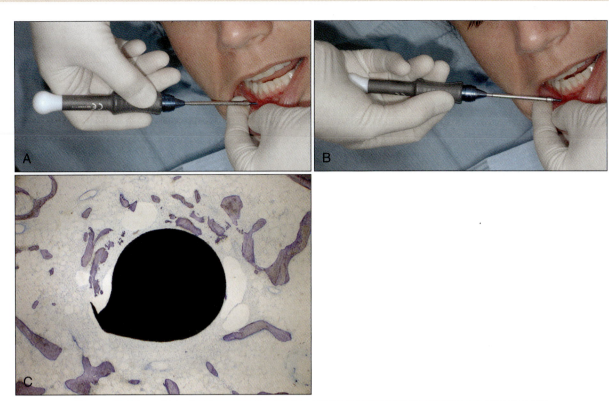

Figure 5-11
A, Incorrect way to hold screwdriver when inserting screw. Holding the screwdriver like a pencil leads to a continuous change in direction and microdamage to the bone. The consequence may be lack of primary stability or early loss of the implant. **B,** Correct way to hold screwdriver. The screwdriver is stabilized by letting the top of the handle rest in the palm of the hand. This leads to a stable insertion direction. **C,** Histological image demonstrating the result of continuous change in direction during insertion; a number of microfractures surround the screw.

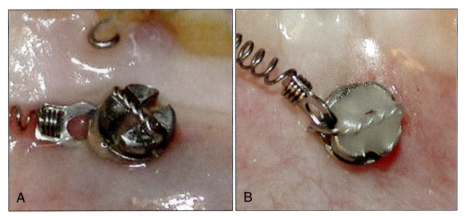

Figure 5-12
A, Incorrect placement of ligature. Placing the ligature around the bracketlike head, as on a tooth, will produce irritation and plaque accumulation. **B,** Correct placement of ligature. The loose end of the ligature is placed on top of the "bracket" and fixed with a light-cured composite gel.

the direction of the screw be kept stable during its insertion. If the screwdriver grabs around the screw, it is important not to apply "wiggling" forces, either during the insertion procedure or when removing the screwdriver.

Solution: Choose a mini-implant in which the screwdriver has a fixed grip on the screw without applying a major force. It is also recommended that the screwdriver handle be removed before the screwdriver itself is removed.

- *Problem:* The risk of infection seemed to be higher when a flap surgery was needed.
Solution: If possible, use a mini-implant system that does not require predrilling.

FAILURE RELATED TO THE PATIENT

- *Problem:* Too little bone is present. In patients with cortical thickness less than 0.5 mm and low trabecular bone density, primary stability cannot be obtained, and the prognosis is poor.
Solution: Recognize the high failure risk, and change the biomechanics so that another insertion site can be used, with the implant as indirect instead of direct anchorage.

- *Problem:* In patients with thick mucosa, the distance between the point where force is applied and the screw's center of resistance is increased; thus a large moment is generated when a force is applied.
Solution: When possible, choose a longer screw; otherwise, consider changing the biomechanics as previously indicated, or recognize that the limits of treatment have been reached.

- *Problem:* Bone remodeling occurs. If a screw is inserted in an area with high bone remodeling related to resorption of a deciduous tooth or healing after extraction, loosening of the screw can occur even after primary stability has been achieved.
Solution: Take this issue into consideration when choosing the implant site.

- *Problem:* The patient has a systemic alteration in the bone metabolism because of disease, medication use, or heavy smoking.
Solution: Accept that some patients are not candidates for skeletal anchorage or implants.

CONCLUSION

Skeletal anchorage will become an integral part of daily orthodontic practice. Careful planning and consideration of the risk factors are important when choosing the patient, the site, and the mini-implant. Skeletal anchorage should be used to widen the spectrum of orthodontics, not replace the rational application of biomechanics.

REFERENCES

1. Weinstein S: Minimal forces in tooth movement, *Am J Orthod* 53(12):881-903, 1967.
2. Ren Y, Maltha JC, Kuijpers-Jagtman AM: Optimum force magnitude for orthodontic tooth movement: a systematic literature review, *Angle Orthod* 73(1):86-92, 2003.
3. Burstone CJ, Koenig HA: Optimizing anterior and canine retraction, *Am J Orthod* 70(1):1-19, 1976.
4. Melsen B, Verna C: Miniscrew implants: the Aarhus Anchorage System, *Semin Orthod* 11:24-31, 2005.
5. Rozencweig G, Rozencweig S: Use of implants and ankylosed teeth in orthodontics: review of the literature, *J Parodontol* 8(2):179-184, 1989.
6. Kofod T, Wurtz V, Melsen B: Treatment of an ankylosed central incisor by single tooth dentoosseous osteotomy and a simple distraction device, *Am J Orthod Dentofacial Orthop* 127(1):72-80, 2005.
7. Heymann GC, Tulloch JF: Implantable devices as orthodontic anchorage: a review of current treatment modalities, *J Esthet Restor Dent* 18(2):68-79, 2006.
8. Roberts WE, Helm FR, Marshall KJ, et al: Rigid endosseous implants for orthodontic and orthopedic anchorage, *Angle Orthod* 59(4):247-256, 1989.
9. Wehrbein H: Endosseous titanium implants as orthodontic anchoring elements: experimental studies and clinical application, *Fortschr Kieferorthop* 55(5):236-250, 1994.
10. Block MS, Hoffman DR: A new device for absolute anchorage for orthodontics, *Am J Orthod Dentofacial Orthop* 107(3):251-258, 1995.
11. Costa A, Raffini M, Melsen B: Miniscrews as orthodontic anchorage: a preliminary report, *Int J Adult Orthod Orthognath Surg* 13(3):201-209, 1998.
12. Park HS, Bae SM, Kyung HM, et al: Micro-implant anchorage for treatment of skeletal Class I bialveolar protrusion, *J Clin Orthod* 35(7):417-422, 2001.
13. Umemori M, Sugawara J, Mitani H, et al: Skeletal anchorage system for open-bite correction, *Am J Orthod Dentofacial Orthop* 115(2):166-174, 1999.
14. De Clerck H, Geerinckx V, Siciliano S: The zygoma anchorage system, *J Clin Orthod* 36(8):455-459, 2002.
15. Sherwood KH, Burch JG, Thompson WJ: Closing anterior open bites by intruding molars with titanium miniplate anchorage, *Am J Orthod Dentofacial Orthop* 122(6):593-600, 2002.
16. Sherwood KH, Burch J, Thompson W: Intrusion of supererupted molars with titanium miniplate anchorage, *Angle Orthod* 73(5):597-601, 2003.
17. Erverdi N, Keles A, Nanda R: The use of skeletal anchorage in open bite treatment: a cephalometric evaluation, *Angle Orthod* 74(3):381-390, 2004.
18. Kanomi R: Mini-implant for orthodontic anchorage, *J Clin Orthod* 31(11):763-767, 1997.
19. Bae SM, Park HS, Kyung HM, et al: Clinical application of micro-implant anchorage, *J Clin Orthod* 36(5):298-302, 2002.
20. Deguchi T, Takano-Yamamoto T, Kanomi R, et al: The use of small titanium screws for orthodontic anchorage, *J Dent Res* 82(5):377-381, 2003.
21. Kyung HM, Park HS, Bae SM, et al: Development of orthodontic micro-implants for intraoral anchorage, *J Clin Orthod* 37(6):321-328, 2003.
22. Maino BG, Bednar J, Pagin P, et al: The spider screw for skeletal anchorage, *J Clin Orthod* 37(2):90-97, 2003.
23. Melsen B: Is the intraoral-extradental anchorage changing the spectrum of orthodontics? In McNamara JA Jr, editor: *Implants, microimplants, onplants and transplants: new answers to old questions in orthodontics*, Ann Arbor, 2004, University of Michigan.
24. Joo BH: A new era of orthodontic anchorage: Mini-anchor-screws (MAS). In McNamara JA Jr, editor: *Implants, microimplants, onplants and transplants: new answers to old questions in orthodontics*, Ann Arbor, 2004, University of Michigan.
25. Carano A, Velo S, Incorvati C, et al: Clinical applications of the Mini-Screw-Anchorage System (M.A.S.) in the maxillary alveolar bone, *Prog Orthod* 5(2):212-235, 2004.

26. Luzi C, Verna C, Melsen B: *The Aarhus Anchorage System: histological and clinical investigation*, Aarhus, Denmark, 2005, University of Aarhus.
27. Melsen B: Mini-implants: where are we? *J Clin Orthod* 39(9):539-547, 2005.
28. Lee JS, Park HS, Kyung HM: Micro-implant anchorage for lingual treatment of a skeletal Class II malocclusion, *J Clin Orthod* 35(10):643-647, 2001.
29. Armbruster PC, Block MS: Onplant-supported orthodontic anchorage, *Atlas Oral Maxillofac Surg Clin North Am* 9(1):53-74, 2001.
30. Bengi AO, Karacay S, Akin E, et al: Use of zygomatic anchors during rapid canine distalization: a preliminary case report, *Angle Orthod* 76(1):137-147, 2006.
31. Gelgör IE, Buyukyilmaz T, Karaman AI, et al: Intraosseous screw-supported upper molar distalization, *Angle Orthod* 74(6):838-850, 2004.
32. Sugawara J, Kanzaki R, Takahashi I, et al: Distal movement of maxillary molars in nongrowing patients with the skeletal anchorage system, *Am J Orthod Dentofacial Orthop* 129(6):723-733, 2006.
33. Kircelli BH, Pektas ZO, Kircelli C: Maxillary molar distalization with a bone-anchored pendulum appliance, *Angle Orthod* 76(4):650-659, 2006.
34. Roberts WE, Marshall KJ, Mozsary PG: Rigid endosseous implant utilized as anchorage to protract molars and close an atrophic extraction site, *Angle Orthod* 60(2):135-152, 1990.
35. Roberts WE: Adjunctive orthodontic therapy in adults over 50 years of age: clinical management of compensated, partially edentulous malocclusion, *J Indiana Dent Assoc* 76(2):33-38, 40, 1997.
36. Bae SM, Park HS, Kyung HM, et al: Ultimate anchorage control, *Texas Dent J* 119(7):580-591, 2002.
37. Sugawara J, Baik UB, Umemori M, et al: Treatment and posttreatment dentoalveolar changes following intrusion of mandibular molars with application of a skeletal anchorage system (SAS) for open bite correction, *Int J Adult Orthod Orthognath Surg* 17(4):243-253, 2002.
38. Melsen B, Garbo D: Treating the "Impossible Case" with the use of the Aarhus Anchorage System, *Orthodontics* 1:13-20, 2004.
39. Kuroda S, Katayama A, Takano-Yamamoto T: Severe anterior open-bite case treated using titanium screw anchorage, *Angle Orthod* 74(4):558-567, 2004.
40. Sugawara J: Orthodontic reduction of lower facial height in open-bite patients with skeletal anchorage system: beyond traditional orthodontics, *World J Orthod* 6(suppl):24-26, 2005.
41. Melsen B: Temporary skeletal anchorage: the Aarhus Anchorage System. In Cope JB, editor: *Temporary anchorage devices in orthodontics*, Dallas, 2005, Under Dog Media.
42. Creekmore TD, Eklund MK: The possibility of skeletal anchorage, *J Clin Orthod* 17(4):266-269, 1983.
43. Jenner JD, Fitzpatrick BN: Skeletal anchorage utilising bone plates, *Aust Orthod J* 9(2):231-233, 1985.
44. Chung KR, Kim YS, Linton JL, et al: The miniplate with tube for skeletal anchorage, *J Clin Orthod* 36(7):407-412, 2002.
45. Sugawara J, Baik UB, Umemori M, et al: Treatment and posttreatment dentoalveolar changes following intrusion of mandibular molars with application of a skeletal anchorage system (SAS) for open bite correction, *Int J Adult Orthod Orthognath Surg* 17(4):243-253, 2002.
46. Park HS, Kwon TG: Sliding mechanics with microscrew implant anchorage, *Angle Orthod* 74(5):703-710, 2004.
47. Yao CC, Wu CB, Wu HY, et al: Intrusion of the overerupted upper left first and second molars by mini-implants with partial-fixed orthodontic appliances: a case report, *Angle Orthod* 74(4):550-557, 2004.
48. Giancotti A, Arcuri C, Barlattani A: Treatment of ectopic mandibular second molar with titanium miniscrews, *Am J Orthod Dentofacial Orthop* 126(1):113-117, 2004.
49. Sugawara J, Daimaruya T, Umemori M, et al: Distal movement of mandibular molars in adult patients with the skeletal anchorage system, *Am J Orthod Dentofacial Orthop* 125(2):130-138, 2004.
50. Costa A, Pasta G, Bergamaschi G: Intraoral hard and soft tissue depths for temporary anchorage devices, *Semin Orthod* 11:10-15, 2005.
51. Jeon YJ, Kim YH, Son WS, et al: Correction of a canted occlusal plane with miniscrews in a patient with facial asymmetry, *Am J Orthod Dentofacial Orthop* 130(2):244-252, 2006.
52. Chae JM: A new protocol of Tweed-Merrifield directional force technology with microimplant anchorage, *Am J Orthod Dentofacial Orthop* 130(1):100-109, 2006.
53. De Clerck HJ, Cornelis MA: Biomechanics of skeletal anchorage. 2. Class II nonextraction treatment, *J Clin Orthod* 40(5):290-298, 2006.
54. Tseng YC, Hsieh CH, Chen CH, et al: The application of mini-implants for orthodontic anchorage, *Int J Oral Maxillofac Surg* 35(8):704-707, 2006.
55. Koudstaal MJ, van der Wal KG, Wolvius EB, et al: The Rotterdam palatal distractor: introduction of the new bone-borne device and report of the pilot study, *Int J Oral Maxillofac Surg* 35(1):31-35, 2006.
56. Kircelli BH, Pektas ZO, Uckan S: Orthopedic protraction with skeletal anchorage in a patient with maxillary hypoplasia and hypodontia, *Angle Orthod* 76(1):156-163, 2006.
57. Keim RG: Answering the questions about miniscrews, *J Clin Orthod* 39(1):7-8, 2005.
58. Feldmann I, Bondemark L: Orthodontic anchorage: a systematic review, *Angle Orthod* 76(3):493-501, 2006.
59. Kesling P: Questions and miniscrews, *J Clin Orthod* 39(9):527-528, 2005.
60. Melsen B, Petersen JK, Costa A: Zygoma ligatures: an alternative form of maxillary anchorage, *J Clin Orthod* 32(3):154-158, 1998.
61. Carano A, Lonardo P, Velo S, et al: Mechanical properties of three different commercially available miniscrews for skeletal anchorage, *Prog Orthod* 6(1):82-97, 2005.
62. Dalstra M, Cattaneo PM, Melsen B: Load transfer of miniscrews for orthodontic anchorage, *Orthodontics* 7:53-62, 2004.
63. Büchter A, Wiechmann D, Gaertner C, et al: Load-related bone modelling at the interface of orthodontic micro-implants, *Clin Oral Implants Res* 17(6):714-722, 2006.
64. Wilmes B, Rademacher C, Olthoff G, et al: Parameters affecting primary stability of orthodontic mini-implants, *J Orofac Orthop* 67(3):162-174, 2006.
65. Motoyoshi M, Hirabayashi M, Uemura M, et al: Recommended placement torque when tightening an orthodontic mini-implant, *Clin Oral Implants Res* 17(1):109-114, 2006.
66. Miyawaki S, Koyama I, Inoue M, et al: Factors associated with the stability of titanium screws placed in the posterior region for orthodontic anchorage, *Am J Orthod Dentofacial Orthop* 124(4):373-378, 2003.
67. Cheng SJ, Tseng IY, Lee JJ, et al: A prospective study of the risk factors associated with failure of mini-implants used for orthodontic anchorage, *Int J Oral Maxillofac Implants* 19(1):100-106, 2004.
68. Fritz U, Ehmer A, Diedrich P: Clinical suitability of titanium microscrews for orthodontic anchorage: preliminary experiences, *J Orofac Orthop* 65(5):410-418, 2004.
69. Kuroda S, Sugawara Y, Deguchi T, et al: Clinical use of miniscrew implants as orthodontic anchorage: success rates and postoperative discomfort, *Am J Orthod Dentofacial Orthop* 131(1):9-15, 2007.

PART III

BIOMECHANICAL CONSIDERATIONS

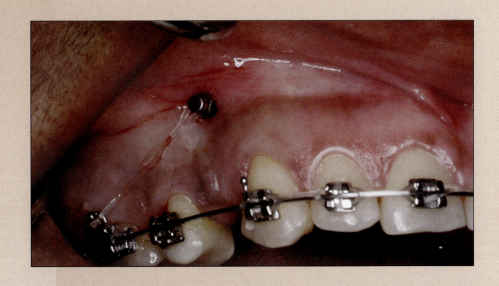

CHAPTER 6

Biomechanical Principles in Miniscrew-Driven Orthodontics

Young-Chel Park and Kee-Joon Lee

Bone-borne temporary anchorage devices (TADs) have opened a new era in clinical orthodontics by revolutionizing the way anchorage is controlled. Previously, various intraosseous TADs have been introduced to move a tooth or segments of teeth, with dramatic results.[1-4] In particular, the surgical miniscrew-type implants have gained much more attention during the past decade than other types of anchorage devices because they are fail-safe, can be easily inserted and removed, cost less, and are stable.[5] Monocortical miniscrews can be placed by the orthodontist, so referral to other specialists is not required. Miniscrews have now become indispensable for the treatment of many clinical cases.

To obtain satisfactory clinical results, however, it is crucial to understand the underlying mechanism of the action of the miniscrew when it is incorporated into orthodontic appliances. This chapter details the fundamental biomechanical principles and their practical application.

OVERVIEW OF MINISCREW IMPLANTS

FORCE SYSTEM

Miniscrews are used to generate a constant, single force with mild to moderate magnitude, regardless of the patient's compliance.[6,7] The actual treatment outcome therefore largely depends on the force system designed by the orthodontist.[8] To achieve predictable results with the miniscrews, two factors are essential: (1) a thorough understanding of the anatomical structure to find appropriate insertion sites and (2) the knowledge of biomechanics to construct a precise force system (Figure 6-1). The force delivered by the miniscrews can be characterized as follows:

1. *Single linear force.* A single miniscrew and the elastic components (elastic chains or nickel-titanium [Ni-Ti] coil springs) engaged to the screw head generate a linear force whose line of action is represented by the direction of the elastic component. It is not yet recommended to apply torsional force on a single miniscrew because it may threaten the miniscrew stability, whether it is a winding or unwinding motion. The line of action is thus determined by the insertion site and the location of the attachments on the tooth or the hooks on the archwire.[9]

2. *Moderate magnitude of force.* A single miniscrew is expected to withstand approximately 200 to 300 grams (g) of force, which appears to be sufficient to move segments of teeth or a single tooth.[5,10] This conversely implies that multiple miniscrews may be indicated to provide anchorage to heavier forces for the movement of a larger segment, such as the posterior segment or the whole arch.

3. *Intrusive component of force.* Conventional orthodontic mechanics tend to extrude the teeth by "jiggling" motion. Because miniscrews are usually placed apical relative to the archwire, the forces from the miniscrews normally always have an intrusive component, causing some intrusion of the reactive dentition.

In conventional mechanics the molars or posterior segments have always served as the anchor, with the rest of the arch as the moving part. The biomechanical principles were complicated because the force system had to be differentially expressed in the moving part and the nonmoving (anchor) part in the same arch. In contrast, when miniscrews are incorporated in the system as the third counterpart, selective movement of the anterior and posterior segments is possible. However, precise planning for the amount of tooth movement desired is thus a prerequisite before active treatment can be initiated.

APPLIANCE DESIGN

Appliances are constructed according to the following step-by-step procedure:

Step 1. Determine the required type of tooth/segment movement (Figure 6-2, *A*).

Step 2. Determine the required force system (Figure 6-2, *B*).

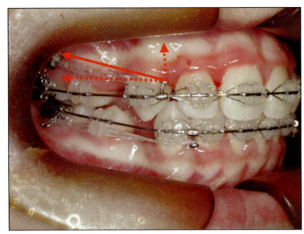

Figure 6-1

Characterization of Force from Miniscrew. Relative to the occlusal plane, the linear force has an intrusive component.

Step 3. Determine the insertion site and point of force application (Figure 6-2, C).

Step 4. Modify the appliance as needed.

Step 1 refers to the type or amount of tooth movement desired, such as tipping or translation. This is the step for deciding "what, where, and how" to move the specific tooth. Step 2 is construction of a suitable force system, including line of force(s) and moment(s), for the desired tooth movement with regard to the estimated center of resistance." Step 3 is the final stage of appliance design. For example, if a line of force passes through the center of resistance of the anterior segment for retraction, the miniscrew position and the archwire hook need to be determined accordingly so that the line connecting the hook and the miniscrew head is identical to the planned line of force. Step 4 is sometimes necessary because of limitations in the insertion sites and appliance design.

Clinical examples for the appliance design are provided later in this chapter.

DRILL-FREE SYSTEM

This chapter describes a system of self-drilling (drill-free) miniscrews in combination with manual guide drills. According to the previous reports, the drill-free system has the following advantages:

- Operative procedure is relatively simple because it does not require costly armamentarium, such as a handpiece, engine, and surgical burs for pilot drilling.
- Manual drilling can provide better tactile sense, enabling the operator to sense probable root contact during insertion.
- Orthodontic loading can be applied immediately after miniscrew insertion. According to a recent study, the machine-threaded implants show relatively constant bone-implant contact, regardless of the orthodontic loading.[12] One to 2 weeks for soft tissue healing may be necessary when the miniscrews are placed on mobile soft tissue.
- The self-drilling type of screw can lead to significantly greater bone-implant contact.[13] Guide drilling may threaten the stability by an increase in localized remodeling or cell death caused by excessive heat generation, when the revolutions per minute (rpm) value is high.[14]

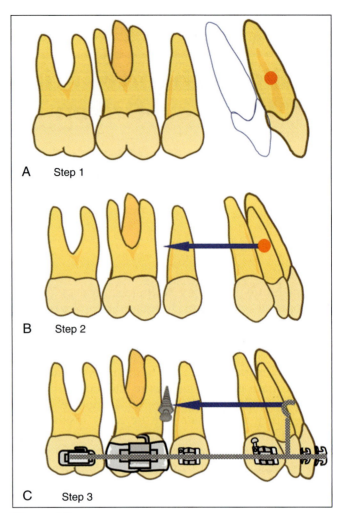

Figure 6-2

Step-by-Step Construction of Miniscrew System. Bodily retraction of upper incisors is induced by appropriate line of force. **A,** Step 1: type of tooth movement required is determined. **B,** Step 2: desirable line of force is determined from a diagram or lateral cephalogram. **C,** Step 3: miniscrews are placed exactly on the planned lines of force. To complete the line of force, the lever arms are extended so that the position of elastics coincides with the planned lines of force.

ORLUS SYSTEM

Implants are supported by the surrounding bones. Unlike the osseointegrated dental implants, orthodontic miniscrews need to exhibit sufficient direct bone-implant contact immediately after insertion for immediate loading. Furthermore, miniscrews are subjected to constant lateral forces, whereas prosthetic implants are subjected to vertical forces. These features provide the basis for adequate miniscrew design. A finite element method (FEM) analysis revealed that a lateral force increases the strain on a miniscrew, mainly around the coronal collar area, which corresponds to the cortical bone in the clinical situation (Figure 6-3).[15] It is therefore crucial to select an insertion site with sufficient cortical bone thickness. Moreover, the miniscrew must be properly designed for effective distribution of the orthodontic load to minimize the strain.

MINISCREW DIMENSIONS: DIAMETER AND LENGTH

According to the FEM, miniscrews with a 1.8-mm collar diameter displayed remarkably reduced strain compared with those with a 1.4-mm collar diameter[15] (Figure 6-4, A). Under 400 centinewtons (cN) of force, the highly strained area is shown as a red spot, which may be detrimental to the initial fixation and long-term stability of the miniscrew. Regarding the length of the miniscrew, a length of 6 mm within the bone remarkably reduced the strain around the miniscrew compared with a length of 4 mm (Figure 6-4, B). Miniscrews with threaded portions greater than 6 mm in length also showed very low strain, but the difference compared with 6-mm miniscrew was minimal. Therefore the threaded portion within the hard tissue should be at least 6 mm long, for better initial stability.

MINISCREW SHAPE: TAPERING

The miniscrew is tapered on the downside, with a sharp, pointed tip at the apex, first used in the Orlus system. This tapered design provides two major advantages. First, the reduced diameter at the apical region can minimize the possible root injury, whereas the larger collar area helps the distribution of stress on the cortical bone. Second, in the self-drilling system, it is essential to maintain initial bone-implant contact regardless of the possible "wobbling" during insertion (Figure 6-5). Because the coronal portion occupies a larger area than the apical portion, the stability of the tapered miniscrews becomes less technique sensitive than the cylindrical miniscrews.

MINISCREW COMPOSITION

The miniscrew is composed of the following parts, from the top through the apical tip (Figure 6-6):

- The button-shaped head portion allows the engagement of elastic components. The negative structure underneath the button is equivalent to the .022 slot, which allows the engagement of .019 × .025 wire or less, for various purposes.
- The nonthreaded, smooth collar portion forms the junction with the overlying soft tissue.
- Reverse-buttress threads around the upper one third of the threaded area contribute to the wide distribution of the stress during the lateral loading.
- Trapezoidal thread design makes the penetration easy without predrilling.
- Corkscrew-like tip is reinforced to facilitate the initial penetration on the cortical surface.
- The overall surface of the threaded portion of the miniscrew is sandblasted and acid-etched to maximize the potential for osseointegration during orthodontic treatment.

MINISCREW TYPES

The Orlus system features three major types of miniscrews, with distinctive shapes and indications, eliminating the need to equip the clinic with a complicated armamentarium (Figure 6-7).

Standard Type (Universal Type)

The standard miniscrew is characterized by a 1.8-mm diameter at the collar region, a threaded portion 6 mm in length for the bone penetration, and a 1-mm smooth (nonthreaded) collar portion (see Figure 6-7, A). This universal type is indicated in the maxillary buccal alveolus, mandibular buccal alveolus, and midpalatal area, where the soft tissue thickness is minimal. The maxillary palatal soft tissue is generally thicker than the corresponding buccal soft tissues.[16] However, the standard type can be also applied on the palatal slope when the overlying gingiva is acceptably thin. The standard type is applicable in most clinical situations, including molar and incisor control.

Wide-Collared Type

The wide-collared miniscrew exhibits wider diameter (2.2 mm) at the coronal region (see Figure 6-7, B). This unique miniscrew is specifically indicated when the host bone quality is rather soft or thin and when the previous miniscrew has failed. This type is also indicated in growing children with immature cortical bone.

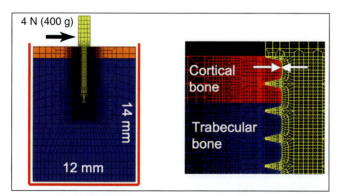

Figure 6-3
Contact (nonlinear) finite element model for the analysis of the stress and strain around a miniscrew under 4 newtons (N) of force.

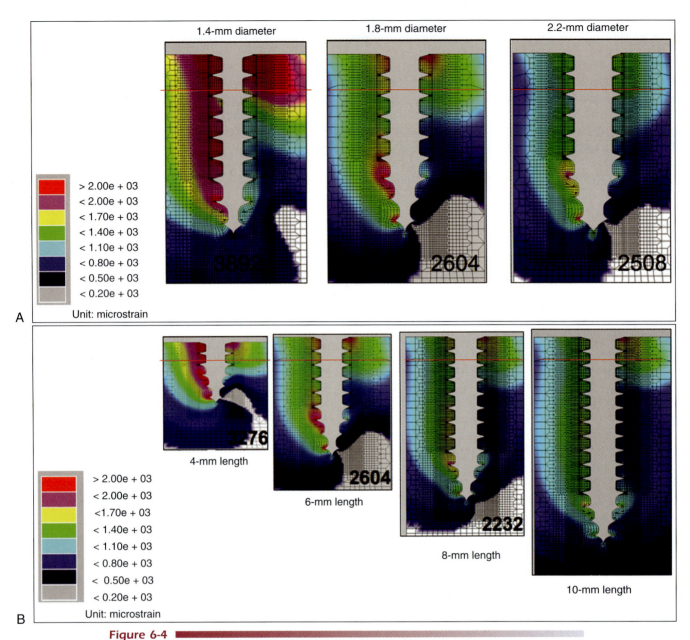

Figure 6-4
Effect of Miniscrew Diameter and Length on Strain. A, Miniscrews with 1.4-mm diameter generated significantly more strain than screws with 1.8-mm and 2.2-mm diameters. **B,** Miniscrews with 6-mm length induced significantly less strain around the bone than 4-mm screws.

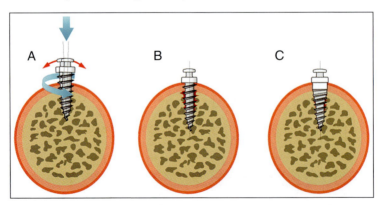

Figure 6-5
A and **B,** Schematic figure of bone-miniscrew relationship during insertion depending on the miniscrew shape. Cylindrical screw core may leave a microgap after insertion in the presence of possible wobbling. **C,** Tapered screw core maintains tight bone-miniscrew contact, regardless of wobbling.

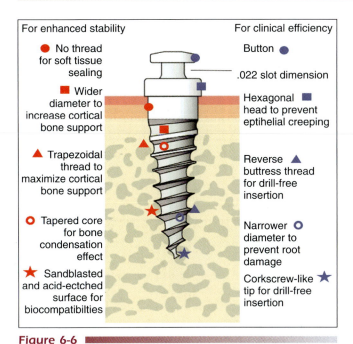

Figure 6-6
Anatomy of Orlus Miniscrew. (This particular design is protected by international patents.)

Long-Collared Type
The long-collared miniscrew is characterized by its long (2-mm to 5-mm) nonthreaded portion, for insertion sites with relatively thick soft tissue (see Figure 6-7, C). The appropriate sites are maxillary palatal slopes and the mandibular retromolar pad area.

ARMAMENTARIUM FOR MINISCREW INSERTION
The armamentarium for this drill-free (self-drilling) system is relatively simple. Insertion sites can be classified into areas requiring either straight (good access) or contra-angle (poor access) screwdrivers. Despite the individual anatomical variation, insertion and removal are rather uniform (Figure 6-8).

Straight and Contra-Angle Screwdriver Handle
The straight screwdriver handle is indicated in the buccal and labial alveolar area and deep areas with relatively good access, including infrazygomatic crest, lower symphyseal area, and mandibular retromolar area. The contra-angle screwdriver is indicated in the areas of poor access, such as palatal slope, midsagittal/parasagittal palate, and lingual slope of the mandibular alveolar bone.

Short/Long Driver Tip
The driver tip is the part that delivers the insertion torque to the miniscrew head. Only one size of driver tip is combined with the straight screwdriver handle, and two different lengths (short and long) are compatible with the contra-angle driver handle. The short driver tip is used for palatal slope, anterior rugae area, and midpalatal region in patients with relatively low palatal vault. The long driver tip is suitable for midpalatal and parasagittal areas. It is essential to keep sufficient (at least 6 mm) clearance between the shank of the screwdriver and the upper incisal edges at the start of insertion to prevent interference during the complete insertion procedure.

Short/Long Manual Guide Drill
Guide drills are provided with the same lengths as the driver tips. Thus, one universal guide drill for the straight screwdriver and two different lengths for the contra-angle screwdriver are available.

Periodontal Probe and Periotest
A periodontal probe is useful to make an indentation for the long axis of the roots or to mark the insertion point. Other instruments used include a dental mirror, pincette, and explorer.

Additional measuring devices, such as torque gauge (MGT50E Torque Gauge, Mark-10 Co, Copiague, NY) and the Periotest (Medizintechnik Gulden, Benshelm, Germany), are helpful in immediately assessing the initial stability of the miniscrew. For example, Periotest values greater than +10 may indicate insufficient initial fixation of the miniscrew, whereas a −3 is a

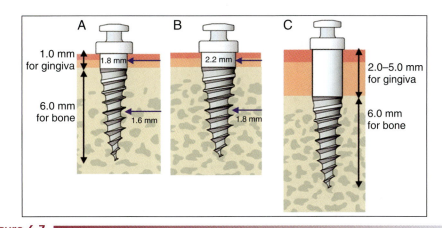

Figure 6-7
Types of Miniscrews. A, Standard (universal) type. B, Wide-collared type. C, Long-collared type.

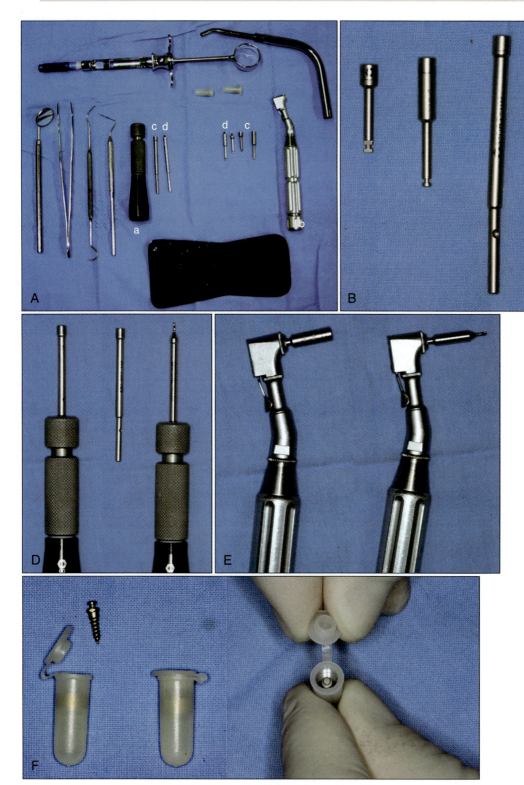

Figure 6-8

A, Armamentarium for miniscrew insertion: *a,* straight screwdriver handle; *b,* contra-angle screwdriver handle; *c,* driver; *d,* manual guide drill. **B,** *From left,* contra-angle short and long driver tips, and manual driver tip. **C,** *From left,* manual guide drill, long and short contra-angle guide drills. **D,** Driver assembly for manual insertion on the buccal side. Long driver tip *(right)* and screwdriver handle with guide drill *(left)*. **E,** Driver assembly for contra-angle insertion on the palatal side with long guide drill *(left)* and long driver tip *(right)*. **F,** Miniscrew assembly: miniscrew supplied in sterilized capsules.

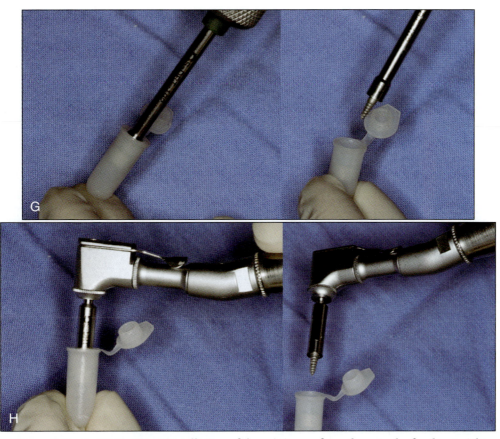

Figure 6-8, cont'd G, Direct installation of the miniscrew from the capsule, for the straight screwdriver. **H,** Direct installation of the miniscrew for the contra-angle screwdriver.

recommended value for success of the osseointegrated dental implants. No definitive guideline exists for the Periotest value in evaluating the success of the orthodontic miniscrews, but orthodontic loading can be deferred for 1 to 2 weeks when the initial Periotest value is relatively high, to determine whether the value is reduced after initial healing.

INSERTION PROCEDURE

Factors shown to influence miniscrew stability include soft tissue incision, predrilling, water irrigation during insertion, and timing of loading. Therefore the insertion procedure is characterized by the following:
- No soft tissue incision or flap reflection
- Direct insertion without (machine-driven) predrilling
- No water irrigation
- Immediate loading

Assessment of Insertion Area

The insertion area is reviewed clinically and radiologically. The quality and quantity of the soft and hard tissues at insertion sites are assessed. Radiological evaluation includes panoramic x-ray films and computed tomography (CT) (Figure 6-9). CT is a valuable tool for three-dimensional (3D) evaluation of the root configuration, cortical bone thickness, and location of anatomical structures such as maxillary sinus and inferior alveolar canal.

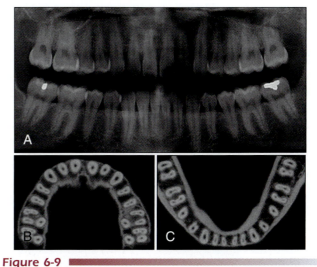

Figure 6-9

Radiographic Assessment of the Insertion Area. A, Panoramic radiograph. **B** and **C,** Axial CT view of the same patient demonstrating the amount of interradicular space.

Local Anesthesia

Local infiltration anesthesia is administered by injecting one fourth of a lidocaine ample per insertion site. The epinephrine content is determined based on the patient's general condition. Although the injection point should be adjacent to the estimated insertion site, an apical and distal injection is ideal considering the trajectory of the neurovascular bundle.

Determining Insertion Sites

The insertion site or insertion point refers to the point where the miniscrew tip first starts penetration into the soft tissue. Determination of a safe insertion site is the critical first step, especially in the tooth-bearing areas (alveolar bone), where dental roots are the major anatomical structure. Therefore, horizontal and vertical positions of the screw must be accurately determined to prevent root damage.

Horizontal Position. The alignment of the roots can be assessed by extending the height of contour from the buccal cusp tip of the clinical crown. Additionally, the depression between the neighboring root contours can be palpated, which represents the configuration of the root alignment and is the major indicator for the insertion site. The safe interdental area is estimated by making a linear indentation with a periodontal probe. When the clinical crown exhibits considerable mesiodistal inclination, the interdental area should be assessed accordingly (Figure 6-10).

When assessing the interdental distance from the panoramic radiograph, the clinician must consider possible distortions (enlargement or shrinkage). For example, the premolar area is generally shrunken and the anterior and molar regions enlarged on the panoramic radiograph.[17]

Vertical Position. A coronally placed miniscrew is likely to be on the firm attached gingiva, but the risk of root damage increases because of the conical shape of the roots. In contrast, apical/subapical insertion may cause soft tissue impingement. A compromised insertion point is therefore the mucogingival junction, where the clinician can minimize possible root damage while preventing soft tissue irritation. If the miniscrew needs to be placed on movable mucosa, a wire extension from the miniscrew head is created at insertion so that the miniscrew head can be covered by soft tissue during initial healing. Elastic components are engaged on the hooked end of the wire extension at the next visit (Figure 6-11).

Marking Insertion Point. The estimated insertion site is marked by punching the soft tissue with a sharp instrument for pinpoint bleeding.

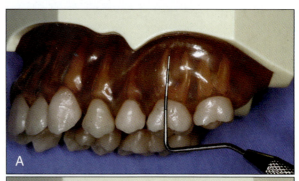
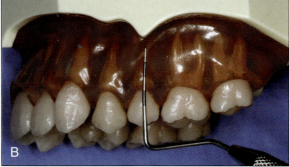
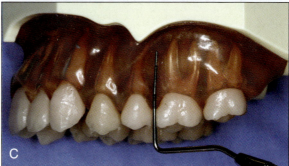

Figure 6-10
Horizontal Position of Interdental Insertion Site. **A** and **B**, Prominent root contours of first molar and second premolar can be detected. **C**, Using a periodontal probe, a linear indentation is formed in the depression area.

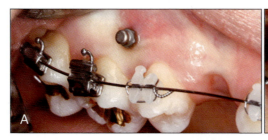
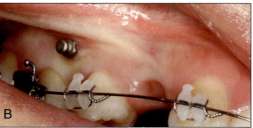

Figure 6-11
A and **B**, Vertical position of insertion site is determined by clinical evaluation and largely influenced by the mucogingival junction. Buccal frenum can often be overlooked when the cheek is fully reflected by the mirror.

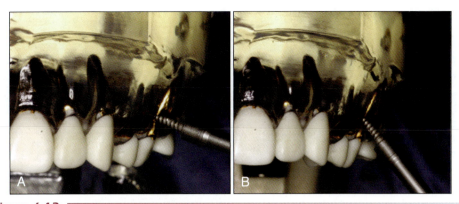

Figure 6-12
Insertion Angulation. Angulation can be adjusted during the initial phase of the cortical bone penetration. **A,** Perpendicular approach. **B,** Angulated approach.

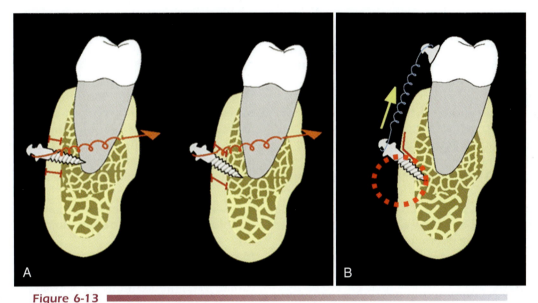

Figure 6-13
Insertion Angle of Miniscrew. A, Oblique insertion is advantageous to avoid possible root damage, but it is sometimes difficult because of possible slippage on the bone surface. **B,** Excessive angulation on the bone surface may weaken the cortical bone structure, and part of the threaded portion may be exposed on the buccal side.

Insertion Angle (Occlusogingival)

It is generally recommended to apically incline the insertion path to avoid possible root injuries and increase cortical bone support. However, the clinician should consider three risk factors. First, excessive angulation on the bone surface may not be easy because the miniscrew tip tends to slip on the bone surface, especially when the buccal alveolar ridge is very thin and lingually inclined with regard to the occlusal plane. Second, the cortical bone on the buccal side is "wedged" by the miniscrew shaft; therefore, the superficial layer of the cortical bone may be weakened. Third, regarding bone-miniscrew contact, the buccal surface of the miniscrew will exhibit less bone contact than the lingual surface, and some part of the threaded portion may be exposed and unsupported by the bone proper because of the angulation of the miniscrew (Figures 6-12 and 6-13).

Therefore, angulation on the bone surface needs to be moderate. A 45-degree angulation relative to the occlusal plane is considered acceptable.

Insertion Path (Mesiodistal)

Even if the insertion site is appropriate, an incorrect insertion path can lead to root damage. Thus a reliable insertion path is as important as the insertion site. A good clinical guideline is the direction of the proximal contact area, since the configuration of the interradicular space reflects the direction of the contact surface viewed from the occlusal surface. The axial cross-sectional CT view, depicting a cut parallel to the occlusal plane and through the roots of the maxillary teeth, show

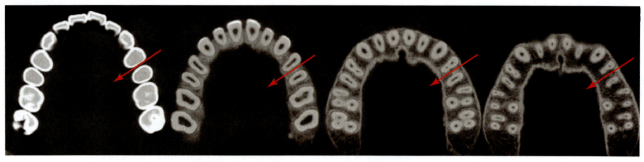

Figure 6-14

Insertion Path of Miniscrew. Proximal contact area is a good reference for determination of the proper insertion path, as shown in this serial sectional view of maxilla. The *arrow* representing the proximal contact area maintains sufficient clearance from adjacent roots regardless of the vertical level.

that the labial cortical bone is not exactly perpendicular to the interproximal contact, especially in the buccal segments (Figure 6-14).

The insertion path should therefore be identical to the proximal contact surface viewed from the occlusal surface throughout the insertion procedure.

Soft Tissue Penetration
An incision is not required for insertion on the firm tissues such as attached gingiva. On movable tissue, however, a minimal incision of 2 to 5 mm is helpful to expose the underlying bone surface for better access and visibility. Soft tissue penetration is performed by gentle pressing of the screw tip against the bone surface.

Cortical Bone Penetration and Establishment of Insertion Path
The miniscrew tip is stabilized on the established insertion point. The first two or three turns require firm pressure against the bone surface, to prevent possible slippage and to establish a stable insertion path by itself. A proper insertion path needs to be carefully maintained during the insertion procedure because an unexpected change in the path may occur. Angulation of insertion path can be changed before one third of the miniscrew has been inserted. Change in the path during the second half of the procedure may lead to miniscrew failure. Insertion is terminated when the shelf on the miniscrew head is lightly touched by the soft tissue surface; hence the whole smooth collar portion is expected to contact the surrounding soft tissue (Figure 6-15).

Manual Predrilling for Guiding Hole
In the areas showing excessive cortical bone, such as midpalatal suture and mandibular buccal alveolar bones in adults, guide drilling is often indicated to facilitate the insertion. Whether to make a guide hole can be determined before or during the insertion procedure. The guiding hole is made using the guide drill installed in the screwdriver or contra-angle driver. Predrilling is normally performed the same way as miniscrew insertion, without engine-driven handpieces.

Use of Engine-Driven Handpiece
An engine-driven handpiece can also be used for predrilling or actual insertion of miniscrews. Guide drills or driver tips with different lengths can be installed on the deceleration contra-angle handpiece (1:256), to maintain about 30 rpm. The advantage of the engine-driven handpiece is not necessarily better stability of miniscrews, but the easiness and comfort during insertion, by ensuring the consistency of the insertion axis.

Management of Soft Tissue
After completing the insertion of the screw, the clinician should carefully examine the surrounding soft tissue. Any elevation of the surrounding soft tissue or circular tension on the movable tissue around the miniscrew head should be relieved using a circular releasing incision around the collar. Postoperative bleeding is negligible or minimal.

REMOVAL PROCEDURE
Removal of Miniscrew (Screw Heads)
In general, local anesthesia is not required if the miniscrew head remains exposed and the miniscrew can be gradually removed from the bone bed by simply unscrewing. Because of the tapered shape of the threaded portion, the greatest removal torque is required at the initial stage of the removal, when the overall threads are simultaneously detached from the bone surface, with no pain. Patients may feel discomfort or even slight pain at the final stage of removal, caused by irritation of the periosteum or gingival soft tissue.

Removal of Miniscrew (Screw Heads Covered by Soft Tissue)
If the screw head was covered by the overlying soft tissue, a minimal incision under infiltration anesthesia

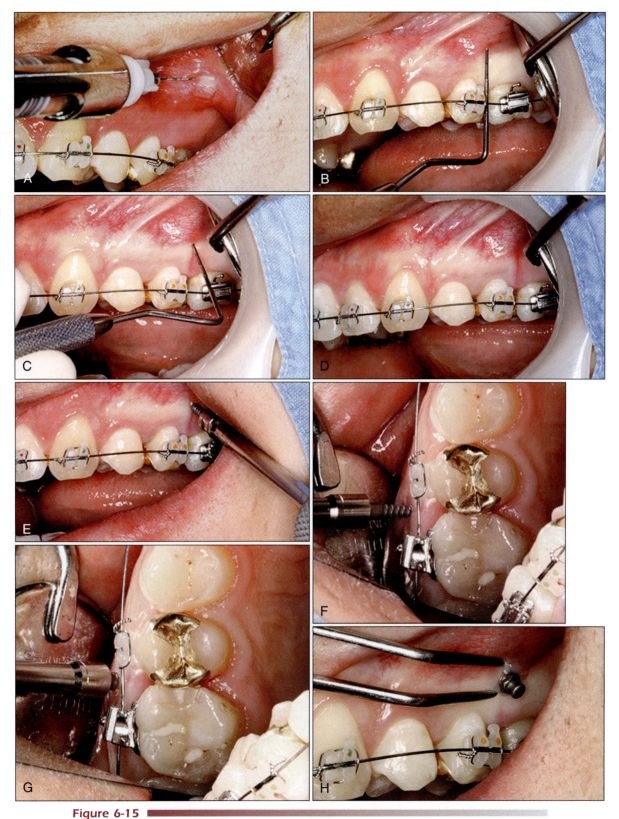

Figure 6-15

Clinical Insertion Procedure. A, Infiltration anesthesia. **B,** Indentation on the interdental depression area. **C,** Marking of the vertical level of insertion point. **D,** Insertion point marked on the gingiva. **E,** Initiation of insertion. **F** and **G,** Maintenance of the insertion path with the interproximal area from the occlusal view as reference. **H,** Manipulation of the surrounding gingival soft tissue.

is indicated to expose the miniscrew head. The removal procedure is the same as previously described. Incision lines greater than 5 mm may require suturing, whereas those less than 5 mm can be left unstitched.

MINISCREW SUCCESS AND FAILURE

The success rate of the miniscrew reportedly ranges from 80% to 100%, depending on the region and the operator, but slightly lower than that of the miniplate.[5,18] Three factors are critical for the prolonged stability of the miniscrew: (1) miniscrew design, (2) proper insertion site, and (3) careful operation. Securing firm initial fixation is the first step toward successful treatment.

IMMEDIATE FAILURE

Immediate failure (loosening) of the miniscrew usually occurs during the initial healing phase. Possible causes include improper insertion site and improper handling during insertion. Insertion sites with rare cortical bone, recent extraction sockets, and redundant overlying soft tissue are defined as improper insertion sites (Figure 6-16). Improper handling includes wobbling or abrupt change in the path of insertion. Percussion test on the miniscrew head or Periotest measurement after insertion is advised, with immediate removal and reinsertion at another site.

DELAYED FAILURE

Even if the initial fixation appeared favorable, miniscrew loosening may take place during active orthodontic treatment. The exact reason for delayed failure is not clear. Possible reasons include excessive loading from the elastic component, sudden impact on the miniscrew head during mastication, possible contact with root surface, and excessive or insufficient bone remodeling around the miniscrew, indicating a possible shift of the miniscrews in the bone.[19] Although the cortical bone thickness is critical for initial fixation, the cortical bone exhibits low bone-remodeling potential compared with trabecular bone.[20] Therefore it is important that the strain around the miniscrew caused by the lateral force is tolerated by sufficient bone remodeling around the miniscrew (Figure 6-17).

A failed miniscrew needs to be removed and a new miniscrew inserted at an adjacent site. Reinsertion at the same site may increase the risk of failure; however, if the particular insertion site is crucial, using a miniscrew with wider diameter or reinsertion 2 to 3 months later is recommended.

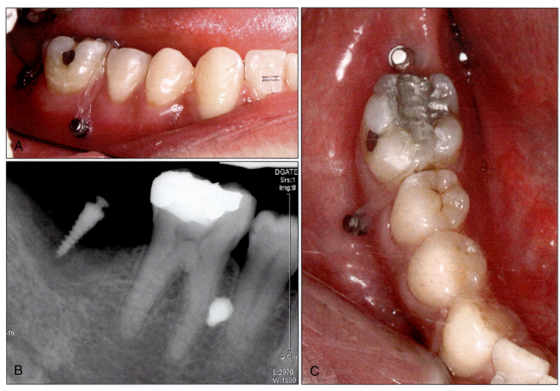

Figure 6-16
A to C, Immediate failure of miniscrew may result from insufficient cortical bone. A miniscrew inserted on a new extraction socket of the second molar displays significant mobility. Periapical radiography showing insufficient bone support for the miniscrew.

OTHER COMPLICATIONS

SOFT TISSUE INFLAMMATION, ULCERATION, ABSCESS, AND COVERAGE

Inflammation or an abscess is relatively rare if the miniscrew is placed on the firm attached gingiva, as long as proper oral hygiene is maintained during treatment. Ulceration or soft tissue coverage is associated with miniscrews placed on or near the buccal frenum (Figure 6-18). The buccal frenum can often pass unnoticed on full reflection of the lips for visibility (see Figure 6-11). An incisional frenectomy can be performed if the insertion is critically indicated in the frenum area (Figure 6-19).

Ulceration on the buccal mucosa or cheek can be managed by application of Orabase and soft utility wax on the miniscrew head during initial healing for 1 to 2 weeks. When the miniscrew head is covered by thin soft tissue, a simple incision and tying of wire ligature is advised, for the engagement of the elastic component. This normally does not affect miniscrew stability.

ROOT DAMAGE

Root damage can be managed depending on the severity of the injury. Serious injury, including root perforation or fracture, is extremely rare in the drill-free system because the obvious difference in the surface hardness between the bone and the root cementum can be readily sensed by the operator. Nevertheless, the anatomical structure must be properly understood before insertion, especially when the miniscrew is placed on the tooth-bearing area. Minor injuries on the cementum area can undergo spontaneous healing after removal of the miniscrew.[21] Invasion of the miniscrew in the periodontal tissue may not cause discomfort or pain to the patient, so obtaining periapical x-ray films routinely after insertion is recommended (Figure 6-20).

Root Contact During Tooth Movement

Adjacent tooth movement toward the miniscrew can result in miniscrew-root contact (Figure 6-21). Root contact by the orthodontic tooth movement remains largely asymptomatic. Thus, probable root contact should be diagnosed clinically: no movement of the tooth, excessive crown tipping toward the miniscrew, and (rarely) miniscrew loosening. Removal and insertion on an adjacent site is recommended for further tooth movement.

MINISCREW FRACTURE

Fracture of a miniscrew is rare if the diameter is greater than 1.5 mm and especially if the miniscrew is tapered. However, guide drilling is advised when the resistance

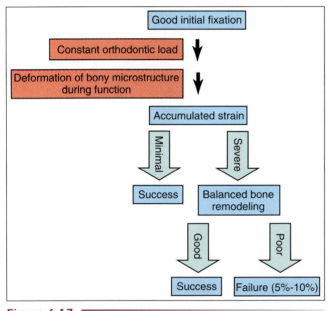

Figure 6-17

Ontogeny of Orthodontic Miniscrew Implants. Bone-remodeling procedure may explain the cause of delayed failure.

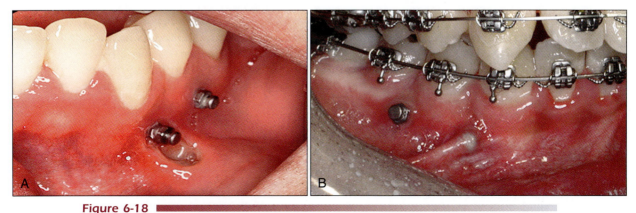

Figure 6-18

Soft Tissue Complications. **A,** Soft tissue ulceration. **B,** Soft tissue coverage by overlying frenum. These complications are not associated with miniscrew failure.

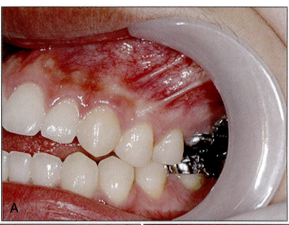
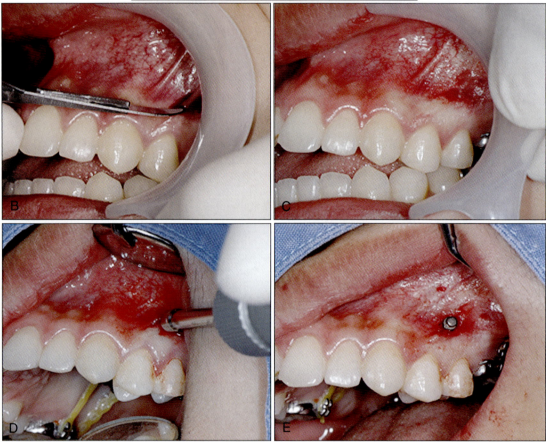

Figure 6-19

A, Buccal frenum running on the insertion site between upper first and second premolar. B, Releasing incision with #12 blade at the coronal end of the frenum. C, After bleeding control, a frenum-free insertion site was established. D, Immediate insertion on the predetermined insertion site. E, After insertion, there is no need for further soft tissue manipulation.

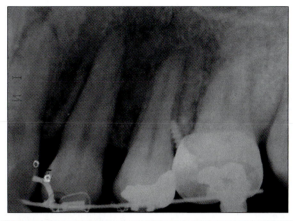

Figure 6-20

Root Contact During Insertion. Periapical radiograph showing intrusion of the miniscrew into the periodontal space.

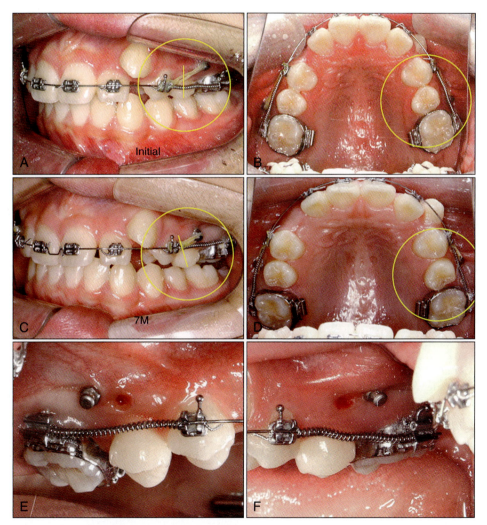

Figure 6-21

Root Contact During Tooth Movement: Signs and Troubleshooting. A and **B,** Initial lateral and occlusal view showing interdental miniscrews between second premolar and first molar *(yellow circles)*, with Class II molar relation. Molar distalization using indirect miniscrew anchorage was initiated. **C** and **D,** After 7 months, all premolars and molars were distalized into overcorrected Class I position. Inadvertent distal tipping of the second premolar was noted, with no symptoms. **E** and **F,** New miniscrews were placed at the interradicular area mesial to the first molar. Treatment was finished with no pathologic changes on the second premolar.

increases significantly during insertion. With miniscrew fracture, removal of the bone around the miniscrew thread is indicated.

PAIN

Pain is a relatively common sequela but usually it is not serious. The pain related to miniscrew operation comes from the nerve endings in the soft tissue and periosteum, not necessarily from the bone proper. Nonsteroidal antiinflammatory drug (NSAID) for 2 days following the procedure is sufficient to manage the postoperative pain in most patients.

BLEEDING AND NUMBNESS

Excessive bleeding or numbness is not associated with miniscrew implantation on the tooth-bearing area or midpalate region. However, care should be taken not to injure the palatine neurovascular bundle. The greater palatine foramen is positioned distal to the upper second molar and midway between the cementoenamel junction (CEJ) and the midpalate. The rest of the masticatory gingiva on the palatal slope is a safe area for implantation.

BIOMECHANICS FOR ANTERIOR RETRACTION

Some conventional biomechanical principles need to be modified for the system incorporating the miniscrews. This section explains the essential factors to help increase the clinical efficiency of treatment.

ANCHORAGE VALUES IN UPPER AND LOWER ARCHES

In extraction cases requiring maximum anchorage, miniscrews are placed in the posterior region for incisor segment retraction. Reinforcement of anchorage is primarily required in the upper arch for the following reasons:
1. The *root surface area* of the upper anterior teeth is larger than that of the lower anterior teeth, which will increase the resistance to posterior movement of the upper anterior segment[22] (Figure 6-22).
2. *Bodily translation* is more frequently planned in the upper arch, especially in Class II cases displaying dental compensations, whereas controlled tipping is indicated in the lower arch. Relatively abundant lingual supporting bone in the upper anterior region, compared to the thin alveolar housing in the lower incisor region, allows translation of the anterior segment. Translation or root movement of the upper anterior region requires a higher anchorage value than tipping.
3. The *trabecular bone structure* in the upper posterior segment may lead to more anchorage movement during retraction than in the lower posterior segment.

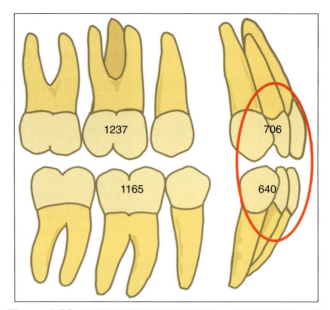

Figure 6-22

Comparison of Root Surface Area. Upper incisors display larger root surface area, necessitating higher posterior anchorage value for incisor retraction. (Redrawn from Proffit WR, Fields HW, Sarver DM: *Contemporary orthodontics*, ed 4, St Louis, 2007, Mosby.)

DETERMINATION OF INSERTION SITE AND SEQUENCE DEPENDING ON ANCHORAGE TYPES

Conventional anchorage is classified into A, B, and C types, representing maximum, moderate, and minimum anchorage, respectively.[23] Miniscrews can be applied strategically depending on the anchorage demand, as follows:
- *Type A anchorage* (Figure 6-23, *A*). When more than 75% of the extraction space is used for the anterior retraction, upper and lower miniscrews are placed between the second premolar and first molar. Lower implants may not be necessary initially and can be added if needed during the retraction phase.
- *Type B anchorage* (Figure 6-23, *B*). Both anterior and posterior segments are reciprocally moved to close

Figure 6-23

Anchorage Classification and Miniscrew Position. A, In type A anchorage, miniscrews are placed in both the upper and the lower buccal segment to provide firm anchorage. Lower miniscrews may not be necessary considering the high anchorage value of the mandibular posterior segment. **B,** In type B anchorage, upper miniscrews may be required in the middle of retraction phase.

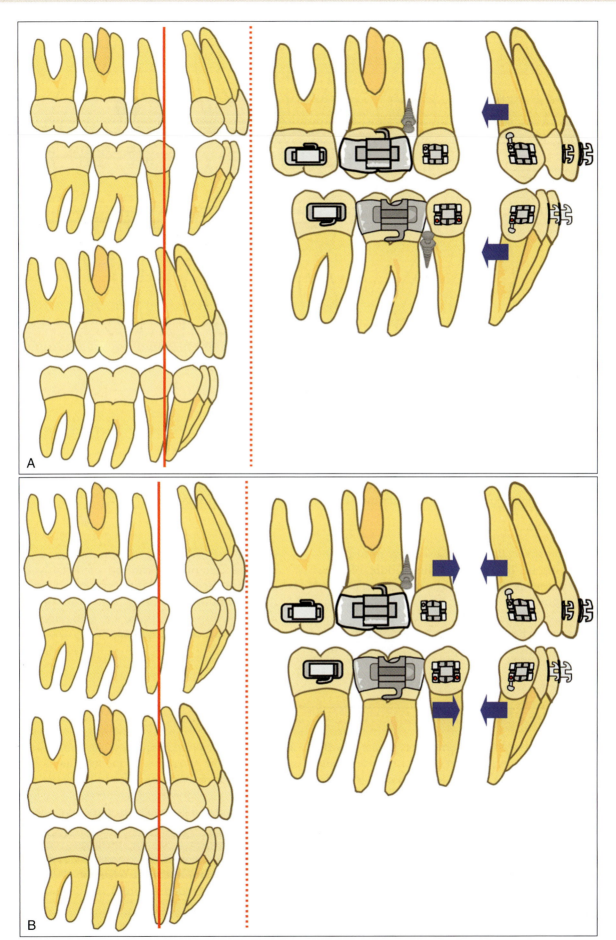

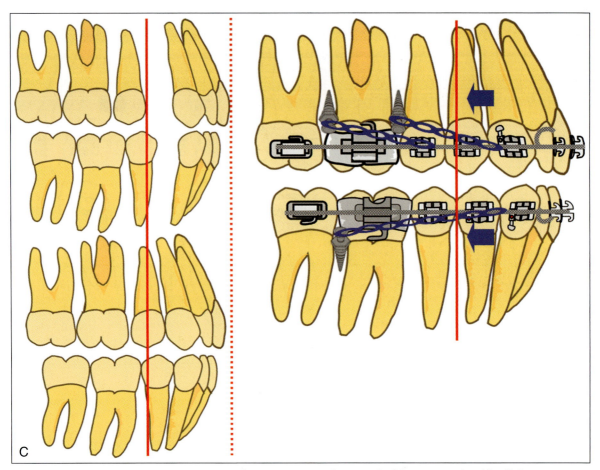

Figure 6-23, cont'd C, Type C anchorage cases may be treated without extraction if sufficient distalization of buccal segments can be achieved using miniscrew implants.

the extraction space. In some cases, upper miniscrew implants may be indicated in the middle of the retraction phase, depending on the movement of the posterior segment.
- *Type C anchorage* (Figure 6-23, C). When more than 75% of the extraction space needs to be closed by the forward movement of the posterior segments or second premolar extraction is indicated. However, because the molars can be predictably distalized using miniscrew implants even in adults, many of the minimum anchorage cases can be treated as nonextraction modalities, or sometimes with the extraction of second molars.

Text continued on p. 116

CASE REPORT 6-1: CLASS II, DIVISION 2 MALOCCLUSION

A 21-year-old woman wanted to correct her anterior crowding and deep bite. Moderate upper anterior crowding was initially noticed, with a Class II molar relationship on both sides, characterizing a typical Class II, Division 2 malocclusion (Figure 6-24).

Because her lip profile was rather flat, compared to the Asian norm, distalization of maxillary molars was indicated following extraction of maxillary second molars, considering that the maxillary third molars were in normal position and inclination. Extraction of the mandibular third molars was done simultaneously. Distalization of the posterior segment was performed using two miniscrews on the right side and a single miniscrew on the left side, according to the amount of distalization required on either side. Subsequent anterior alignment and retraction were performed using the same miniscrews as orthodontic anchorage (Figure 6-25).

At the completion of the treatment, cephalometric superimposition showed distal bodily movement of both molars, establishing a Class I relationship. Incisors were simultaneously intruded to form an acceptable incisor relationship (Figure 6-26).

CASE REPORT 6-1: CLASS II, DIVISION 2 MALOCCLUSION—cont'd

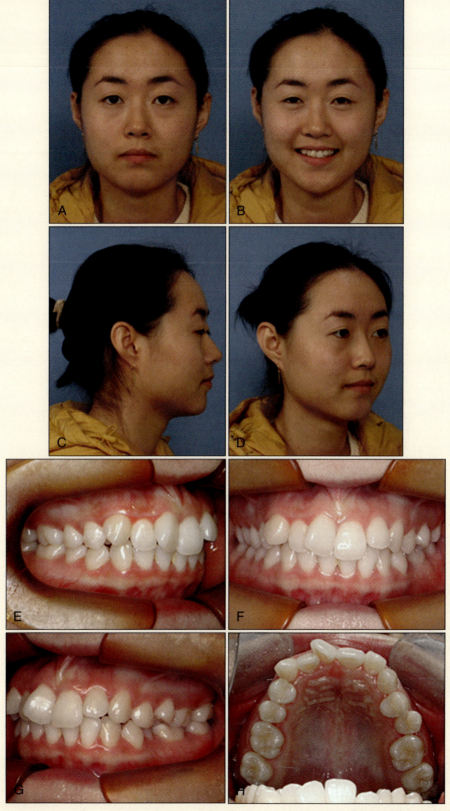

Figure 6-24 Class II, Division 2 Malocclusion. Pretreatment photographs: **A** to **D**, extraoral; **E** to **I**, intraoral.

Continued

CASE REPORT 6-1: CLASS II, DIVISION 2 MALOCCLUSION—cont'd

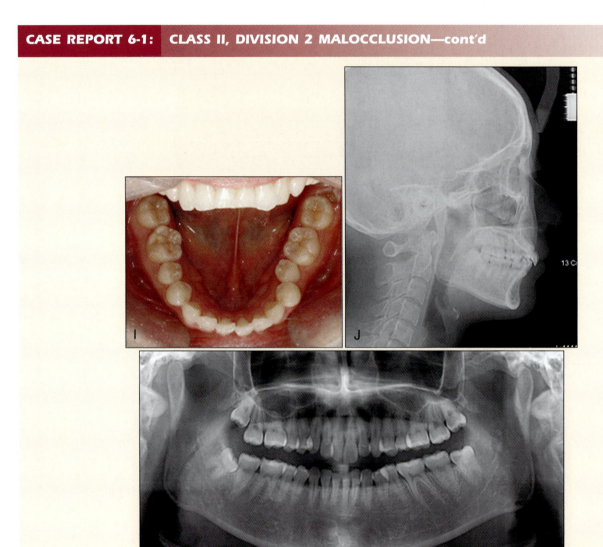

Figure 6-24, cont'd I, intraoral. J and K, Cephalometric radiograph and analysis. L, Panoramic radiograph.

CASE REPORT 6-1: CLASS II, DIVISION 2 MALOCCLUSION—cont'd

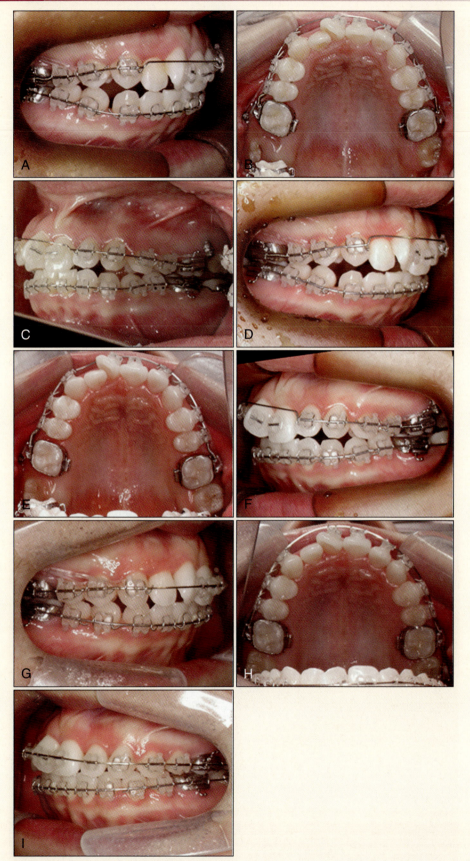

Figure 6-25 **Treatment Progress.** **A** to **C,** After upper second molar was extracted, upper-arch distalization was started. **D** to **F,** After 2 months, space between upper first molar and second premolar was seen. **G** to **I,** After 5 months, upper-arch alignment was started.

Continued

CASE REPORT 6-1: CLASS II, DIVISION 2 MALOCCLUSION—cont'd

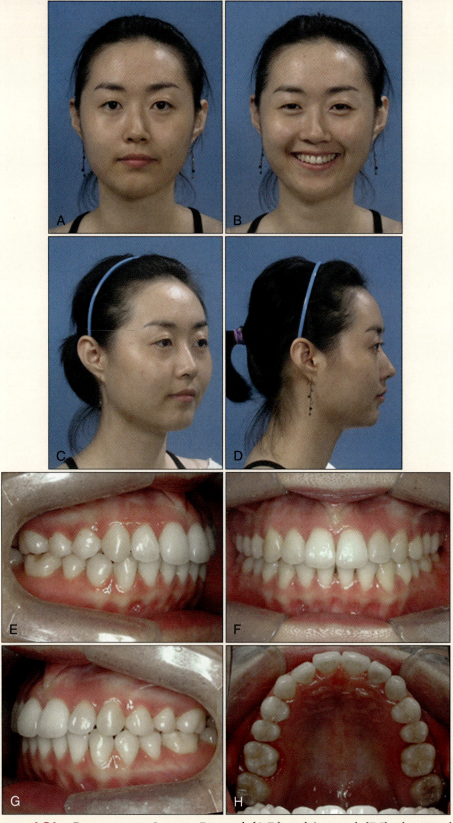

Figure 6-26 Posttreatment Images. Extraoral (A-D) and intraoral (E-I) photographs. J and K, Cephalometric and panoramic radiographs. L, Superimposition of pretreatment and posttreatment cephalometric radiographs.

CASE REPORT 6-1: CLASS II, DIVISION 2 MALOCCLUSION—cont'd

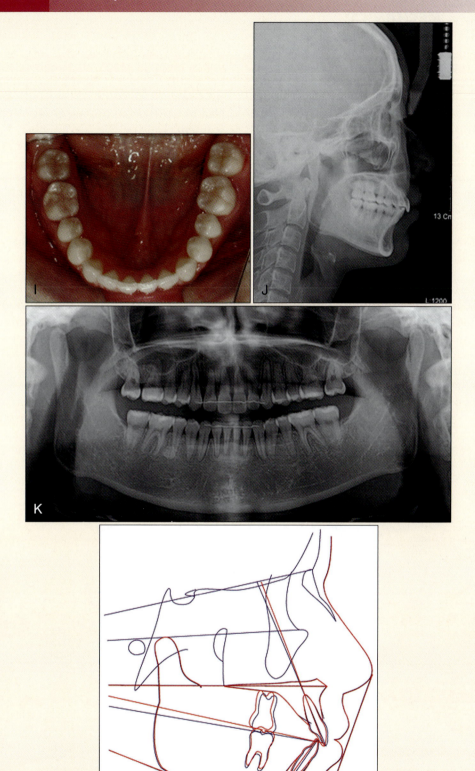

Figure 6-26, cont'd For legend see opposite page.

APPLIANCE CONSTRUCTION: THE DIFFERENCE FROM CONVENTIONAL MECHANICS

Sliding Mechanics vs Loop Mechanics

Loop (friction-free) mechanics and sliding (friction) mechanics have been the two most common retraction techniques used in conventional orthodontics (Figure 6-27). Despite the inherent friction, sliding mechanics is considered biomechanically advantageous over loop mechanics in miniscrew-assisted orthodontics. Incorporation of the loop might complicate the precise interpretation of the force system, because of the discontinuous structure between anterior and posterior regions. In sliding mechanics, however, whole-arch integrity is maintained throughout the retraction procedure, and the resulting tooth movement is determined by the relation of the center of resistance of the dental arch and the line of force running through the miniscrew.[24,25]

Rotation of Occlusal Plane from a Lateral View

Is the Compensating/Reverse Curve of Spee Necessary? In conventional mechanics, either a compensating or a reverse curve of Spee is incorporated in the archwire to reinforce the posterior anchorage units and counteract the reactive mesial tipping of the molars.[26] In contrast, when the retraction force is provided by the miniscrews, reactions in the posterior segment depend on the movement of the anterior segment. For example, in the anterior segment the line of force below the center of resistance of the incisors tends to cause lingual tipping of the incisors. This lingual tipping can be resisted by the stiffness of the steel archwire. However, under frequent reactivation and relatively heavy force on a stiff archwire, the rigid continuous arch might subsequently displace the posterior segment. This can lead to either distal tipping or intrusion of the posterior segment, causing a posterior open bite, as shown in Figure 6-28. A compensating curve or a reverse curve of Spee may exacerbate this side effect, causing even more distal tipping of the molars. In miniscrew-assisted sliding mechanics, therefore, a compensating curve is not necessary on a routine basis. This can be demonstrated not only theoretically but also clinically (Figure 6-29). The archwire was not engaged to the upper second molar when constant force was applied from the miniscrews to the archwire. Retraction using miniscrews resulted in a significant marginal ridge discrepancy between the first and the second molars on both sides, indicating the clockwise rotation of the occlusal plane. Force magnitude, reactivation period need to be appropriately adjusted in order not to induce the occlusal plane canting (Figure 6-30).

Accordingly, practical guidelines for effective maintenance of the occlusal plane are as follows:
- Use a stiff stainless steel wire for active retraction
- Apply a moderate level of force
- Avoid frequent reactivation of the appliance

Are the Toe-In Bends Necessary? In the same context, conventional toe-in bends may result in a distal-in

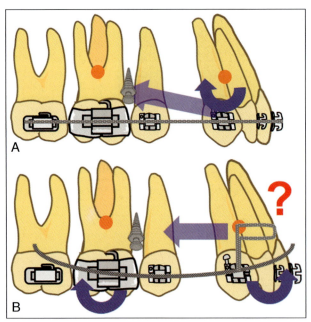

Figure 6-27

Comparison of Sliding Mechanics and Loop Mechanics. Straight, rigid archwire is used to construct a simple appliance in which the type of movement is determined by the relationship between the line of force and the centers of resistance. **A,** Sliding mechanics: less wire bending, more predictable force system, and minimal discomfort. **B,** Loop mechanics: more wire bending, less predictable force system, and more discomfort.

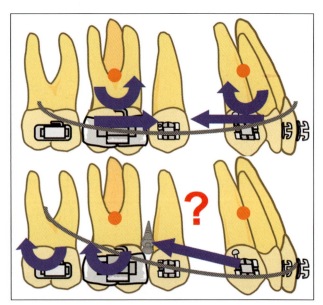

Figure 6-28

Role of Gable/Compensation Bend in the Sliding Mechanics. Gable bends or reverse curve of Spee in combination with miniscrews may induce excessive tip-back of the buccal segment, leading to posterior open bite.

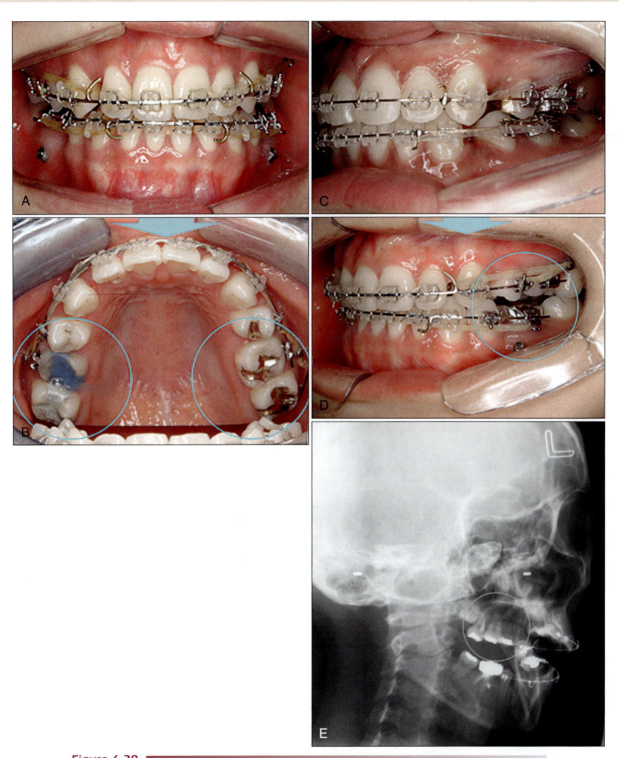

Figure 6-29
Clinical Example of Occlusal Plane Steepening. A to **D**, Sliding mechanics in combination with miniscrews. **E**, Oblique lateral radiographic view shows excessive marginal ridge discrepancy between upper first and second molars and posterior open bite *(circle)*, possibly caused by the tip-back and intrusion of the upper molar. (Courtesy Dr JY Lee.)

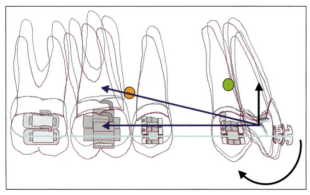

Figure 6-30
Occlusal Plane Change in the Anteroposterior Direction. Initial lingual tipping of the incisors may affect the posterior segment by the rigid rectangular wire connecting the two parts. Displacement of the incisor segment is expressed upward movement of the posterior segment, leading to posterior open bite. (Courtesy Dr JY Lee.)

rotation of the posterior unit and thus are not necessary for the anterior retraction. Plain archwire with minimal curvature is suitable for miniscrew-assisted sliding mechanics.

Unlike the conventional intraarch mechanics, miniscrews transduce a linear force originating from the points above the archwire. Therefore, unexpected changes in the overall occlusal plane might occur. From the sagittal plane, as shown in Figure 6-30, the line of force is expected to pass below the center of resistance of the whole dentition, which is expected to induce the clockwise rotation of the occlusal plane.

Rotation of Occlusal Plane: Frontal View

Asymmetric vertical position of the miniscrews may cause transverse canting of the occlusal plane. Therefore, it is important to place the miniscrews at the same vertical position on both sides and to establish the same vertical component of force. Careful monitoring of the occlusal plane during retraction is essential (Figure 6-31).

PREDICTABLE CONTROL OF TYPE OF TOOTH MOVEMENT

The type of tooth movement can be classified as controlled tipping, uncontrolled tipping, bodily movement, and root movement.[11] In conventional mechanics, the type of tooth movement affects the posterior anchorage unit. For example, bodily movement or root movement of the anterior segment requires a higher anchorage value than controlled/uncontrolled tipping. Using the miniscrews, any type of anterior teeth movement can be achieved, regardless of the anchorage requirement of the posterior segment. However, some discrepancies between theory and clinical reality must be clarified.

First, although the eventual type of tooth movement is determined by the moment/force (M/F) ratio in the anterior unit, the exact M/F ratio in the target tooth or segment of teeth cannot be measured in the practical situation, unless precalibrated appliances are used (e.g., segmented-arch technique).

Second, the type of tooth movement can be adjusted by establishing the line of force below, through, or above the center of resistance of the object. This can be achieved by extending lever arms from the anterior segment or by modifying the height of the insertion sites in the posterior region (Figure 6-32). In the posterior region, however, because of the height of the attached gingiva and the buccal frenum, it is often not practical to place the miniscrew on the desired height. Even if there is no impingement around the insertion site, the elastic component extending from the miniscrew head may often cause constant irritation on the buccal frenum (see Figure 6-11). Similar problems are anticipated in the anterior region when the lever arm is excessively extended from the main archwire.

Therefore, alternatively, movement of the anterior segment can be effectively controlled by applying an "equivalent force system." An additional moment is provided by adjusting the torque in the rectangular archwire, and the resultant type of tooth movement would be determined by the M/F ratio on the anterior segment. This can be summarized as follows:

- **Controlled tipping.** Short hooks are attached on the archwire, and a regular retraction force of 150 to 250 g/side is applied. The line of force runs below the center of resistance of the anterior segment, and thus controlled tipping is anticipated, when the working wire passively fits the anterior brackets (Figure 6-33).
- **Root movement.** The force magnitude is reduced to less than 100 g, whereas additional labial crown torque is applied to the archwire in the incisor

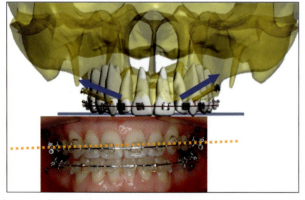

Figure 6-31
Occlusal Plane Canting During Anterior Retraction. From a frontal plane evaluation, unequal level of miniscrews on both sides may induce asymmetric change in the posterior segment, leading to occlusal plane canting.

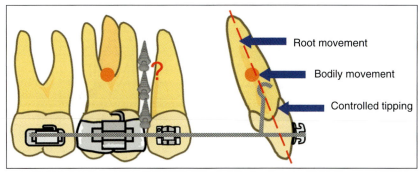

Figure 6-32
Limitations in Construction of Line of Force. Both the insertion site and the length of the lever arm are limited on the labial/buccal side of the arch because of the soft tissue impingement.

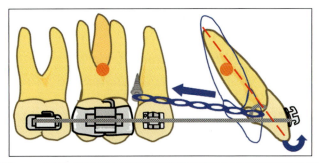

Figure 6-33
Appliance Construction for Controlled Tipping. For controlled tipping, short hooks are attached on the archwire, and the line of force is below the center of resistance. Thus the resultant tooth movement is expected to be tipping of incisors.

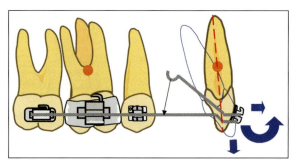

Figure 6-35
Side Effects of Conventional Root Spring. Conventional torque spring tends to extrude and flare the incisors by the resulting force system.

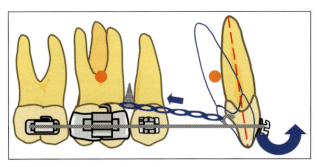

Figure 6-34
Appliance Construction for Root Movement. For root movement, retraction force is reduced to the minimum level, and the moment is increased by torquing the anterior archwire. The lever arm usually cannot be extended above the level of the center of resistance of the anterior segment. A light, constant force from the miniscrew helps maintain the position of incisor tip during root torquing.

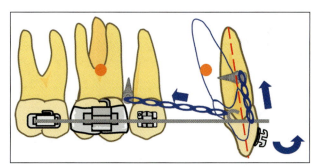

Figure 6-36
Appliance Construction for Intrusion and Root Movement. For active intrusion of incisor segment, an additional miniscrew can be placed in the anterior segment. This system enables effective correction of the Class II, Division 2 cases exhibiting anterior deep bite and upright upper incisors.

segment (Figure 6-34). The main difference from the conventional torque spring is that a constant, light intrusive force from the miniscrews prevents extrusion or labial flaring of the incisors, securing "pure" root movement while maintaining the position of the incisor tip[27] (Figures 6-35 and 6-36).

- **Translation.** Lever arms are extended from the archwire to bring the line of force closer to the center of resistance of the anterior segment. Additional labial crown torque is recommended on the archwire because the lever arm from the archwire does not reach the level of the center of resistance in most cases (Figures 6-37 and 6-38).

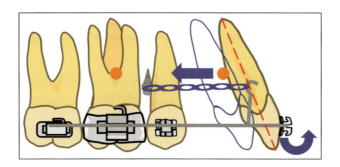

Figure 6-37
For bodily retraction of incisors, lever arms are extended from the main arch, and the line of force becomes closer to the center of resistance. Additional torque on the archwire is required for the maintenance of proper moment/force (M/F) ratio in the force system.

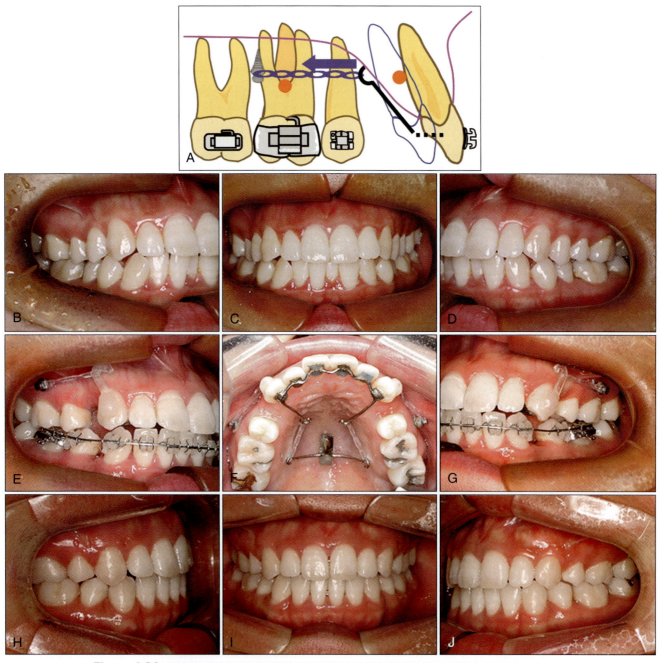

Figure 6-38
Appliance Construction for Bodily Movement in Lingual Orthodontics. A, In lingual orthodontics, bodily retraction of incisors can easily be achieved by extending the lever arms from the main arch. Miniscrews are placed on the palatal slope to establish the line of force. **B to D,** Pretreatment intraoral photographs. **E to G,** Extension of lever arms for bodily retraction. **H to J,** Posttreatment intraoral photographs.

BIOMECHANICS FOR MOLAR INTRUSION

Intrusion ofovererupted molars is primarily indicated for prosthetic purposes, eliminating the need for occlusal reduction or an additional prosthesis. Molar intrusion was considered difficult with conventional mechanics but now is a routine practice using miniscrews.[9,28,29] As with incisor control, insertion point and construction of a proper force system are essential for a successful outcome.

Vertical change in the molar position may affect the alveolar bone height. Thus the existing infrabony pockets can be aggravated by molar intrusion while elevation of the alveolar bone contour around the target tooth can be leveled along with the leveling of the crown. It is therefore important to check the alveolar bone level before intrusion.

INTRUSION OF SINGLE MOLAR

An extruded molar requires pure molar intrusion along its long axis of the tooth without the extrusion of the adjacent teeth (Figure 6-39). It is crucial to provide a line of force passing through the center of resistance (Cres) both on the lateral view and on the frontal view, to prevent possible buccolingual or mesiodistal tipping during intrusion. The Cres of the upper first molar, is expected to be at the center of the occlusal table, close to the palatal root. The line of force should pass through the approximate Cres of the molar, along the central axis on the occlusal table. The recommended insertion points of miniscrews are therefore the mesial interdental area on the buccal surface and the distal interdental area on the palatal side, or vice versa. In this way, the combined bilateral force from the buccal and palatal sides will produce a line of force passing through the

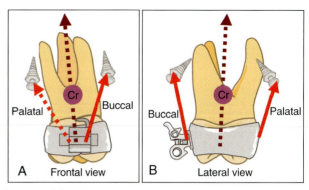

Figure 6-39
Force System for Single-Molar Intrusion. The resultant line of force goes through the center of resistance of the molar in both **A**, frontal view, and **B**, lateral view.

Cres of the molar, inducing pure intrusion without tipping (Figure 6-40). Additional miniscrews can be placed on either side of the alveolar slope to enhance the adjustability of force direction. Three or four miniscrew implants are useful to prevent or correct the tipping of the molars, especially if the molar is severely extruded (Figure 6-41).

INTRUSION OF ADJACENT MOLARS

Two adjacent molars can be efficiently intruded with two miniscrews inserted in the interproximal buccal and palatal area (Figure 6-42). The center of resistance is expected to be localized below the proximal contact, close to the molar.[30] Two miniscrews placed at the interproximal interdental area produces a line of force close to the Cres of the neighboring molars, leading to the segmental intrusion without additional miniscrew(s).

Text continued on p. 126

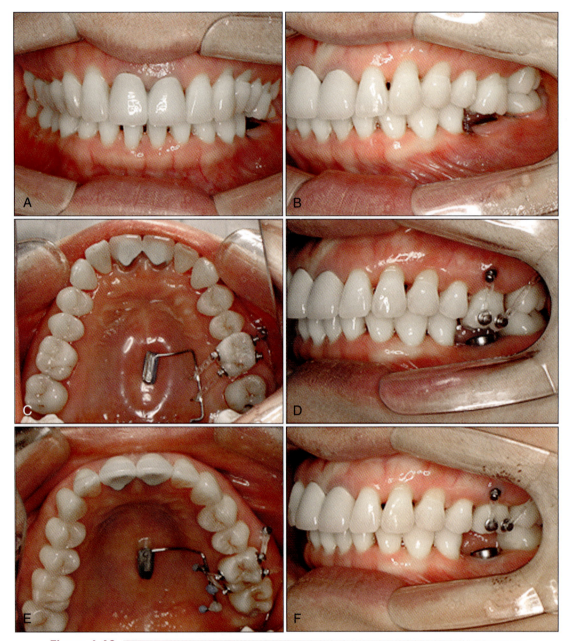

Figure 6-40

Miniscrew Application from Buccal and Palatal Sides for Single-Molar Intrusion. A and B, Pretreatment intraoral photographs. C and D, Miniscrews applied to the palate and the buccal side. E and F, Intrusion completed in 6 months.

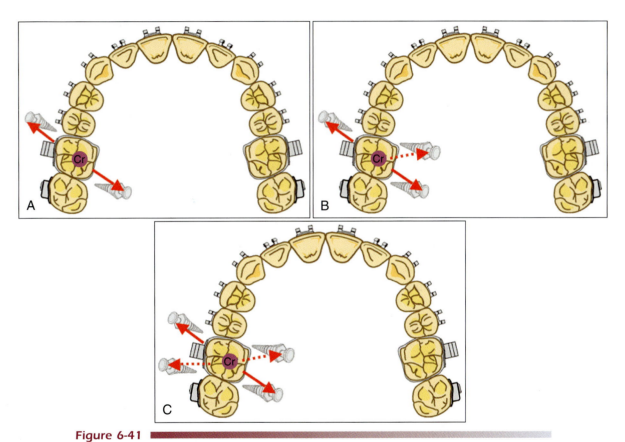

Figure 6-41
Various Insertion Sites and Number of Miniscrews. The force should be balanced buccolingually and mesiodistally during active intrusion. **A,** Two miniscrews. **B,** Three miniscrews. **C,** Four miniscrews.

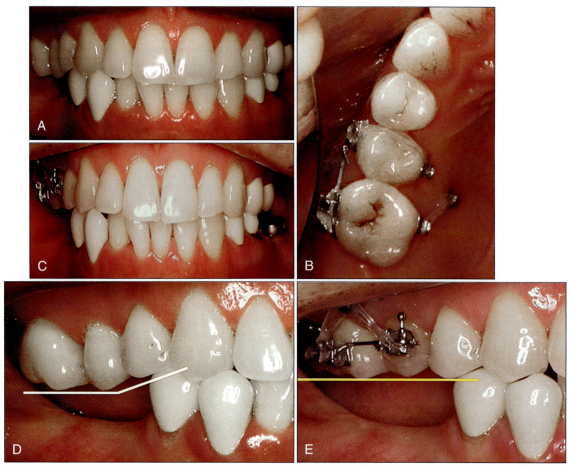

Figure 6-42

Miniscrew Position for Intrusion of Neighboring Two Molars. **A** and **B**, Pretreatment photographs. **C**, The resultant force is expected to induce controlled intrusion of the two molars. **D** and **E**, Treatment completed in 5 months.

CASE REPORT 6-2: EXTRUDED MOLARS

A 50-year-old male was referred from the prosthodontics department to correct the extruded molars (#16, #17) (Figure 6-43, A). His upper-left first and second molars showed overeruption (Figure 6-43, B). The treatment plan was to intrude these molars. Miniscrews were inserted on the midpalate and the buccal gingival area (Figure 6-43, C). First-order control was performed by applying forces from both the buccal and the palatal side. Molar angulation was maintained by applying the parallel intrusive force on the mesial and distal sides of the molar. Figure 6-43, C, shows the treatment progress after 5 months (D) and 8 months (E). The upper first and second molars were intruded enough that prosthodontic treatment could be done (Figure 6-43, F).

CASE REPORT 6-2:   EXTRUDED MOLARS—cont'd

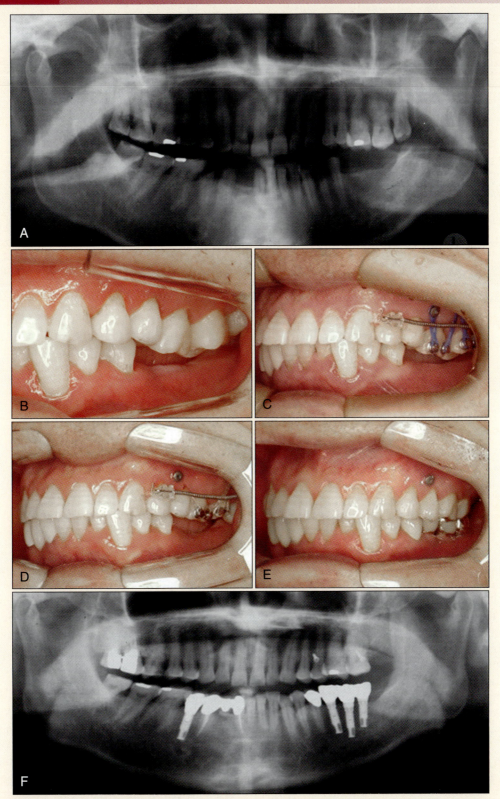

Figure 6-43 Extruded Molars. **A,** Pretreatment panoramic radiograph. **B,** Pretreatment intraoral photograph. **C,** Initiation of molar intrusion. **D,** After 5 months. **E,** After 8 months. Debonded, and prosthodontic treatment complete. **F,** Posttreatment panoramic radiograph.

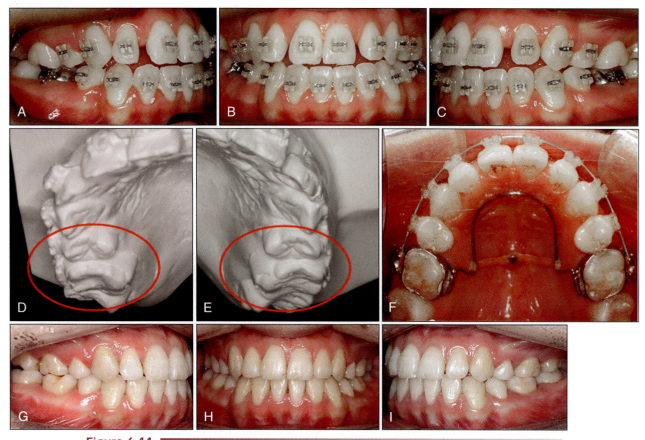

Figure 6-44

Midpalatal Miniscrew for Intrusion of First Molars. A to **C**, Anterior openbite caused by extrusion of maxillary first molars. **D** to **F**, To eliminate the significant marginal ridge discrepancy between the second premolar and first molar via intrusion of molars, a horseshoe-shaped TPA was tied to the midpalatal miniscrew with elastic chain. **G** to **I**, Marginal ridge discrepancy was corrected and anterior overbite was normalized by pure intrusion of molars.

INTRUSION OF MOLARS ON BOTH SIDES

When the molars on both sides need to be symmetrically intruded, a single miniscrew on the midpalate can be sufficient[31] (Figure 6-44). The intrusive force is delivered through the transpalatal bar connecting both molars. The transpalatal arch (TPA) needs to be slightly expanded to prevent the molars from tipping palatally. If the buccolingual position cannot be controlled during intrusion, additional miniscrews on the buccal side may be necessary. In terms of anterior-posterior (A-P) position, the miniscrew should be on the line connecting the central fossa of both molars.

BIOMECHANICS FOR MOLAR DISTALIZATION AND UPRIGHTING

In terms of molar distalization, the main advantage of using the miniscrew over the conventional headgear is that the patient's compliance is not required. Moreover, unlike the conventional noncompliance appliances such as pendulum or distal jet, there is no undesired reaction in the anterior segment. The miniscrews can reduce the side effects and increase the predictability of molar distalization.[32]

To achieve distal translation of the molars, the line of force needs to be established at the vertical level of the Cres of the molar. Insertion sites and type of appliance need to be carefully chosen.

MIXED DENTITION

Molar distalization frequently is a part of the treatment plan in the mixed-dentition phase, to establish a Class I molar relationship or to regain space for nonextraction treatment. In the mixed-dentition phase the premolar germs are present underneath the deciduous molars, so neither the buccal nor the palatal slope is considered as an insertion site because of possible injury to the developing tooth germs. Available insertion sites are limited to the midpalatal and anterior rugae area. The midpalatal area displays sufficient cortical layer for miniscrews because the nasal floor is elevated toward the midline in an anatomic structure known as the

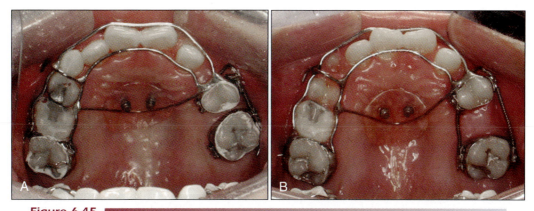

Figure 6-45
Unilateral molar distalization using Nance holding button fixed with miniscrews. **A,** Before distalization. **B,** After distalization.

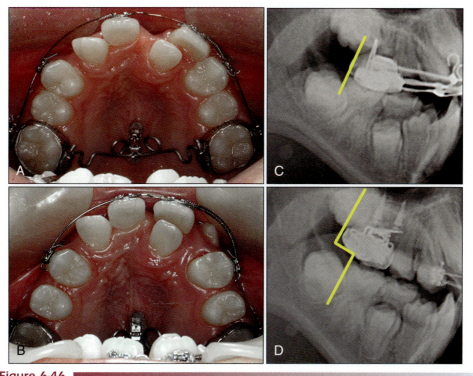

Figure 6-46
Bilateral molar distalization using fixed pendulum on the midpalate. **A** and **C,** Before distalization. **B** and **D,** After distalization.

nasal crest.[33,34] The most central suture area may not be tightly closed during prepubertal growth,[34] so it is helpful to place the miniscrew on the parasagittal area about 2 to 3 mm apart from the central suture line, to utilize the nasal crestal bone. The success rate of the miniscrew during prepubertal stage is not as high as that of postpubertal stage. This is one limiting factor of miniscrew application in adolescent patients.

Possible appliance designs are as follows:
- Miniscrew-reinforced Nance holding arch (Figure 6-45)
- Bone-borne pendulum appliance (Figure 6-46)

These appliances initially induce distal tipping of the molars; therefore, subsequent root movement of the molars is required. Bracket positioning and alignment with archwires need to be followed.

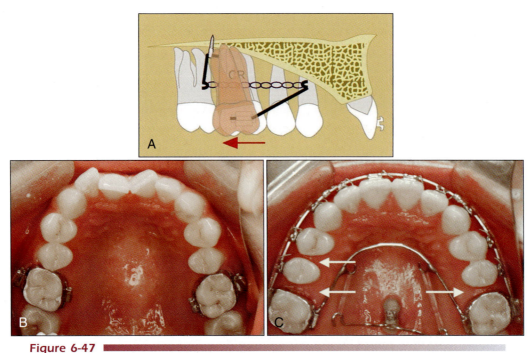

Figure 6-47
Combination of Transpalatal Arch and Lever Arms from the Midpalatal Miniscrews for Distal Translation of Molars. **A,** The line of force goes through the center of resistance of the first molar. **B,** Before distalization. **C,** After distalization.

Permanent Dentition

When the premolars are fully erupted, both buccal and palatal alveolar slope can be used for miniscrew insertion, and thus a variety of appliances are available for precise molar distalization. Regardless of the appliance type, the line of force should be established at the adequate level of the Cres of the molar.

The molar distalization appliances incorporating miniscrews are as follows:

- Midpalatal miniscrew combined with transpalatal lever arm and the horseshoe-type transpalatal bar (Figure 6-47). Two miniscrews are inserted along the midpalatal suture, and a lingual sheath is bonded on the head, with light-cured resin.[35] A transpalatal lever arms made of 0.9-mm stainless steel wire is inserted from behind. A horseshoe-type TPA with soldered hooks connecting both molars is retracted by elastic chains engaged to the hooks of the transpalatal lever arm. This system generates a constant line of force that runs through the Cres of the molars, inducing translation without tipping.
- Miniscrews on the palatal slope and a horseshoe-type TPA. The transpalatal components are replaced by the two miniscrews on the palatal slope (Figure 6-48). The height of the insertion site is determined from the lateral cephalogram, by drawing a line through the Cres of the molars. Midpalatal miniscrews often generate a force above the level of Cres, leading to a root movement rather than translation.
- Miniscrews on the buccal alveolar bone combined with an archwire and an open coil spring (Figure 6-49). Miniscrews are inserted between the second premolar and the first molar. Distalizing force is applied indirectly by the open coil spring between the premolars and molars, while the forward tipping is prevented by the elastic chain engaged to the first premolar.

FORCE SYSTEM FOR MOLAR UPRIGHTING

Molar uprighting is frequently indicated for mesially impacted second molars (Figure 6-50). The anchorage segment in the conventional appliances can be replaced by a single miniscrew, which makes the whole appliance remarkably simple.[36] The clinician can select the insertion site on either the mesial side or the distal side of the target molar, depending on the severity and the biomechanical principles described next.

Mild Mesial Tipping

A single miniscrew is inserted between the first molar and the second premolar. A 0.016-inch stainless steel sectional wire with an open-coil spring (miniscrew-assisted push spring [MAPS]) is engaged from the miniscrew head to provide distally directed linear force. In cases of mild mesial tipping, the distance from line of force to the center of resistance of the second molar is

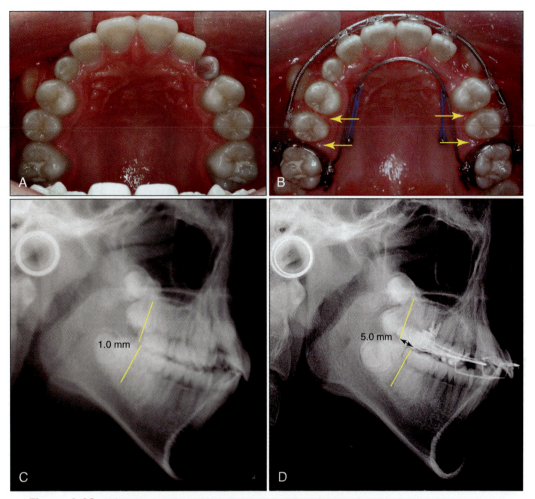

Figure 6-48
Transpalatal arch in combination with miniscrews on the palatal slope for distalization of molars. **A** and **C**, Before distalization. **B** and **D**, After distalization.

sufficient to generate a high enough "moment of force" for the distal tip-back of the second molar (Figure 6-51).

Moderate Tipping
A single miniscrew is placed between the first molar and the second premolar. The open-coil spring can be used initially to "unlock" the second molar from the distal contour of the first molar but not necessarily for uprighting because of the reduced moment of the force. A molar uprighting spring (miniscrew-assisted uprighting spring [MAUS]) is then hooked on the miniscrew head to deliver a tip-back moment. A moment is considered to be more effective for moderate tipping than a single force because the linear force is not expected to produce a high enough moment due to the short distance to the center of resistance (Figure 6-52).

Severe Tipping
When a molar is severely tipped and blocked by the adjacent molars, it is often impossible to attach tubes or brackets on the buccal surface. Miniscrews inserted in the retromolar area can provide a distally oriented uprighting force. Considering the thick soft tissue overlying this area, the long-collared miniscrews at least 8 mm in length are appropriate for this purpose. In case the third molar is in the way while moving the second molar, the third molar is removed before second molar uprighting (Figure 6-53).

Text continued on p.134

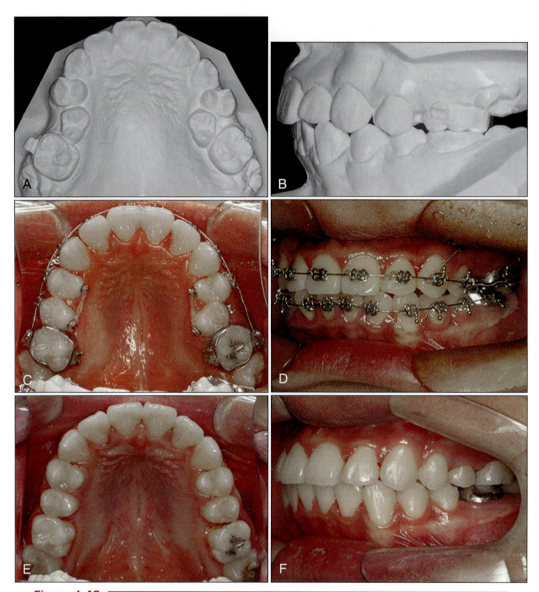

Figure 6-49
Molar Distalization Using Buccal Miniscrew. A and **B,** Pretreatment casts. **C** and **D,** System in place. Premolar movement is prevented by the ligature tie from the miniscrew, while distalization is being performed by the open coil spring. **E** and **F,** Posttreatment intraoral photographs showing a Class I molar.

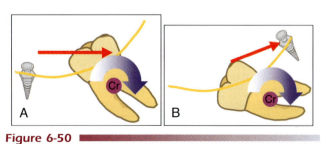

Figure 6-50
Mesioangulated lower second molar can be corrected using a single mesial or distal miniscrew, depending on the severity of mesial inclination. **A,** Mild to moderate tipping, pushing from the mesial side. **B,** Severe tipping, pulling from the distal side.

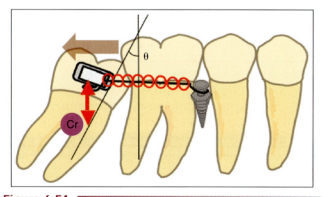

Figure 6-51
Correction of Mild Mesioangulation. Distally directed single force provides a sufficient moment of the force for uprighting the molar.

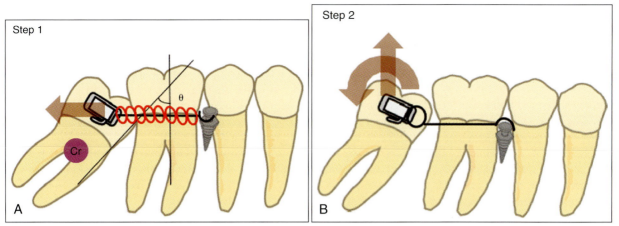

Figure 6-52

Correction of Moderate Mesioangulation. A, Step 1: distalized single force first frees the second molar from the distal height of contour of the first molar. There is sufficient moment of force for the uprighting of the molar. **B,** Step 2: uprighting spring then is applied to give a tip-back moment.

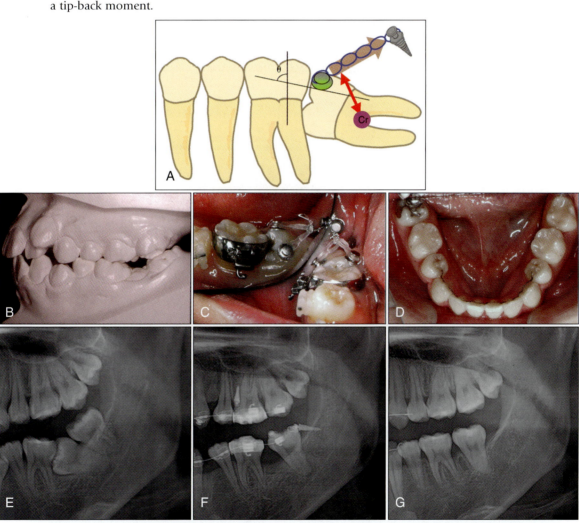

Figure 6-53

A, Force system for severe mesioangulation of tooth #37. A button is bonded to the distal surface of the second molar, and a miniscrew is placed distal in the ramus. An elastic chain is placed to deliver a single distal force that unlocks the tooth. The high moment of the force tips the crown distally. **B,** Preoperative view of the left mandibular second molar impacted between the first and third molars. **C,** Clinical view of the applied mechanics. **D,** Final position of the second molar from an occlusal view. **E,** Radiograph showing the preoperative inclination of #37. **F,** Radiograph showing the second molar in upright position after extraction of #38. **G,** Radiograph showing the final position of the second molar.

CASE REPORT 6-3: IMPACTED LOWER-LEFT SECOND MOLAR

A 13-year-old girl was transferred from a private clinic for her impacted lower-left second molar. Moderate mesioangulation of the second molar was found both clinically and radiologically, with evidence of caries on the distal surface of the first molar (Figure 6-54).

The patient did not want comprehensive treatment and asked for no visible appliances. A single miniscrew was placed between the second premolar and the first molar. The uprighting procedure consisted of a distal "unlocking" step followed by an "uprighting" step. An open coil spring on the .016 stainless steel wire was the first appliance to release the locked second molar. In the second step the uprighting cantilever spring was engaged to deliver uprighting moment (Figure 6-55).

The treatment was finished in 5 months. The mandibular third molar was removed after completion of the restoration on the first and second molars (Figure 6-56).

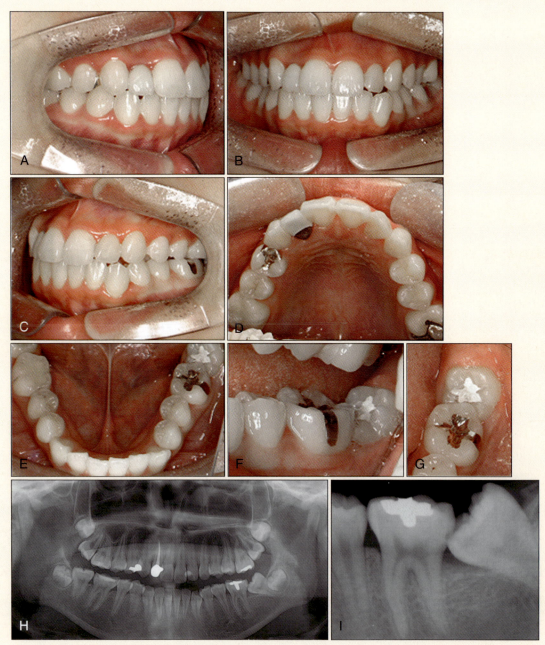

Figure 6-54 Impacted Molar. A to G, Pretreatment intraoral photographs show moderate tipping and "locking" of the lower-left second molar. H and I, Pretreatment panoramic and periapical radiographs showing the locked molar.

CASE REPORT 6-3: IMPACTED LOWER-LEFT SECOND MOLAR—cont'd

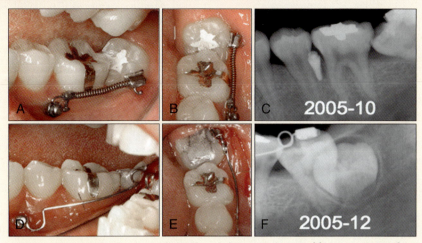

Figure 6-55 Treatment Progress. **A** to **C**, Miniscrew is inserted between second premolar and first molar. Distal force is applied with open-coil spring initially to "unlock" the second molar. **D** to **F**, Molar uprighting spring is engaged to deliver the tip-back moment, which is required to complete the uprighting of the second molar.

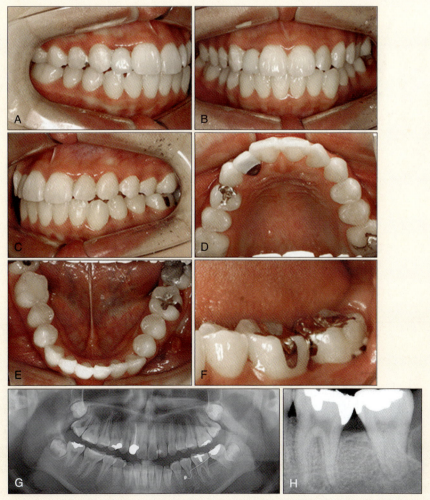

Figure 6-56 Posttreatment Images. **A** to **F**, Intraoral photographs. **G** and **H**, Panoramic and periapical radiographs. Treatment time was 5 months.

BIOMECHANICS FOR MOLAR PROTRACTION

Edentulous spaces resulting from a missing molar, as well as residual extraction spaces, can be closed using miniscrews via molar protraction. Because of the density of cortical bone, molar protraction is more frequently required in the lower arch than in the upper arch. The increased density of the mandibular bone generally hinders the anterior movement of the molars in the mandible.

FORCE SYSTEM FOR PURE TRANSLATION

Pure forward translation of the molar is indicated in cases of congenitally missing premolars or incomplete closure of extraction spaces. Miniscrews can be inserted between the first and second premolars, and elastic chains are engaged to protract the molars. Without lever arms, the line of force generates the mesial tipping moment of the molar (Figure 6-57, A), which may lead to the bowing of the arch in the premolar area.[9] To achieve constant translation of the molars in maintaining the arch shape, a lever arm made of rigid stainless steel wire is placed on the molar so that the line of force from the miniscrew will go through the Cres of the molar (Figure 6-57, B). Figure 6-58 provides an example of protraction of a lower molar.

FORCE SYSTEM FOR ROOT MOVEMENT

Root movement of the molar(s) is often indicated when adjacent molars are already mesially inclined because of a missing, impacted, or ankylosed tooth. The required force system is a tip-back moment of the molar, together with mild mesial linear force, to prevent distal tipping of the clinical crown. One miniscrew is inserted on the mesial interdental space relative to the target molar. MAUS in combination with a passive elastic chain can effectively induce the mesial root movement by the mesiogingivally directed force from the miniscrew head as the counterpart for the extrusive force from the uprighting spring. Mesial root movement helps establish proper occlusion, preserves periodontal health by formation of

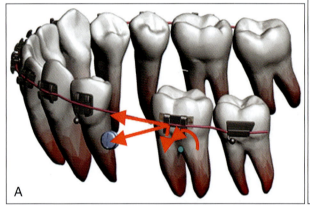 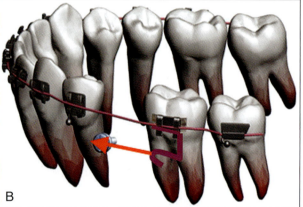

Figure 6-57

Proper Force System for Protraction of Molars. To avoid the unwanted mesial tipping of a molar, a lever arm is extended to lower the level of the line of force. **A,** Protraction with a single force can result in unwanted tipping. **B,** Protraction with a single force plus the use of a cantilever avoids unwanted tipping.

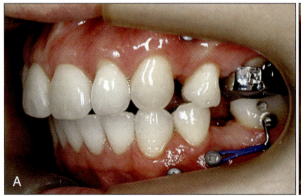 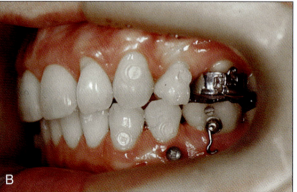

Figure 6-58

Miniscrews combined with a lever arm are used for protraction of a lower molar. **A,** Molar before protraction. **B,** Molar after protraction.

the alveolar bone, and eliminates the need for additional prostheses (Figure 6-59).

FORCE SYSTEM FOR ROOT MOVEMENT PLUS TRANSLATION

Mesial inclination of the second molar sometimes necessitates mesial root movement together with translation. Especially when the first molar is present but diagnosed as hopeless because of severe caries or a periodontal problem, mesial translation of the second molar can replace the hopeless molar with the adjacent sound molar. To prevent unwanted extrusion of the molar during protraction, two miniscrews are placed on the buccal interdental space. The root spring (miniscrew-assisted root spring [MARS]) is engaged on the dual miniscrew to deliver a moment for root movement while preventing an intrusive force vector to eliminate the possible occlusal interference. This approach is useful when the patient does not want comprehensive treatment, because the miniscrew-anchored root spring can induce highly selective movement of the second molar without other attachments (Figure 6-60). Figure 6-61 provides an example of replacement of a mandibular first molar by protraction of a second molar.

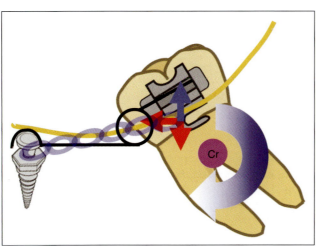

Figure 6-59
Proper Force System for Pure Root Movement of Molars. A miniscrew-assisted uprighting spring (MAUS) in combination with passive elastic tie can induce pure root movement. Blue arrows indicate the extrusive force and tipback moment generated by uprighting spring. Red arrows indicate the mesiogingival force vector counteracting the extrusion and distal crown movement, thus leading to pure root movement.

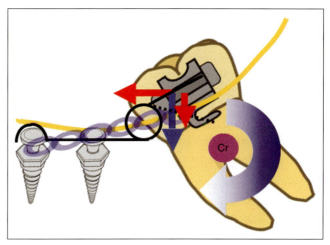

Figure 6-60
Proper Force System for Root Movement plus Protraction of Molars. A miniscrew-assisted root spring (MARS) in combination with two miniscrews can induce pure root movement and intrusion of molars. A tipback moment and an intrusive force (blue arrows) are generated by the root spring, because of the presence of the second miniscrew. The dotted line indicates the spring shape before insertion (preactivation form). Additional mesialization force is given by a light elastic chain (red arrows). Molar extrusion during uprighting can be strictly prevented with this method.

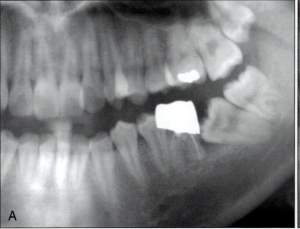
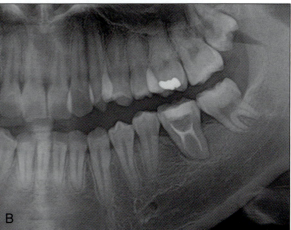

Figure 6-61
Replacement of mandibular first molar by protraction of the mesially inclined second molar. Alveolar bone support was also remarkably improved with the forward movement of the second molar. **A**, Initial radiograph. **B**, Area after 14 months.

MOVEMENT OF WHOLE SEGMENTS

Movement of the whole arch, including the anterior and posterior segments, can be achieved with miniscrews.[37] As previously shown, the inadvertent canting or tipping of the whole occlusal plane may occur during anterior retraction with miniscrews, which conversely means that intentional change of the occlusal plane is also feasible. In extraction cases demanding minimal anchorage, a nonextraction modality is applicable through distalization of the whole arch.

The whole-arch movement is indicated for the "camouflage" of generalized Class II, Class III, or open-bite problems, where movement is attempted in both vertical and horizontal planes.

The advantages of whole-arch movement are simple appliance construction and minimal appliance change. Treatment efficiency is greatly improved because the segments of teeth move simultaneously. For example, nonsurgical correction of an open bite requires simultaneous intrusion of all buccal segments. This can be performed using multiple miniscrews on the buccal and palatal slopes.

EN MASSE MOVEMENT FOR OPEN-BITE CORRECTION

To achieve effective intrusion of the whole buccal segment, the intrusive force needs to be delivered simultaneously to the individual tooth in the buccal segment. To balance the intrusive force from the buccal miniscrews, the palatal miniscrews are regularly placed on the opposing palatal slope or midpalatal suture. The force direction is adjusted by selectively activating the buccal and the lingual forces. Careful monitoring of any residual prematurity on the posterior segment is necessary, since it may hinder the bite closure.

Text continued on p. 143

CASE REPORT 6-4: ANTERIOR OPEN BITE

A 20-year-old woman presented with anterior open bite. The initial clinical and radiological examination revealed that she displayed a high gonial angle with a skeletal open bite. She was diagnosed as "skeletal Class II" with anterior open bite (Figure 6-62).

Two occlusal planes are present between posterior teeth and anterior teeth. Intrusion of upper posterior teeth was planned for the treatment of the open bite with miniscrews. To prevent buccolingual tipping, miniscrews can be implanted on both the buccal and the lingual side, or only on the buccal side with cross-arch splinting, such as a TPA. In this case, a rapid palatal expander was used for maxillary expansion and cross-arch splinting. After 8 months, as the upper posterior teeth were intruded, the anterior negative overbite was eliminated (Figure 6-63).

After completion of the intrusion, brackets were placed on the teeth. After 28 months, the appliance was removed (Figure 6-64). After 1 year of retention, there was no sign of relapse (Figure 6-65). Cephalometric superimposition reveals that the mandible was rotated upward and forward, with the chin moving forward to the true vertical line. With the decrease in anterior facial height, the facial profile was improved.

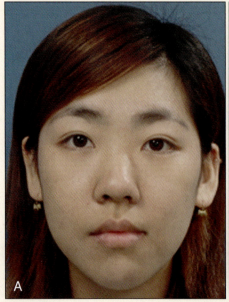
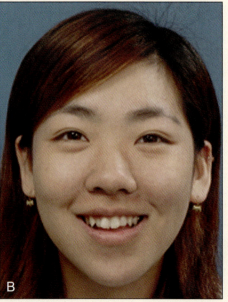

Figure 6-62 Anterior Open Bite. Pretreatment extraoral (A-D) and intraoral (E-I) photographs.

CASE REPORT 6-4: ANTERIOR OPEN BITE—cont'd

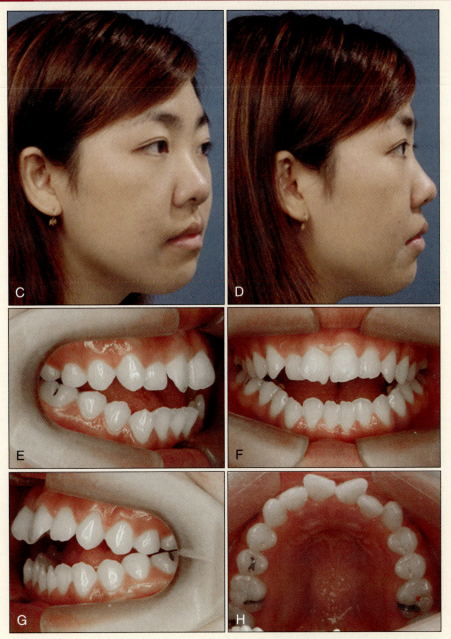

Figure 6-62, cont'd For legend see opposite page.

Continued

CASE REPORT 6-4: ANTERIOR OPEN BITE—cont'd

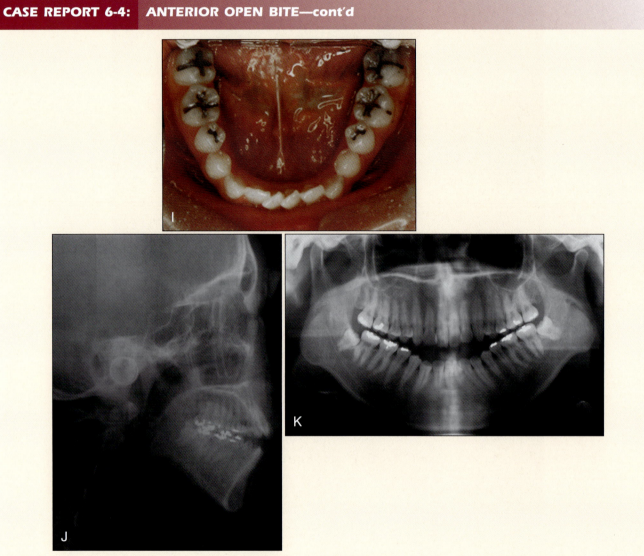

Figure 6-62, cont'd Anterior Open Bite. Pretreatment intraoral (**I**) photograph. Pretreatment cephalometric (**J**) and panoramic (**K**) radiographs.

CASE REPORT 6-4: ANTERIOR OPEN BITE—cont'd

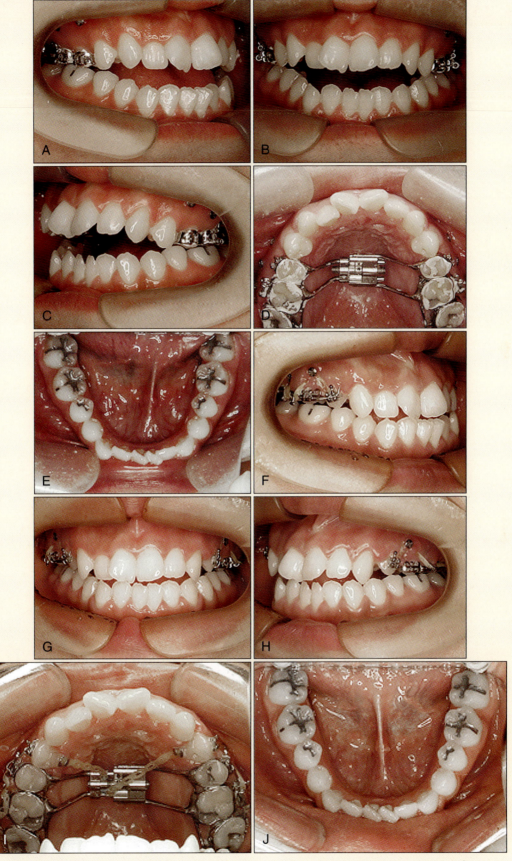

Figure 6-63 Treatment Progress. A to E, Beginning of molar intrusion. F to J, After 8 months, intrusion is complete.

Continued

140 PART III Biomechanical Considerations

CASE REPORT 6-4: ANTERIOR OPEN BITE—cont'd

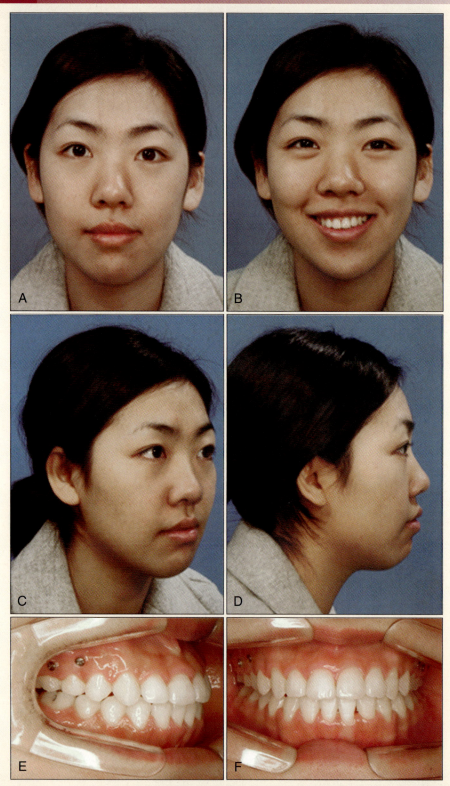

Figure 6-64 Posttreatment Images. Extraoral **(A-D)** and intraoral **(E-I)** photographs. Cephalometric **(J)** and panoramic **(K)** radiographs.

CASE REPORT 6-4: ANTERIOR OPEN BITE—cont'd

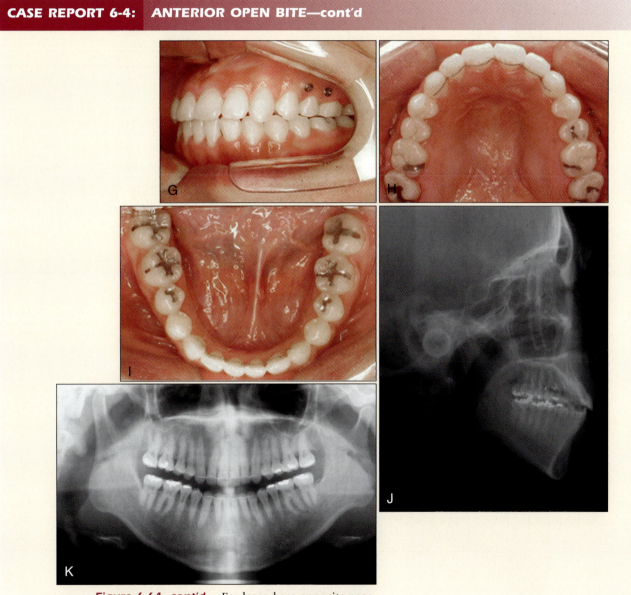

Figure 6-64, cont'd For legend see opposite page.

Continued

CASE REPORT 6-4: ANTERIOR OPEN BITE—cont'd

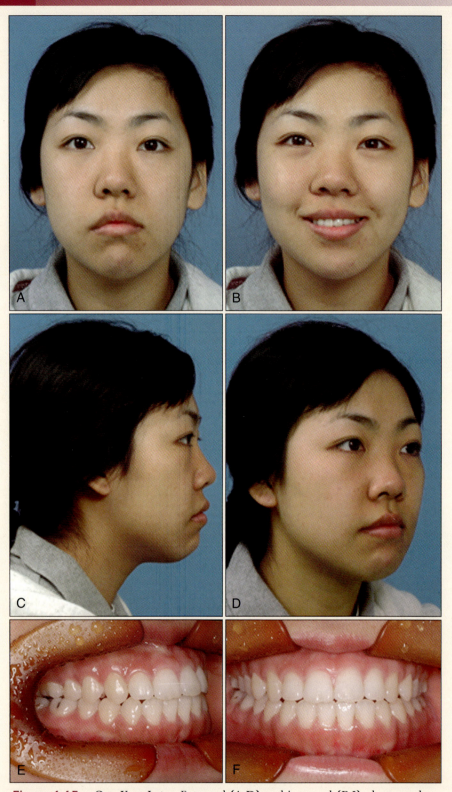

Figure 6-65 One Year Later. Extraoral (A-D) and intraoral (E-I) photographs.

CASE REPORT 6-4: ANTERIOR OPEN BITE—cont'd

Figure 6-65, cont'd   For legend see opposite page.

CONCLUSION

Previously viewed as just another new device to reinforce anchorage, miniscrews have introduced a new era of orthodontic treatment modalities. Miniscrews can reduce treatment time and simplify the appliance while increasing the predictability of the treatment outcome. Many surgical or extraction cases are now treated through nonsurgical and nonextraction modalities using miniscrews. Alternative approaches are also feasible, such as the combination of the esthetic appliance and the miniscrews. Miniscrews are powerful tools reestablishing conventional orthodontic concepts and might become indispensable in future orthodontics practice.

REFERENCES

1. Roberts WE, Nelson CL, Goodacre CJ: Rigid implant anchorage to close a mandibular first molar extraction site, *J Clin Orthod* 28:693-704, 1994.
2. Linkow LI: The endosseous blade implant and its use in orthodontics, *Int J Orthod* 7:149-154, 1969.
3. Kanomi R: Mini-implant for orthodontic anchorage, *J Clin Orthod* 31:763-767, 1997.
4. Creekmore TD, Eklund MK: The possibility of skeletal anchorage, *J Clin Orthod* 17:266-269, 1983.
5. Miyawaki S, Koyama I, Inoue M, et al: Factors associated with the stability of titanium screws placed in the posterior region for orthodontic anchorage, *Am J Orthod Dentofacial Orthop* 124:373-378, 2003.
6. Chung YK, Lee YJ, Chung KR: The experimental study of early loading on the miniplate in the beagle dog, *Kor J Orthod* 33:307-317, 2003.
7. Yoon BS, Choi BH, Lee WY, et al: A study on titanium miniscrew as orthodontic anchorage: an experimental investigation in dogs, *Kor J Orthod* 31:517-523, 2001.
8. Egolf RJ, BeGole EA, Upshaw HS: Factors associated with orthodontic patient compliance with intraoral elastic and headgear wear, *Am J Orthod Dentofacial Orthop* 97:336-348, 1990.
9. Kyung SH, Choi JH, Park YC: Miniscrew anchorage used to protract lower second molars into first molar extraction sites, *J Clin Orthod* 37:575-579, 2003.
10. Buchter A, Wiechmann D, Koerdt S, et al: Load-related implant reaction of mini-implants used for orthodontic anchorage, *Clin Oral Implants Res* 16:473-479, 2005.
11. Tanne K, Koenig HA, Burstone CJ: Moment to force ratios and the center of rotation, *Am J Orthod Dentofacial Orthop* 94:426-431, 1988.
12. Linkow LI, Miller RJ: Immediate loading of endosseous implants is not new, *J Oral Implantol* 30:314-317, 2004.
13. Kim JW, Ahn SJ, Chang YI: Histomorphometric and mechanical analyses of the drill-free screw as orthodontic anchorage, *Am J Orthod Dentofacial Orthop* 128:190-194, 2005.
14. Cordioli G, Majzoub Z: Heat generation during implant site preparation: an in vitro study, *Int J Oral Maxillofac Implants* 12:186-193, 1997.

15. Lee JS, Park YC: A contact finite element analysis for initial stability of orthodontic miniscrew, Orthodontics Department, Yonsei University, Seoul, 2004.
16. Kim HJ, Yun HS, Park HD, et al: Soft-tissue and cortical-bone thickness at orthodontic implant sites, *Am J Orthod Dentofacial Orthop* 130:177-182, 2006.
17. Schnelle MA, Beck FM, Jaynes RM, Huja SS: A radiographic evaluation of the availability of bone for placement of miniscrews, *Angle Orthod* 74:832-837, 2004.
18. Park HS: Clinical study on success rate of microscrew implants for orthodontic anchorage, *Kor J Orthod* 33:151-156, 2003.
19. Liou EJ, Pai BC, Lin JC: Do miniscrews remain stationary under orthodontic forces? *Am J Orthod Dentofacial Orthop* 126:42-47, 2004.
20. Davies JE: Understanding peri-implant endosseous healing, *J Dent Educ* 67:932-949, 2003.
21. Asscherickx K, Vannet BV, Wehrbein H, Sabzevar MM: Root repair after injury from mini-screw, *Clin Oral Implants Res* 16:575-578, 2005.
22. Proffit WR, Fields HWJ: *Contemporary orthodontics*, St Louis, 2000, Mosby.
23. Burstone CJ: Rationale of the segmented arch, *Am J Orthod* 48:805-822, 1962.
24. Burstone CJ, Koenig HA: Force systems from the ideal arch, *Am J Orthod Dentofacial Orthop* 65:270-289, 1974.
25. Park HS, Kwon OW, Sung JH: Microscrew implant anchorage sliding mechanics, *World J Orthod* 6:265-274, 2005.
26. Burstone CJ, Koenig HA: Creative wire bending-the force system from step and V bends, *Am J Orthod Dentofacial Orthop* 93:59-67, 1988.
27. Issacson RJ, Lindauer SJ, Rubenstein LK: Moments with edgewise appliance: incisor torque control, *Am J Orthod Dentofacial Orthop* 103:428-423, 1993.
28. Park YC, Lee SY, Kim DH, Jee SH: Intrusion of posterior teeth using mini-screw implants, *Am J Orthod Dentofacial Orthop* 123:690-694, 2003.
29. Park HS, Kwon TG, Kwon OW: Treatment of open bite with microscrew implant anchorage, *Am J Orthod Dentofacial Orthop* 126:627-636, 2004.
30. Nanda R: *Biomechanics and esthetic strategies in clinical orthodontics*, St Louis, 2005, Mosby-Elsevier.
31. Kyung SH: A study on the treatment of anterior open bite with midpalatal miniscrews, *Kor J Orthod* 34:13-21, 2004.
32. Park HS, Bae SM, Kyung HM, Sung JH: Simultaneous incisor retraction and distal molar movement with microimplant anchorage, *World J Orthod* 5:164-171, 2004.
33. Wehrbein H, Merz BR, Diedrich P, Glatzmaier J: The use of palatal implants for orthodontic anchorage: design and clinical application of the Orthosystem, *Clin Oral Implants Res* 7:410-416, 1996.
34. Wehrbein H, Merz BR: Aspects of the use of endosseous palatal implants in orthodontic therapy, *J Esthet Dent* 10:315-324, 1998.
35. Kyung SH, Choi HW, Kim KH, Park YC: Bonding orthodontic attachments to miniscrew heads, *J Clin Orthod* 39:348-353 (quiz, 369), 2005.
36. Lee KJ, Park YC, Hwang WS, Seong EH: Uprighting mandibular second molars with direct miniscrew anchorage, *J Clin Orthod* 41:627-635, 2007.
37. Park HS, Lee SK, Kwon OW: Group distal movement of teeth using microscrew implant anchorage, *Angle Orthod* 75:602-609, 2005.

CHAPTER 7

Skeletal Anchorage Based on Biomechanics

Flavio Andres Uribe and Ravindra Nanda

The new millennium has ushered in great interest in skeletal anchorage. Loss of anchorage is a major orthodontic problem that often leads to compromised treatment results not only in extraction cases but also in cases requiring molar distalization or protraction. Skeletal anchorage has the potential to provide reliable solutions to such anchorage-related situations. It has also allowed clinicians to achieve tooth movements once considered impossible with conventional orthodontic methods, such as significant molar intrusion and distalization of lower molars.

EVALUATING SKELETAL ANCHORAGE

As with any other new clinical technique, skeletal anchorage should be evaluated under three broad categories: (1) need, (2) supporting evidence, and (3) cost effectiveness.[1]

There is a definite need for skeletal anchorage in orthodontics, although the specific situations where it is absolutely necessary have yet to be defined. Any new technique carries an inherent risk of overutilization. For example, many thought that distraction osteogenesis would solve the extraction/nonextraction debate, but time and clinical research led to refined applications for this technique, and its use is now limited to specific clinical situations.[2] Thus, clinicians should carefully evaluate those clinical situations where temporary anchorage devices (TADs) offer a clinical advantage over efficient and well-established orthodontic treatment protocols.

The evidence to support TADs is still in development. Most published literature is based on case reports depicting application of TADs to correct a range of orthodontic problems, including crossbite,[3] "absolute" anterior-posterior (A-P) anchorage,[4] and space closure of long edentulous spans.[5,6] In addition, TADs have facilitated orthodontic tooth movement with distalization of molars,[7] intrusion of incisors and molars,[8,9] and protraction of molars.[5] However, more evidence is needed from well-controlled, prospective clinical trials; more importantly, long-term data are essential.

Analyzing *cost effectiveness* in orthodontic treatment leads to certain key questions. Is the appliance being used best suited for the problem? Does the cost in terms of treatment time (office visits, duration of treatment) and materials justify use of the appliance? Are side effects prevented with the appliance? For example, in some patients, absolute A-P anchorage is required for space closure. Do TADs provide any clinical advantage (superior outcome) over intraoral anchorage obtained through techniques such as differential moments or differential forces in the noncompliant patient? The clinician should determine whether a TAD is necessary in such patients.

Cost effectiveness is also relevant in the patient with a long edentulous span. The clinician has two options for skeletal anchorage: the restorable implant (conventional endosseous dental implant) and a nonrestorable TAD. The TAD will serve as anchorage to achieve significant molar protraction. On the other hand, the conventional endosseous dental implant will partially or completely occupy the edentulous space, and thus less space closure is needed. The dental implant could also be used as a TAD to achieve the desired movements of the adjacent teeth to be restored later prosthetically. Thus the patient would save on treatment time, but the cost in materials and procedures could be increased. When considering skeletal anchorage for a patient, the clinician should include cost and time in the informed consent.

Cost efficiency is also important. "Efficiency" can be defined in orthodontics as achievement of the delineated objective in the least amount of time with the least amount of side effects. Although not yet evaluated with TADs, skeletal anchorage may reduce treatment time.[10,11] Side effects may be negated in the anchorage unit but still need to be controlled in the active unit when using TADs, because forces are not applied precisely through the center of resistance of the teeth in all the planes of space.

Anchorage control is significantly enhanced with the use of skeletal hardware.[4,12] Biomechanical concepts essential for anchorage control would then seem less relevant or even obsolete with TADs; however, we see in this chapter that this is not always true. Over the past few years, various case reports have detailed creatively designed appliances that effectively apply biomechanics.[13-15] Understanding biomechanics allows the clinician to determine ideal cost effectiveness (minimal amount of skeletal TADs and maximal mechanical advantage) as well as the proper sites for TADs.[16] Biomechanical principles also assist the clinician in preventing side effects of TADs and in selecting the most appropriate device from the many systems now available.

This chapter describes different clinical scenarios in which skeletal anchorage may provide an advantage to conventional treatment mechanics. The biomechanical concepts reviewed are useful in determining the best site for TAD placement (least amount of undesired reactive forces or most advantageous location to use reactive forces) and thus the most appropriate skeletal anchorage system for a particular orthodontic movement.

DIRECT AND INDIRECT ANCHORAGE

Anchorage from TADs can be obtained directly or indirectly.[17] *Direct anchorage* is the application of a force directly from the skeletal anchorage device to a tooth or group of teeth; thus it can be described as a TAD-tooth interaction. The line of force is usually at an angle to the occlusal plane, resulting in an ever-present intrusive force when direct intraarch anchorage is applied. On the other hand, *indirect anchorage* is a tooth-tooth interaction. The anchor unit or reactive unit (tooth or group of teeth) is attached rigidly to the skeletal anchor device; therefore the force is generally applied along the occlusal plane. The indirect approach can be easily integrated to the straight-wire technique or any other traditional orthodontic technique.

The most common example of the indirect anchorage approach is the Orthosystem implant (Straumann, Waldenburg, Switzerland) in the palate. This mini-implant, once osseointegrated in approximately 10 weeks, is connected by a rigid palatal bar to the anchor teeth (usually the molars). However, even with a .032 × .032 transpalatal arch (TPA) used as a connector to the palatal implant, approximately 1 mm of anchorage loss is evident in cases where maximum anterior retraction is desired.[18] Thus a more rigidly casted bar may provide less anchorage loss and more patient comfort (Figure 7-1).

FORCE SYSTEMS

Biomechanical concepts are more applicable to direct anchorage from TADs. Force systems must be understood to plan properly for the system and TAD placement site. The line of action of the force and its direction, the point of force application, force vector addition, and equivalent force systems are important concepts that can help the clinician optimize skeletal anchorage.

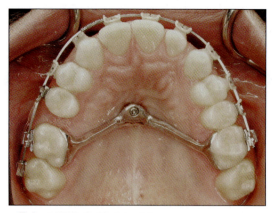

Figure 7-1
Transpalatal bar connecting the palatal implant to the first molars for indirect anterior-posterior (A-P) anchorage. Oval shape and proximity of the bar to the soft tissue contribute to patient comfort. The larger dimension of the casted bar imparts stiffness to the appliance and thus the anchorage unit.

The *line of action* of the force and its direction describe how a body (tooth or group of teeth) will move. The line of action and its direction need to be traced to the point of application to describe precisely the force vector. Moreover, the relationship between the line and point of force application to the center of resistance of the tooth (or group of teeth) needs to be analyzed to predict the three-dimensional (3D) movement of the body.

This relationship can be analyzed using *equivalent force systems*. Briefly, a force can be replaced from its point of force application by the same force plus its rotational moment produced around an arbitrary point in the same plane.[19] To understand tooth movement, the selected arbitrary point is at the center of resistance of the tooth or group of teeth. In Figure 7-2, *A-D*, a force from a miniscrew is applied buccal to the center of resistance of the tooth. From an occlusal view the center of resistance is close to the central fossa. As the force is applied in the buccal direction, the equivalent force system at the center of resistance results in a mesial force and a rotational moment (mesial-in, lingual direction) in the lower-right first molar. From a lateral view, the line of force in Figure 7-2, *E*, is close to the center of resistance of the molar (generally found at the furcation area) and parallel to the occlusal plane. This force system results in a translatory movement of the molar. However, the distance from the arm to the miniscrew precludes achieving a good activation force. Figure 7-2, *F* to *H*, shows the extension arm bent distally to achieve more activation in the spring. Bending the arm distally results in a more coronal point of force application. The line

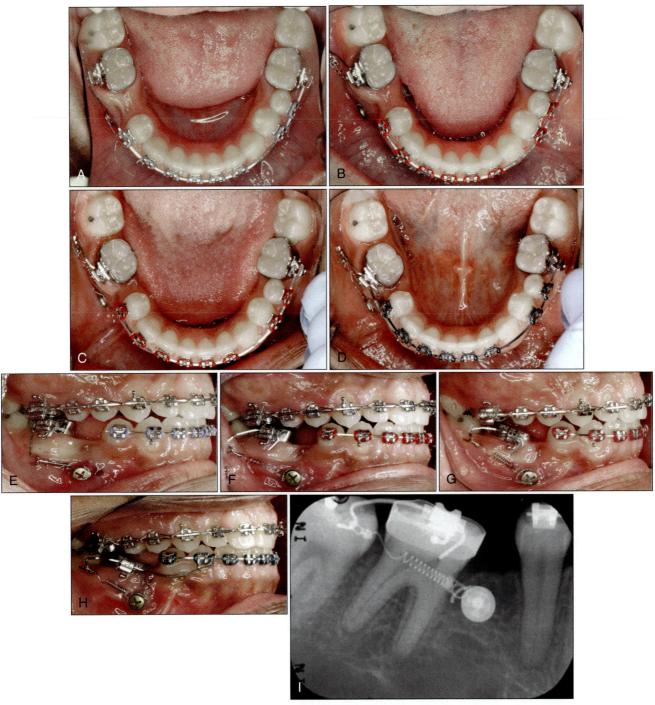

Figure 7-2

Lower-Right First Molar Protracted to Close Space of Congenitally Missing Second Premolar. Equivalent force systems can be used to predict tooth movement. **A to D,** Force applied buccal to the center of resistance of the first molar. Equivalent force system of the applied buccal force at the center of resistance describes the resulting tooth movement from the occlusal plane. Mesial rotation and molar protraction result from the applied force. **E,** Lateral view of force applied close to the center of resistance of the molar. An extension arm was dropped from the lower first molar to conform to the line of force that produces translatory movement. The arm was extended distally to increase the distance of spring activation to the temporary anchorage device (TAD). **F,** To increase the spring activation, the arm was activated distally, resulting in a line of force slightly above the center of resistance and with an intrusive component in addition to the A-P component. **G,** The arm is extended more distally, and the line of force is more occlusal to the molar's center of resistance. **H,** Clinical result is a molar that is tipped anteriorly and slightly intruded. **I,** Radiograph showing molar tipped anteriorly.

of force is slightly above the center of resistance (Figure 7-2, *I*) and at an angle to the occlusal plane. In addition to the horizontal component of the force, a vertical component is generated that results in intrusion with the mesial movement of the molar. Figure 7-2, *G*, depicts a line of force more occlusal to the center of resistance and a greater intrusive component. The equivalent force system at the center of resistance results in the same force in a mesial direction, with an intrusive component and a moment of the force in a clockwise direction. Analyzed in the sagittal plane, these force systems result in a tooth that has tipped mesially and intruded from the occlusal plane (Figure 7-2, *H*).

FORCE MAGNITUDE

Tooth movement relies on the application of forces, and Newton's Third Law (for every action there is an equal and opposite reaction) applies. In skeletal anchorage, however, the reactive force is dissipated by the implant-bone interface, which does not remodel because the periodontal ligament is absent. Nonetheless, miniscrews have some mobility when loaded, although this movement is minimal in magnitude, generally not exceeding 1 mm.[20]

Force magnitude is important not only for tooth movement but also for the stability of TADs. The maximum load that can be applied to the skeletal anchorage unit needs to be above the range of minimal forces required for the different tooth movements. Miniscrews have been shown to withstand up to 300 grams (g) of force without compromising their stability.[16,20] Among the types of tooth movement, molar intrusion needs the greatest amount of force; approximately 200 g is needed to achieve molar intrusion,[8,21] much less than the tolerance level of the miniscrew. However, newer applications for skeletal anchorage may require a significant increase in the load resistance of the screw, including the delivery of orthopedic forces through TADs. In a recent clinical report, protraction headgear from miniplates was used in the maxilla.[22] Another application reported was intermaxillary bone-bone–borne, fixed functional appliances from the posterior region of the maxilla to the anterior region of the mandible.[23] In this latter situation, plates also need to be considered because the forces generated are considerably higher.[24]

SYSTEM SELECTION AND TOOTH MOVEMENT

The many TAD types and brands make selection of the most appropriate system difficult. Important factors to consider are simplicity in design and placement technique, stability, cost, interval between placement and loading, ability to be placed in many sites intraorally, and versatility in the attachment head to apply different force systems. Most TADs meet one or more of these requirements. Ultimately, choosing the most appropriate TAD for any clinical situation is based on a force system approach, with the other factors secondary.

When a TAD is part of the patient's treatment, the clinician must first define which type of dental movement is desired. With molar intrusion, for example, the clinician must decide what forces are needed to produce intrusion, and the line of action and point of force application for a tooth or group of teeth. This information enables selection of the TAD site, which can be determined by simply following the line of action of the force. Careful evaluation of the site is then needed to avoid damage to important anatomical structures, such as the roots of teeth, maxillary sinus, nasal floor, and nerves. If one of these structures is located in the planned site, the clinician must decide between slightly changing the line of force or using a system that allows the selection of the surgical site in order to reduce the risk of damaging structures. A power arm is then extended to conform precisely to the selected line of action of the force (Figure 7-3).

Analyzing the placement site also involves the TAD's relationship to the tooth's anticipated final location. The clinician needs to ensure that the TAD does not interfere with the tooth's final position or its path. Thus, TADs that can be placed at a distance from the roots of the teeth also offer the advantage of greater tooth movement in A-P or vertical direction, without the need for TAD replacement.

The types of orthodontic tooth movement can be divided into seven broad categories: intrusion, extru-

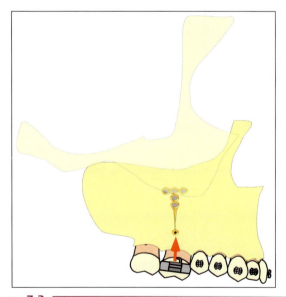

Figure 7-3

Placement of the TAD should conform to the planned line of force. Translatory molar intrusion can be obtained by placing the attachment head of the plate at the furcation area of the upper first molar.

sion, retraction, protraction, rotation, expansion, and constriction. All these movements are generally described in relation to the crown. However, these tooth movements can be further classified as *translatory*, *tipping* (controlled and uncontrolled), and *root movement*. TADs provide a mechanical advantage that may be more evident for certain types of orthodontic tooth movement.

The following sections describe the different types of tooth movements in relationship to the applicability of TADs to help accomplish these movements. The most common force systems delivered with a TAD are described from both theoretical and technical perspectives. The expected side effects and their control are also addressed.

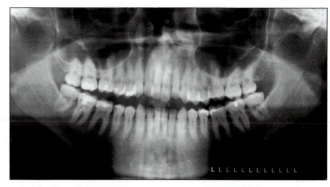

Figure 7-4
Panoramic radiograph showing there is no interradicular space in the maxillary buccal segments for placement of a miniscrew in the labial surface.

MOLAR INTRUSION

Intrusion is one tooth movement most likely to require a TAD. Historically, molar intrusion in orthodontics has been difficult to achieve.[25] This tooth movement has primarily been obtained by holding the molars against vertical growth.[26] Clinical reports of attempted molar intrusion in adult patients show small amounts of molar movement, which is difficult to verify in lateral cephalometric superimpositions. The clinical appearance of intrusion in many cases has resulted from extrusion of the adjacent teeth.[23]

Many adult patients requiring multidisciplinary care are referred by the dentist/prosthodontist for correction of altered occlusal planes and distribution of edentulous spaces preprosthetically. The correction of the occlusal plane in these patients usually requires intrusion of molars that have overerupted into an edentulous space in the opposing arch. A pure translatory intrusive force is usually necessary to achieve this correction. To accomplish this translatory movement, the line of force must be perpendicular to the occlusal plane, in a gingival direction, and passing through the center of resistance of the molar. This type of force is better delivered through a direct rather than an indirect anchorage method. The TAD needs to be placed apical to the crown of the molar to be intruded in an effort to deliver an intrusive force from either the buccal or the lingual side.

A problem is usually encountered when a miniscrew needs to be placed on the buccal aspect. Root divergence in the molar buccal roots (Figure 7-4) and no interradicular space preclude placement of a miniscrew in the buccal mucosa in many cases. Therefore, if a miniscrew will be used, the force needs to be delivered from the palatal aspect because of this anatomical limitation.

Once the location of the TAD is selected, an attachment to the tooth's crown can be soldered to a band or bonded to the buccal or lingual side. It usually is attached on the same side as the TAD if direct anchorage is used. Regardless of the TAD type and attachment location (buccal or lingual), the line of action of the intrusive force will displace the crown gingivally. However, the moment of the intrusive force will tip the crown either buccally or lingually. In most cases this moment is unwanted, although it can be controlled in various ways.

Passive or active appliances can be used to control the moment of the intrusive force. The recommended passive appliance is a large, stainless steel transpalatal arch.[25,27] However, the moment of the intrusive force may be difficult to counteract despite the rigidity of the TPA. Therefore, it may be better to place a soldered archwire of heavier dimensions, as done with a Hyrax palatal expander. This expander can also actively control the side effects of buccal tipping if cemented with the screw open. Slow constriction of the screw (when necessary) may be able to counteract the buccal tipping. However, rigid cross-arch splinting may inhibit the efficiency of molar intrusion in patients in whom this type of movement is desired unilaterally.

A second active solution to control the moment of the intrusive force is to place an additional TAD on the opposite side of the tooth. The intrusive force applied to the new TAD should be of equal magnitude to achieve a pure translatory movement of the molar (Figure 7-5, A). A third option to control the moment of the intrusive force does not require an additional bone anchor but must be used with a TAD already placed on the buccal side; it consists of a .036 × .036 Beta-Titanium transpalatal arch. This TPA applies a buccal crown torque couple in the stationary molar and ties the other end of the arch occlusally or gingivally to the lingual attachment of the tooth to be moved. An intrusive lingual force is generated that counteracts the moment of the intrusive force in the buccal area. Not engaging the slot of the bracket ensures that a single-force, one-couple system is generated. Another option to prevent a couple in the active side is to round off the TPA on

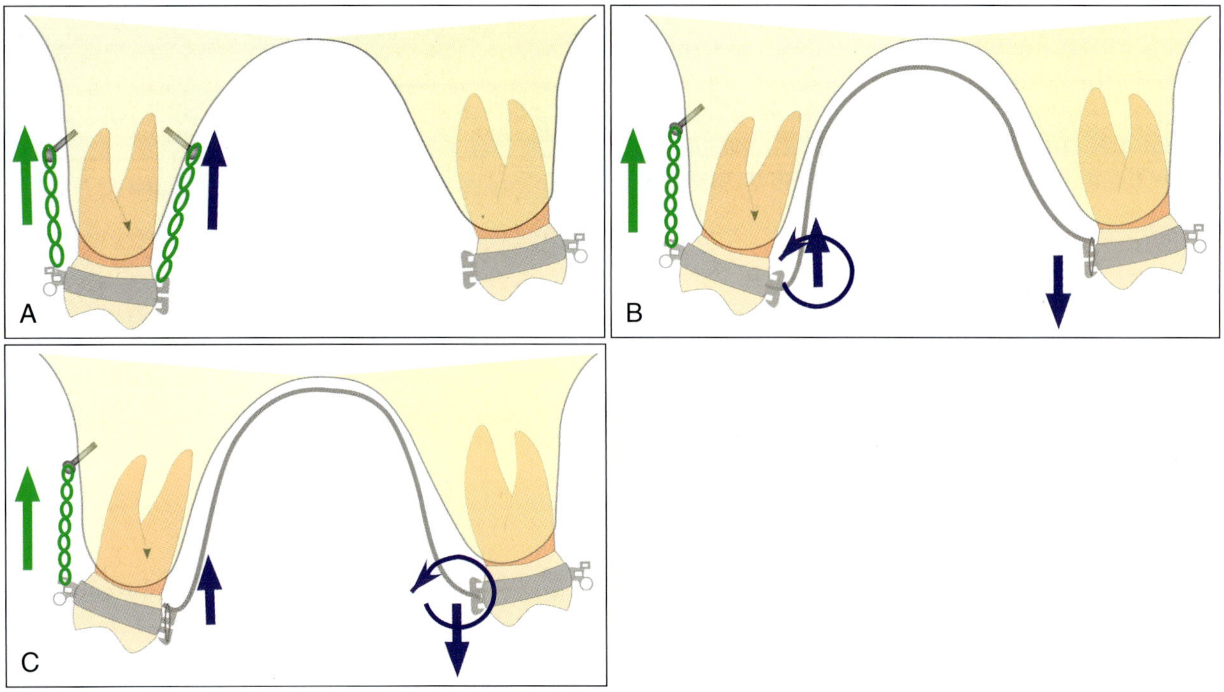

Figure 7-5

Active Applications to Control Moment of Intrusive Buccal Force. A, Miniscrew is added to the lingual side and an intrusive force with the same magnitude is applied. **B,** A .036 × .036 Beta-Titanium transpalatal arch (TPA) is placed with buccal crown torque on the contralateral upper molar. The other end of the arch is tied gingival to the tube of the bracket, thereby delivering an intrusive force that will counteract to certain extent the moment of the buccal force. **C,** Same force system but reversed generates a moment on the molar where the moment of the buccal force needs to be controlled. In addition, an intrusive force also counteracts this same buccal moment.

the intrusive force side and then engage it in the slot of the lingual bracket (Figure 7-5, *B*). Thus, a couple cannot be generated in the active side, and only the desired intrusive force will be acting in that molar from the lingual side. Finally, the same force system can be reversed, with the couple side producing buccal root torque on the active tooth to intrude. With this method the lingual intrusive force can be lower in magnitude than the buccal force, because the buccal root moment is also counteracting the moment of the buccal force (Figure 7-5, *C*). The only side effect is the extrusive force at the other end of the TPA. However, if a low intrusive force is maintained, the resultant extrusive force will be the same in magnitude and likely counteracted by the occlusal forces.

Overall, the best TADs for molar intrusion are the miniplates and miniscrews. However, miniscrew use often faces anatomical limitations to achieve the exact line of action of the force needed for molar intrusion. The miniplate can be placed directly on top of the furcation area of the molar, whereas the miniscrew must be placed mesially or distal to the center of resistance of the molar, creating a tip-back or tip-forward movement on the molar when force is applied. Although placing a miniscrew in the furcation area would be technically possible, the clinician must consider the amount of molar intrusion needed. Extensive molar intrusion would probably entail placement of the miniscrew high in the buccal vestibule. A high placement of the TAD usually results in problems with soft tissue irritation (Figure 7-6). Therefore, a miniplate offers the possibility of a distant placement site (zygomatic buttress) without the soft tissue irritation, because the extension arm with the attachment head is placed close to the attached gingiva.

Another alternative to achieve molar intrusion from a distant site using a direct anchorage force system involves a miniscrew or a mini-implant in the palate.[21] Although either system could be used for molar intrusion, an extension arm must be fabricated to achieve a more vertical vector in the line of action of the force. In the Orthosystem, a casting from the mini-implant extends close to the tissue along the palate, ending gingival to the crown of the molar to be intruded. An active spring or elastic is then used from the free end of the casting to deliver a more vertical force vector (Figure 7-7).

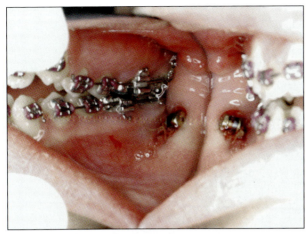

Figure 7-6
Irritation seen around the attachment head of a TAD due to its location deep in the sulcus and in unattached gingiva. The attachment head is buried in the soft tissue, making the TAD unusable.

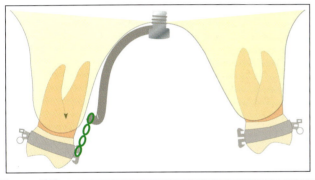

Figure 7-7
Rigid framework extended along the palate to deliver an intrusive force from a mini-implant placed distant from the molar to be intruded. The same framework can be extended using a miniscrew placed in a similar location in the hard palate.

BUCCAL SEGMENT INTRUSION

Patients with anterior open bite caused by an excess of dentoalveolar posterior segments have been successfully treated with TADs.[28-30] The anterior open bite is often found with the occlusal planes diverging anteriorly from the first premolars. Intrusion of the buccal segments not only corrects the occlusal problem but also reduces the lower anterior facial height and facial convexity as the mandible autorotates anteriorly and superiorly in a counterclockwise direction (Figure 7-8).

The intrusion of the buccal segment or occlusal plane can be either a *level* or a *canted* intrusion.[31] If the occlusal planes diverge from the molar anteriorly, a canted intrusion is indicated and accomplished by differentially intruding a larger amount posteriorly. On the other hand, if the occlusal planes diverge anteriorly from the canine, a level intrusion may be indicated.

The force systems necessary to achieve level and canted intrusions are different. In level intrusion a force passing through the center of resistance of the buccal segment is necessary to produce translation. In canted intrusion a force passing distal to the center of resistance is needed to intrude differentially more on the molar than the premolar. In general, the center of resistance of the buccal segment (first molar to first premolar) is estimated between the first molar and the second premolar.[32]

Intrusion of a buccal segment is easier to accomplish with a plate system than with miniscrews; especially if a canted intrusion of the buccal segment is desired. A miniscrew could interfere with the movement of the teeth, and the line of action of the force is more difficult to adjust once the tooth movement ensues. The plate system, however, gives the clinician more versatility; the buccal segment can be moved in any direction without concerns of root damage to the teeth. Moreover, the line of action of the force can easily be altered by adding a power arm to a miniplate system (Figure 7-9).

Miniscrews are a viable option if a level intrusion of the occlusal plane is to be corrected. Because the interradicular space is limited, however, any force not passing through the estimated center of resistance will cause a moment that might tip the roots into the miniscrew. To prevent this, the miniscrew should be used initially to intrude the molar separately. Thereafter, the premolars can be intruded directly or indirectly after rigidly connecting the molar to the miniscrew. Another alternative is adding another miniscrew between the roots of the premolars. This would allow controlling the cant of the buccal segment as the intrusive forces from the two adjacent miniscrews are applied.

Pure translatory intrusion of the buccal segment can be challenging. From a sagittal view, as the force is applied to the buccal segment distal to its center of resistance, a clockwise rotation of the segment is observed. To control this rotation, some have proposed adding a miniscrew more anteriorly.[24,33] However, the clinical effect is caused by the line of action of the force. By altering this line, the cant can be controlled. An alternative is to apply the line of action closer to the center of resistance of the segment. Another option is to ligate one of the ends of the molar, fixing the vertical distance to the TAD and applying a force to the other end of the buccal segment after extending an arm from the TAD (Figure 7-10).

TECHNICAL ASPECTS

Intrusion of the buccal segments in a patient with an anterior open bite resembles a three-piece maxillary impaction. The upper anterior segment remains in the same vertical position. The objective is intrusion of the buccal segment to close the anterior open bite through posterior intrusion instead of incisor extrusion. The upper arch is set up by placing a rigid .017 × .025 stain-

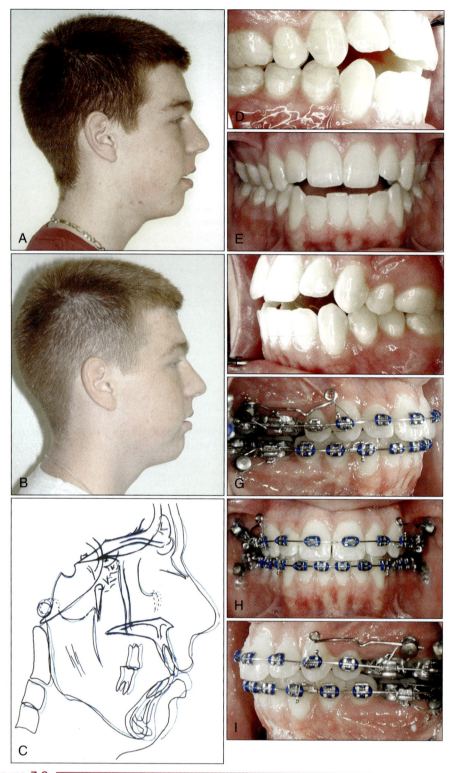

Figure 7-8

Facial and dental changes with intrusion of the buccal posterior segments. **A**, Pretreatment profile view. **B**, Posttreatment profile view. **C**, Superimposition shows 2-year period, including 1½ years of observation. **D to F**, Pretreatment intraoral views of the anterior open bite. **G to I**, Mini-plates used to achieve dentoalveolar intrusion of the posterior segments. Arms extending anteriorly from the attachment head of the plate with locking mechanism allows controlled delivery of the line force.

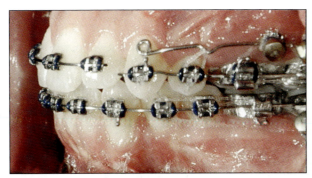

Figure 7-9
Extension arm (cantilever) is used from the attachment head to deliver an intrusive line of force to the canine and premolar.

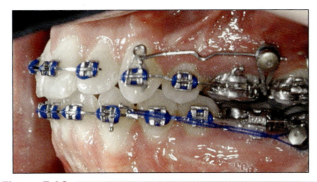

Figure 7-10
Canting of the buccal segment is controlled by maintaining the vertical position of the molar and by adding an intrusive force to the most anterior tooth in the segment by extending an arm from the attachment head.

less steel wire segment bilaterally from the second molar to the first premolar. The anterior segment includes the upper incisors with the same wire dimensions. The canine is included on either the anterior or the posterior segment, depending on the vertical relationship to the adjacent teeth and its estimated final vertical position. In many cases the canine should not be connected to either segment initially, but rather connected to the archwire after the buccal segment has intruded. Connecting the canine to the buccal segment may cause extrusion of the canine if the intrusive force is applied to the first or second molar. This effect is more clinically evident with a large buccal segment that extends from the second molar to the canine and is a result of the moment of the intrusive force applied at the molar level (Figure 7-11).

The same mechanics are applied to the lower arch if the occlusal plane significantly diverges anteriorly from the premolar. Severe divergence in the lower arch is uncommon, however, so a continuous archwire can be placed from the beginning before placing the active intrusive force.

Although significant intrusion can be accomplished in only one of the buccal segments, compensatory erup-

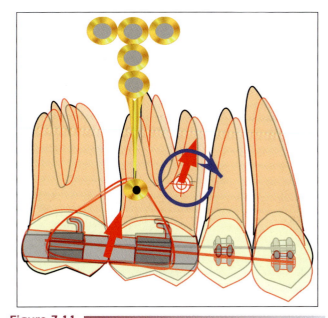

Figure 7-11
Having a posterior buccal segment extending to the canine may cause canting of the segment with extrusion of the canine as a result of the moment of the molar intrusive force. Reducing the size of the buccal segment not to include the canine may aid in obtaining a more leveled intrusion.

tion of the antagonist teeth has been reported.[34] Therefore, if intrusion of the dentoalveolar segments is only desired in one arch, the TAD needs to be placed in the antagonist arch to stop the buccal segments from overerupting.

Once the treatment plan for buccal segment intrusion is defined, the plates can be placed. Although the leveling stage to a .017 × .025 stainless steel archwire would generally take significantly longer than the 2 weeks of healing after plate placement, the intrusive forces can be delivered during the buccal segment leveling stages.

Finally, the same buccal tipping side effect of molar intrusion is observed with the intrusion of the buccal segments. A rigid TPA is needed to prevent this tipping movement. As previously mentioned, the moment of the force may overcome the rigidity of the TPA. In this case a bonded acrylic expander not only helps with the rigidity but also can be used to place the buccal attachment in the acrylic, increasing the distance to the TAD. Thus, a more constant force through a nickel-titanium (Ni-Ti) spring may be delivered. Furthermore, the acrylic plate may also aid in the vertical control, preventing the described compensatory eruption of the lower segment after intrusion of the upper buccal segment.[34]

Active applications may also be used to control for the tipping of the buccal segment. If significant upper premolar buccal tipping occurs, intrusion should be continued from the lingual side by fixing the molar to the TAD with a ligature wire and applying a force to the

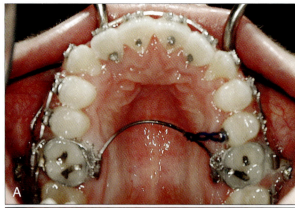

Figure 7-12
A, Cant of the buccal segment and Brodie bite tendency can be controlled by tying the molar to the TAD on the buccal aspect and extending a wire anteriorly from a TPA in the lingual aspect. **B,** Line of force will intrude the premolars, and moment of the force will incline the crowns lingually.

lingual side of the premolar from a welded spur on the TPA (Figure 7-12).

INCISOR INTRUSION

Temporary anchorage devices for intrusion of any of the teeth in the anterior segment can be considered impractical and unnecessary. Additionally, anatomical limitations exist for placement of miniscrews in the anterior region. The labial frenum can be easily irritated if a miniscrew is placed in proximity. Therefore, if miniscrews are absolutely needed, two would need to be placed distal to the lateral incisor.

Numerous studies have shown the efficiency of incisor intrusion using a *cantilever* system.[35-37] This force system can deliver the same incisor intrusive force as that obtained from a miniscrew placed anteriorly. Furthermore, the cantilever permits easy adjustment of the line of force. The inability of the cantilever to deliver a high force magnitude without significant side effects, as possible with a miniscrew, may be the only difference between both systems. However, incisor intrusion does not require a great magnitude of force; values can be kept under 60 g for the four incisors and 30 g for each canine and still achieve incisor intrusion.[38,39]

It has also been recommended, for en masse upper anterior retraction, to place a miniscrew in the anterior region in conjunction with TADs placed mesial to the molar.[40] This additional miniscrew in the anterior region is intended to control the extrusive tendency of the incisors that results from the retraction force from a miniscrew placed in the molar region. However, the incisor extrusion observed as the anterior segment is retracted can be controlled with the same cantilever system provided by an intrusion arch or two cantilevers extended from the molars. Overall, incisor intrusion with TADs is not cost-effective because the mechanics described earlier can accomplish the same results.

However, TADs can be used to achieve incisor intrusion in adult patients with a severe brachyfacial pattern, convergent occlusal planes, and 100% impinging deep bite, in whom correction of the vertical problem of the malocclusion is complex (Figure 7-13, *A*). The solution relies on either extruding the posterior buccal segments (very unstable orthodontic movement in adults)[41,42] or intruding the anterior teeth. Many adults also present with minimal upper incisor display, which means the vertical problem can be resolved only by lower incisor intrusion. The convergence of the occlusal planes allows for about 2 to 3 mm of intrusion in the lower arch (Figure 7-13, *B*). To achieve more incisor intrusion, the lower occlusal plane needs to rotate clockwise around the crown of the lower first molars, thus intruding the premolars slightly. TADs could be used simultaneously with a lower intrusion arch, as previously described. The real use of TADs in this clinical situation would be to obtain the clockwise cant of the lower occlusal plane at the level of the premolars as the lower incisors are intruded by the cantilever system (Figure 7-13, *C*).

ANTERIOR-POSTERIOR MOVEMENTS
DISTALIZATION

Molar distalization with TADs is generally accomplished by indirect anchorage. A TAD is placed anterior to the molar, and two equal and opposite forces are applied between the first molar and the first or second premolars.[43] The molar is thus distalized, and the premolars remain stationary as the molar is fixed rigidly to the TAD. Once the molar is distalized, the TAD is fixed to the molars, and the anterior segment is retracted. Any type of TAD can be used for this purpose; however, the Orthosystem (palatal mini-implant) was one of the first systems to deliver this type of indirect anchorage.[44]

Direct anchorage for molar distalization has been previously described for a mini-implant in the palate.[7] This approach has a mechanical advantage because it offers translatory movement of the molars. A similar approach has been described using one or two screws placed in the same location in the palate, from which a framework is connected and direct anchorage provided.[14,40,45]

This same mini-implant or a miniscrew can be used for direct anchorage for distalization in the lower arch if placed in the retromolar pad.[46,47] However, a plate system offers a more hygienic alternative. Furthermore,

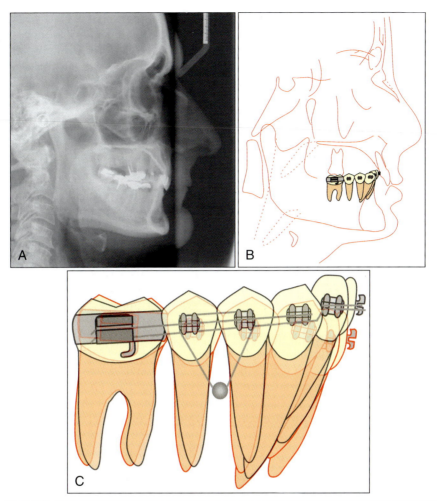

Figure 7-13
A, Brachyfacial pattern in adult patient. **B,** Control of the buccal segments is critical. The convergent occlusal planes need to diverge anteriorly. **C,** Intrusion of the premolars in the lower buccal segments is needed before the intrusion of the lower incisors with an intrusion arch.

the miniplate may be better for lower molar distalization because the surgeon has easier access to the placement site. In addition, the more anterior location of the attachment head of the plate allows the orthodontist easier access to deliver the forces (Figure 7-14). The plate system can also be used for upper molar distalization with direct anchorage.[48]

Although miniscrews placed in the buccal aspect can be used as direct anchorage for molar distalization, the greatest drawback is that the screws need to be placed initially between the roots of the premolars, later to be removed and replaced mesial or distal to the distalized molar to allow distal movement of the premolars and anterior teeth.[40]

As the molars are distalized, two common side effects are observed, depending on the location of the line of action of the force. When the line of action from a sagit-

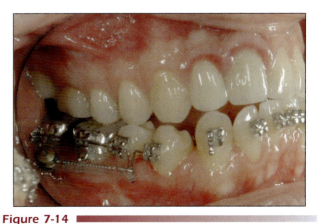

Figure 7-14
Plate system provides an attachment head more easily accessed by the orthodontist to deliver the mechanics and by the patient to maintain hygiene.

tal aspect does not cross through the center of resistance, the molar will tip mesially or distally. Most frequently, the line of force passes below the center of resistance, and because the force is distal, the molar will tip distally. The point of application of the force from the TAD is usually from the alveolar bone, and thus a greater translatory movement tendency with direct anchorage should be observed compared with traditional distalizing tooth-borne appliances using indirect anchorage. From the occlusal aspect the molar will rotate mesial-out or distal-in, depending on the location of the distalizing force (buccal side for mesial-out, lingual side for distal-in). Preventing this rotational tendency is usually more difficult in the first order than in the second order because of anatomical constraints. A rigid TPA may help prevent this rotational tendency.

Overall, distalization with TADs can be considered an adequate alternative when the incisors need to be slightly to moderately retracted or maintained in the same A-P position, and posterior segments need to be moved posteriorly approximately 3 to 4 mm. In addition, these systems can be used to correct midlines by differentially distalizing one of the buccal segments. Research studies of upper and lower molar distalization with miniplate systems have shown an average of 3 mm of distalization at the coronal level and 2 mm at the apical level.[48,49]

MESIALIZATION

TADs have made "mesialization" a popular term. One of the major indications for TADs is the mesial movement of teeth in the buccal segments in patients with missing molars or premolars. It is a cost-effective procedure because the patient does not require fixed partial dentures or implants. Additionally, if implant placement is considered, grafting procedures, which may be necessary to reconstruct atrophic ridges, are obviated. Space closure through mesial movement of the posterior teeth can generate new bone in the defect and spare the patient from costly dental procedures.[50] The mesialization of the posterior segment is usually indicated for one missing molar or premolars. Using a screw to mesialize posterior teeth is usually not recommended because the amount of time required to protract would be significant if the edentulous space is more than the mesio-distal width of a molar.[47,51] Mesial movement of the posterior segments is another indication in patients with congenitally missing maxillary lateral incisors and a Class I molar occlusion. Although a bridge or implants may be used to replace the missing teeth in these patients, limited finances may indicate canine substitution. To completely move the buccal segments anteriorly in these patients, TADs are highly indicated.

The different TADs and force systems necessary for mesialization are similar to those described for distalization. Both direct anchorage and indirect anchorage are possible mechanisms of force delivery. Generally, a pull-type force system is indicated, which makes insertion of the TAD easier because the placement site is more anterior. Although push systems can be applied, the TADs and the appliances to deliver such forces need to be placed in areas that not only have difficult access for placement, but also are uncomfortable and difficult to maintain for the patient (e.g., ramus of mandible).

SPACE CLOSURE

Orthodontics has always been in search of obtaining "perfect" anchorage. This perfect anchorage has usually been described in the A-P dimension as the resistance of the molars to anterior movement when the anterior teeth are retracted. TADs have been suggested as the replacements for headgear.[12,17] Although the intention of maintaining perfect anchorage may be the goal, orthodontic correction with anchor loss of only 1 to 2 mm (Group A anchorage) can be obtained without using TADs. Therefore the question to be asked is: By how much and to what degree would this affect esthetic results?

In general, anteroposterior lip changes to incisor movement have been considered unpredictable; no perfect algorithm exits. Furthermore, the relationship of upper lip response to incisor retraction is usually less than 50%. If this assumption were correct, would a difference of 1 mm or less (50% of 2 mm) in A-P position of the upper lip be noticeable? Unpublished data suggest no significant difference in the final incisor edge position using Tweed mechanics compared to retraction with mini-implants in patients undergoing premolar extractions.[52]

The biomechanics in space closure with direct anchorage differ from indirect anchorage. Indirect anchorage is delivered through conventional mechanics, where the mesial force to the molar is negated by the connection to the TAD. In direct anchorage the force is usually delivered from the TAD in an occlusal direction. Therefore, the distal force also has an intrusive component with direct anchorage. If the canine is being retracted separately along the archwire, the normal force in the second order is increased. Therefore, depending on the stiffness of the wire, the deflection will generate two side effects: extrusion of the incisors and friction.

To control for the extrusion side effect during retraction, a miniscrew placed anteriorly in the maxilla is recommended.[40] As mentioned, this extrusion can be easily controlled with a cantilever system such as the intrusion arch. The other side effect, additional friction, may reduce the efficiency in canine retraction. To limit this effect, an extension arm can be attached to the canine, achieving a more translatory movement of the canine and thus less friction (Figure 7-15). The wire may still serve for rotational control in the first order. Another alternative is to use a frictionless system (loops) for anterior retraction, extending a force from

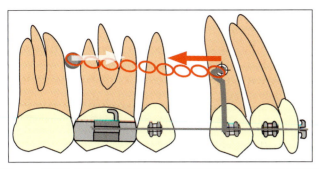

Figure 7-15
Line of force for canine retraction passing through the center of resistance ensures a more translatory movement of this tooth.

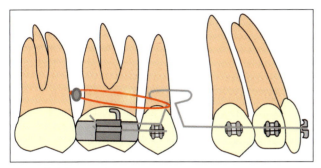

Figure 7-16
Direct anchorage achieved by adding a force from an elastic chain or thread to the loop in a frictionless system for en masse retraction.

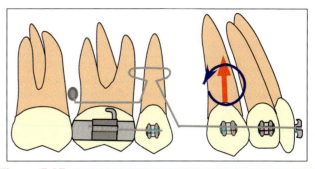

Figure 7-17
Direct Anchorage with Frictionless System for En Masse Retraction. Distal leg of the loop is connected to the TAD. Anterior leg is gabled to achieve torque and intrusion as the segment is retracted.

the TAD to the loop system[40] (Figure 7-16). This last anchorage approach is more indirect however; the force delivered from the miniscrew is not driving the appliance.

When en masse retraction is planned, the line of the force applied from the TAD may have a predominant horizontal component by attaching it to the lateral incisors. In this case, however, friction is still an issue. Extrusion of the incisors would also occur, although to a lesser extent than just with canine retraction, because the moment of the retraction force is reduced.

Miniscrews in the upper anterior region have been advocated with en masse retraction to control vertical incisor position. Instead, the same cantilever system described earlier should be added. Another alternative is to add a loop system to deliver a moment and an intrusive force from the TAD (Figure 7-17). However, the loop system may be more appropriate for indirect anchorage because it would probably impinge on the soft tissues if delivered from a TAD.

TRANSVERSE EXPANSION

Miniscrews have been used to assist in the correction of a transverse discrepancy.[3] From a force system perspective, this is the least of the indications for TADs. Expansion can be easily obtained from a force system exerting

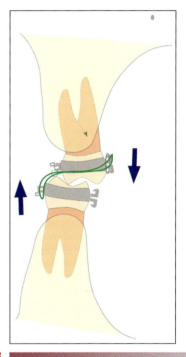

Figure 7-18
Extrusive component of the force delivered by a cross-elastic to correct a dental crossbite.

equal and opposite forces, delivered by an orthopedic device (e.g., palatal expander) or by conventional orthodontic force delivered through an expanded archwire. Placement of a TAD would be indicated only in a patient with unilateral crossbite, along with an anterior open-bite tendency. The extrusive component usually encountered by traditional crossbite mechanics consists of a cross-elastic, which would accentuate the anterior open-bite tendency (Figure 7-18). Even in these patients, however, other alternatives to obtain unilateral expansion without an extrusive force instead of TADs have been described.[53,54] For example, on the side where no expansion is desired, a TPA with a moment is added with buccal root torque direction. Concurrently, an equal and opposite force is delivered through a TPA with an expansion force (Figure 7-19).

COUPLE SYSTEMS

Skeletal anchorage can be used to produce one-couple and two-couple force systems for tooth movement. One-couple systems provide the advantage of high predictability in tooth movement.[55,56] The classic example of a one-couple system is the cantilever (Figure 7-20). This is a versatile system having two discernible units with two different effects. On one end of the system, there is only a directional force in that plane of space to be applied at a single point. On the other end, there is a force of the exact magnitude and in the opposite direction in the same plane of space. Additionally, this side has a moment or couple produced by the spring engaging a tube or bracket. This system is in equilibrium, so the sum of the forces and moments equals zero. This type of force system makes tooth movement predictable. It can be well applied to the biomechanics of TADs. Either side of the force system can be used (force and moment side or single force side) to achieve desired tooth movements with TADs.

Using the single force from a cantilever spring has a major advantage, especially when TADs are used for direct anchorage. This force can be applied in almost any direction and along the entire longitudinal axis of the tooth or group of teeth to be moved; the only limitation is soft tissue discomfort. Also, the force can be delivered from a distant point, offering the advantage of more constant force delivery. Further, the single force provided by a cantilever system is cost-effective when using TADs because fewer of these will need to be placed.

The clinician must consider two important technical elements when applying a one-couple system from a TAD. If the second-order couple side of the wire will be attached to a TAD, a slot for the wire needs to be present in the attachment head to create the couple. However, most miniscrew systems available do not have this feature in the attachment head. Some systems may have a slot, but it is usually round and sometimes with a large dimension, up to 0.045 inch in diameter. Although a round wire can be used to apply a single force with a cantilever system, intraoral stability in the couple side can be compromised, especially if the cantilever system is unilateral instead of bilateral (intrusion arch). Furthermore, a large dimension slot needs a wire with a similar dimension to ensure stability, which would probably deliver unnecessarily high force values and discomfort to the patient.

The direction of the force of the cantilever may create another potential problem in TADs with a round slot in the attachment head. For example, if the TAD is placed on the ridge parallel to the long axes of the adjacent teeth and the slot is perpendicular to the screw in a buccolingual direction, an intrusive or extrusive force cannot be delivered because of the absence of a second-order couple in a round wire (Figure 7-21). Solutions include bonding the wire to the head of the screw using flowable composite to create a rigid junction between the TAD and the wire, thus producing a second-order couple in the TAD. This rigid union will generate the intrusive or extrusive force needed. A second solution is to bond a bracket to the attachment head of the TAD, also with flowable composite, although the adhesive strength to the screw head might be questionable (Figure 7-22). A rectangular sectional wire also needs to be used with this option to ensure the stability of the cantilever system. A third solution is to cement an acrylic coping on top of the screw head with a wire extension. Thus, the couple can be resisted by the height of the screw head (Figure 7-23, *A*). To use this third option, the head must have sufficient resistance form to prevent the cemented acrylic coping from loosening or becoming dislodged. The arm is connected to the teeth by a force delivered through a coil spring or an elastic chain or

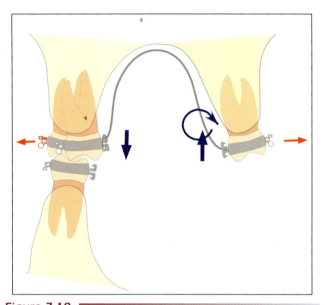

Figure 7-19

Force System from TPA to Achieve Unilateral Expansion. Couple on the molar at left counteracts the expansive force. A slight extrusive force is evident in the molar at right as it tips buccally. This extrusive force is of low magnitude and usually counteracted by the occlusal forces.

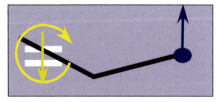

Figure 7-20

One-Couple or Cantilever System. One side is engaged on a tube or bracket to generate a couple. This same side has a force in the direction of the vertex of the V bend. The other end of the system is a point of application of the force in the opposite direction to the force in the couple side.

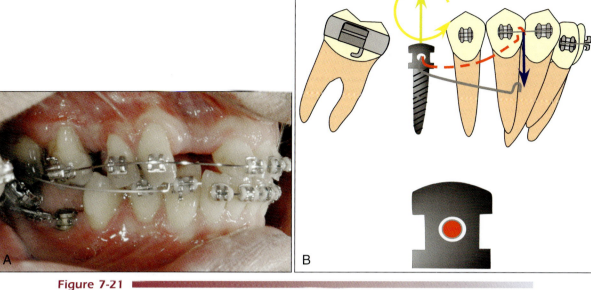

Figure 7-21
A, Miniscrew placed on the edentulous ridge distal to the second premolar. **B,** A couple cannot be generated from this TAD when the attachment head has a round slot perpendicular to the extrusive of intrusive force of the cantilever.

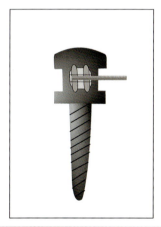

Figure 7-22
Bracket can be bonded to the attachment head to produce a couple and generate the necessary force at the other end of the system.

thread (Figure 7-23, *B*). In this case the dimensions of the extension wire should be high enough to resist deformation from the force. Figure 7-23 shows the extension wire with a bracket spot welded to it, which serves as an attachment to the force-producing mechanism and also allows delivery of a two-couple system if needed.

Most miniplate systems offer the alternative of bonding a tube to the plate or have a locking mechanism to attach a wire. Figure 7-8, *I*, shows a locking mechanism that acts as rigid junction. Also, in this particular situation, the applied force and the slot of the

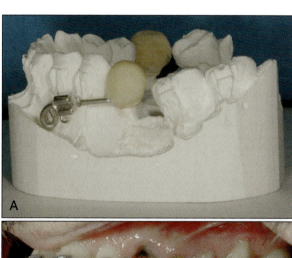
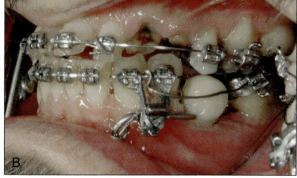

Figure 7-23
A and **B,** Acrylic coping with an extension arm is cemented to the attachment head of the miniscrew. A force can be delivered from the arm to achieve intrusion of the canine and the premolar.

attachment head are in the same plane. Although the slot in the attachment head is round, the locking mechanism provides a rigid junction, and the second-order couple is resisted by the width of the slot. Moreover, when the force and the couple are in the same plane, intraoral stability of the sectional wire is not compromised, provided a tight fit exists between the slot of the attachment head and the wire.

The second important consideration when using a one-couple system is the magnitude of the force. The higher the magnitude of the force, the larger will be the moment generated in the couple side, as described at the miniscrew level. The magnitude of this moment is not a problem when it is resisted by the longitudinal axis of the tooth, as shown in Figure 7-24, *A*. However, the magnitude can become an issue when the moment generated by the force is in a plane perpendicular to the longitudinal axis of the screw. In this case the moment will act as torque to the screw head in a clockwise or counterclockwise rotation, depending on the direction of the force (Figure 7-24, *B*).

Miniscrews reportedly can withstand an average removal torque of 11,000 g/mm.[57] This means that for an average distance of 30 mm for a given cantilever, the force delivered can be up to 366 g/mm. This force level is well above the force levels of 200 g needed to intrude a molar. However, these results must be evaluated with caution because removal torque values varied greatly, from 200 to 22,000 g/mm.[57]

This same clinical scenario can be encountered when a TAD is placed on top of the ridge. When an A-P force is applied, a rotational moment on the TAD in a clockwise or counterclockwise direction is generated. However, because the soft tissue limitation is evident, the moment arm will generally be small. Thus, significant force well above 1000 g needs to be applied to generate a moment of 11,000 g/mm.

One-couple systems can also be used so that the couple acts on the teeth to be moved and the force is applied to the TAD. This force system can be useful in molar uprighting and correction of root inclinations. The most important aspect when using this type of system is that the same magnitude of force being applied to the TAD will be acting on the tooth in the opposite direction. Thus, if a lower molar is being uprighted and a high force magnitude is delivered to the TAD, the tooth will tend to overerupt and possibly cause traumatic occlusion (Figure 7-25).

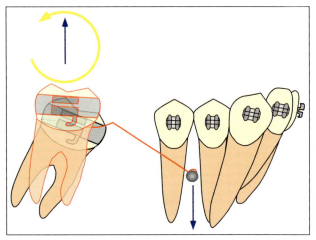

Figure 7-25
Miniscrew can be used to receive the single-force side of a one-couple system. This system can be used to upright molars.

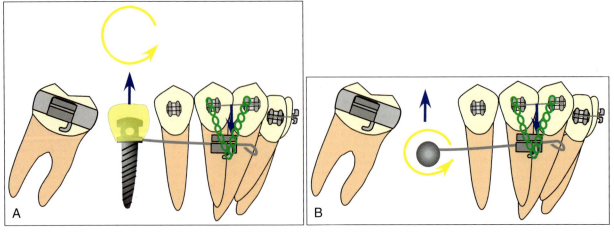

Figure 7-24
A, One-couple system or cantilever delivered from the acrylic coping. The attachment head requires enough retention form to withstand the couple. *B*, If the miniscrew's longitudinal axis is perpendicular to the force, the couple will screw or unscrew the TAD, depending on the magnitude of the force and its distance to the attachment head.

TROUBLESHOOTING

In cases where the TAD is placed in a less-than-ideal position, the clinician must seriously consider replacing the device. An alternative is to design an appliance that will most benefit from the TAD before its removal. Figure 7-26 shows improper TAD placement in the edentulous area where the mandibular molar was to be moved. Ideally, the molar should be bodily translated to contact distal to the lower-right second premolar. However, this translatory movement would be interrupted halfway during the space closure effort. To maximize use of the miniscrew, the TAD was used to accomplish the most difficult type of movement, root movement. The line of force was directed from the miniscrew to an arm almost to the full depth of the buccal sulcus, promoting translation of the molar. To obtain root movement, a cantilever was added to the molar until it almost contacted the mini-implant. The miniscrew would then be removed and a crown-tipping movement obtained with conventional mechanics.

Figure 7-27 shows a similar problem in which the implant was placed too distal to the canine in an effort to prevent root damage. In this patient the miniscrew was placed too close to the apical third of the premolar to be moved anteriorly. The TAD can be used to tip the second premolar and first molar mesially almost completely through the edentulous space and then can be removed to correct the root inclination of the buccal segment.

A common clinical problem is inability to deliver the desired line of force from the TAD. This usually results from placement of the TAD close to the free gingival margin. This site is often necessary to prevent burying the TAD, mainly seen when placed in unattached gingiva. To achieve the desired line of force, an arm is extended from the TAD or from the tooth to be moved. This is usually difficult to achieve in the second-molar region because of the soft tissue limitation. Additionally, the appliances may impair access to hygiene, a critical factor to miniscrew attachment head clearance.

A problem related to the line of force is encountered when the TAD is close to the tooth to be moved. The solution is to extend arms along the line of force from the TAD or the attachment of the tooth to be moved. Figure 7-2, *E*, shows a molar to be moved anteriorly and in proximity to the TAD. The arm was placed from the distal aspect to increase the distance. Because the tissue was growing around the TAD, no arm could be extended from it. Thus, the distance was further increased by

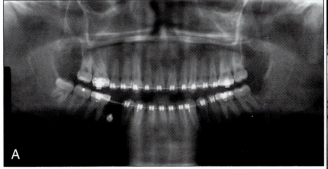
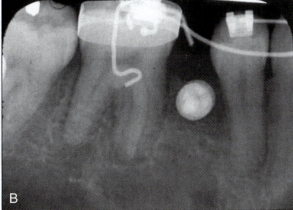
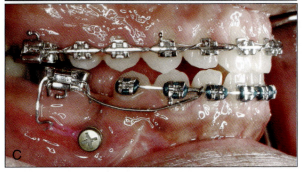

Figure 7-26
Miniscrew placed in the middle of edentulous site. The molar can be only protracted partially. Root correction is attempted to achieve the most difficult type of movement with the TAD. The TAD will then be removed to tip the crown mesially. **A,** Panoramic radiograph. **B,** Periapical radiograph. **C,** Clinical photograph.

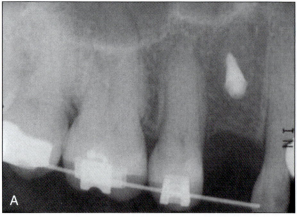
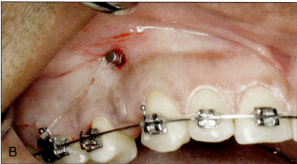

Figure 7-27
Miniscrew placed in the middle of the edentulous site to where the buccal segment needs to be moved. Because the miniscrew was placed close to the apices of the adjacent teeth, mesial tipping of the posterior segment to close the edentulous area can be accomplished without contacting the TAD. The TAD later is removed and the teeth roots are then corrected. **A,** Periapical radiograph. **B,** Photograph.

bending the arm distally instead (see Figure 7-2, *F*), almost maintaining the same line of force.

Troubleshooting with TADs especially occurs in the initial phases of becoming familiar with the system. An understanding of the biomechanics involved allows the clinician to be creative and find solutions to the side effects and possible complications still found with TADs. In some cases the TADs need to be removed and the desired tooth movements reassessed so that if required a new TAD site or skeletal anchorage system can be selected.

CONCLUSION

Temporary anchorage devices have become increasingly popular, and most orthodontists are incorporating TADs into the armamentarium of their daily practice. As with any device in orthodontics, TADs remain as a tool to achieve a treatment objective. The clinician should always determine whether these devices are the most cost-effective way to achieve the desired objectives. Overall, TADs expand the range of tooth movements achievable. Two such types of tooth movement are molar intrusion and significant tooth displacement in the A-P direction. Other applications, such as anchorage control and incisor intrusion, may be obtained by other orthodontic methods that do not rely on patient compliance. The biomechanical applications with TADs generally use the same principles that govern traditional orthodontic tooth movement.

REFERENCES

1. Prahl-Anderson B: Review of article. Implants for cleft lip and palate patients: myth or reality, Edward H. Angle Society of Orthodontics, North Atlantic Component, Naples, Fla, 2005.
2. Yu JC, Fearon J, Havlik RJ, et al: Distraction osteogenesis of the craniofacial skeleton, *Plast Reconstr Surg* 114:1E-20E, 2004.
3. Park HS, Kwon OW, Sung JH: Uprighting second molars with micro-implant anchorage, *J Clin Orthod* 38:100-103 (quiz, 192), 2004.
4. Park HS, Bae SM, Kyung HM, Sung JH: Micro-implant anchorage for treatment of skeletal Class I bialveolar protrusion, *J Clin Orthod* 35:417-422, 2001.
5. Melsen B: Miniscrew implants: the Aahrus Anchorage System, *Semin Orthod* 11:24-31, 2005.
6. Melsen B: Mini-implants: where are we? *J Clin Orthod* 39:539-547 (quiz, 531-532), 2005.
7. Keles A, Erverdi N, Sezen S: Bodily distalization of molars with absolute anchorage, *Angle Orthod* 73:471-482, 2003.
8. Yao CC, Wu CB, Wu HY, et al: Intrusion of the overerupted upper left first and second molars by mini-implants with partial-fixed orthodontic appliances: a case report, *Angle Orthod* 74:550-557, 2004.
9. Ohnishi H, Yagi T, Yasuda Y, Takada K: A mini-implant for orthodontic anchorage in a deep overbite case, *Angle Orthod* 75:444-452, 2005.
10. Cornelis MA, De Clerck HJ: Biomechanics of skeletal anchorage. Part 1. Class II extraction treatment, *J Clin Orthod* 40:261-269 (quiz, 232), 2006.
11. Carano A, Velo S, Leone P, Siciliani G: Clinical applications of miniscrew anchorage system, *J Clin Orthod* 34:9-24, 2005.
12. Kyung HM, Park HS, Bae SM, et al: Development of orthodontic micro-implants for intraoral anchorage, *J Clin Orthod* 37:321-328 (quiz, 314), 2003.
13. Chung KR, Kim SH, Kook YA: The C-orthodontic micro-implant, *J Clin Orthod* 38:478-486 (quiz, 487-478), 2004.
14. Park HS: A miniscrew-assisted transpalatal arch for use in lingual orthodontics, *J Clin Orthod* 40:12-16, 2006.
15. Park YC, Chu JH, Choi YJ, Choi NC: Extraction space closure with vacuum-formed splints and miniscrew anchorage, *J Clin Orthod* 39:76-79, 2005.
16. Favero L, Brollo P, Bressan E: Orthodontic anchorage with specific fixtures: related study analysis, *Am J Orthod Dentofacial Orthop* 122:84-94, 2002.
17. Celenza F, Hochman MN: Absolute anchorage in orthodontics: direct and indirect implant-assisted modalities, *J Clin Orthod* 34:397-402, 2000.
18. Wehrbein H, Feifel H, Diedrich P: Palatal implant anchorage reinforcement of posterior teeth: a prospective study, *Am J Orthod Dentofacial Orthop* 116:678-686, 1999.

19. Smith RJ, Burstone CJ: Mechanics of tooth movement, *Am J Orthod* 85:294-307, 1984.
20. Liou EJ, Pai BC, Lin JC: Do miniscrews remain stationary under orthodontic forces? *Am J Orthod Dentofacial Orthop* 126:42-47, 2004.
21. Lee JS, Kim DH, Park YC, et al: The efficient use of midpalatal miniscrew implants, *Angle Orthod* 74:711-714, 2004.
22. Kircelli BH, Pektas ZO, Uckan S: Orthopedic protraction with skeletal anchorage in a patient with maxillary hypoplasia and hypodontia, *Angle Orthod* 76:156-163, 2006.
23. Erverdi N: *Bone anchorage in orthodontics*, New York; 2005, North Eastern Society of Orthodontics.
24. Sung JH, Kyung HM, Bae SM, et al: Clinical examples of microimplant anchorage. In *Microimplants in orthodontics*, Daegu, South Korea, 2006, Dentos, pp 83-163.
25. Sugawara J: A bioefficient skeletal anchorage system. In Nanda R, editor: *Biomechanics and esthetic strategies in clinical orthodontics*, St Louis, 2005, Mosby, pp 295-309.
26. Uribe F, Nanda R: Management of open bite malocclusion. In Nanda R, editor: *Biomechanics and esthetic strategies in clinical orthodontics*, St Louis, 2005, Mosby, pp 156-176.
27. Everdi N, Keles A, Nanda R: Orthodontic anchorage and skeletal implants. In Nanda R, editor: *Biomechanics and esthetic strategies in clinical orthodontics*. St Louis, 2005, Mosby, pp 278-294.
28. Umemori M, Sugawara J, Mitani H, et al: Skeletal anchorage system for open-bite correction, *Am J Orthod Dentofacial Orthop* 115:166-174, 1999.
29. Sherwood KH, Burch J, Thompson W: Intrusion of supererupted molars with titanium miniplate anchorage, *Angle Orthod* 73:597-601, 2003.
30. Erverdi N, Keles A, Nanda R: The use of skeletal anchorage in open bite treatment: a cephalometric evaluation, *Angle Orthod* 74:381-390, 2004.
31. Torres M: Treatment objectives and treatment planning, *Dent Clin North Am* 25:27-41, 1981.
32. Van Steenbergen E, Burstone CJ, Prahl-Andersen B, Aartman IH: The role of a high pull headgear in counteracting side effects from intrusion of the maxillary anterior segment, *Angle Orthod* 74:480-486, 2004.
33. Jeon YJ, Kim YH, Son WS, Hans MG: Correction of a canted occlusal plane with miniscrews in a patient with facial asymmetry, *Am J Orthod Dentofacial Orthop* 130:244-252, 2006.
34. Kuroda S, Katayama A, Takano-Yamamoto T: Severe anterior open-bite case treated using titanium screw anchorage, *Angle Orthod* 74:558-567, 2004.
35. Ng J, Major PW, Heo G, Flores-Mir C: True incisor intrusion attained during orthodontic treatment: a systematic review and meta-analysis, *Am J Orthod Dentofacial Orthop* 128:212-219, 2005.
36. Van Steenbergen E, Burstone CJ, Prahl-Andersen B, Aartman IH: The influence of force magnitude on intrusion of the maxillary segment, *Angle Orthod* 75:723-729, 2005.
37. Weiland FJ, Bantleon HP, Droschl H: Evaluation of continuous arch and segmented arch leveling techniques in adult patients: a clinical study, *Am J Orthod Dentofacial Orthop* 110:647-652, 1996.
38. Burstone CR: Deep overbite correction by intrusion, *Am J Orthod* 72:1-22, 1977.
39. Nanda R, Marzban R, Kuhlberg A: The Connecticut Intrusion Arch, *J Clin Orthod* 32:708-715, 1998.
40. Sung JH, Kyung HM, Bae SM, et al: Biomechanical considerations in microimplant anchorage. In *Microimplants in orthodontics*, Daegu, South Korea, 2006, Dentos, pp 63-82.
41. Engel G, Cornforth G, Damerell JM, et al: Treatment of deep bite cases, *Am J Orthod* 77:1-13, 1980.
42. Dermaut LR, De Pauw G: Biomechanical aspects of Class II mechanics with special emphasis on deep bite correction as part of the treatment goal. In Nanda R, editor: *Biomechanics in clinical orthodontics*, Philadelphia, 1997, Saunders, pp 86-98.
43. Gelgor IE, Buyukyilmaz T, Karaman AI, et al: Intraosseous screw-supported upper molar distalization, *Angle Orthod* 74:838-850, 2004.
44. Crismani AG, Bernhart T, Bantleon HS, Cope JS: Palatal implants: the Straumann Orthosystem, *Semin Orthod* 11:16-23, 2005.
45. Kinzinger G, Wehrbein H, Byloff FK, et al: Innovative anchorage alternatives for molar distalization: an overview, *J Orofac Orthop* 66:397-413, 2005.
46. Paik CH, Nagasaka S, Hirashita A: Class III nonextraction treatment with miniscrew anchorage, *J Clin Orthod* 40:480-484, 2006.
47. Roberts WE, Marshall KJ, Mozsary PG: Rigid endosseous implant utilized as anchorage to protract molars and close an atrophic extraction site, *Angle Orthod* 60:135-152, 1990.
48. Sugawara J, Kanzaki R, Nanda R, et al: Distal movement of maxillary molars in nongrowing patients with the skeletal anchorage system, *Am J Orthod Dentofacial Orthop* 129:723-733, 2006.
49. Sugawara J, Daimaruya T, Umemori M, et al: Distal movement of mandibular molars in adult patients with the skeletal anchorage system, *Am J Orthod Dentofacial Orthop* 125:130-138, 2004.
50. Roberts WE: Bone physiology of tooth movement, ankylosis, and osseointegration, *Semin Orthod* 6:173-182, 2000.
51. Roberts WE, Arbuckle GR, Analoui M: Rate of mesial translation of mandibular molars using implant-anchored mechanics, *Angle Orthod* 66:331-338, 1996.
52. Takano-Yamamoto T: Clinical application of mini-screw implants as an orthodontic anchorage, World Mini Implant Congress, Las Vegas, 2006.
53. Burstone CJ: Precision lingual arches: active applications, *J Clin Orthod* 23:101-109, 1989.
54. Van Steenbergen E, Nanda R: Biomechanics of orthodontic correction of dental asymmetries, *Am J Orthod Dentofacial Orthop* 107:618-624, 1995.
55. Kuhlberg A: Cantilever springs: force system and clinical applications, *Semin Orthod* 7:150-159, 2001.
56. Lindauer SJ, Isaacson RJ: One-couple orthodontic appliance systems, *Semin Orthod* 1:12-24, 1995.
57. Chen YJ, Chen YH, Lin LD, Yao CC: Removal torque of miniscrews used for orthodontic anchorage: a preliminary report, *Int J Oral Maxillofac Implants* 21:283-289, 2006.

PART IV

ANCHORAGE DEVICE SYSTEMS AND CLINICAL APPLICATIONS

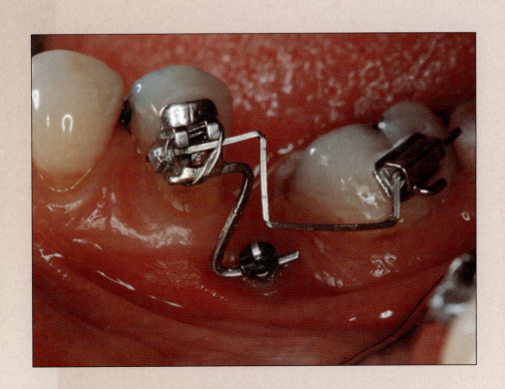

CHAPTER 8

Appliances, Mechanics, and Treatment Strategies Toward Orthognathic-Like Treatment Results

Eric Jein-Wein Liou and James Cheng-Yi Lin

Orthodontic miniscrews have been applied as osseous anchorage for the treatment of various malocclusions.[1-18] Without any limitations in anchorage, it is now possible to move teeth maximally by using miniscrews and mimicking treatment results of orthognathic surgery in certain types of malocclusion,[13,15-18] such as Class I and II dentoalveolar protrusion, Class III dentoalveolar protrusion, anterior open bite, and Class II mandibular retrognathism. This chapter defines "orthognathic-like orthodontics" as the orthodontics that mimics results of orthognathic surgical treatment, but without surgery, by moving teeth maximally with miniscrews as the osseous anchorage.

Treatment strategies toward orthognathic-like orthodontics can be developed after the following two issues regarding migration of the miniscrew and biological boundary of orthodontic tooth movement are clarified:

1. Do the orthodontic miniscrews remain stationary throughout the entire treatment, and if the miniscrews migrate, where would the appropriate insertion sites be located?
2. Is there a biological boundary of orthodontic tooth movement, and if there is a biological boundary, what strategies would be used toward orthognathic-like orthodontics?

STATUS OF MINISCREWS DURING TREATMENT

MINISCREW MIGRATION UNDER ORTHODONTIC LOADING

Both dental implants and orthodontic miniscrews have revealed a certain degree of migration under loading, although both types were clinically stable and had no detectable mobility.[19-21]

For example, endosseous implants had been reported to migrate 0.5 mm in an edentulous ridge with low bone density.[19] Also, the miniscrews in infrazygomatic (IZ) crests of the maxilla clinically migrated up to 1.5 mm under orthodontic loadings.[20,21] Both the predrilling and the self-drilling miniscrews migrated under loading,[21] although experimentally the self-drilling miniscrew had much less mobility and more bone-to-metal contact than the predrilling miniscrew.[22] The migration direction of miniscrews reflected the force direction, and the patterns of migration were extrusion and controlled tipping, extrusion and bodily movement, and extrusion and uncontrolled-tipping. The force magnitude did not correlate with the migration, but the longer the loading period, the greater the miniscrew migration. The miniscrew migration may be a progressive process throughout the loading period rather than a temporary process.[21]

Migration of a dental implant was found to result from microfracture of the periimplant microcalli and vigorous bone remodeling and resorption on the tension and compression sides.[19] The same might apply to the miniscrew migration, although the exact mechanism is not clear. Factors such as the premature loading and bone density at the implant site may also contribute to miniscrew migration.

A waiting period generally is not necessary after miniscrew insertion because the mechanical retention is sufficient to sustain a loaded miniscrew without compromising its stability.[2-4,23] However, a layer of fibrous tissue was found interposed between the implant and bone contacts when the dental implant was loaded prematurely,[24] which also explains migration of a loaded miniscrew or dental implant.

Dental implants can migrate in low-bone–density edentulous ridges.[19] This may even apply to miniscrews, especially in the maxillary or mandibular interdental

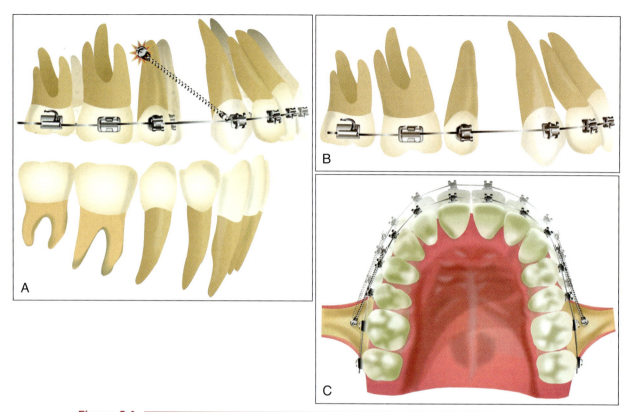

Figure 8-1

A, Both the miniscrews and the teeth might be subjected to migrate and move causing root injury during orthodontic treatment. **B,** Root injury can be avoided by keeping a 2.0-mm safety clearance between the miniscrew and dental roots. **C,** Root injury can also be avoided by inserting miniscrews in the non–tooth-bearing area.

areas where bone density is the least.[25,26] Although miniscrew migration in the interdental areas has not been reported before, it does not mean that it does not happen. The fact that the miniscrew is inserted perpendicular to the bone surface[10] or 30 to 40 degrees to the long axis of teeth in the interdental area[7,8] makes miniscrew migration difficult to reveal on a lateral or posteroanterior (PA) cephalometric radiograph.

APPROPRIATE MINISCREW INSERTION SITE WHEN A LOADED MINISCREW MIGRATES

Miniscrew migration in non–tooth-bearing areas may not be a serious problem, but miniscrews also may migrate and hit adjacent dental roots in tooth-bearing areas (Figure 8-1, *A*). On the other hand, teeth themselves might move and hit the miniscrews, even if the screws remain stationary in the tooth-bearing areas. The interdental areas therefore are not appropriate insertion sites when buccal teeth need to be distalized or protracted. Miniscrews should be inserted in non–tooth-bearing areas with no foramina, major nerves, or blood vessels or in tooth-bearing areas by keeping a safety clearance of 2.0 mm between the miniscrew and dental root[20,21] (Figure 8-1, *B*). The non–tooth-bearing areas, such as the IZ crest of maxilla, palate, and oblique ridge of mandible, are the recommended insertion sites for orthognathic-like orthodontics (Figure 8-1, *C*).

Maxillary Infrazygomatic Crest

The IZ crest is a palpable pillar of cortical bone between the zygomatic process of maxilla and the alveolar process (Figure 8-2). In younger individuals the IZ crest is between the maxillary second premolar and the first molar, whereas it is above the maxillary first molar in adults. It has been used as osseous anchorage for maxillary canine retraction, anterior retraction, en masse anterior retraction, or intrusion of the maxillary posterior teeth.* Its thickness ranges from 5.5 to 8.8 mm in adults.[31] The IZ crest consists of two cortical plates—the buccal cortical plate and the floor or lateral wall of maxillary sinus—with cancellous bone between the plates. These plates provide bicortical fixation and possibly better primary miniscrew stability when the miniscrew penetrates into the maxillary sinus.

The maxillary sinuses must be free of infection before screw insertion. Maxillary sinusitis is a contraindication. Therefore, the clinician must check the patient's medical history, palpate the buccal cheeks for tenderness, and check the clarity of the maxillary sinuses on panoramic

---

*References 2, 6, 10, 13-18, 20, 27-30.

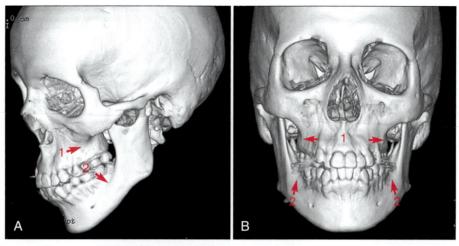

Figure 8-2
Lateral view **(A)** and frontal view **(B)** of non–tooth-bearing areas for miniscrew insertion in orthognathic-like miniscrew orthodontics; the infrazygomatic crest in the maxilla **(1)** and oblique ridges in the mandible **(2)**.

and PA radiographs before insertion of miniscrews in the IZ crests of maxilla.

Mandibular Oblique Ridge

The mandibular oblique ridge is a thick pillar of cortical bone extending from the ascending ramus down to the body of mandible and merging into the alveolar process distally and laterally to the mandibular first molar in adult patients (see Figure 8-2). The mergence of mandibular oblique ridge and alveolar process is palpable clinically when the fingers feel right and left along the ridge. The risk of hitting the dental roots during insertion of the miniscrew in the mandibular oblique ridge is almost nonexistent when the miniscrew is inserted perpendicular to the ridge's surface.

MINISCREWS FOR ORTHOGNATHIC-LIKE ORTHODONTICS

Whether self-drilling or predrilling, an orthodontic miniscrew must be (1) durable without breakage during insertion or removal, (2) compatible and user-friendly with the current edgewise system, and (3) sustained well throughout the loading period.

To be durable without breakage during insertion or removal, an orthodontic miniscrew made of titanium (Ti) alloy has a higher tensile and compressive strength than the pure-Ti miniscrew. Titanium alloy has been the material of choice in most orthodontic miniscrews.

To be compatible with the current edgewise system, an orthodontic miniscrew with a bracket or bracketlike head, auxiliary rectangular tube, hook, and platform is more user-friendly. The platform is between the screw body and head; its thickness provides an elevation for the elastics or coil springs from the gingiva or oral mucosa and prevents the screw head from embedding into the soft tissue. For example, the LOMAS (Lin/Liou Orthodontic Mini Anchor System, Mondeal Medical System GMBH, Tuttlingen, Germany) is a self-drilling miniscrew of Ti alloy that has a platform and bracket head rather than bracketlike structure.[10,14,32] The LOMAS hook screw works like a molar hook, and the LOMAS Quattro screw has a Lewis bracket and an auxiliary rectangular tube for the direct application of a rectangular or round archwire or auxiliary lever arm (Figure 8-3). The advantage of the auxiliary rectangular tube (vs. round hole) is three-dimensional (3D) control of a rectangular archwire.

The *diameter* rather than the length of a miniscrew determines its stability.[33] To be sustained well throughout the entire loading period, a miniscrew therefore should be thick rather than long. We recommend a miniscrew that is thicker than 1.5 mm for the tasks in orthognathic-like orthodontics. In the IZ crest and mandibular oblique ridge, a miniscrew of 2.0 mm in diameter and 9 mm in length is recommended.[32]

MINISCREW INSERTION IN INFRAZYGOMATIC CREST OF MAXILLA AND MANDIBULAR OBLIQUE RIDGE

Bone Surface Hardness–Guided Technique

We developed a technique guided by bone surface hardness for miniscrew insertion in the IZ crest of maxilla and mandibular oblique ridge.[10,32] Before insertion, bone hardness (density) is evaluated on computed tomography (CT) images, using Hounsfield units (HU),[25,26] or by tissue punch, to remove the overlying soft tissue and examine the bone surface hardness of the insertion site (Figure 8-4). The punch is made through the soft tissue and periosteum and firmly into the cortical surface of the insertion site. The bone surface hardness is D3/D4 when the tissue punch makes an indent and bites into the cortical bone; if not, it is D1/D2 (Table 8-1).

A self-drilling miniscrew can be driven directly into surface hardness of D3/D4, whereas a pilot-drilling hole is necessary with D1/D2, regardless whether the

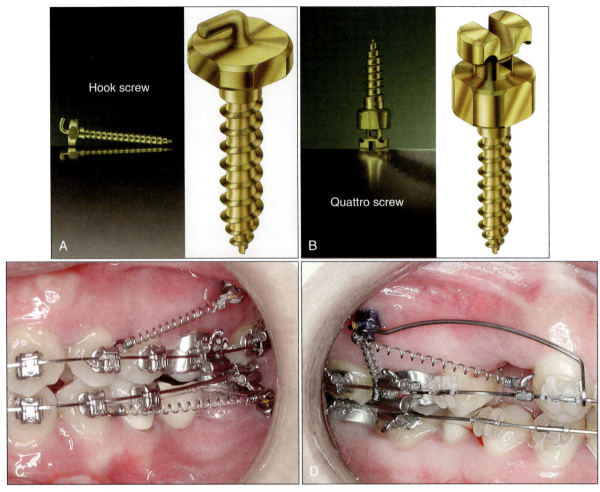

Figure 8-3
A, LOMAS hook screw. **B,** LOMAS Quattro screw. **C,** Hook of LOMAS hook miniscrew used for direct attachment of nickel-titanium (Ni-Ti) coil springs. **D,** LOMAS Quatrro screw is used to hold an auxiliary rectangular archwire (e.g., intruding lever arm). Ni-Ti coils are directly attached to the end of the intruding lever arm. Miniscrew is 2 × 9 mm.

TABLE 8-1	Misch Bone Density, Hounsfield Unit, and Corresponding Surface Hardness	
Misch Bone Density	Hounsfield Units	Tissue Punch into Bone Surface
D1	>1250	Surface indent
D2	850-1250	Indent but no biting
D3	350-850	Indent with biting
D4	150-350	Indent with biting

miniscrew is self-drilling or predrilling (Figure 8-5). The pilot drill should be at least 75% less in size than the selected miniscrew size.[34] The drilling speed should be 500 to 800 rpm under thorough normal-saline irrigation to avoid overheating and necrotic bone.[35,36]

Infrazygomatic Crest of Maxilla
The bone surface hardness of the IZ crest of maxilla is usually D3 to D4, whereas that of the mandibular oblique ridge is usually D1 to D2. In the IZ crest of maxilla a self-drilling miniscrew can be inserted directly without pilot drilling.[10,32] To avoid injury to the mesiobuccal root of the maxillary first molar, the miniscrew is inserted 14 to 16 mm above and 55 to 70 degrees to the maxillary occlusal table[31] (Figure 8-6). Because the miniscrew is inserted at an angle rather than perpendicular to the bone surface of the IZ crest, pilot-drilling an indent hole in the cortical bone is helpful for holding the tip of the miniscrew and avoiding miniscrew slippage and bone stripping during insertion.[32]

Mandibular Oblique Ridge
In the mandibular oblique ridge, whether the miniscrew is self-drilling or predrilling, it is always necessary to drill a pilot hole through the cortical bone.[10,32] This helps to prevent cracks in the cortical plate and breakage of the miniscrew during insertion. A 1.5-mm drill is recommended for a 2.0-mm miniscrew. For ease of insertion and application of orthodontic appliances, the miniscrew should be inserted 1 to 2 mm behind the mergence of the oblique ridge and alveolar process so that the mini-

8 Appliances, Mechanics, and Treatment Strategies Toward Orthognathic-Like Treatment Results

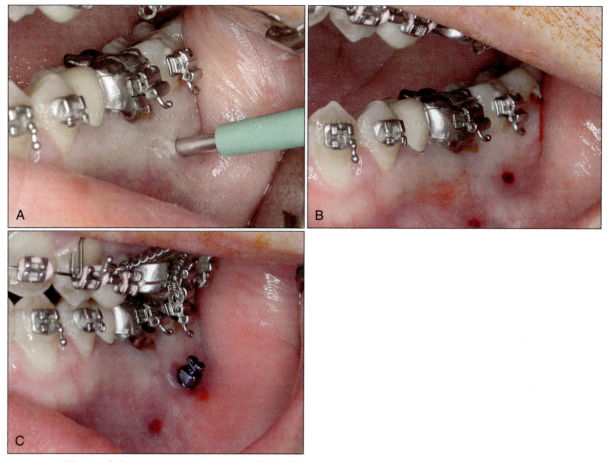

Figure 8-4
A, Tissue punch inserted into the soft tissue. **B,** Miniscrew insertion site. **C,** Miniscrew inserted.

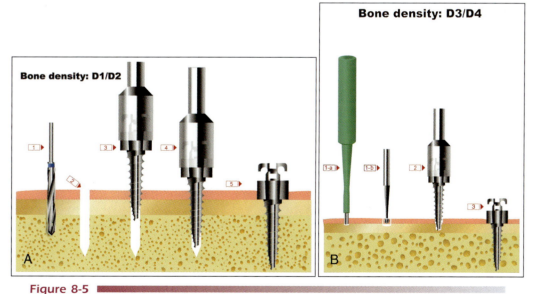

Figure 8-5
Miniscrew Insertion Technique Guided by Bone Surface Hardness. A, When the bone surface hardness is D1/D2 the insertion procedure is to remove the soft tissue with a tissue punch and to pilot-drill a hole through the cortical bone (*1* and *2*), then drive the miniscrew into the insertion site with a screw driver (*3, 4,* and *5*). **B,** When the bone surface hardness is D3/D4 the procedure is to remove the soft tissue with a tissue punch (*1-a*), to make a small indent in the cortex with a rotary bur when it is necessary (*1-b*), then drive the miniscrew into the insertion site with a screw driver (*2* and *3*).

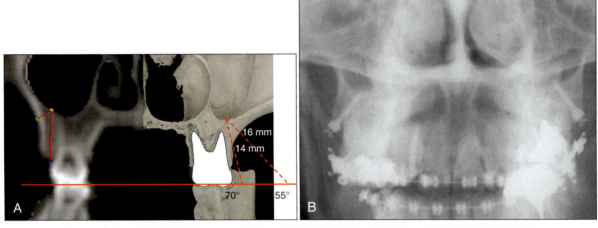

Figure 8-6
Miniscrew Insertion in Infrazygomatic Crest of Maxilla. A, Safe zone for placement of the miniscrew in reference to the occlusal plane. **B,** Posteroanterior cephalometric radiograph showing the angulation of the miniscrew in relation to the buccal alveolar bone of the maxillary buccal segment.

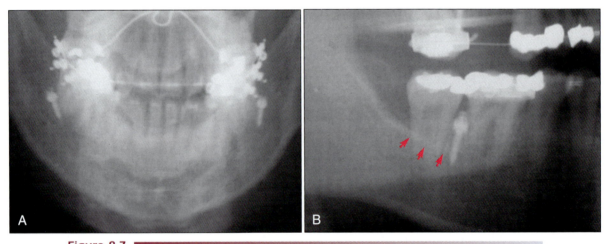

Figure 8-7
Miniscrew Insertion in Mandibular Oblique Ridge. A, Posteroanterior cephalometric radiograph showing the insertion angle of the miniscrew in the mandibular oblique ridge and the relation to the alveolar bone in the mandibular buccal segment. **B,** Radiograph from a lateral view showing the anteroposterior relationship of the miniscrew to the mandibular oblique ridge *(arrows)* and the mandibular molars.

screw is kept in the ridge without infringing on the buccal mucosa. The insertion site is usually between the mandibular first and second molars in adults.[32] The drilling and miniscrew insertion angle is perpendicular to the surface of the mandibular oblique ridge (Figure 8-7).

General Guidelines
Regardless of where an orthodontic miniscrew penetrates into the IZ crest or mandibular oblique ridge, the emergence of an orthodontic miniscrew is better kept at the attached gingiva or at the mucogingival junction (Figure 8-8). The emergence of a miniscrew through the oral mucosa frequently causes soft tissue irritation.[37]

Only topical anesthesia or local infiltration of 0.3 to 0.5 mL anesthesia is necessary for miniscrew insertion in the IZ crest of maxilla or in the mandibular oblique ridge.[32,38] It is extremely important not to use a complete nerve block so that the patient is aware of any pain or soreness as the miniscrew approaches the periodontal ligament of a dental root. Pain or soreness means the miniscrew must be removed immediately and redirected to avoid dental root injury.

Postoperative Care
A postoperative PA cephalometric radiograph is obtained to ensure that the miniscrew is not impinging on any dental root. Antibiotics may be unnecessary after miniscrew insertion when preoperative disinfection has been performed intraorally and extraorally. However, 2% chlorhexidine is still recommended for postoperative care.[32]

A periodontal dressing around the miniscrew for 1 week adapts the soft tissue and periosteum of the

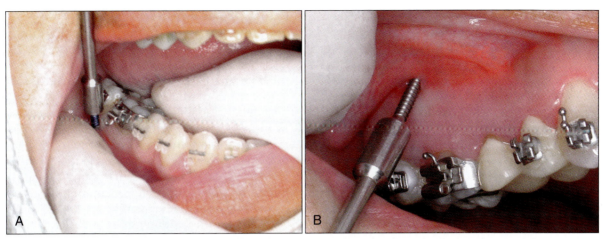

Figure 8-8
A, Orthodontic miniscrew penetrating mandibular oblique ridge. **B**, Orthodontic miniscrew penetrating infrazygomatic crest.

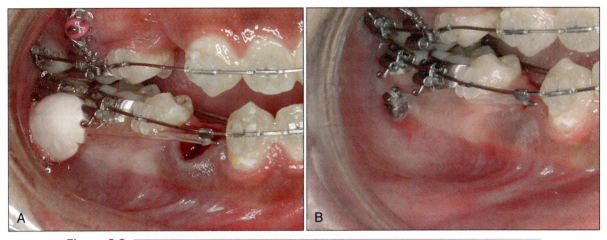

Figure 8-9
A, Postoperative periodontal dressing around a miniscrew. **B**, The head of the miniscrew is not embedded into the soft tissue.

insertion site back to the bone surface and prevents the head of miniscrew from embedding into soft tissue[39] (Figure 8-9). The periodontal dressing material can also help alleviate soft tissue inflammation around the miniscrew site during orthodontic treatment.[39]

Clinical Evaluation

In a review of 77 LOMAS screws inserted in the IZ crest of maxilla, the 1-year success rate was 91.9%.[40] We also found a learning curve in miniscrew insertion[41]; the learning period was approximately 8 months. The failure rate was higher in the first few months of miniscrew insertion, then decreased and leveled off after the eighth month.

BIOLOGICAL BOUNDARY OF ORTHODONTIC TOOTH MOVEMENT

For any orthodontic tooth movement, the tooth should remain within the anatomical boundaries of the dentoalveolar process to survive and function. For distalization or retraction of maxillary teeth, the boundaries are the palatal cortical plate and the posterior wall of the maxillary tuberosity. For distalization or retraction of mandibular teeth, the boundaries are the lingual plate of the alveolar ridge and the ascending ramus. For maxillary intrusion, the boundaries are the floors of the nasal cavity and maxillary sinus. For protraction of maxillary or mandibular incisors, the boundaries are the labial plate of the maxilla and mandible.

The phrase "alveolar bone traces tooth movement" has been one explanation for the biological and physiological mechanisms for unlimited orthodontic tooth movement. Such movement assumes that the osseous housing can fully reconstitute itself in any direction of tooth movement. Actually, clinicians are barely able to move teeth in this way because of the limits in conventional anchorage and patient compliance.

The osseous response of alveolar bone during orthodontic tooth movement, such as maxillary or mandibular anterior retraction, should be the same regardless of whether conventional or miniscrew anchorage is used. Clinical studies in conventional anchorage have indicated limitation in anterior-posterior incisor movement. Patients with narrow alveolar width, such as both labial and lingual to the mandibular incisors, and lingual to the maxillary incisors in individuals with high mandibular plane angle (MPA), are most likely to demonstrate limitation in orthodontic correction.[42]

ALVEOLAR OSSEOUS REACTIONS
During Incisor Retraction

The osseous reactions of the labial and the palatal alveolus during retraction of maxillary incisors are different. The labial alveolus is the tension side of the retraction where bone deposits. It follows incisor retraction, and its thickness remains unchanged[43] or increases.[44] The thickness of the superior and inferior labial maxillary alveolus increases 28% and 65%, respectively, when the incisors are retracted with lingual root torque.[44] The tension side of tooth movement in maxilla follows the postulate of "bone traces tooth movement," and the alveolar thickness remains unchanged or even increases (Figure 8-10).

The palatal alveolus is the pressure side of the retraction where bone resorbs. Alveolar bone remodeling occurs at the margin and midroot levels[43] but has a definite limit in remodeling where the root apex abuts against the palatal cortex.[45,46] The alveolar thickness decreases after the retraction.[43] The pressure side of tooth movement in maxilla remodels but decreases in alveolar thickness, and the root apex should remain inside the alveolus (see Figure 8-10).

The osseous reaction of the labial and lingual alveolus in mandible during incisor retraction is similar to that in maxilla (see Figure 8-10). The tension side, labial alveolus, follows the postulate of "alveolar bone traces tooth movement," and its thickness remains unchanged, except at the crest level, which may decrease significantly.[43] The pressure side, lingual alveolus, remodels, but its width significantly decreases after incisor retraction.[43] The root apex also should be left inside the alveolus.

The maxillary and mandibular alveolus remodels and decreases in thickness on the pressure side,[43-46] and excessive incisor retraction causes loss of alveolar bone and exposure of the root.[42,44,47-57] Similarly, excessive transverse tooth movement also causes dehiscence and fenestration on the pressure side.[53-55,58,59] Clinical studies[46] and autopsy findings[53-55] revealed the fenestration and dehiscence on the pressure side could be reestablished by a thin layer of bone, but experimental studies indicated that the thin layer of bone was insufficient to cover the root completely.[48,60,61] Clinically we observed relapse of the root and apex back into alveolus when maxillary incisors were overretracted, and apparently the palatal plate was repaired because of the tension-side reaction when the incisors relapsed labially (Figure 8-11).

During Molar Intrusion

The osseous reactions on the pressure side during intrusion are similar to those of incisor retraction. The nasal floor cortex remodeled and the mucosal membrane lifted intranasally to encompass the intruded tooth root apices when maxillary premolars were experimentally intruded remarkably into nasal cavity in dogs (4.2 mm of intrusion in 7 months).[62] However, the nasal floor remodeled into a thin layer of newly formed bone sufficient to cover the tooth root. In the mandible the inferior alveolar neurovascular bundles repositioned inferiorly when the mandibular molars were experimentally intruded, remarkably (3.4 mm of intrusion in 7 months), to reach the inferior alveolar neurovascular bundles in dogs.[63]

THE PRESSURE SIDE IS A BIOLOGICAL BOUNDARY

The tension side of tooth movement follows the postulate of "bone traces tooth movement," and the alveolar thickness remains unchanged or even increases,[43,44] whereas the pressure side of tooth movement is a biological limit for orthodontic tooth movement.[43-46] The biological limits set by the pressure side are thinning of alveolus, loss of alveolar bone, fenestration, dehiscence, and limited capability of reestablishing the cortex, whether the tooth movement is incisor retraction, buccolingual movement, or molar intrusion.[42-62] A thin layer of alveolar cortical bone compromises periodontal support, health, and posttreatment stability.

Because of the inherent biological limits set by the pressure side of tooth movement, the range of orthodontic tooth movement will be limited even with miniscrews as the osseous anchorage.

TREATMENT STRATEGIES

Orthognathic-like orthodontics strives to mimic the surgical results of orthognathic surgery by moving teeth to their limit with miniscrews but without the complications of fenestration and dehiscence on the pressure side and moving root apex out of alveolus. Unfortunately, miniscrews preserve anchorage but do not prevent fenestration and dehiscence.

A thicker alveolus on the pressure side allows greater range of tooth movement. To move teeth maximally without fenestration and dehiscence on the pressure side and without moving the root apex out of the alveolus, one strategy is to increase the alveolar thickness on the pressure side by selective decortication and onlay bone graft. The advantage of this approach is that the rate of tooth movement also could be accelerated.[64,65] The disadvantage is that the extensive full-thickness mucoperiosteal flap surgery and the transient burst of severe bone resorption after flap surgery[66,67] might neutralize the osteogenic effect of the onlay bone graft.

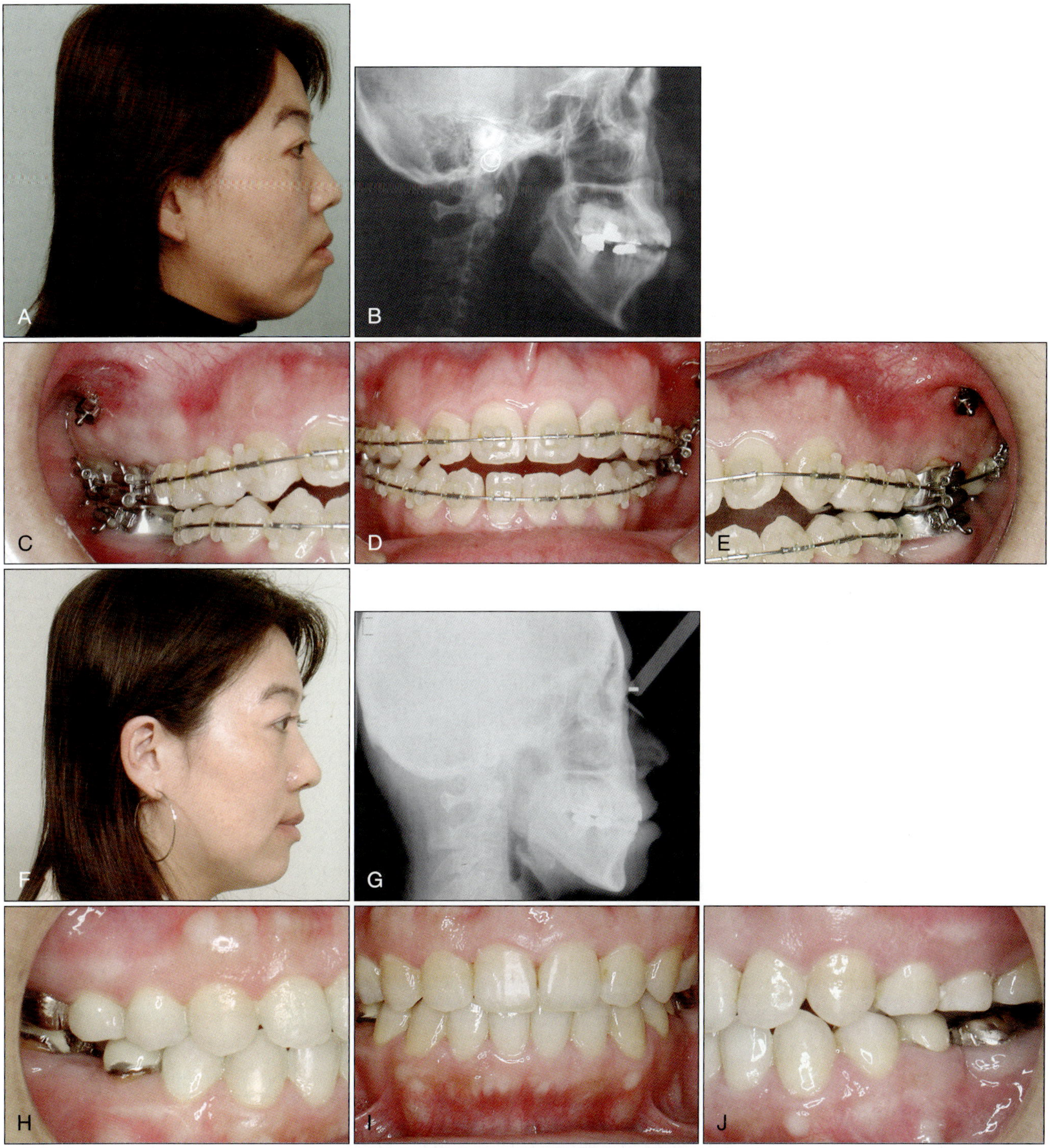

Figure 8-10
Orthognathic-Like Treatment Results for Anterior Open Bite Using Miniscrews and Non-extraction. The maxillary dentition was distalized and intruded, and the mandible rotated upward and forward. The maxillary and mandibular labial plates traced the movement incisors and their thickness remained unchanged, while the maxillary and mandibular lingual plates remodeled but their thickness decreased. Pretreatment: **A**, facial photograph; **B**, cephalometric radiograph; **C** to **E**, intraoal photographs. Posttreatment: **F**, facial photograph; **G**, cephalometric radiograph; **H** to **J**, intraoral photographs.

Continued

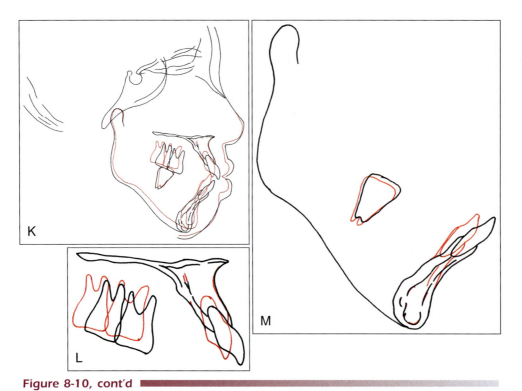

Figure 8-10, cont'd
K to M, Superimpositions showing pretreatment findings *(black line)* and posttreatment results *(red line)*.

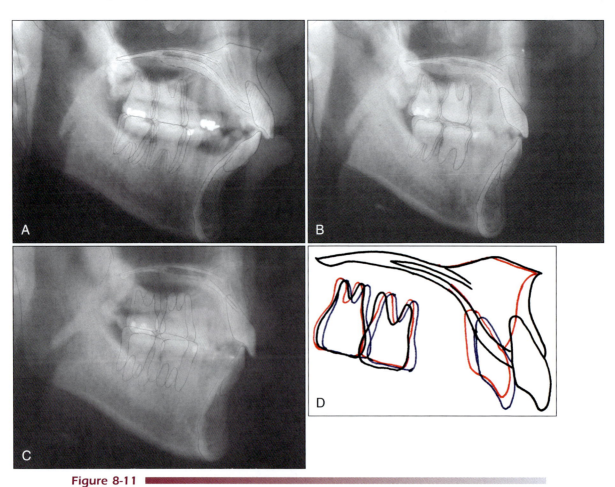

Figure 8-11
Relapse of Root and Apex Back into Alveolus from Overretracted Maxillary Incisors.
A, Pretreatment radiograph. B, Posttreatment radiograph. C, Posttreatment radiograph 2 years later. D, Superimposition showing pretreatment findings *(black line)*, posttreatment results *(red line)*, and posttreatment findings at 2 years *(blue line)*.

DENTOALVEOLAR PROTRUSION

The dentoalveolar process is tapered in shape, thinner at the tooth level, and thicker at the basal bone level. Apparently, intrusion of anterior teeth allows a greater range of anterior retraction because they are intruded into the basal bone level, where the bone is thicker, and because the limit of alveolar bone remodeling, where the root apex abuts against the palatal cortex, is moved apically (see Figure 8-10).

The treatment strategy for dentoalveolar protrusion is therefore *en masse anterior retraction-and-intrusion,* to mimic the maxillary or mandibular anterior subapical osteotomy, in which the first premolars are extracted and the entire anterior segment is set back and repositioned apically. It is indicated in the following types of protrusion:

Class I bimaxillary dentoalveolar protrusion (Figure 8-12). The maxillary and mandibular first premolars are extracted and the miniscrews inserted in the IZ crests of maxilla and/or mandibular oblique ridges. The amount of intrusion depends on the extent of anterior retraction. The more severe the dentoalveolar protrusion, the more the intrusion is needed.

Class II maxillary dentoalveolar protrusion (Figure 8-13). The maxillary first premolars are extracted and the miniscrews inserted in the IZ crests of maxilla. The maxillary anterior teeth must be intruded as much as possible for overbite reduction and maximal anterior retraction. The maxillary posterior teeth may be intruded as well, during intrusion of the anterior teeth, for upward and forward rotation of the mandible, increasing the chin prominence and chin-throat length. These steps mimic the maxillary anterior subapical osteotomy, Le Fort I impaction of the maxilla, and upward and forward rotation of the mandible.

Class III mandibular dentoalveolar protrusion (Figure 8-14). The mandibular first premolars are extracted and the miniscrews inserted in the mandibular oblique ridges. The mandibular anterior teeth must be intruded as much as possible for maximal anterior retraction. The maxillary anterior teeth may be extruded as well, when appropriate, to tilt the maxillary occlusal plane downward anteriorly and thus rotate the mandible downward and backward to improve the lateral facial profile. These steps mimic the mandibular anterior subapical osteotomy and Le Fort I anterior downward repositioning of maxilla.

Class III mandibular prognathism with retroclined mandibular incisors, thin mandibular anterior dentoalveolus, high MPA, or long face should be treated with surgical orthodontics. Orthognathic-like orthodontics is only indicated in cases of Class III mandibular dentoalveolar protrusion with enough thickness of the dentoalveolus lingual to the mandibular incisors and average to low mandibular plane angle and anterior facial height.

MECHANICS AND APPLIANCES

Four basic types of mechanics have been developed for the orthognathic-like orthodontics: (1) en masse anterior retraction, (2) anterior intrusion, (3) posterior intrusion, and (4) posterior intrusion-and-distalization. Each type of mechanics can work independently for a single purpose or can be selectively combined into advanced mechanics for multiple purposes[10,14-18,20,21,32] (Table 8-2 and Figures 8-15 to 8-19).

The design of these mechanics follows the concept of "one miniscrew in one insertion site for multiple mechanics" so that the number of miniscrews is kept as low as possible. The following orthodontic appliances have been developed for the mechanics toward orthognathic-like orthodontics:

- *Appropriate size of stainless steel archwires with palatal/lingual root torque at the anterior teeth and attachment of crimpable hooks for the en masse anterior retraction or retraction-and-intrusion.* The palatal/lingual crown torque avoids excessive palatal or lingual tipping of the anterior teeth during retraction. The crimpable hook can be attached 3 mm distal to the bracket of maxillary canine or mandibular second premolar on the stainless steel archwire.

- *Medium-force nickel-titanium (Ni-Ti) closed-coil springs.* The springs are attached between the miniscrews and the crimpable hooks on the archwire for the en masse anterior retraction-and-intrusion, posterior teeth intrusion, or posterior intrusion-and-distalization.

- *0.032-inch β-Ti transpalatal arch and lingual-holding-arch with 0 to 6 degrees of mesial angulation and 0 to 10 degrees of buccal root torque.* They are removable, adjustable, and could be inserted into the weldable/bondable lingual sheaths. They allow bodily intrusion and prevent buccal version of the posterior teeth during intrusion. The material of stainless steel is not resilient enough for the purposes.

- *0.019 × 0.025 β-Ti intruding/extruding lever arms with 70 degrees of tip-back bend.* These removable, adjustable arms can be inserted into the auxiliary molar tube or in the rectangular auxiliary tube of the LOMAS Quattro screw to provide en masse intrusion or extrusion of the anterior teeth.

ANTERIOR OPEN BITE

Intrusion of the posterior teeth and upward rotation of the mandible using miniscrews or miniplates is one treatment strategy for anterior open bite.[13,17,27] However, this strategy may not be appropriate for all cases. For example, the lateral facial profile may be worsened by upward rotation of mandible in patients with Class III anterior open bite.

Class III Anterior Open Bite with Mandibular Dentoalveolar Protrusion

Class III anterior open bite with retroclined mandibular incisors and high MPA is not an indication for miniscrew orthodontics. The strategy for Class III anterior

Text continued on p. 188

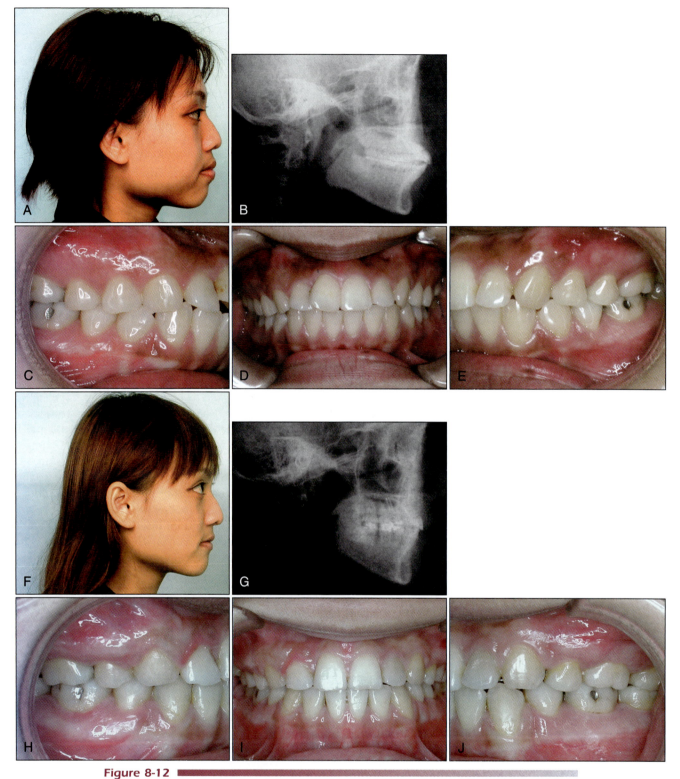

Figure 8-12

Orthognathic-Like Treatment Results for Class I Bimaxillary Dentoalveolar Protrusion Using Miniscrews. Maxillary incisors were retracted and intruded to mimic maxillary anterior subapical osteotomy. The mandibular incisors were tipped lingually. The root apexes of maxillary and mandibular incisors remained inside the alveolus. Pretreatment: **A**, facial photograph; **B**, cephalometric radiograph; **C** to **E**, intraoral photographs. Posttreatment: **F**, facial photograph; **G**, cephalometric radiograph; **H** to **J**, intraoral photographs.

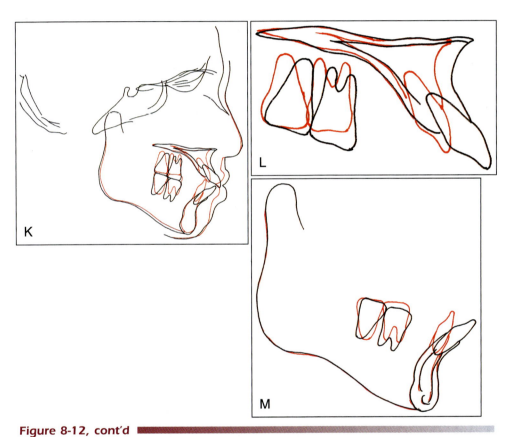

Figure 8-12, cont'd
K to M, Superimpositions showing pretreatment findings *(black line)* and posttreatment results *(red line)*.

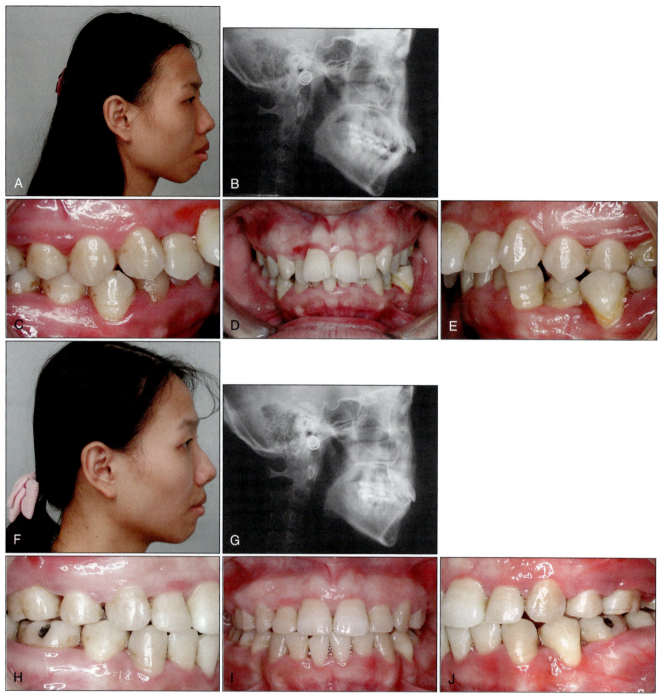

Figure 8-13

Orthognathic-Like Treatment Results for Class II Bimaxillary Dentoalveolar Protrusion Using Miniscrews. Maxillary incisors were retracted and intruded to mimic maxillary anterior subapical osteotomy, and the entire maxillary dentition was intruded to mimic LeFort I impaction of maxilla. The mandibular molars were held without extrusion, and the mandibular incisors were intruded for maximizing mandibular upward rotation and chin prominence. The root apexes of maxillary and mandibular incisors were remained inside the alveolus. Pretreatment: **A**, facial photograph; **B**, cephalometric radiograph; **C** to **E**, intraoral photographs. Posttreatment: **F**, facial photograph; **G**, cephalometric radiograph; **H** to **J**, intraoral photographs.

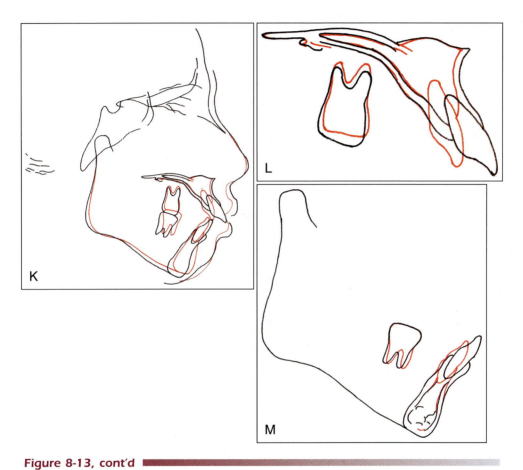

Figure 8-13, cont'd
K to M, Superimpositions showing pretreatment findings *(black line)* and posttreatment results *(red line)*.

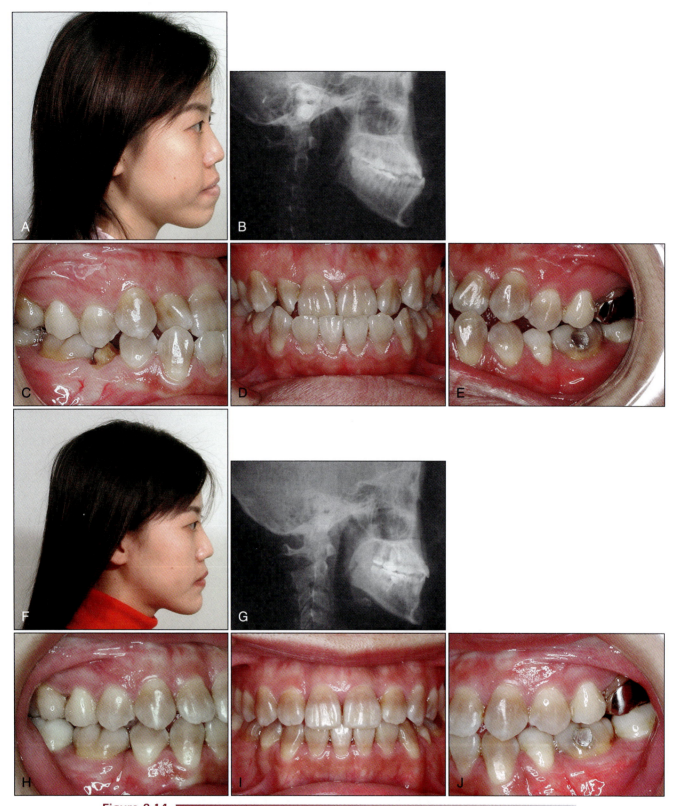

Figure 8-14
Orthognathic-Like Treatment Results for Class III Dentoalveolar Protrusion Using Miniscrews. Mandibular incisors were retracted bodily to mimic mandibular anterior subapical osteotomy. Pretreatment: **A**, facial photograph; **B**, cephalometric radiograph; **C** to **E**, intraoral photographs. Posttreatment: **F**, facial photograph; **G**, cephalometric radiograph; **H** to **J**, intraoral photographs.

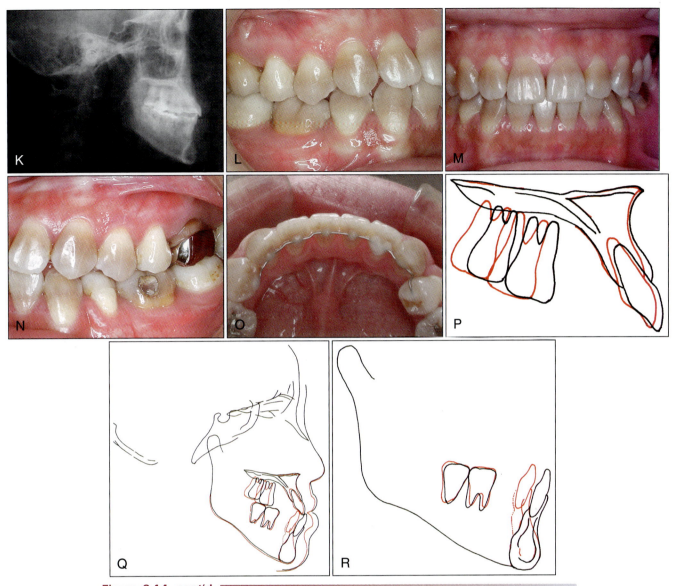

Figure 8-14, cont'd
Although the mandibular incisors overretracted without intrusion and the root apices were not left inside the alveolus, the 2-year posttreatment cephalometric radiograph (**K**) and clinical examination (**L-O**) revealed sound periodontal support around the incisors. **P** to **R**, Superimpositions showing pretreatment findings *(black line)* and posttreatment results *(red line)*.

TABLE 8-2 Select Mechanics for Anchorage in Orthognathic-like Treatment

Mechanics	Miniscrew	Insertion Site	Appliance
En masse anterior retraction Posterior intrusion	Hook or Quattro screw	IZ crest Oblique ridge	Ni-Ti coil spring
En masse anterior retraction Posterior intrusion-and-distalization	Hook or Quattro screw	IZ crest Oblique ridge	Ni-Ti coil spring
En masse anterior retraction-and-intrusion	Quattro screw	IZ crest Oblique ridge	Ni-Ti coil spring Intruding lever arm
En masse anterior retraction-and-intrusion Posterior intrusion	Quattro screw	IZ crest Oblique ridge	Ni-Ti coil spring Intruding lever arm
En masse anterior retraction-and-intrusion Posterior intrusion-and-distalization	Quattro screw	IZ crest Oblique ridge	Ni-Ti coil spring Intruding lever arm

IZ, Infrazygomatic; *Ni-Ti*, nickel-titanium.

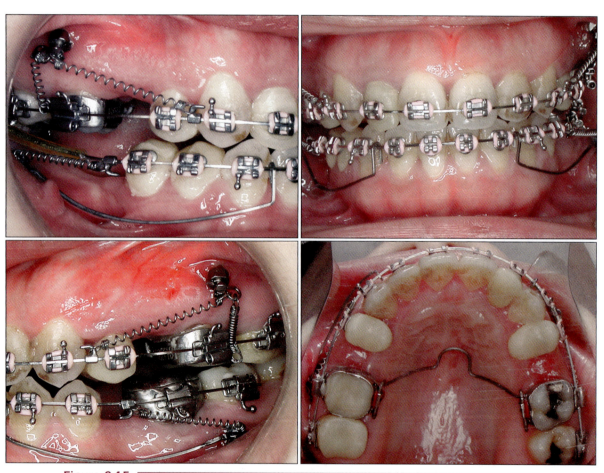

Figure 8-15
Intraoral photographs demonstrating advanced mechanics of en masse anterior retraction and posterior intrusion for orthognathic-like orthodontics.

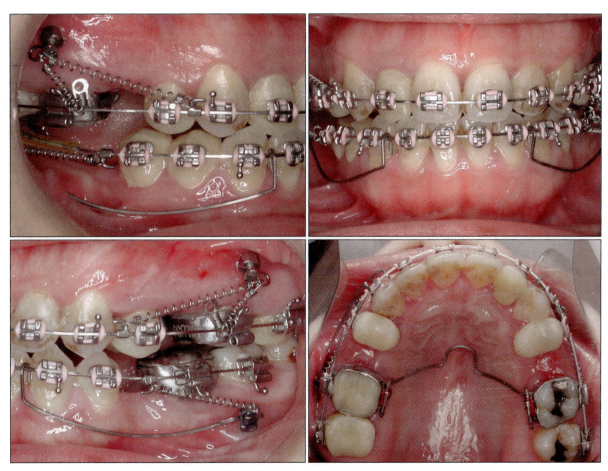

Figure 8-16
Intraoral photographs demonstrating advanced mechanics of en masse anterior retraction and posterior intrusion-and-distalization for orthognathic-like orthodontics.

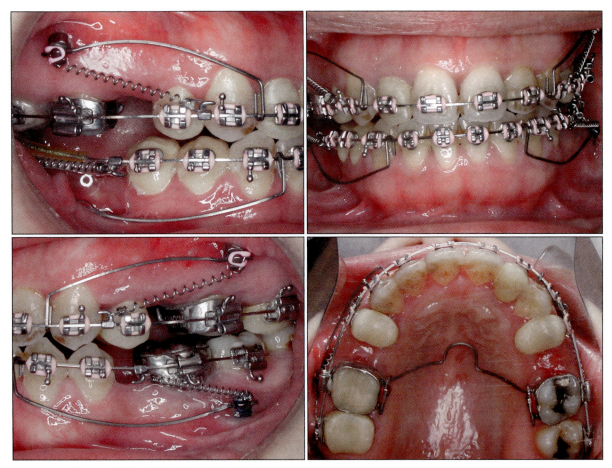

Figure 8-17
Intraoral photographs demonstrating advanced mechanics of en masse anterior retraction-and-intrusion for orthognathic-like orthodontics.

8   Appliances, Mechanics, and Treatment Strategies Toward Orthognathic-Like Treatment Results

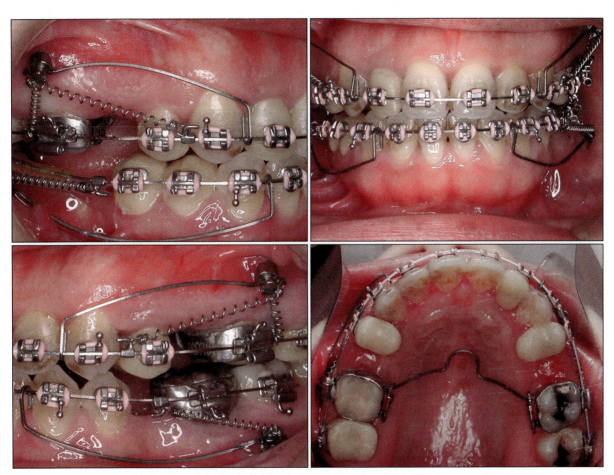

Figure 8-18
Intraoral photographs demonstrating advanced mechanics of en masse anterior retraction-and-intrusion and posterior intrusion for orthognathic-like orthodontics.

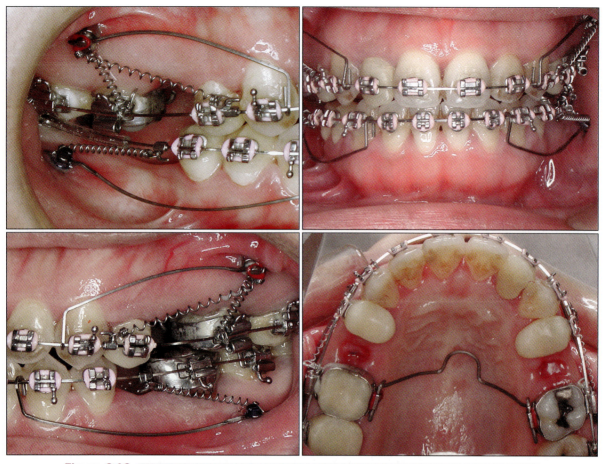

Figure 8-19
Intraoral photographs demonstrating advanced mechanics of en masse anterior retraction-and-intrusion and posterior intrusion-and-distalization for orthognathic-like orthodontics.

open bite with dentoalveolar protrusion is (1) to correct the anterior crossbite by maximal anterior retraction-and-intrusion of the mandibular anterior teeth and (2) to correct the anterior open bite and prevent upward rotation of the mandible by anterior downward tilting of the maxillary occlusal plane.[32] This mimics the mandibular anterior subapical osteotomy, in which the anterior segment is set back and repositioned apically, and Le Fort I osteotomy with anterior downward fracture of the maxilla (Figure 8-20).

- *Maximal anterior retraction-and-intrusion of the mandibular anterior teeth to mimic mandibular anterior subapical osteotomy:* This is accomplished by extraction of the mandibular first premolars and anterior retraction-and-intrusion of the lower anterior teeth using miniscrews, Ni-Ti coil springs, and a pair of β-Ti intruding lever arms. The miniscrews are inserted in the mandibular oblique ridges. The intrusion of the mandibular incisors does not increase overbite, but it allows maximal anterior retraction without excessive mandibular incisor shown.
- *Anterior downward tilting of maxillary occlusal plane to mimic Le Fort I osteotomy with anterior downward fracture of the maxilla:* This is accomplished by extraction of the maxillary second premolars and palatal tipping and extrusion of the maxillary incisors by a pair of β-Ti extruding lever arms. The extrusion and palatal tipping of the maxillary incisors increase the overbite and tilt the maxillary occlusal plane downward anteriorly, preventing upward rotation of the mandible.

The posttreatment overbite and mandibular posture are maintained by the relapse (extrusion) of mandibular anterior teeth and the "reciprocal relapse" (intrusion) of maxillary anterior teeth.

Class II Anterior Open Bite with High Mandibular Plane Angle

Intrusion of the maxillary or mandibular molars with upward rotation of mandible is used to treat cases of Class II anterior open bite with high MPA. In some cases, however, we noted that intrusion of the maxillary or mandibular molars alone did not rotate the mandible upward because of the "compensating" molar eruption and extrusion of incisors in the antagonistic dentition (Figure 8-21). For adequate upward rotation of mandible and chin prominence, the antagonistic dentition should be held in place or even intruded with miniscrews to avoid the compensating eruption. Both

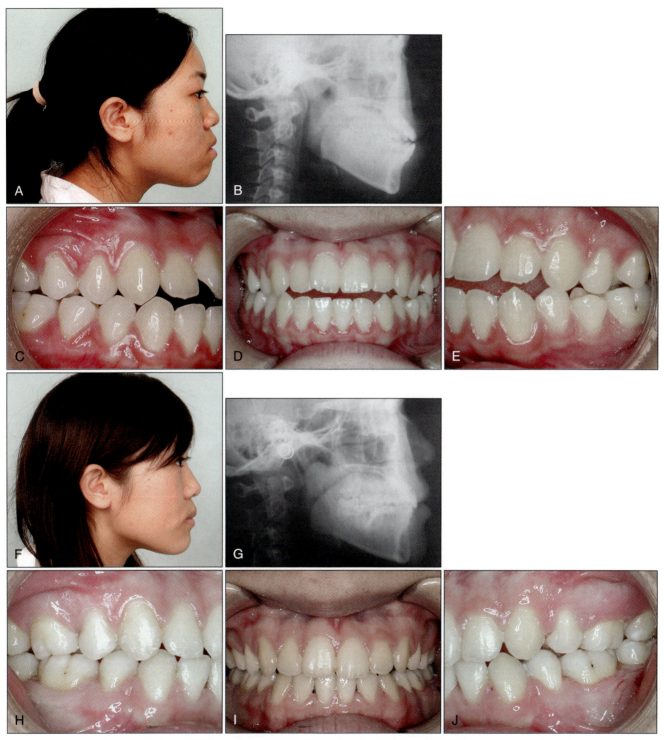

Figure 8-20
Orthognathic-Like Treatment Results for Class III Anterior Open Bite Using Miniscrews. Mandibular incisors were retracted to mimic mandibular anterior subapical osteotomy, and the palatal tipping and extrusion of the maxillary incisors was accomplished to mimic LeFort I osteotomy with anterior downward repositioning of the maxilla in which the maxillary incisors were tipped palatally and extruded to prevent upward rotation of the mandible. The root apices of mandibular incisors were left inside the alveolus. Pretreatment: **A,** facial photograph; **B,** cephalometric radiograph; **C** to **E,** intraoral photographs. Posttreatment: **F,** facial photograph; **G,** cephalometric radiograph; **H** to **J,** intraoral photographs.

Continued

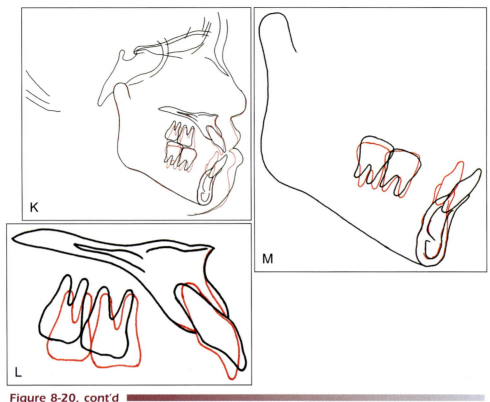

Figure 8-20, cont'd

K to M, Superimpositions showing pretreatment findings *(black line)* and posttreatment results *(red line)*.

the entire maxillary and the entire mandibular dentition should be intruded for maximal upward and forward rotation of the mandible and chin prominence.

The strategy for the treatment in Class II anterior open bite with high MPA is (1) to correct the maxillary dentoalveolar protrusion by maximal anterior retraction-and-intrusion and (2) to correct the anterior open bite by intrusion of the maxillary and mandibular molars and intrusion-and-lingual-tipping of the mandibular incisors. This mimics Le Fort I impaction and maxillary anterior subapical osteotomy.

- *Maximal maxillary anterior retraction-and-intrusion and intrusion of the maxillary molars to mimic maxillary anterior subapical osteotomy and Le Fort I impaction.* This is accomplished by extraction of the maxillary first premolars, anterior retraction-and-intrusion at the maxillary anterior teeth, and posterior intrusion using miniscrews, Ni-Ti coil springs, and a pair of β-Ti intruding lever arms. The miniscrews are inserted in the IZ crests of maxilla. The intrusion of the maxillary anterior teeth does not increase overbite but does allow maximal amount of anterior retraction and avoids an excessively "gummy" smile.
- *Intrusion of mandibular molars and intrusion-and-lingual-tipping of mandibular incisors.* This is accomplished by extraction of mandibular second/first premolars or en masse distalization-and-intrusion of the entire mandibular dentition by using miniscrews, Ni-Ti coil springs, and a pair of β-Ti intruding lever arms. The miniscrews are inserted in the mandibular oblique ridges. The intrusion of the entire mandibular dentition enhances upward rotation of the mandible.

The posttreatment overbite would be maintained by the relapse (extrusion) of the maxillary and mandibular molars and the "compensating relapse" (extrusion) of the maxillary and mandibular anterior teeth.

Class I Anterior Open Bite with Dentoalveolar Protrusion

The strategy for the treatment of Class I anterior open bite lies between the strategies for Class I bimaxillary dentoalveolar protrusion and Class II anterior open bite (Figure 8-22). This may involve a selective combination of bimaxillary anterior retraction, anterior retraction-and-intrusion, or intrusion of maxillary and mandibular molars. The bimaxillary anterior retraction or retraction-and-intrusion is for the correction of dentoalveolar protrusion and anterior open bite. This mimics the anterior subapical osteotomy. The intrusion of the maxillary and mandibular molars provides upward and forward rotation of the mandible in cases of high MPA. This simulates the Le Fort I posterior impaction and the consequent upward rotation of mandible.

- *Bimaxillary anterior retraction or retraction-and-intrusion to mimic anterior subapical osteotomy.* This is

8 Appliances, Mechanics, and Treatment Strategies Toward Orthognathic-Like Treatment Results

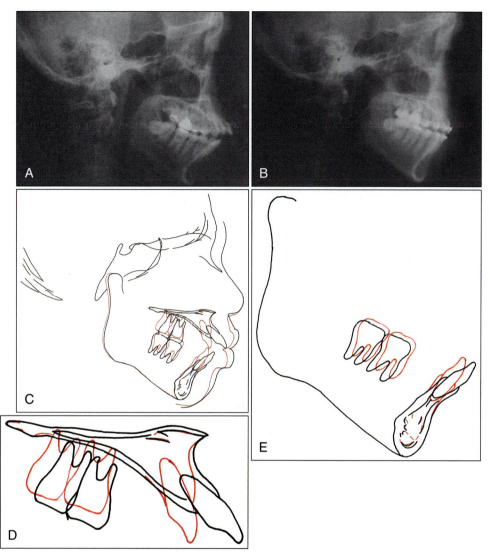

Figure 8-21

Class II Anterior Open Bite with High Mandibular Plane Angle. Although the entire maxillary dentition was intruded to mimic LeFort I impaction for the correction of anterior open bite and upward rotation of the mandible, the mandible did not rotate upward because of the "compensating" eruption of the mandibular molars. The mandibular dentition should be held in place or even intruded with miniscrews to allow adequate upward rotation and chin prominence in the correction of Class II anterior open bite. **A,** Pretreatment cephalometric radiograph. **B,** Cephalometric radiograph during treatment. **C to E,** Superimpositions showing pretreatment findings *(black line)* and posttreatment results *(red line)*.

accomplished by extraction of the maxillary and mandibular first premolars and anterior retraction or retraction-and-intrusion using miniscrews, Ni-Ti coil springs, and β-Ni-Ti intruding lever arms. The miniscrews are inserted in the IZ crests of maxilla and mandibular oblique ridges.

- *Intrusion of maxillary and mandibular molars to mimic Le Fort I posterior impaction and upward rotation of mandible.* This is accomplished by posterior intrusion and miniscrews in the IZ crests and mandibular oblique ridges.

CLASS II MANDIBULAR MICROGNATHIA

Surgical advancement of the mandible is the treatment of choice for the correction of Class II mandibular micrognathia. However, surgical advancement of the mandible is contraindicated in patients with degenerative temporomandibular joint (TMJ) arthritis and small mandibular condyles. Mandibular surgery may provoke severe condylar resorption postoperatively in such cases, resulting in anterior open bite and recessive chin.

The treatment strategy for Class II mandibular micrognathia with degenerative TMJ arthritis should be con-

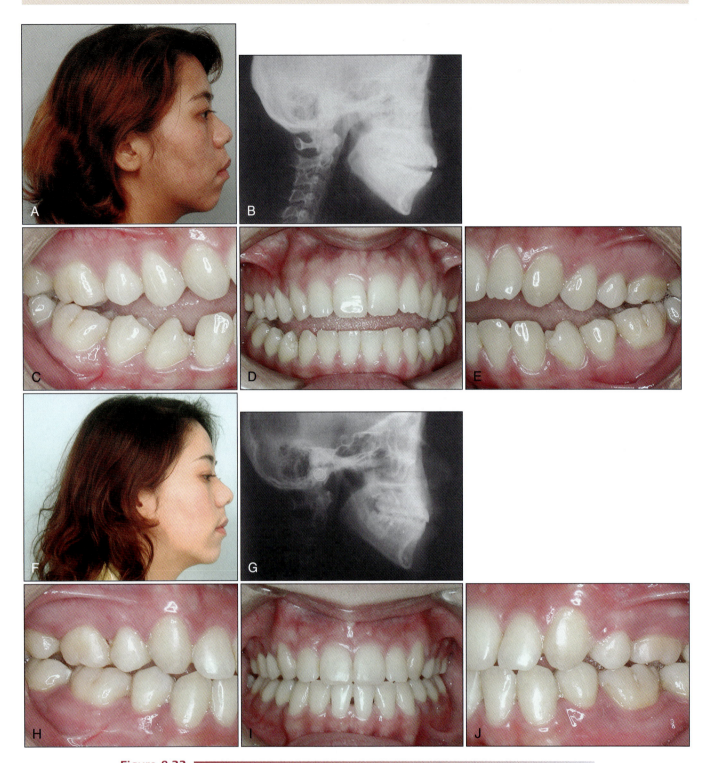

Figure 8-22

Orthognathic-Like Treatment Results for Class I Anterior Open Bite Using Miniscrews. Maxillary incisors were retracted to mimic anterior subapical osteotomy, and the maxillary molars were intruded to mimic LeFort I posterior impaction. The mandibular molars were held without compensating eruption and the mandibular incisors were intruded for maximizing upward rotation of mandible and chin prominence. Pretreatment: **A,** facial photograph; **B,** cephalometric radiograph; **C** to **E,** intraoral photographs. Posttreatment: **F,** facial photograph; **G,** cephalometric radiograph; **H** to **J,** intraoral photographs.

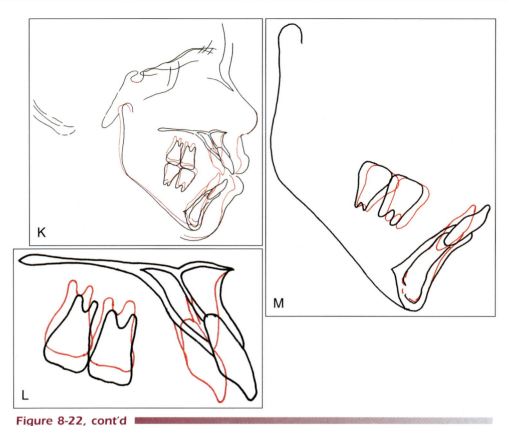

Figure 8-22, cont'd K to M, Superimpositions showing pretreatment findings *(black line)* and posttreatment results *(red line)*.

servative. It could be the same as for patients with Class II anterior open bite and high MPA in whom both mandibular and maxillary dentitions are intruded for maximal upward and forward rotation of mandible and chin prominence (Figure 8-23).

CLINICAL EVALUATION

It is a misconception that miniscrews accelerate the rate of orthodontic tooth movement and shorten the orthodontic treatment period. With or without miniscrews makes no difference in bone physiology. The osteoblasts and osteoclasts in periodontal ligament respond the same way toward mechanical stretch and compression regardless of whether the anchorage is a tooth or a miniscrew.

In 30 cases of bimaxillary dentoalveolar protrusion treated by extraction of the first premolars and miniscrews, treatment averaged 167.8 days, significantly longer than the 20 cases treated without miniscrews.[68] The anterior teeth were retracted and intruded in both groups of patients. The average amount of anterior retraction in the patients treated with miniscrews was 8.2 mm and 3.0 mm at the incisal tip and root apex, respectively, significantly more than the patients treated without miniscrews (6.5 mm at incisal tip and 1.3 mm at root apex). More time was spent on complete closure of the extraction space in patients treated with miniscrews because of no loss of anchorage (mesial migration of the molars), and all the extraction space was saved for the anterior retraction-and-intrusion. In some cases the molars were distalized because of the archwire friction during anterior retraction, and consequently a space wider than a premolar's width had to be closed.

The apical root resorption of maxillary incisors varied greatly in patients treated with or without miniscrews.[68] The apical root resorption of the maxillary incisors was 16.5% to 19.8% of their pretreatment length in the patients treated with miniscrew, significantly more than the patients treated without miniscrews (5.4%). This could be a result of the longer treatment period in patients treated with miniscrews.

On cephalometric evaluation of the maxillary incisors at 1 year posttreatment, the component of relapse in retraction was 10% to 15%, and the component of relapse in intrusion was 25% to 30%.[69] The relapse of anterior teeth intrusion was twice the relapse of retraction, and therefore the overbite became deeper when there was no intrusion of the posterior teeth. To maintain the posttreatment overbite, it is helpful to intrude the posterior teeth as well in patients with dentoalveolar protrusion. The relapse of molar intrusion compensates for the relapse of anterior intrusion. This is the concept of "compensating relapse" mentioned earlier. However,

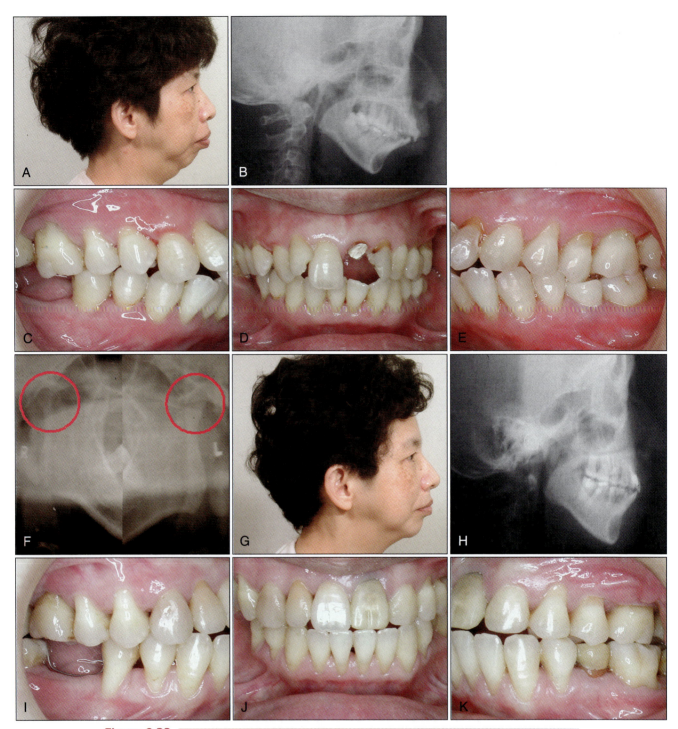

Figure 8-23

Orthognathic-Like Treatment Results in a Case of Class II Mandibular Micrognathia by Using Miniscrews. Orthognathic surgery was excluded from the treatment planning because of the patient's small mandibular condyles. The entire maxillary dentition was intruded and distalized to mimic LeFort I impaction and anterior subapical osteotomy. The mandibular molars and incisors were intruded for maximizing mandibular upward rotation and chin prominence. **A** to **E**, Pretreatment photographs: facial (A); cephalometric radiograph (B); intraoral (C-E). **F**, Radiograph showing the flattened morphology of the condyles *(circles)*, consistent with degenerative joint disease. Posttreatment: **G**, facial photograph; **H**, cephalometric radiograph; **I** to **K**, intraoral photographs.

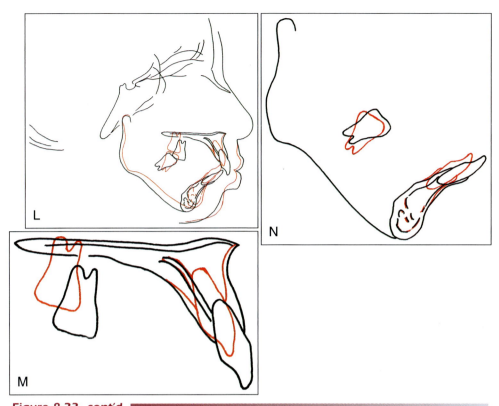

Figure 8-23, cont'd
M and N, Superimpositions showing pretreatment findings *(black line)* and posttreatment results *(red line)*.

the relapse of anterior retraction can be managed only with overcorrection.

Relapse of molar intrusion in patients with anterior open bite has been reported to be 27.2% at the mandibular first molars and 30.3% at the mandibular second molars,[70] similar to the relapse of anterior teeth intrusion in our patients. This is one reason why, in the treatment of Class II anterior open bite, both the maxillary and the mandibular anterior and posterior teeth need to be intruded for the maintenance of overbite through the posttreatment compensating and reciprocal relapses.

CONCLUSION

The role of the miniscrew in orthodontics is more than a replacement for Class II/III elastics, headgear, or patient compliance. It expands the spectrum of orthodontics to orthognathic-like orthodontics, new territories, where clinicians need to be aware of the migration of miniscrew, biological boundaries that encompass risk of fenestration and dehiscence, treatment period, apical root resorption, and posttreatment relapse.

REFERENCES

1. Kanomi R: Mini-implant for orthodontic anchorage, *J Clin Orthod* 31:763-767, 1997.
2. Costa A, Raffainl M, Melsen B: Miniscrews as orthodontic anchorage: a preliminary report, *Int Adult Orthod Orthog Surg* 13:201-209, 1998.
3. Melsen B, Verna C: A rational approach to orthodontic anchorage, *Prog Orthod* 1:10-22, 1999.
4. Costa A, Dalstra M, Melsen B: L'Aarthus Anchorage System, *Ortognatodonzia Italiana* 9:487-496, 2000.
5. Kanomi R, Takada K: Application of titanium mini-implant system for orthodontic anchorage. In Davidovitch Z, Mah J, editors: *Biological mechanics of tooth movement and craniofacial adaptation*, Boston, 2000, Harvard Society of the Advancement of Orthodontics, pp 253-258.
6. Melsen B, Costa A: Immediate loading of implants used for orthodontic anchorage, *Clin Orthod Res* 3:23-28, 2000.
7. Park HS, Bae SM, Kyung HM, Sung JH: Micro-implant anchorage for treatment of skeletal Class I bialveolar protrusion, *J Clin Orthod* 35:417-422, 2001.
8. Lee JS, Park HS, Kyung HM: Micro-implant for lingual treatment of a skeletal Class II malocclusion, *J Clin Orthod* 35:643-647, 2001.
9. Park HS, Kyung HM, Sung JH: A simple method of molar uprighting with micro-implant anchorage, *J Clin Orthod* 36:592-596, 2002.
10. Lin JCY, Liou EJ: A new bone screw for orthodontic anchorage, *J Clin Orthod* 37:676-682, 2003.
11. Park HS, Kwon TG, Sung JH: Non-extraction treatment with miniscrew implant, *Angle Orthod* 74:539-549, 2004.
12. Lee JS, Kim DH, Park YC, et al: The efficient use of midpalatal miniscrew implants, *Angle Orthod* 74:711-14, 2004.
13. Kuroda S, Katayama A, Takano-Yamamoto T: Severe anterior open-bite case treated using titanium screw anchorage, *Angle Orthod* 74:558-567, 2004.

14. Lin JC, Liou EJ, Yeh CL: Intrusion of overerupted maxillary molars with miniscrew anchorage, *J Clin Orthod* 40:378-383, 2006.
15. Lin JCY, Liao JJL, Liou EJW: Bidentoalveolar protrusion treated with premolar extraction and maximum retraction. In Cope JB, editor: *OrthoTADs: the clinical guide and atlas*, Dallas, 2007, Under Dog Media, pp 279-283.
16. Liao JJL, Lin JCY, Liou EJW: Bialveolar protrusion treated by first premolar extraction and maximum retraction. In Cope JB, editor: *OrthoTADs: the clinical guide and atlas*, Dallas, 2007, Under Dog Media, pp 317-321.
17. Liao JJL, Lin JCY, Liou EJW: Canted occlusal plane and anterior open bite treatment. In Cope JB, editor: *OrthoTADs: the clinical guide and atlas*, Dallas, 2007, Under Dog Media, pp 327-331.
18. Liou EJW, Lin JCY: Adult Class II subdivision malocclusion treated with extraction of decayed maxillary second premolars. In Cope JB, editor: *OrthoTADs: the clinical guide and atlas*, Dallas, 2007, Under Dog Media, pp 322-326.
19. Trisi P, Rebaudi A: Progressive bone adaptation of titanium implants during and after orthodontic load in humans, *Int J Periodont Restor Dent* 22:31-43, 2002.
20. Liou EJ, Pai BC, Lin JCY: Do miniscrews remain stationary under orthodontic forces? *Am J Orthod Dentofacial Orthop* 126:42-47, 2004.
21. Wang YC, Liou EJ: Comparison of the loading behavior of the self-drilling and pre-drilling miniscrews throughout orthodontic loading, *Am J Orthod Dentofacial Orthop* 133:38-43, 2008.
22. Kim JW, Ahn SJ, Chang YI: Histomorphometric and mechanical analyses of the drill-free screw as orthodontic anchorage, *Am J Orthod Dentofacial Orthop* 128:190-194, 2005.
23. Deguchi T, Takano-Yamamoto T, Kanomi R, et al: The use of small titanium screws for orthodontic anchorage, *J Dent Res* 82:377-381, 2003.
24. Majzoub Z, Finotti M, Miotti F, et al: Bone response to orthodontic loading of endosseous implants in the rabbit calvaria: early continuous distalizing forces, *Eur J Orthod* 21:223-230, 1999.
25. Misch CE: Bone character: second vital implant criterion, *Dent Today* 7:39-40, 1998.
26. Misch CE, Kircos LT: Diagnostic imaging and techniques. In Misch CE, editor: *Contemporary implant dentistry*, ed 2, St Louis, 1999, Mosby, pp 73-87.
27. Umemori M, Sugawara J, Mitani H, et al: Skeletal anchorage system for open-bite correction, *Am J Orthod Dentofacial Orthop* 115:166-174, 1999.
28. Melsen B, Peterson JK, Costa A: Zygoma ligatures: an alternative form of maxillary anchorage, *J Clin Orthod* 32:154-158, 1998.
29. Clerck H, Geerinckx V, Siciliano S: The zygoma anchorage system, *J Clin Orthod* 36:455-459, 2002.
30. Chung KR, Kim YS, Linton Lee J, Lee YJ: The miniplate with tube for skeletal anchorage system, *J Clin Orthod* 36:407-412, 2002.
31. Liou EJ, Chen RP, Wang YC, Chang PM: A CT-image study on the thickness of the infrazygomatic crest of the maxilla and its clinical implications for miniscrew insertion, *Am J Orthod Dentofacial Orthop* 131:352-6, 2007.
32. Liou EJW, Lin JCY: The LOMAS System. In Cope JB, editor: *OrthoTADs: the clinical guide and atlas*, Dallas, 2007, Under Dog Media, pp 213-230.
33. Miyawaki S, Koyama I, Inoue M, et al: Factors associated with the stability of titanium screws placed in the posterior region for orthodontic anchorage, *Am J Orthod Dentofacial Orthop* 124:373-378, 2003.
34. Heidemann W, Gerlach KL, Grobel KH, Kollner HG: Influence of different pilot sizes on torque measurements and pullout analysis of osteosynthesis screws, *J Craniomaxillofac Surg* 26:50-55, 1998.
35. Matthews J, Hirsch C: Temperature measured in human cortical bone when drilling, *J Bone Joint Surg* 45A:297-308, 1972.
36. Misch CE: Density of bone: effect on surgical approach and healing. In *Contemporary implant dentistry*, ed 2, St. Louis, 1999, Mosby, pp 374-375.
37. Cheng SJ, Tseng IY, Lee JJ, Kok SH: A prospective study of the risk factors associated with failure of mini-implants used for orthodontic anchorage, *Int J Oral Maxillofac Implants* 19:100-106, 2004.
38. Mah J, Bergstrand F, Graham JW: Temporary anchorage devices: a status report, *J Clin Orthod* 39:132-136, 2005.
39. Liou EJ, Lin JC: Periodontal dressing for the miniscrew postoperative care, *J Clin Orthod* (submitted for publication).
40. Yang LI, Liou EJ: Clinical evaluation on the factors related to orthodontic miniscrew failure. In *Proceedings of the Third Asia Implant Orthodontics Conference*, 2004, Taipei, Taiwan.
41. Yang LI, Liou EJ: Learning curve in orthodontic miniscrew insertion, *Am J Orthod Dentofacial Orthop* (submitted for publication).
42. Handelman CS: The anterior alveolus: its importance in limiting orthodontic treatment, *Angle Orthod* 2:95-110, 1996.
43. Sarikaya S, Haydar B, Ciger S, Ariyurek M: Changes in alveolar bone thickness due to retraction of anterior teeth, *Am J Orthod Dentofacial Orthop* 122:15-26, 2002.
44. Vardimon AD, Oren E, Ben-Bassat Y. Cortical bone remodelling/tooth movement ratio during maxillary incisor retraction, *Am J Orthod Dentofacial Orthop* 114:520-529, 1998.
45. Edward JC: A study of the anterior portion of the palate as it relates to orthodontic therapy, *Am J Orthod* 69:249-273, 1976.
46. Mulie RM, Ten Hoeve A: The limitations of tooth movements within the symphysis studied with laminography and standardized occlusal films, *J Clin Orthod* 10:882-899, 1976.
47. Ten Hoeve A, Mulie RM: The effect of antero-postero incisor repositioning on the palatal cortex as studied with laminagraphy, *J Clin Orthod* 10:804-822, 1976.
48. Wingard CE, Bowers GM: The effect of facial bone from facial tipping of incisors in monkeys, *J Periodontol* 47:450-454, 1976.
49. De Angelis V: Observations on the response of alveolar bone to orthodontic force, *Am J Orthod* 58:284-294, 1970.
50. Remmelink HJ, van der Molen AL: Effects of anteroposterior incisor repositioning on the root and cortical plate: a follow up study, *J Clin Orthod* 18:42-49, 1984.
51. Meikle MC: The dentomaxillary complex and overjet correction in Class II division 1 malocclusion: objectives of skeletal and alveolar remodeling, *Am J Orthod* 77:184-197, 1980.
52. Bimstein E, Crevoisier RA, King DL: Changes in the morphology of the buccal alveolar bone of protruded permanent mandibular incisors secondary to orthodontic alignment, *Am J Orthod Dentofacial Orthop* 97:427-430, 1990.
53. Wehrbein H, Fuhrmann RAW, Diedrich PR: Human histologic tissue response after long-term orthodontic tooth movement, *Am J Orthod Dentofacial Orthop* 107:360-371, 1995.
54. Wehrbein H, Bauer W, Diedrich PR: Mandibular incisors, alveolar bone, and symphysis after orthodontic tooth movement: a retrospective study, *Am J Orthod Dentofacial Orthop* 110:239-246, 1996.
55. Wehrbein H, Fuhrmann RAW, Diedrich PR: Periodontal conditions after facial root tipping and palatal root torque of incisors, *Am J Orthod Dentofacial Orthop* 106:455-462, 1994.
56. Batenhorst K, Bower GM, Williams IE: Tissue changes resulting from facial tipping and extrusion in monkeys, *J Periodontol* 46:660-668, 1974.
57. Steiner G: Changes of marginal periodontium as a result of labial tooth movement in monkeys, *J Periodontol* 52:314-320, 1981.
58. Wainwright WM: Faciolingual tooth movement: its influence on the root and cortical plate, *Am J Orthod* 64:278-302, 1973.
59. Vardimon AD, Graber TM, Voss LR, Lemke J: Determinants controlling iatrogenic external root resorption and repair during and after palatal expansion, *Angle Orthod* 61:113-124, 1991.
60. Engelking C, Zachrisson BU: Die auswirkung der schneidezahnretraktion auf das parodontium von affen nach vorausgegangener protrusion durch die kortikalis, *Inf Orthod Kieferorthop* 2:127-46, 1983.

61. Karring T, Nyman S, Thilander B, Magnusson I: Bone regeneration in orthodontically produced alveolar bone dehiscence, *J Periodontal Res* 17:309-315, 1982.
62. Daimaruya T, Takahashi I, Nagasaka H, et al: Effects of maxillary molar intrusion on nasal floor and tooth root using the skeletal anchorage system in dogs, *Angle Orthod* 73:158-166, 2003.
63. Daimaruya T, Nagasaka H, Umemori M, et al: The influences of molar intrusion on the inferior alveolar neurovascular bundle and root using the skeletal anchorage system in dogs, *Angle Orthod* 71:60-70, 2001.
64. Wilcko WM, Wilcko T, Bouquot JE, Ferguson DJ: Rapid orthodontics with alveolar reshaping: two case reports of decrowding, *Int J Periodont Restor Dent* 21:9-19, 2001.
65. Wilcko WM, Ferguson DJ, Boouquot JE, Wilcko T: Rapid orthodontic decrowding with alveolar augmentation: case report, *World J Orthod* 4:197-205, 2003.
66. Frost HM: The biology of fracture healing, *Clin Orthop* 248:283-293, 1989.
67. Yaffee A, Fine N, Binderman I: Regional accelerated phenomenon in the mandible following mucoperiosteal flap surgery, *J Periodontol* 65:79-83, 1994.
68. Chang PM, Liou EJ, Huang CS, Chen PKT: The apical root resorption of maxillary incisors in orthognathic-like orthodontics, Department of Orthodontics and Craniofacial Dentistry, Graduate Institute of Craniofacial Medicine, Chang Gung University, 2007 (master's thesis).
69. Hsu SSP, Liou EJ: Stability evaluation of the en masse maxillary retraction-intrusion by using miniscrews: one year follow up. In *Proceedings of the 2005 Annual Meeting of the Taiwan Association of Orthodontists*, Kaohsiung, Taiwan.
70. Sugawara J, Baik UB, Umemori M, et al: Treatment and posttreatment dentoalveolar changes following intrusion of mandibular molars with application of a skeletal anchorage system (SAS) for open bite correction, *Int J Adult Orthod Orthognath Surg* 17:243-253, 2002.

CHAPTER 9

Controlled Occlusal Plane Changes Using Temporary Anchorage Devices

George Anka

Management of the occlusal plane is critical in the control of orthodontic treatment. The recent development of temporary anchorage devices (TADs) has enabled us to better predict this difficult clinical undertaking (i.e., vertical control of posterior buccal segments). In a growing patient, control of the occlusal plane may also be obtained by other means, such as dentoavleolar modeling of the erupting buccal segments. In the adult, nongrowing patient, however, skeletal anchorage is the major orthodontic adjunct if an occlusal plane alteration is desired.

The type of device described in this chapter is a screw-type TAD. From a practitioner's perspective, this type of TAD is chosen because of its ease of management in terms of placement and infection control. From a patient's perspective, the TAD provides relative comfort. From a biomechanical perspective, the miniscrew provides excellent versatility for the correction of occlusal plane problems. This type of TAD should be placed, if possible, on the attached gingiva; therefore, the palatal alveolar area is often an ideal site for placement.

The occlusal plane can be divided into upper and lower planes. Although usually correlated, in some clinical situations the two planes dissociate from each other. For example, upper and lower occlusal planes can be separated in an open bite, medially or laterally deviated in a crossbite, or overlapping, as clinically evident in a Brodie bite.

In treating a malocclusion, control of all three dimensions of tooth movement is necessary. Each occlusal plane location within the craniofacial structure should be identified separately and the objectives of the three-dimensional (3D) movement adequately planned. It is important to note that dentoalveolar approaches do not correct the skeletal problem itself; rather the goal of treatment is to compensate for the problem and help the patient function better.

THREE DIMENSIONS OF OCCLUSAL PLANE IN SPACE

Changing the occlusal plane entails its control in all the three dimensions of space, which are (1) sagittal space, (2) vertical space, and (3) transverse space.

The upper and the lower occlusal planes and the supporting structures should be examined and compared using both normal cephalographic views and frontal posteroanterior (PA) views. Information from 3D scans, magnetic resonance imaging (MRI) for temporomandibular joint (TMJ) evaluation, and myography for muscle evaluation can supplement a thorough clinical evaluation and study models. I prefer to mount models in a semiadjustable articulator (Sam II articulator) because better information is obtained with the models mounted three-dimensionally in space. When there is a canted occlusal plane, I have the patient bite on a tongue blade while taking the frontal photograph so that the cant can be easily visualized. During treatment I also take PA cephalograms with the patient biting on a tongue blade with a wire taped to it. This makes it easy to diagnose the underlying problem and evaluate treatment progress.

A problem list is created before initiating treatment, and a treatment plan is formulated. Treatment usually begins in the maxilla. Correction of the maxillary occlusal plane can affect the jaw position (because of occlusal contacts), so it is important to determine the effect of changing the upper occlusal plane in relation to the lower jaw. During treatment, it is mandatory to reevaluate the case periodically and check if the tooth movement is occurring in the right direction.

FORCE APPLICATION

When using TADs, force can be applied in the following two ways:
- Direct force; this is used when the TAD is connected directly to the tooth or teeth that are going to move (Figure 9-1, A).

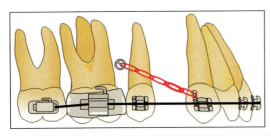

Figure 9-1
Direct application of force.

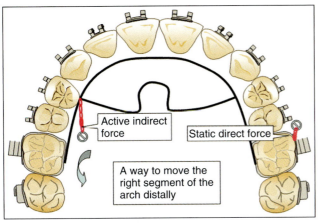

Figure 9-2
Transpalatal Bar Plus Hooks. Left first molar is tied with a ligature wire to the miniscrew, which is the area that should not move. The right segment should move distally, so an elastic chain is threaded from the hook behind the first bicuspid on the transpalatal bar. The end result is distalization of the whole right segment in the distal direction.

- Indirect force; this is used when the TAD is attached to a tooth or group of teeth and a force is delivered from the tooth (or group) instead of the TAD (Figure 9-1, *B*).

A combination of the two ways of applying force is often needed (Figure 9-2).

SAGITTAL OCCLUSAL PLANE CONTROL

When attempting to move a tooth or group of teeth in the anterior-posterior or the vertical direction, it is imperative to determine the center of resistance so that forces can be applied accordingly and proportionately. Otherwise, uncontrolled movement can easily occur. The direction of force, as dictated by the placement of the miniscrew relative to the teeth, often does not provide good control of the movement, primarily because of two factors. First, the miniscrew is usually placed below the gingival mucosa of the teeth and not parallel with the crown of the teeth. Second, the placement of the miniscrew often is not a matter of free choice; it must be limited, as much as possible, to available alveolar bone.

SAGITTAL CONTROL IN MANDIBLE

The optimal site on the mandible for placement of the miniscrew, to maximize the efficiency of the method described here, is on the buccal side of the alveolar process between the second premolar and the first molar. However, depending on the needs of the individual patient, all the alveolar bone process from the canine to the second molar may be used. The placement is usually about 8 mm below the cervical gingival line. The common point of implantation is on the attached gingiva, near the mucogingival junction.

The available interradicular space in the buccal aspect of the mandibular alveolar bone is one of the most crucial criteria to be considered before implantation. When insufficient space is available, space should be created or another placement site sought. Many times, leveling and aligning should be done first to create the necessary space. In general, I prefer to place the fixed appliances first and start moving the teeth, then place the miniscrew later once the arch has become aligned.

The possibility for immediate loading depends on the quality of the alveolar bone at the specific site of implantation. This bone quality can be clinically determined by the torque value in the last turn of the screw at the time of implantation. When the torque gauge is 10 Ncm or greater, immediate loading is acceptable. The choice of immediate loading also depends on the practitioner's preference and the type of miniscrew being used, whether an osseointegrated or a mechanical retention type. In osseointegrated miniscrew types, a prudent waiting period of 6 to 8 weeks is advised before applying a loading force.

Distalization

Once the TADs are placed, the delivery of the distalizing forces is obtained through the "lingual arch with extended arms" appliance. A lingual arch is placed, which is important in preventing rotation of the molars during long-distance molar distalization, (≥3 mm). Extended arms are soldered onto the molar band of the first molars, from which forces can be delivered anteriorly to complement the appliance. The distalization process can be done simultaneously, and once the molars start to move, the whole arch can be moved as a group.

Construction of the device is shown in Figure 9-3, *A*. The main lingual arch and the "extended arms" are made of 0.036-inch stainless steel wire. The extended arms are soldered to the buccal surface of the molar bands of the first molar, anterior to the buccal tube. Elastic chains from the miniscrew to the hook of the extended arm provide the necessary force to distalize the molars.

In mandibular unilateral distalization, the extended arms are maintained, and the lingual arch is removed (Figure 9-3, *B* and *C*).

SAGITTAL CONTROL ON MAXILLA

The main device used to control the maxillary occlusal plane is the "transpalatal bar with hooks" type appliance (Figure 9-4).

The position and distance of the miniscrew from the cervical gingival line is an important consideration. Selection of this location determine how much intrusion can be obtained. However, anatomical limitations, such as the depth of the mucobuccal fold, need to be evaluated. The width of the alveolar process area can be estimated using a panoramic radiograph. A 3D scan provides more informative data but may not always be available.

Distalization

When using distalization approaches, the location of the third molar should be assessed. Adequate space for distalization should be prepared, and for most cases the third molars should be removed at an early age. This is an important consideration since the distance between the upper first molar and the pterygomaxillary fossa is approximately 21 mm (SD, 1.6 mm),[1] and the width of the second molar averages 12 mm. This leaves about 8 to 9 mm of space between the second molars and the pterygoid plates. Theoretically, the upper molars can be distalized about 5 to 6 mm, assuming the absence of third molars, yielding a possible 3 to 4 mm of anterior teeth retraction in nonextraction cases.

The transpalatal bar plus hooks appliance can be used to achieve bilateral as well as unilateral distalization. Unilateral distalization can be achieved by converting the transpalatal arch to an extended arm, as illustrated in Figure 9-5. An additional miniscrew on the buccal side is recommended when considerable unilateral distalization is needed to prevent the molars from rotating during the distal movement.

If no alveolar bone is available to place the miniscrew, such as in the narrow interradicular space, the midpalatal area may be selected. In adults the midpalatal suture is a good site for miniscrew placement. The cortical bone is dense and thick and thus is ideal for immediate loading. Sometimes, in such dense bone, predrilling is advocated. I recommend predrilling when more than 20 Ncm of insertion torque is applied. This can be easily measured with a torque gauge during the implantation.

Figure 9-6 shows an example of midpalatal placement in which the plan is to move the first and second molars together distally by connecting the miniscrew to the omega loop of the transpalatal bar with an elastic chain. The major advantage of this design is that only one screw is needed. However, control of the tooth movement on both the distalizing segments is not as good as the standard transpalatal bar plus hooks appliance, as seen in Figure 9-4.

Figure 9-7 shows a modification of the distalizing appliance with a single midpalatal screw that can be used to incorporate an intrusive force. The "hooks" in the transpalatal bar are placed close to the gingival margin. An elastic or a closed-coil spring can be placed between the hook and the TAD to intrude the maxillary buccal segments. The amount of force required to

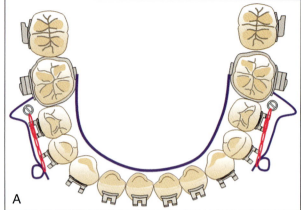
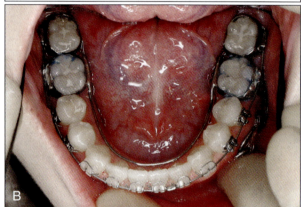
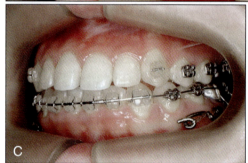

Figure 9-3

A, Lingual arch plus extended arms. Elastic is used to distalize the molar from the hook to the miniscrew. **B** and **C,** Clinical views of the lingual arch plus extended arms in place. A lingual arch and extended arms are soldered on the molar bands of the first molar teeth.

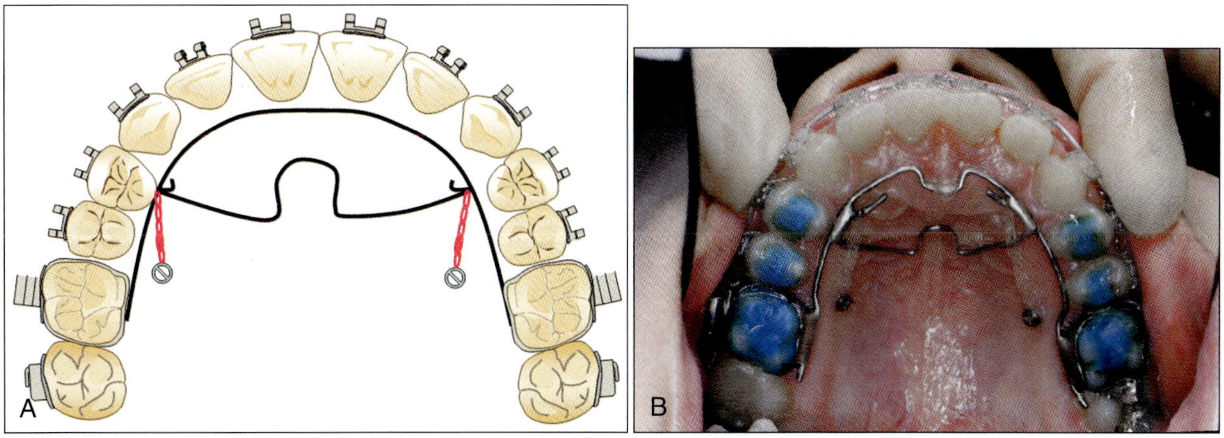

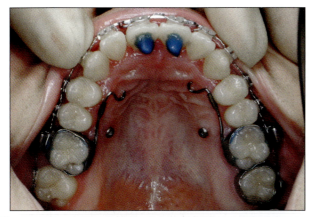

Figure 9-4

A, Transpalatal bar plus hooks. **B,** Clinical view of appliance in place. The miniscrews are placed on the lingual side of the alveolar bone between the second bicuspids and the first molar.

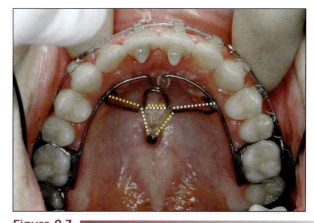

Figure 9-5

Transpalatal bar plus hooks that has been converted to an extended-arm device.

Figure 9-7

Miniscrew connected to hooks, resulting in long-range intrusion effect, combined with some distalization. The dotted lines represent the elastics placed from the single miniscrew to the hooks in the palatal arch.

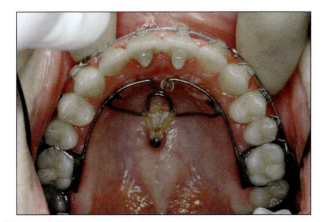

Figure 9-6

Transpalatal bar plus hooks and midpalatal miniscrew.

intrude the buccal segments is reportedly about 400 g per side. This modification to the appliance provides the opportunity not only to distalize the buccal segments but also to intrude them.

Mesialization

The approach for mesial movement of the buccal segments is similar to the distalization approach. One variation in the appliance is the soldering of a hook on the band for easy engagement to the miniscrew (Figure 9-8). Another variation in the appliance, more specifically for the maxilla, is the addition of a buccal miniscrew between the canine and first bicuspid, for better control of posterior segment rotation as it is being protracted anteriorly.

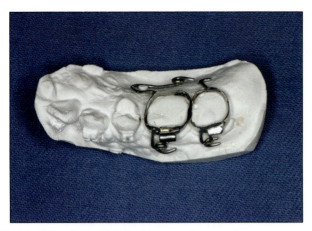

Figure 9-8
Hooks on the band facilitate engaging the miniscrew.

The ability to drive molars distally or mesially and the entire arch distally has opened a new dimension of decision making about whether to extract or not. The following case reports illustrate the management of the buccal segments using miniscrew anchorage.

CASE REPORT 9-1: CLASS II MALOCCLUSION

The patient in Figure 9-9 presented with a Class II molar occlusion on the left and an end-to-end Class II relationship on the right. Maxillary protrusion and crowding in the upper and lower arches was also evident. The patient agreed to have all remaining wisdom teeth extracted, but not her bicuspids as recommended. The crowding was approximately 10 mm in the upper jaw and 6 mm in the lower jaw. The treatment plan was to expand and move all teeth posteriorly.

The results show an improvement in the profile after significant distalization of molars with the transpalatal bar plus hooks appliance (Figure 9-10). Distal movement of the left maxillary first molar was 4.45 mm, and of the right maxillary molar, 5.60 mm. Distal movement of the mandibular first molars was less. In the transverse dimension the intermolar width was increased 3.42 mm in the maxilla but was maintained in the mandible. The vertical dimension increased slightly with the distal movement of the molars.

This case, involving a nongrowing adult patient, shows that significant molar distalization is achievable. The benefit of such movement was the Class II correction and the improved patient profile; however, treatment time was almost 3 years.

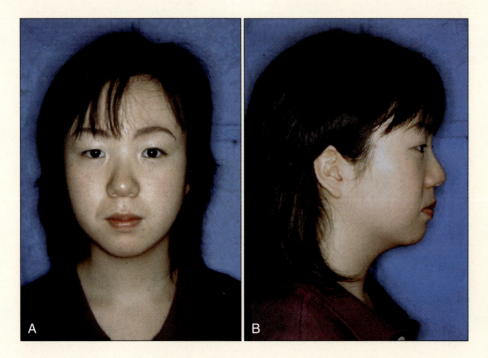

Figure 9-9 Class II Malocclusion: Pretreatment. **A** and **B**, Facial photographs.

CASE REPORT 9-1: CLASS II MALOCCLUSION—cont'd

Figure 9-9, cont'd **C** to **G**, Intraoral photograhs. **H**, Panoramic radiograph.

Continued

CASE REPORT 9-1: CLASS II MALOCCLUSION—cont'd

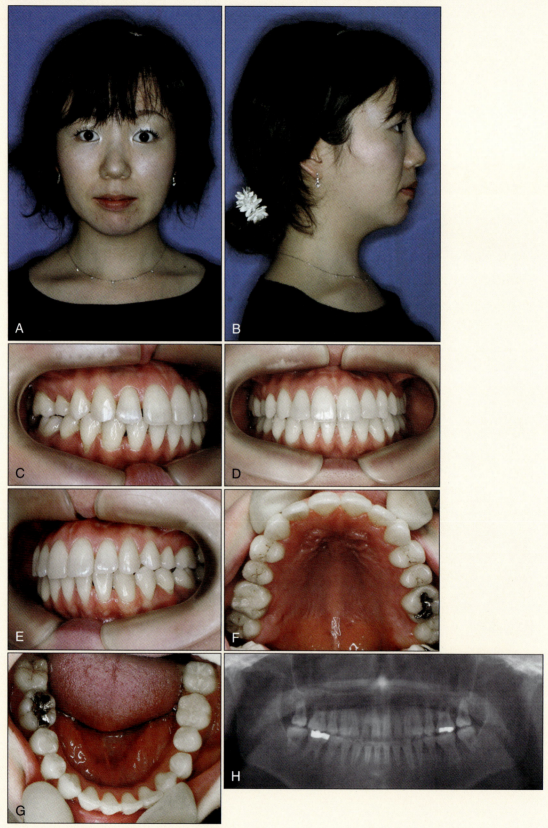

Figure 9-10 Class II Malocclusion: Posttreatment. **A** and **B**, Facial photographs. **C** to **G**, Intraoral photographs. **H**, Panoramic radiograph.

CASE REPORT 9-1: CLASS II MALOCCLUSION—cont'd

Facial angle	85.4	82.6
Convexity	10.5	10.7
A-B plane	-5.2	-7.2
Y-axis	64.1	66.7
FH to SN	7.4	6.7
∠SNA	83.0	81.1
∠SNB	78.9	76.1
∠ANB	4.1	4.9
N-Pog to SN	77.9	75.9
Nasal floor to SN	10.2	10.6
Nasal floor to FH	2.8	3.9
Mandibular pl. to SN	38.8	41.6
Mandibular pl. to FH	31.3	34.8
Ramus pl. to SN	92.9	93.9
Ramus pl. to FH	85.4	87.1
Gonial angle	125.9	127.7
U1 to SN	107.7	99.1
U1 to FH	115.2	105.8
L1 to mandibular pl.	93.3	92.3
Interincisal angle	120.2	127.0
Occlusal pl. to SN	16.8	25.5
Occlusal pl. to FH	9.4	18.8

Figure 9-10, cont'd **I**, Superimposition before *(black line)* and after *(red line)* treatment, on SN of last cephalograph. **J**, Cephalometric values before *(left)* and after *(right)* treatment.

CASE REPORT 9-2: CLASS III MALOCCLUSION

A 28-year-old woman with a Class III skeletal relationship consulted to have her teeth straightened without orthognathic surgery. Her records showed a Wits appraisal of −7.3 mm, still within "dentoalveolar compensation" by orthodontic means (Figure 9-11).

The treatment plan was to extract the lower second molars because the patient, a dental professional herself, believed that the left second molar had a poor prognosis. This tooth was carious, and the curve in the roots would make root canal treatment difficult. Extraction of the upper right third molar was also indicated. Miniscrews were implanted on the mandibular buccal shelf in the area of the second molars to protract the third molars, which were successfully moved mesially approximately 12 mm. The treatment result was a dentoalveolar compensation of the anterior teeth; the occlusal plane was not affected, and very slight bite opening was observed (Figure 9-12).

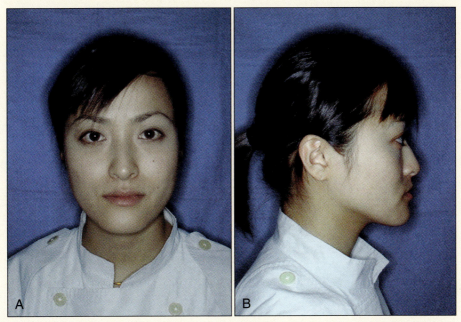

Figure 9-11 Class III Malocclusion: Pretreatment. **A** and **B**, Facial photographs.

Continued

CASE REPORT 9-2: CLASS III MALOCCLUSION—cont'd

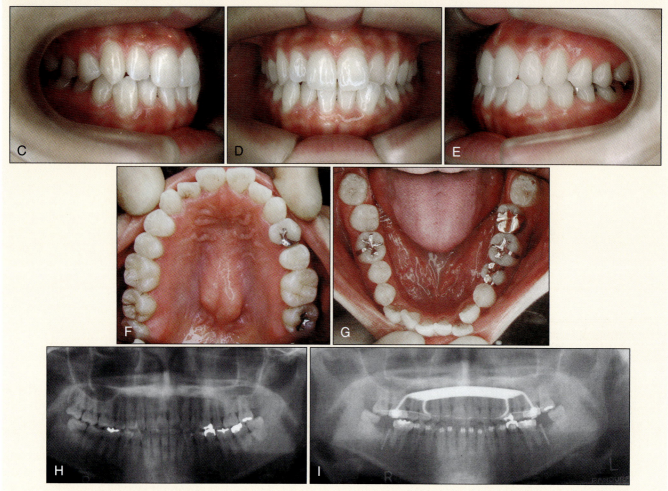

Figure 9-11, cont'd C to G, Intraoral photographs. H, Panoramic radiograph. I, Panoramic radiograph during treatment.

CASE REPORT 9-2: CLASS III MALOCCLUSION—cont'd

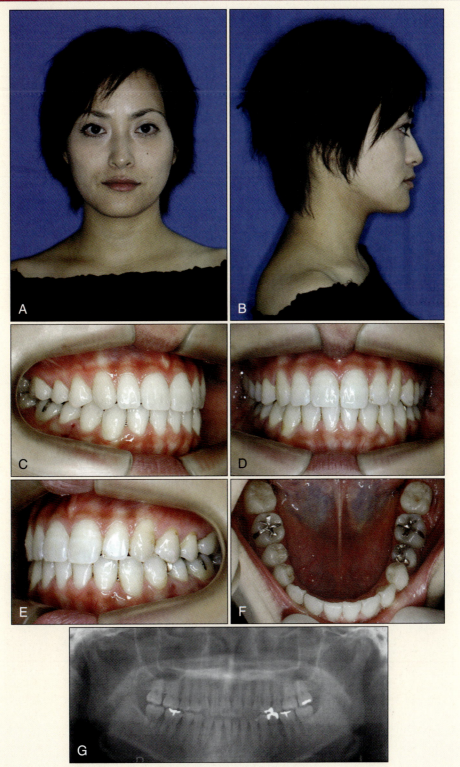

Figure 9-12 Class III Malocclusion: Posttreatment. A and B, Facial photographs. C to F, Intraoral photographs. G, Panoramic radiograph.

Continued

CASE REPORT 9-2: CLASS III MALOCCLUSION—cont'd

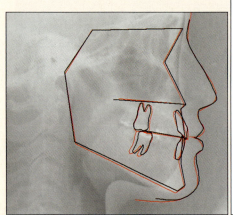

Facial angle	95.4	94.0
Convexity	-4.7	-3.8
A-B plane	-0.9	-2.8
Y-axis	55.6	57.8
FH to SN	5.8	4.3
∠SNA	87.3	87.8
∠SNB	87.9	87.5
∠ANB	-0.6	0.3
N-Pog to SN	89.6	89.7
Nasal floor to SN	5.0	6.0
Nasal floor to FH	-0.7	1.7
Mandibular pl. to SN	25.3	25.7
Mandibular pl. to FH	19.5	21.4
Ramus pl. to SN	85.5	85.1
Ramus pl. to FH	79.8	80.8
Gonial angle	119.7	120.6
U1 to SN	105.9	113.7
U1 to FH	111.7	118.0
L1 to mandibular pl.	80.4	86.6
Interincisal angle	148.4	134.0
Occlusal pl. to SN	11.3	9.8
Occlusal pl. to FH	5.5	5.4

Figure 9-12, cont'd H, Superimposition before *(black line)* and after *(red line)* treatment, on SN of posttreatment cephalograph. I, Cephalometric values before treatment *(left)* and 2.5 years after treatment *(right)*.

CASE REPORT 9-3: CLASS III TENDENCY AND OPEN BITE

An 11-year-old girl presented with an anterior open bite and a Class III tendency (Figure 9-13). The Wits appraisal of −5.2 mm indicated protrusion of the mandibular denture base. The patient had a high mandibular plane angle (35 degrees). The hyperdivergent facial pattern appeared to be related to a habitual tongue posture and a nasal problem at an early age. Orthodontic treatment was initiated with the goal of eliminating the tongue habit through myofunctional therapy.

Four miniscrews were placed; one in each quadrant. The posterior segments were intruded and distalized to correct the anterior open bite and relieve the crowding, respectively. The treatment resulted in a better facial profile. The anterior open bite was closed while the overjet was maintained (Figure 9-14).

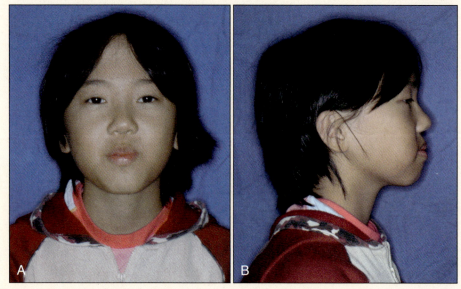

Figure 9-13 Class III Tendency and Open Bite: Pretreatment. A and B, facial photographs.

CASE REPORT 9-3: CLASS III TENDENCY AND OPEN BITE—cont'd

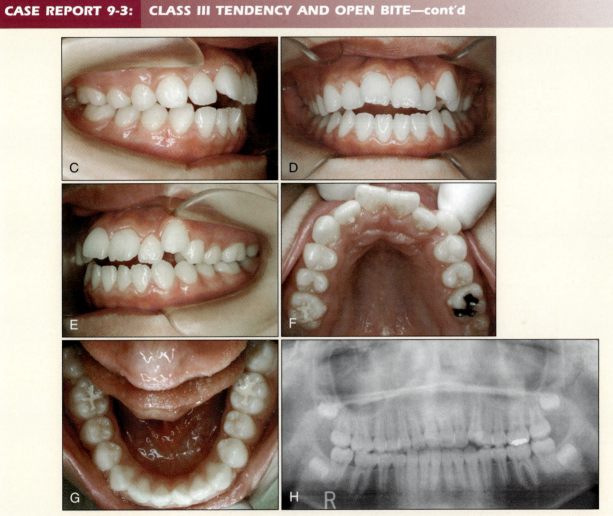

Figure 9-13, cont'd C to G, Intraoral photographs. H, Panoramic radiograph.

Continued

CASE REPORT 9-3: CLASS III TENDENCY AND OPEN BITE—cont'd

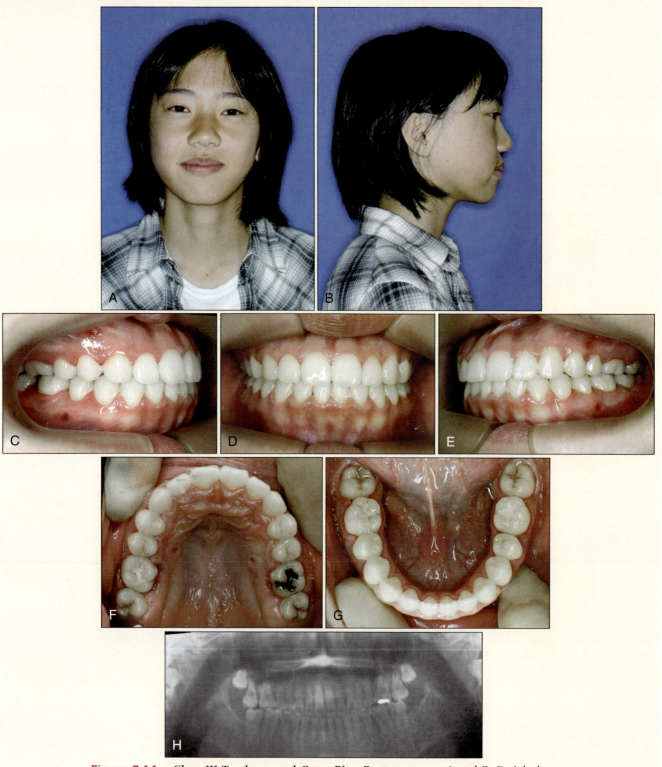

Figure 9-14 Class III Tendency and Open Bite: Posttreatment. **A** and **B**, Facial photographs. **C** to **G**, Intraoral photographs. **H**, Panoramic radiograph.

CASE REPORT 9-3:	CLASS III TENDENCY AND OPEN BITE—cont'd

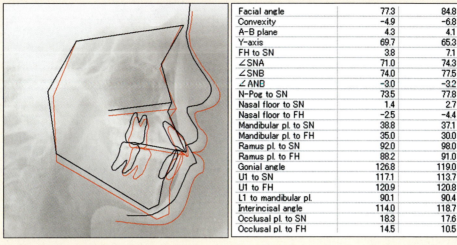

Facial angle	77.3	84.8
Convexity	-4.9	-6.8
A-B plane	4.3	4.1
Y-axis	69.7	65.3
FH to SN	3.8	7.1
∠SNA	71.0	74.3
∠SNB	74.0	77.5
∠ANB	-3.0	-3.2
N-Pog to SN	73.5	77.8
Nasal floor to SN	1.4	2.7
Nasal floor to FH	-2.5	-4.4
Mandibular pl. to SN	38.8	37.1
Mandibular pl. to FH	35.0	30.0
Ramus pl. to SN	92.0	98.0
Ramus pl. to FH	88.2	91.0
Gonial angle	126.8	119.0
U1 to SN	117.1	113.7
U1 to FH	120.9	120.8
L1 to mandibular pl.	90.1	90.4
Interincisal angle	114.0	118.7
Occlusal pl. to SN	18.3	17.6
Occlusal pl. to FH	14.5	10.5

Figure 9-14, cont'd I, Superimposition before (*black line,* age 11) and after (*red line,* age 14 years, 3 months) treatment, on SN. **J,** Cephalometric values before *(left)* and after *(right)* treatment.

VERTICAL DIMENSION: CONTROL OF MOLARS

EXTRUSION

Molar Extrusion in Mandible

Extrusion of the molars may be indicated in patients with canted occlusal planes with or without a lateral open bite. Extrusion is generally only necessary unilaterally, and TADs can be used to provide an extrusive force. The major advantage of this method is that the patient's compliance is not needed, unlike vertical intermaxillary elastics, in which a patient's cooperation is crucial. However, stability is important after molar extrusion because relapse is frequent, especially in nongrowing patients. Figure 9-15 illustrates the method to deliver the extrusive force, with a spring attached from the miniscrew to the first molar. This method can also be used for a segmental extrusion of the molar and the premolar.

Extrusion may require as much as twice the time of intrusion. If these mechanics are to be executed for a long period, it is advisable to integrate a lingual arch to prevent lingual tipping. This technique is very effective and can be used for one tooth or an entire buccal segment. In some cases, however, two screws may be recommended to achieve more control of the extrusive movement. Finally, overcorrection is also advisable because relapse is likely.

Molar Extrusion in Maxilla

Extrusion of the molars in the maxilla can be achieved through different modifications of the transpalatal bar plus hooks appliance. Figure 9-16 shows distalization and extrusion of the molars. Pure molar extrusion is shown in Figure 9-17. These same mechanics can be used to extrude an entire buccal segment distal to the canines. To achieve extrusion of both maxillary buccal segments, a total force of 400 g is applied.

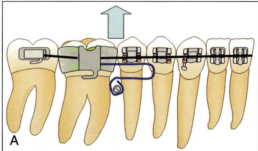

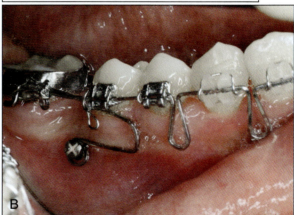

Figure 9-15
A, Extrusion as recommended by Dr. Y.C. Park. **B,** A .016 × .016 wire is used as a spring to extrude the right molar and the second bicuspid together.

Bilateral extrusion may be indicated in some cases. However, an occlusal cant visualized from the frontal plane is best treated with combined unilateral extrusion of contralateral quadrants in the opposing arches. During unilateral extrusion, careful evaluation of the side effects is necessary. For example, an extrusive force

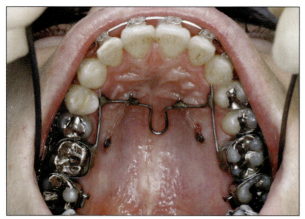

Figure 9-16

Molar Distalization and Extrusion. Transpalatal bar with hooks placed away from the cervical line so that elastic chains can extrude when it is connected to the miniscrew.

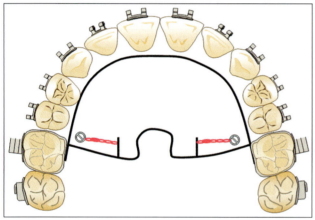

Figure 9-17

Pure Molar Extrusion. Transpalatal bar is placed and soldered on the mesial lingual side of the molar bands to permit a pure extrusion of the posterior molars, as the hooks are placed farther from the cervical area.

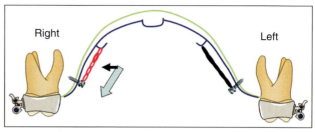

Figure 9-18

One-Sided Molar Extrusion. Large arrow shows direction of extrusion of the molars, and small arrow indicates direction in which the arch is drifting. When this is not desirable, a ligature wire is placed on the left side between the miniscrew and the hook to counter the effect.

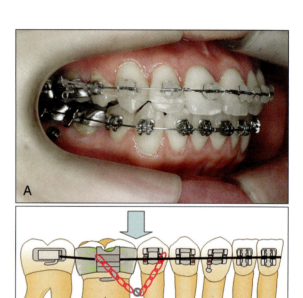

Figure 9-19

A, Intrusion of the first molar and second bicuspid. The miniscrew is placed on the alveolar buccal process between the first molar and the second bicuspids. **B,** TAD placed in the area between the first and second molars provides a better intrusion effect in adults with a severe open bite.

with a buccal component delivered from the lingual side can skew the arch in the transverse plane (Figure 9-18).

INTRUSION

Intrusion of molars became popular with the introduction of TADs, especially in the treatment of anterior open bites. The moderately severe open-bite cases, which are 1 standard deviation (SD) outside the norm for the mandibular plane angle, are generally easier to manage using TADs. Severe open bites combined with skeletal problems are difficult to correct, but a surgical option is still a better alternative to treat these patients.

Intrusion on Mandible

Intrusion of the mandibular molars is mainly indicated in open bites with a Class III occlusal relationship. Open bites with Class II malocclusions are better addressed with maxillary molar intrusion.

Figure 9-19, *A*, shows intrusion of the mandibular first and second bicuspids with miniscrews placed on the alveolar buccal process between the first molar and the second bicuspids. However, the area between the first molar and the second molar allows the mechanical advantage of delivering an intrusive force more posteriorly in an adult patient with a severe open bite (Figure

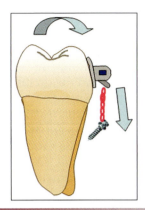

Figure 9-20
Miniscrew placement on the buccal side. The applied force tends to tip the molars toward the buccal aspect.

9-19, *B*). A full-size wire and a lingual arch are generally necessary to prevent buccal tipping of the lower molars (Figure 9-20).

Intrusion on Upper Arch
Success in managing an occlusal plane cant observed from the frontal or sagittal view depends on the ability to control the upper occlusal plane. The ability to control and direct the line of force in a desirable direction is the key to a successful treatment.

Often the intrusion procedure is combined with distalization of the molars. The transpalatal bar plus hooks offers the possibility of delivering such force vector. The mini-implant is placed at a distance from the gingival margin while the hooks are on the area close to the gingival margin between the canine and the first bicuspid. The resultant line of force will pass through or above the center of resistance causing distalization and intrusion of the molars (Figure 9-21). Occlusal plane rotation and extrusion can be accomplished by changing the location of the miniscrew on the alveolar process in the vertical dimension. Alternatively, the hooks can be placed at different levels in the transpalatal bar (Figure 9-22).

The intrusion of the posterior teeth alone may cause the anterior teeth to tip posteriorly and inferiorly. If extrusion of the anterior teeth is a concern, as in excessive gingival display at smile, two additional miniscrews need to be added on the buccal side. The following three placement sites may be used for these miniscrews to counteract the extrusive tendency of the maxillary incisors:

1. *Between the upper canine and the first bicuspid.* This placement helps intrude the entire upper anterior segment, including the canines, and also accomplishes some retraction (Figure 9-23). The amount of retraction, however, is limited by the interradicular distance.

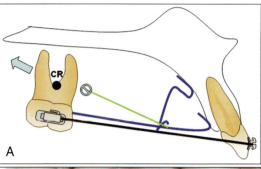

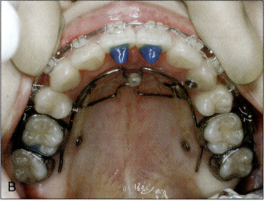

Figure 9-21
A and *B*, Distalization and intrusion of the molars.

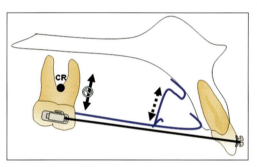

Figure 9-22
Variation of miniscrew and hook location. Two vertical lines show the varying locations of the miniscrews and hooks that effect extrusion or intrusion.

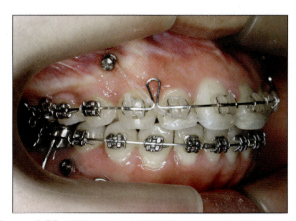

Figure 9-23
Placement of miniscrew between the upper canine and first bicuspid. Elastic is wrapped and hanging from the right to the left miniscrew, causing intrusion of the four anterior teeth.

2. *Between the canine and the lateral.* Placement in this region allows for intrusion of the anterior teeth. Depending on the inclination of the anterior teeth and the slot-to-wire-size ratio, proclination may be observed with intrusion. An advantage of placement in this site is the possibility of significant distalization without the miniscrew interfering in the process.
3. *Between the lateral and center anterior teeth.* This is generally selected when other spaces are not available. The major disadvantage of this placement is the discomfort to the patient's lip.

Placement between the central incisors is seldom attempted because of potential discomfort to the patient and anatomical limitations such as the labial frenum.

The placement decision depends on three factors: (1) available space, (2) the inclination of the anterior teeth, and (3) whether retraction is needed. When placing TADs in the anterior maxillary region, available space is the most vital consideration. The interradicular space availability can be checked on a recent panoramic radiograph.

MYOFUNCTIONAL THERAPY AND THE "PEARL"

Although effective for controlling the vertical dimension, a discussion of myofunctional therapy is beyond the scope of this chapter. One of the easiest ways to keep the tip of the tongue in the upward position is the use of the "pearl," which is integrated to the lingual arch or the transpalatal bar[2,3] (see Figure 9-21, *B*).

CANT OF OCCLUSAL PLANE

One of the most difficult tasks in clinical orthodontics is correcting a tilted or canted occlusal plane. However, with the introduction of the TAD, this task can now be accomplished more easily. The solution to this problem using orthodontics alone, without surgery, lies in maximizing the use of TADs.

A tilted occlusal plane can be adequately diagnosed with the Ricketts-Grummons analysis[4,5] by making measurements for all four quadrants. When there is still potential for growth, it is often necessary to focus on quadrants 1 and 2, which are on the maxilla. Determining the occlusal plane of the maxilla in relationship to the interorbital axis helps determine the most suitable location for correction in these patients. The various options to correct the occlusal plane are as follows:

1. Intrusion of both posterior maxillary quadrants (1 and 2), in an anterior open-bite case.
2. Extrusion of both posterior maxillary quadrants (1 and 2), in a nonextraction brachyfacial case.
3. Intrusion of one quadrant (e.g, quadrant 1), leaving the others alone, when only one side of the alveolar bone is overerupted and the occlusal plane is canted, such as in a growing patient.
4. Extrusion of one quadrant, leaving the others alone; the same situation as 3, except one quadrant is underdeveloped and needs some extrusion.
5. Intrusion of one quadrant (e.g., quadrant 1) and extrusion of the opposite quadrant (e.g., quadrant 2), in a nongrowing patient with a canted occlusal plane.
6. All four quadrants need either extrusion or intrusion, in a nongrowing patient with a tilted occlusal plane.

The devices used to correct occlusal plane inclinations are the extrusion or intrusion devices previously described in Figures 9-17 and 9-18.

Figure 9-24 shows an example of intrusion of quadrant 1 and extrusion of quadrant 2, to correct a canted occlusal plane. A tongue blade with a wire taped on top was used to assess the upper occlusal plane. The occlusal plane changed 5 degrees, as reflected on superimposed PA films.

TRANSVERSE CONTROL

In many cases, both the left and the right need to be expanded equally bilaterally, but in some cases, expansion is required only unilaterally.

BILATERAL EXPANSION

Some of the most popular fixed expansion appliances are the "Quad Helix" and the "Hyrax" screw. In all these tooth-borne devices, buccal tipping of the molars is observed. To decrease this tipping effect, the fixed expansion device, such as the Hyrax in Figure 9-25, can be bonded directly to the miniscrew. This might provide better control over the alveolar bone expansion.

UNILATERAL EXPANSION

Achieving unilateral expansion is difficult. Unilateral expansion may be attempted by anchoring the expansion device on the TAD on one side and attaching it to a tooth on the other side. Figure 9-26, *A*, shows a surgical cast of a patient with skeletal Class III malocclusion in which the objective was unilateral expansion of the right posterior region. The unilateral expansion was done by using the miniscrew on one side and the teeth on the other.

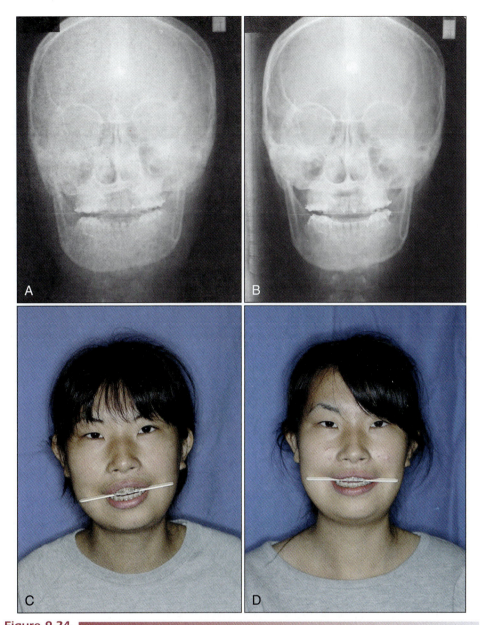

Figure 9-24
Canted Occlusal Plane: Quadrant 1 Intrusion; Quadrant 2 Extrusion. A, Initial AP radiograph. **B,** Radiograph 7 months after treatment. **C** and **D,** Frontal photographs (with tongue blade on area of first molar) show the changes resulting from treatment.

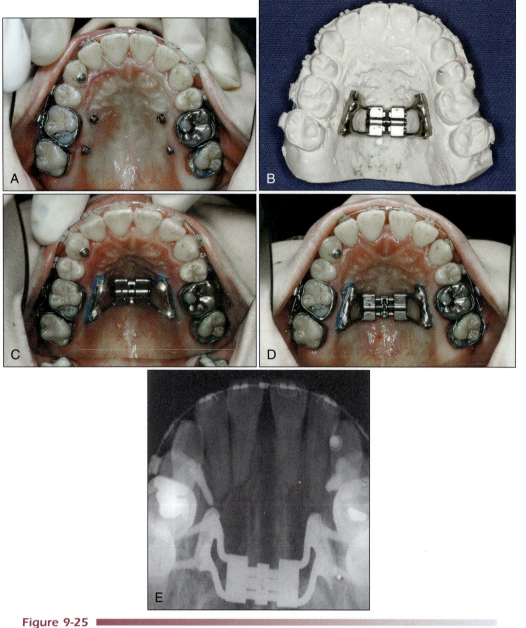

Figure 9-25

Transverse Control: Bilateral Expansion. A, Four miniscrews implanted on the palatal alveolar bone. **B,** Four arms of the Hyrax are soldered to a stainless steel, U-shaped plate. **C,** Hyrax was bonded on top of four miniscrews. **D,** Rapid expansion of 7 mm was accomplished in 1 week. **E,** Radiograph shows the expansion of the maxillary midpalatal suture area.

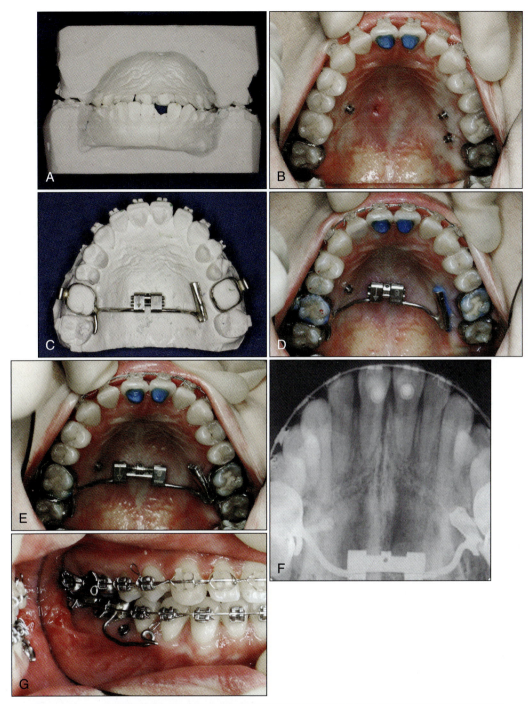

Figure 9-26
Transverse Control: Unilateral Expansion. A, Model before expansion, showing right crossbite of the right second molars. Model was trimmed at the middle of the second molars. **B,** Preparation of upper arch with three miniscrews, two for actual expansion and the third for extrusion after expansion to correct the tilted occlusal plane. **C,** Hyrax expansion screw on model. **D,** Hyrax is cemented on the maxilla. **E,** Maxilla after 7 mm of expansion. **F,** Occlusal radiograph shows that expansion is mainly in the posterior region. **G,** Intraoral photograph after 1 month of expansion on the right side shows that the posterior crossbite has been corrected.

CASE REPORT 9-4: THREE-DIMENSIONAL TREATMENT PLAN FOR OPEN BITE

A female patient age 16 years, 4 months presented with significant anterior open bite (Figure 9-27, A and B). A cephalograph and the profilogram depicting the norm for individuals of the same age, race, and gender are superimposed on the SN (Figure 9-27, C). The differences highlight the deviation of the patient from the norm and guide the clinician in determining the proper treatment plan. Additionally, the PA cephalogram aides in a 3D evaluation of the occlusal planes (Figure 9-27, D).

The lateral cephalogram revealed that the relationship of the Frankfort horizontal plane to the occlusal plane was 15.3 degrees. Intrusion of the maxillary molars was necessary to correct the anterior open bite. Additionally, the vector of the force on the maxillary molars needed to

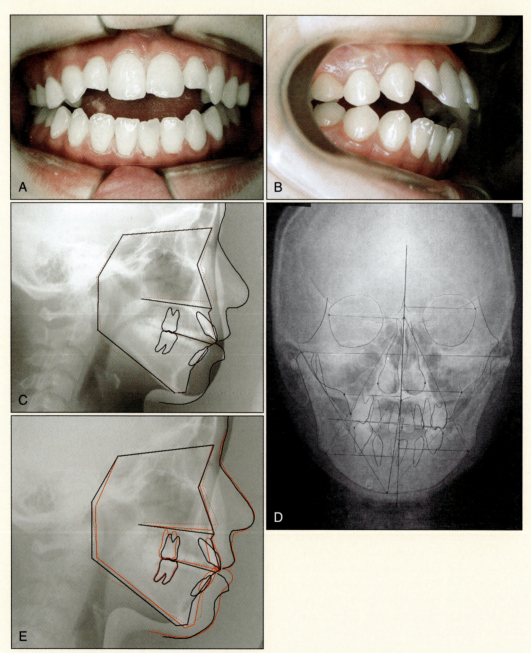

Figure 9-27　Open Bite: Three-Dimensional Evaluation. A and B, Initial intraoral photos. C, Initial cephalogram and average profilogram *(dotted line)* are superimposed on SN. D, 3D image using acquired information. E, Cephalogram after debonding of fixed appliance.

CASE REPORT 9-4: THREE-DIMENSIONAL TREATMENT PLAN FOR OPEN BITE—cont'd

include a distal component to correct the Class II occlusion. Intrusion of the maxillary occlusal plane would not only result in mandibular autorotation and vertical correction but also reduce the anteroposterior discrepancy (overjet) between the two arches for Class II correction.

This patient was treated using the appliance in Figure 9-21, A. This appliance directed an intrusive and posterior force that adequately matched the treatment objectives.

The occlusal and facial outcomes in this patient were favorable. The anterior vertical height was decreased by 5 mm, and the bite was closed (Figure 9-27, E and F).

The upper posterior teeth were retracted and intruded to correct the Class II molar relationship to a Class I. The mandibular midline was corrected to match the maxilla, although both midlines were positioned to the left side by about 1 mm (Figure 9-27, G). Mandibular autorotation improved the chin projection too.

Overall, the facial changes in this patient were significant (Figure 9-28). The amount of the intrusion accomplished at the first molar level was approximately 2 mm. The intermolar width also increased, from 59 to 61 mm in the maxilla and from 55 to 57 mm in the mandible (Figure 9-29).

Age	16y4m	18y10m
Facial angle	82.0	82.4
Convexity	13.8	10.7
A-B plane	-8.2	-5.4
Y-axis	68.0	68.0
FH to SN	5.8	5.1
∠SNA	83.0	82.6
∠SNB	76.8	78.4
∠ANB	6.2	4.3
N-Pog to SN	76.2	77.4
Nasal floor to SN	12.6	11.6
Nasal floor to FH	6.8	6.5
Mandibular pl. to SN	41.5	42.0
Mandibular pl. to FH	35.7	36.9
Ramus pl. to SN	100.2	95.6
Ramus pl. to FH	94.4	90.5
Gonial angle	121.2	126.4
U1 to SN	119.1	103.1
U1 to FH	124.9	108.1
L1 to mandibular pl.	98.3	89.6
Interincisal angle	101.2	125.3
Occlusal pl. to SN	21.1	20.0
Occlusal pl. to FH	15.3	14.9

F

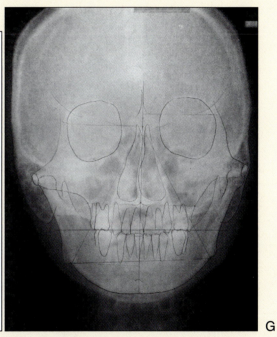

G

Figure 9-27, cont'd **F,** Cephalometric values before *(left)* and after *(right)* treatment. **G,** 3D image showing the upper posterior teeth retracted and intruded to correct the Class II molars to Class I. The mandible midline was corrected to be more proportional to the maxilla.

Continued

CASE REPORT 9-4: THREE-DIMENSIONAL TREATMENT PLAN FOR OPEN BITE—cont'd

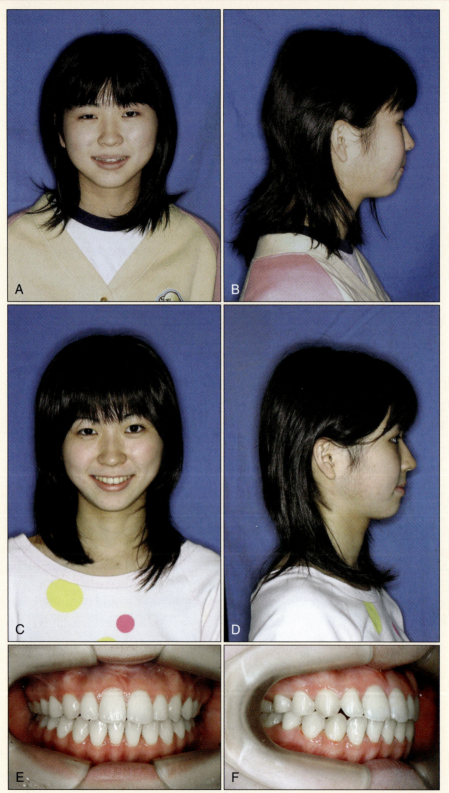

Figure 9-28 Open Bite: Facial Changes. A and B, Pretreatment facial photographs. C and D, Posttreatment facial photographs. E and F, Posttreatment intraoral photographs.

| CASE REPORT 9-4: | THREE-DIMENSIONAL TREATMENT PLAN FOR OPEN BITE—cont'd |

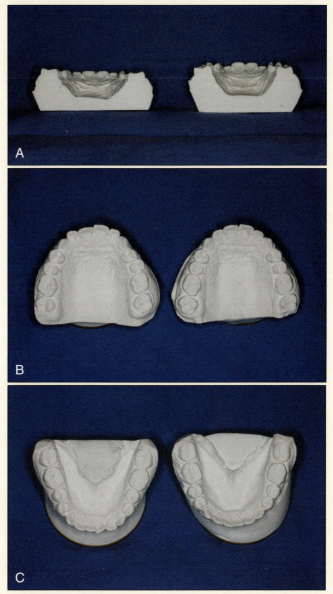

Figure 9-29 Open Bite: Differences on Models. **A,** Intrusion of posterior teeth. **B** and **C,** Difference in posterior arch width.

CONCLUSION

Diagnosis and treatment planning of occlusal plane problems depend on a thorough analysis in the three planes of space: sagittal, vertical, and transverse. Management of the occlusal plane may now be accomplished with TADs. Orthodontic movements of the posterior segments (intrusion, distalization, mesialization) are predictably achieved through skeletal anchorage. Thus, TADs are becoming an indispensable tool for the clinician.

A basic appliance design for three-dimensional management of the occlusal planes consists of an arch that connects the first molar bands of the maxilla or the mandible. This arch has attachments in the form of hooks or arms, to which forces with different vectors are delivered from the miniscrews. The device provides enough versatility to control the occlusal plane in three dimensions by varying the direction of force. It can also be modified in many ways to achieve specific tasks during treatment.

REFERENCES

1. Ricketts RM: *Provocations and perceptions in craniofacial orthopedics,* Denver, 1989, RMO.
2. Ritto AK: The lingual pearl, *Ortodoncia* 1:68-71, April 2000.
3. Ritto AK, Leitão P: The lingual pearl, *J Clin Orthod* 32(5):318-327, 1998.
4. Ricketts RM, Grummons D: Frontal cephalometrics: practical applications. Part 1, *World J Orthod* 4(4):297-316, 2003.
5. Grummons D, Ricketts RM: Frontal cephalometrics: practical applications. Part 2, *World J Orthod* 5(2):99-119, 2004.

ADDITIONAL READING

Anka G: [The management of noncompliant Class II extraction cases: use of Gurin lock and anterior fixed bite plate], *Portuguese Orthod J (Orthodontia),* December 2004.

Dawson PE: *Evaluation, diagnosis and treatment of occlusal problems,* ed 2, St Louis, 1989, Mosby.

Dawson PE: New definition for relating occlusion to varying conditions of the temporomandibular joint, *J Prosthet Dent* 74(6):619-627, 1995.

Dawson PE: A classification system for occlusions that relates maximal intercuspation to the position and condition of the temporomandibular joints, *J Prosthet Dent* 75(1):60-68, 1996.

Grummons D: Nonextraction emphasis: space-gaining efficiencies. Part 1, *World J Orthod* 2(1):21-32, 2001.

Grummons D: Nonextraction emphasis: space-gaining efficiencies. Part 2, *World J Orthod* 2(2):177-189, 2001.

Kanomi R: Mini-implant for orthodontic anchorage, *J Clin Orthod* 31(11):763-767, 1997.

Sugawara J, Daimaruya T, Umemori M, et al: Distal movement of mandibular molars in adult patients with the skeletal anchorage system, *Am J Orthod Dentofacial Orthop* 125(2):130-138, 2004.

Umemori M, Sugawara J, Mitani H, et al: Skeletal anchorage system for open-bite correction, *Am J Orthod Dentofacial Orthop* 115(2):166-174, 1999.

CHAPTER 10

Management of Missing Teeth Using Temporary Anchorage Devices

George Anka

Orthodontic treatment focuses primarily on a full complement of teeth. However, patients may present with missing teeth, and their treatment can be challenging. The orthodontist needs to consider the following factors throughout the treatment-planning process:

- Extractions should not be done on the side where teeth are already missing.
- An extraction on the contralateral side of the arch of the missing tooth is likely needed to create balance between the quadrants.
- A nonextraction approach involving space closure might result in a discrepancy between the facial and dental midlines.
- Replacement of the missing teeth with a dental implant may be needed, and space appropriation may be obtained with preprosthetic orthodontics.

CONGENITAL VS. ACQUIRED

Missing teeth generally have a genetic or an acquired etiology.

The phenomenon of congenitally missing teeth may involve *hypodontia*, with up to six missing teeth; *oligodontia*, more than six missing teeth; or *anodontia*, when all teeth are missing. However, the term *agenesis* more accurately describes the developmental disorder involved. The reported incidence of dental agenesis (missing any tooth) ranges from as low as 0.3% to as high as 36.5% in different communities.[1] The prevalence of agenesis in North America is higher in female (4.6%) than male (3.2%) populations, with a combined total prevalence of 3.9%.[2] Of those affected by agenesis, 41% lack the most frequently missing tooth, the lower second bicuspid; this is followed by the upper lateral (22.9% of those affected) and the upper second bicuspid (21.2%).

Missing teeth also may be classified as *acquired* (after birth). Two major reasons explain the loss of teeth after their eruption. The first is trauma, which is the usual cause of early permanent-tooth loss in the anterior maxillary region. Traumatic injury to the teeth can vary according to age, gender, and participation in activities such as sports; however, teeth in protrusive positions generally are at higher risk of trauma.[3] The second is caries and other dental-related pathology, such as cysts and periodontal disease, which can also result in missing-tooth problems.

Patients with congenitally missing teeth or teeth lost to trauma or pathology can benefit greatly from orthodontic treatment. Use of a temporary anchorage device (TAD) allows more accurate design and execution of the treatment plan and contributes to a good outcome. The TAD can help effect tooth movement of considerable range, as well as move the whole dentition of each arch from left to right, and vice versa. Thus, TADs are useful tools to correct the problem of malocclusion associated with missing teeth.

MESIALIZATION

Mesialization is an important orthodontic movement in which good mechanical control is necessary, especially if reciprocal movement of the anchor unit is unwanted. Additionally, mesial movement of the molars is a common approach to correct problems related to congenitally missing premolars.

MAXILLA

Mesialization of the posterior teeth in the maxilla is best done with TADs placed in the alveolar process of the palatal area. The midpalate provides an alternative if reduced alveolar space is observed. The palate has intact keratinized gingiva that reduces the risk of infection of the soft tissue surrounding the TAD.[4]

Transpalatal Bar Modification
If the missing teeth are the second maxillary bicuspids, or if these teeth must be extracted to match missing lower second premolars, a transpalatal bar can be used

and two TADs placed between the canine and the first bicuspid of the alveolar palate (Figure 10-1, *A*). The function of the transpalatal bar is to prevent rotation of the molar during mesialization. Bodily molar movement can be provided by adjusting the elastic's position so that the hook is placed closer to the center of resistance of the molars. Although the majority of the movement can be accomplished in this way, some independent, unilateral movement might be necessary for a short distance; this can be done by cutting the transpalatal bar and using it as a hook (Figure 10-1, *B* and *C*). This step is important to correct the midline and cusp tip-to-fossa relationship during the finishing phase. If one side of the maxilla is the only area where tooth movement is required, the hook can be soldered to the band itself. In a long-distance movement, however, rotation can occur as a side effect; therefore an additional TAD is placed on the buccal side. Force can be generated by using either an elastic chain or closed-coil nickel-titanium (Ni-Ti) spring.

MANDIBLE

In performing mesialization in the mandible, the clinician can move the molars with the same technique used for the maxilla; however, the active components of the appliance are placed on the buccal side only (Figure 10-2). TAD placement on the lingual side should be avoided because this tends to irritate the tongue, causing patient discomfort.

To accomplish mesialization, the screw must be placed off the trajectory of the moving molar. If this factor is not considered, as the molar moves mesially, the root of the tooth will touch the TAD immediately, and reimplantation of the screw will be necessary. Alternatively, the area of the retromolar pad may be selected as the TAD placement site. A device known as a "push-open coil spring-arm" can be used to deliver the mesially directed forces from the retromolar area. This strategic area can be used to move the quadrants of teeth in sequence. This stepwise approach to tooth movement allows for better control, although at the expense of a longer treatment time, as discussed later.

SHIFTING WHOLE ARCH: CLOCKWISE OR COUNTERCLOCKWISE ROTATION

In attempting to mesialize the posterior teeth, it is also important to ascertain whether there is any midline deviation.

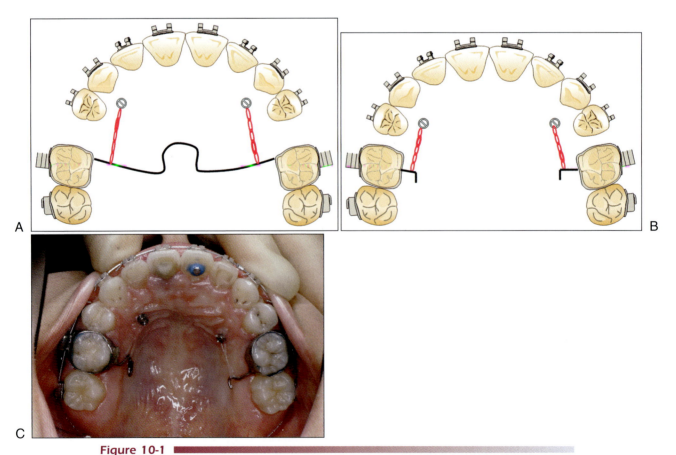

Figure 10-1

A, Transpalatal bar and two temporary anchorage devices (TADs). **B**, Bands with hooks. **C**, Hooks on palatal side of bands to move the molars mesially.

MOVING TEETH IN MAXILLA

In selecting the site for TAD placement, care should be taken not to disturb or irritate the patient's tongue or interfere with speech. The design varies but often integrates a transpalatal bar (Figure 10-3, *A*) or even a small expansion device such as Hyrax (Figure 10-3, *B*).

In doing the rotation movement of the whole arch, the transpalatal bar or expansion device (e.g., Hyrax) is necessary to preserve the integrity of the arch. I prefer to keep the arch as one solid structure, to maintain control of the occlusal plane throughout treatment. Expansion is usually needed during molar movement; otherwise, a crossbite on the posterior region can be created. The upper and lower molar relationship should be checked on each visit and expanded when necessary. The ligature tie on the molar brackets attaching the transpalatal bar should be kept as loose as possible; rotation of the involved molars is expected and will be corrected only after removal of the transpalatal bar. Moving the entire maxillary dentition around the *y* axis using this technique is easy because TAD placement in the maxilla can be done on both the buccal and the palatal side.

Push-Open Coil Spring-Arm

As already noted, the method using a pulling force may be difficult to deliver from a screw because it may interfere with the mesial movement path of the molar. Exerting a *pushing* force may be more desirable. The pushing device is quite simple and consists of a wire and an open-coil spring (Figure 10-4, *A*). Connecting the device to the TAD is also simple; most TADs have a neck around which the wire can be wrapped or a "plus" head form on top on which the wire can be bonded. The best choice of a wire in this case is a .016 × .016–inch stainless steel wire. Stainless steel is optimal because it can be bent to adapt to the configuration of the arch from

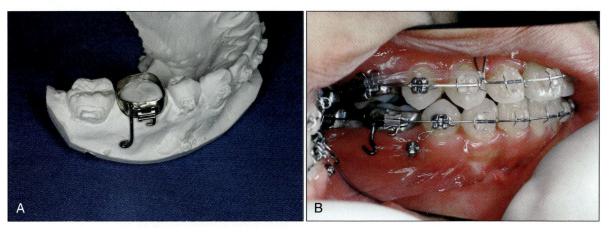

Figure 10-2
Band with a hook and TAD on the buccal side, on a model (**A**) and in place (**B**).

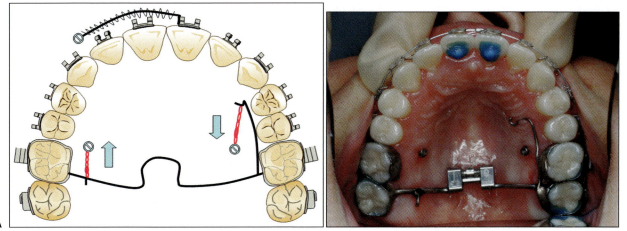

Figure 10-3
A, Transpalatal bar with a hook on the right side and extended arm soldered on the left to facilitate rotation of the upper arch. On the anterior side, a push-open coil spring-arm is used to move the midline to the left side. **B,** Hyrax expander used with a hook and an extended arm soldered on it to facilitate rotational movement of the whole upper arch.

the TAD to the selected tooth. The open-coil spring can be Ni-Ti or stainless steel. The force used can be adjusted to meet the needs of the specific case but is usually about 200 g.

An appropriate length of .030-inch Ni-Ti or stainless steel coil spring is measured (Figure 10-4, B). One end of the main wire is crimped onto the TAD and should be able to rotate freely along the axis of the TAD head; this flexibility is vital to prevent excessive strain on the TAD. At the other end, the wire is connected to the tooth targeted for movement. Brushing and food accumulation may easily dislodge the device. It is recommended to secure the device with a ligature wire to the bracket, instead of relying on the hook to secure the system. Rarely, activation is needed, in which case a stop can be easily added to the sectional wire, close to the attachment head of the screw. The area connected to the TAD may invite accumulation of food, leading to compromised oral hygiene. Cleaning this area is essential to keep the gingival tissue healthy.

MOVING TEETH IN MANDIBLE

Compared with the maxilla, moving the whole arch in the mandible is difficult because it is preferable to limit TAD placement to the buccal side only.

Once the decision has been made to move the whole arch, the usual strategy is to move the anterior part first. The midline is shifted in one direction, and then the molars are mesialized. The push-open coil spring device is very effective for this movement. This device can be adjusted in accordance with the configuration of the arch; it is fairly easy to place the force in the desired direction to deliver a constant force, resulting in the movement of the quadrant as desired. Two steps usually suffice to shift the whole mandibular arch a certain distance to correct the midline (Figure 10-5). In accomplishing sizable movements, it may be necessary to repeat the TAD placement two or even three times, although in actual practice this repeated implantation is rare.

CONGENITALLY MISSING TEETH

As mentioned, the tooth most often missing is the lower second bicuspid, followed by the upper lateral incisor and the upper second bicuspid. As the number of missing teeth increases, the degree of complexity of treatment also increases.

MISSING MANDIBULAR SECOND BICUSPID

The absence of a mandibular second bicuspid can be unilateral or bilateral. Treatment can be accomplished in the following two ways:

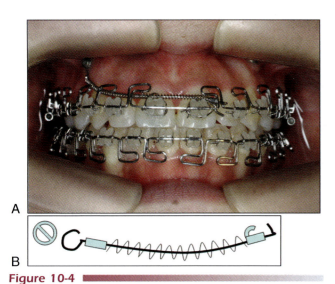

Figure 10-4

A, Push-open coil spring-arm, used to correct midline in the maxilla, moves the anterior teeth to the left side. **B**, Push-open coil spring-arm construction.

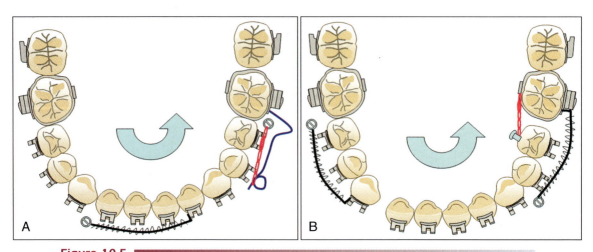

Figure 10-5

Two-step strategy to distalize the mandibular dentition on the left side (**A**) and move the lower midline to the left (**B**).

1. Maintain space for a future dental implant while correcting the rest of the malocclusion.
2. Close the space so that the patient will not need to receive a dental implant in the future.

The choice depends on the preference and philosophy of the primary clinician. Important issues include financial considerations, quality and quantity of alveolar bone, and duration of the orthodontic treatment with space closure versus dental implantation.[5,6]

CASE REPORT 10-1

A patient age 7 years, 6 months presented with congenitally missing lower second bicuspids and lower-right first bicuspid, as shown in the panoramic radiograph (Figure 10-6, A). All the maxillary teeth were present. A Class II, Division 1 deep bite was observed, with maxillary midline deviated to the right (Figure 10-6, B-F). The right upper lateral was in linguoversion. The general practitioner had referred the patient for an interdisciplinary consult to address the missing teeth.

The treatment plan was to align the upper and lower teeth and correct the Class II relationship. The missing teeth were limited to the mandible, so it was necessary to extract two teeth in the upper arch. In the maxilla the plan was to remove the upper second bicuspid and close all spaces except for the area of the lower-right first bicuspid, which was to receive a dental implant in the future.

A fixed appliance was placed only to align the upper anterior teeth, after which it was removed. The patient was

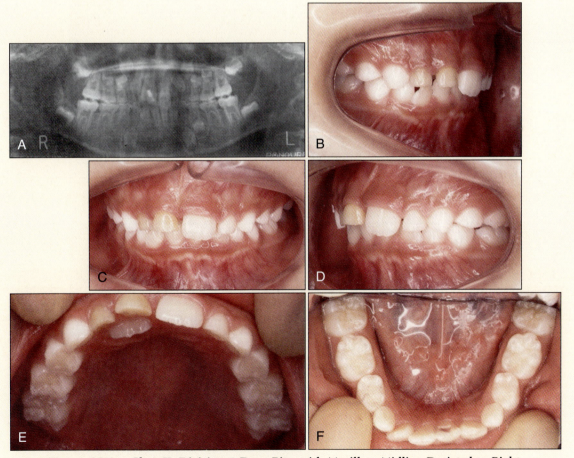

Figure 10-6 Class II, Division 1 Deep Bite, with Maxillary Midline Deviated to Right. Missing teeth: lower-right second bicuspid (#45), lower-right first bicuspid (#44), and lower-left second bicuspid (#35). **A,** Initial panoramic radiograph. **B** to **F,** Initial intraoral photographs.

Continued

CASE REPORT 10-1—cont'd

13 years old when the second phase was initiated. All spaces were closed except for the lower-right first bicuspid area, where a miniscrew was placed (Figure 10-6, *G*). A temporary acrylic crown was built on top of the screw to help restore function and serve as a "space maintainer," which would also prevent the opposing tooth from over-erupting (Figure 10-6, *H* and *I*). This is called a "primary implant" because it is a provisional device that can be applied before the permanent implant is placed. The nonosseointegrating orthodontic screw implant was 2 mm in diameter and 8 mm in length. Although the screw has the advantage of easy removal in the future, it may not withstand severe bruxism, and failure may occur. In the patient with severe bruxism the author recommends placing two screws, splinted together with an acrylic temporary crown, or soldering a space maintainer (e.g., wire) to the molar band (Figure 10-6, *J*).

At completion of the fixed-appliance phase, the patient was 15 years, 10 months old (Figure 10-6, *K* to *O*). The primary implant was in the area of the lower-right first bicuspid. The panoramic radiograph shows a single screw with a provisional crown attached (Figure 10-6, *P*). The dental implant was placed at age 18 years, 4 months, when the patient entered college. The results are shown in Figure 10-6, *Q* and *R*.

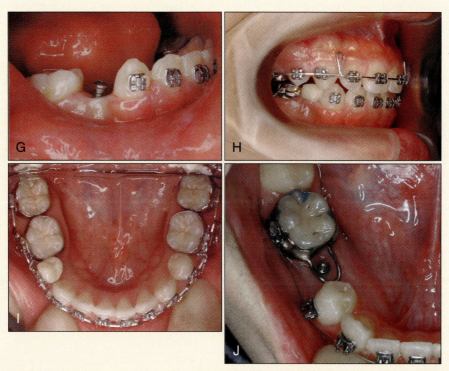

Figure 10-6, cont'd G, Miniscrew placement. **H** and **I,** Crown built on top of screw. **J,** Wire soldered to molar band. **K** to **O,** Patient condition on removal of fixed appliance. **P,** Panoramic radiograph showing a single screw with provisional crown on it. **Q** and **R,** Intraoral photographs showing final treatment results.

CASE REPORT 10-1—cont'd

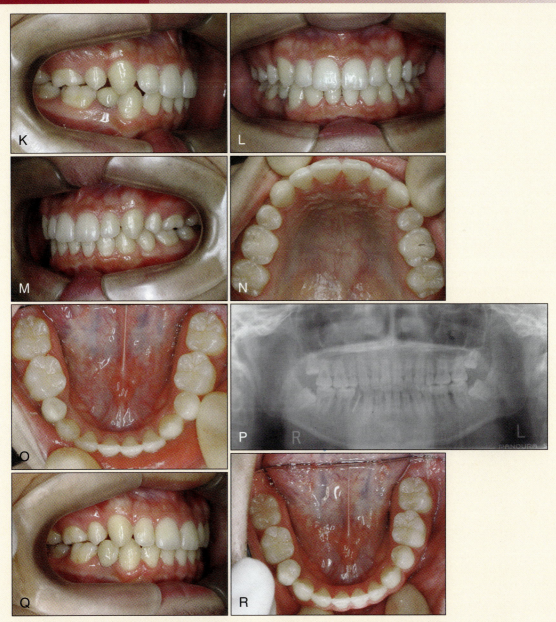

Figure 10-6, cont'd For legend see opposite page.

MISSING UPPER LATERAL INCISOR

The greatest problem with missing upper lateral incisors is the esthetic impact; therefore, treatment should start as early as possible. Indeed, treatment usually is sought by parents, who bring their child at age 8 or 9 years for an orthodontic evaluation after noticing that the lateral incisor is absent. Two treatment options are available, as for any other missing tooth: the space can either be preserved for a future prosthodontic restoration,[7-9] or the space can be closed.[10]

Case Report 10-2 illustrates the management of a patient with congenitally missing maxillary lateral incisors for whom a combination of the two treatment options was used.

CASE REPORT 10-2

A female patient age 9 years, 5 months presented with a large diastema between her central incisors and complained about her appearance. She had an orthognathic skeletal profile and Class I molar relationship. The missing teeth were the upper-right and upper-left lateral incisors and the lower-left lateral incisor. Additionally, the maxillary central incisors were wider than normal (Figure 10-7, A to F).

The diastema was closed in the first phase of treatment using fixed appliances, whereas the space for lateral incisors was maintained with a fixed type of resin-bonded bridge through the retention phase. The patient returned at age 16 to resume treatment, dissatisfied with the esthetics of the resin-bonded bridges. The patient was reevaluated, and the treatment plan included closure of the maxillary right lateral space and prosthetically replacing the left lateral incisor. Space was to be gained for the lateral incisor, partially by interproximal reduction of the wide central incisors. The remaining space would be obtained through distalization of the maxillary buccal segments (Figure 10-7, G to L).

Two TADs were used on the palate and two on the buccal side to retract the maxillary posterior teeth (Figure 10-7, M). Two additional TADs were placed in the posterior mandibular region between the first molar and the second bicuspid on the left, and between the bicuspids on the right (Figure 10-7, N). The specific goal was to shift the lower anterior dentition to the left. The panoramic view shows the exact location of the TADs (Figure 10-7, O).

The results of treatment are seen in Figure 10-7, P to W. On the upper-left side, sufficient lateral space remained for a future prosthetic restoration. Bone support was also adequate for a dental implant. A retainer with a denture tooth was delivered for space maintenance, until the patient decided on the desired type of permanent prosthetic restoration.

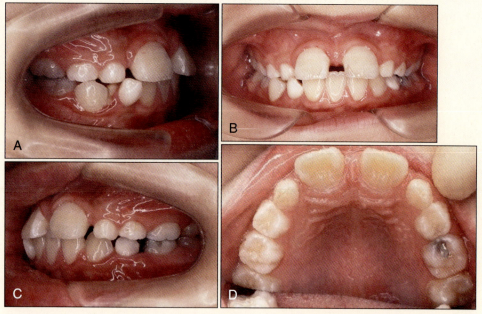

Figure 10-7 **Class I Skeletal and Class I Molar Relationship.** Missing teeth: upper-right lateral (#12), upper-left lateral (#22), and lower-left lateral (#32). **A to E,** Initial intraoral photographs at start of first phase of treatment (age 9 yr, 5 mo). **F,** Initial panoramic radiograph, first phase of treatment. **G to K,** Initial intraoral photographs at start of second treatment phase (age 16 yr, 9 mo). **L,** Initial panoramic radiograph, second phase of treatment. **M,** Two TADs on palate and two on buccal side. **N,** Two TADs on posterior region of mandible between the first molar and the second bicuspid on the left and between the bicuspids on the right.

CASE REPORT 10-2—cont'd

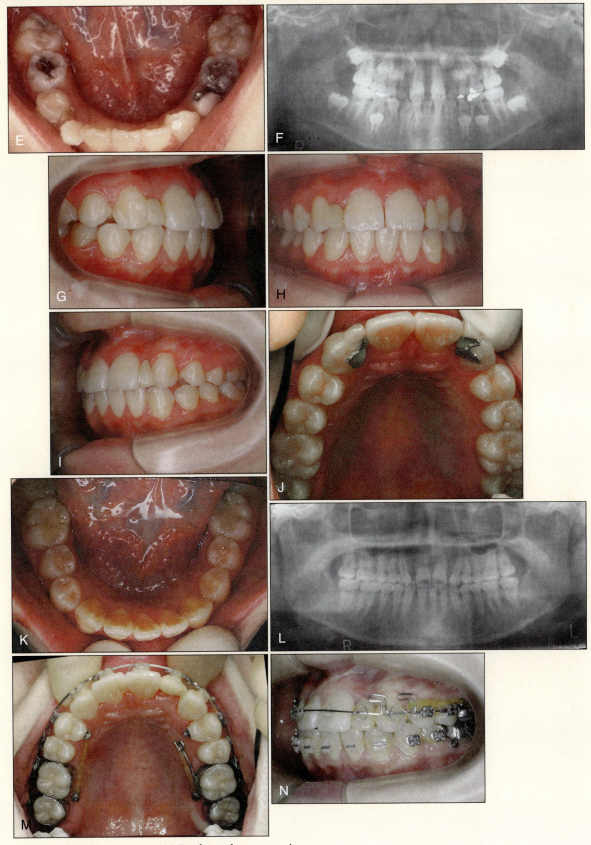

Figure 10-7, cont'd For legend see opposite page.

Continued

CASE REPORT 10-2—cont'd

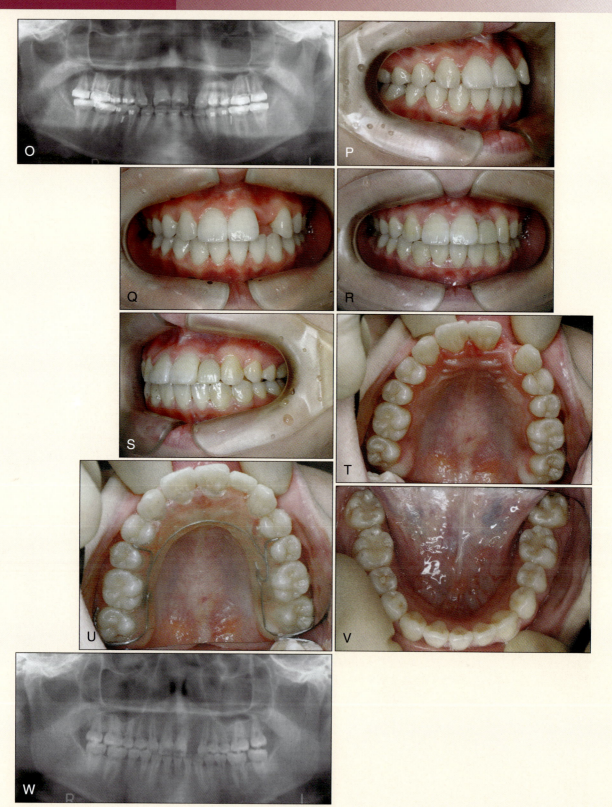

Figure 10-7, cont'd **O**, Panoramic view showing precise location of the TADs. **P** to **W**, Final treatment results.

MISSING UPPER SECOND BICUSPID

The upper second bicuspid is the third most common congenitally missing tooth. The treatment is usually straightforward. Case Report 10-3 describes the space management in a patient missing a maxillary second premolar. Although the absent premolar did not have a genetic etiology, the case illustrates the space management considerations in similar clinical situations.

CASE REPORT 10-3

A male patient age 12 years, 2 months presented with a crowded dentition that his parents wanted addressed. During the radiological examination, a large cyst in the area of the upper-left second bicuspid was detected. The cyst had prevented the eruption of the related tooth and extended to the apices of the adjacent first molar and first bicuspid. He also had an ectopic upper-right canine, which was transposed and located between the central and the lateral incisors. The presence of the deciduous canine may have contributed to his malocclusion (Figure 10-8, A). His skeletal pattern showed a Class II tendency with bimaxillary dentoalveolar protrusion (Figure 10-8, B; intraoral photos, C-F).

After discussing the malocclusion with the general dentist and the oral surgeon, it was decided to perform a total removal of the cyst with the associated tooth and close all spaces. Treatment began by tipping distally the transposed maxillary canine. In the posterior region the plate type of anchorage, or skeletal anchorage system (SAS), was used to move the right maxillary molar forward (Figure 10-8, G and H).

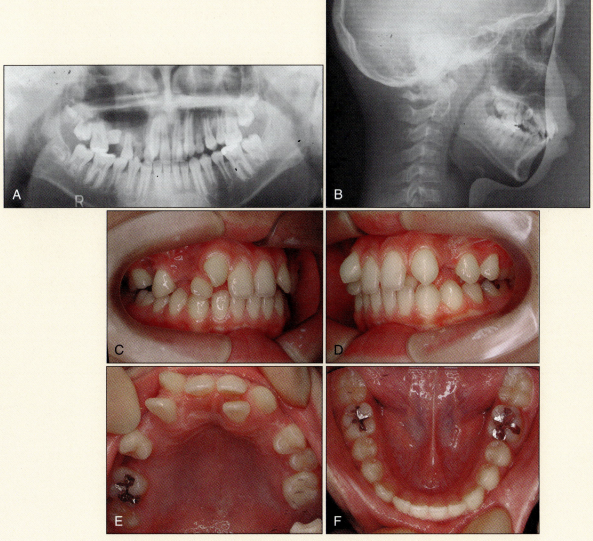

Figure 10-8 **Large Cyst in Area of Upper-Left Second Bicuspid. A,** Panoramic radiograph of initial record. **B,** Cephalograph of initial record. **C to F,** Initial intraoral photographs.

Continued

CASE REPORT 10-3—cont'd

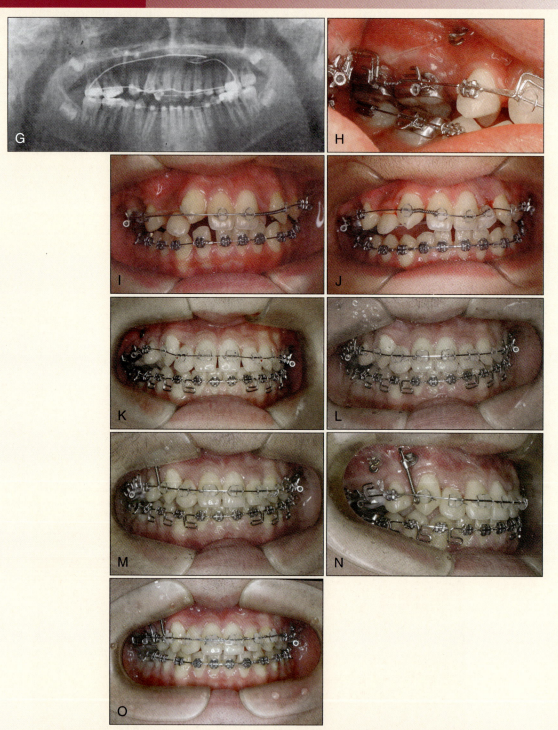

Figure 10-8, cont'd G, Panoramic radiograph, and H, intraoral photograph, showing the skeletal anchorage system in use to move the molar forward. I to O, Sequence of treatment, showing upper-right canine pushed upward during an attempt to correct the reversed teeth. Upper-right canine is extruded and moved mesially, using push-open coil spring-arm device, also used to correct the midline.

CASE REPORT 10-3—cont'd

The upper-right canine was pushed gingivally during the attempt to correct the transposition, resulting in an inclined maxillary plane in the anterior region. Thus, extrusion of the upper-right canine using a push-open coil spring-arm device was necessary to control the side effect. The same device was also used to correct the midline because the upper midline deviated to the right at the completion of alignment of the anterior teeth. The treatment sequence is shown in Figure 10-8, *I* to *O*.

The right maxillary molar protraction proved to be difficult. A redesigned band on the molar with a hook on the lingual aspect of the first and second molar was applied to deliver a force closer to the center of resistance (Figure 10-8, *P-S*). The molars began movement as predicted, and the extraction space, once occupied by the cyst, was closed.

The fixed-appliance treatment achieved good occlusion and function (Figure 10-8, *T-X*). The case shows that a molar mesial movement of considerable distance can be predictably accomplished using TADs (Figure 10-8, *Y* and *Z*).

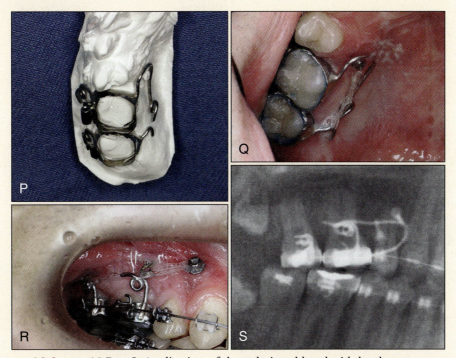

Figure 10-8, cont'd **P** to **S**, Application of the redesigned band with hook.

Continued

CASE REPORT 10-3—cont'd

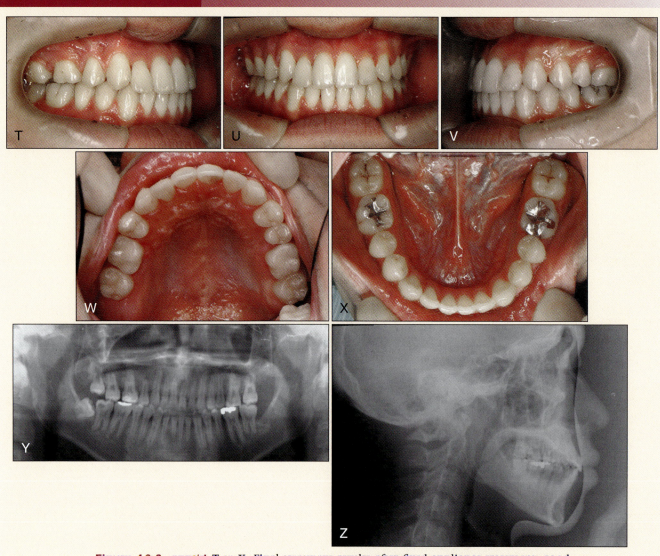

Figure 10-8, cont'd T to X, Final treatment results after fixed-appliance treatment; good occlusion and function were achieved. Y, Posttreatment panoramic radiograph. Z, Posttreatment cephalograph.

CONCLUSION

Problems involving missing teeth are complex and require an interdisciplinary approach. Multiple missing teeth can be especially difficult to manage, particularly when both anterior and posterior teeth are missing. Protraction of posterior teeth is difficult because side effects such as tipping of the occlusal planes often occur. Excellent biomechanical control is needed to achieve this movement in the three planes of space. TADs have helped to widen the range of tooth movements possible, increasing the treatment options for missing teeth.

REFERENCES

1. Mahaney MC, Fujiwara TM, Morgan K: Dental agenesis in Dariusleut Hutterite brethren: comparisons to select Caucasoid population surveys, *Am J Phys Anthropol* 82(2):165-177, 1990.
2. Polder BJ, Van't Hof MA, Van der Linder FP, et al: A meta-analysis of the prevalence of dental agenesis of permanent teeth, *Community Dent Oral Epidemiol* 32(3):217-226, 2004.
3. Kania MJ, Keeling SD: Risk factors associated with incisor injury in elementary school children, *Angle Orthod* 66(6):423-432, 1996.

4. Park H, Jeong S, Kwon O: Factors affecting the clinical success of screw implants used as orthodontic anchorage, *Am J Orthod Dentofacial Orthop* 130(1):18-25, 2006.
5. Fowler PV: Long-term treatment planning for single tooth implants: an orthodontic perspective, *Ann R Australas Coll Dent Surg* 15:120-121, 2000.
6. Wexler G: Missing upper lateral incisors: orthodontic considerations in young patients, *Ann R Australas Coll Dent Surg* 15:136-140, 2000.
7. Millar BJ, Taylor NG: Lateral thinking: the management of missing upper lateral incisors, *Br Dent J* 179(3):99-106, 1995.
8. Kokich VO Jr, Kinzer GA: Managing congenital missing lateral incisors. I. Canine substitution, *J Esthet Restor Dent* 17(1):5-10, 2005.
9. Kinzer GA, Kokich VO Jr: Managing congenitally missing lateral incisors. III. Single-tooth implants, *J Esthet Restor Dent* 17(4):202-210, 2005.
10. Garg AK: Treatment of congenital missing maxillary lateral incisors: orthodontics, bone grafts, and osseointegrated implants, *Dent Implantol Update* 13(2):9-14, 2002.

ADDITIONAL READING

Balshi TJ: Osseointegration and orthodontics: modern treatment for congenital missing teeth, *Int J Periodont Restor Dent* 13(6):494-505, 1993.

Hyomoto M, Kawakami M, Inoue M, et al: Clinical conditions for eruption of maxillary canines and mandibular premolars associated with dentigerous cysts, *Am J Orthod Dentofacial Orthop* 124(5):515-520, 2003.

Kinzer GA, Kokich VO Jr: Managing congenital missing lateral incisors. II. Tooth-supported restorations, *J Esthet Restor Dent* 17(2):76-84, 2005.

Kokich VG: Maxillary lateral incisor implants: planning with the aid of orthodontics, *J Oral Maxillofac Surg* 62(9, suppl 2):48-56, 2004.

Rasmussen P, Kotsaki A: Inherited primary failure of eruption in the primary dentition: report of five cases, *J Dent Child* 64(1):43-47, 1997.

Savarrio L, McIntyre GT: To open or to close space—that is the missing lateral incisor question, *Dent Update* 32(1):16-25, 2005.

Sugawara J, Daimaruya T, Umemori M, et al: Distal movement of mandibular molars in adult patients with the skeletal anchorage system, *Am J Orthod Dentofacial Orthop* 125(2):130-138, 2004.

CHAPTER 11

Skeletal Anchorage: Different Approaches

A. Korrodi Ritto

The need for skeletal anchorage has increased with the growing number of adult and edentulous patients. The use of stable anchorage in orthodontics may help avoid unwanted movements of the anchorage teeth. This approach replaces traditional procedures that use extraoral elements (headgear) or intraoral appliances such as Nance buttons or other complicated appliance designs, which need patient cooperation. This means that the orthodontist no longer depends on patient compliance, which will increase treatment for adults. This anchorage system gives the orthodontist an added benefit because the orthodontic forces, applied continuously, might even shorten the overall treatment time. Moreover, patients without enough tooth support (posterior edentulous areas) can be treated using skeletal anchorage as artificial teeth.

Endosseous implants made from a variety of materials and designs have been used in orthodontic treatment for anchorage for many years.[1,2] Endosseous implants osseointegrate after unloaded healing periods. After achieving osseointegration, these implants can be used for orthodontic purposes. Conventional implants are limited by space and can be placed only in retromolar or edentulous areas. Furthermore, the surgical procedure, cost, and delay between implantation and orthodontic force application are major drawbacks.

Various methods for bone anchorage have been tested: cobalt-chromium (Vitallium) screws,[1] vitreous carbon, bioglass-coated aluminum oxide implants, stainless steel plates and screws, Branemark implants,[3,4] retromolar implants,[3] onplants,[5] zygomatic wires,[6] ankylosed teeth,[7] palatal implants,[8] miniplates,[9,10] and microimplants.[11-28]

Microscrews and miniplates have advantages over cylindrical endosseous implants and disk-shaped onplants, including ease of manipulation, ability to withstand immediate force loading, price, and minimal irritation of the oral tissues.[9,11-28]

CHARACTERISTICS OF MICROIMPLANTS

Microimplants should have the following characteristics (Figure 11-1):

- Simple to use (orthodontist should be able to comfortably insert and remove the implant).
- Immediately loadable.
- Inexpensive.
- Small dimensions (small enough to place in any area of alveolar bone, even apical bone).
- Withstand orthodontic forces.
- Stay immobile during treatment.
- Biocompatible.
- Not require compliance.
- Provide superior results than traditional anchorage.

A microimplant can be divided into three parts: head, neck, and body (Figure 11-2). The head should be designed to be used with auxiliary devices such as coil springs or ligature wires. A long-head type can prevent gingival impingement, particularly in posterior areas. A bracket head type allows concurrent use of orthodontic wires attached to the microimplant.

The neck of the microimplant has two forms. The small neck is used in most cases, and the long, smooth neck is used when the mucosa is thick (palatal mucosa).

For the body of the microimplant, a tapered shape is more common and safer than a parallel shape because the end part is thinner, with less risk of touching the root surface. Although microimplants are available as self-drilling and self-tapping, the threaded part of the body (see Figure 11-2, *D*) should start at the tip. A cut edge is also important for self-drilling types.

NOMENCLATURE

Skeletal anchorage system (SAS) includes all the devices fixed to the bone with the goal of increasing anchorage for orthodontic purposes. Temporary anchorage device (TAD) refers to all variations of implants, screws, pins, and onplants placed specifically to provide orthodontic anchorage and removed on completion of biomechanical therapy. The terms used in the literature include mini-implant, miniscrew, microscrew, micro-implant, anchor screw, anchor implant, mini-implant screw, mini–dental screw, mini–dental implant, micro-anchorage system, micro–anchor implant, ortho–anchor

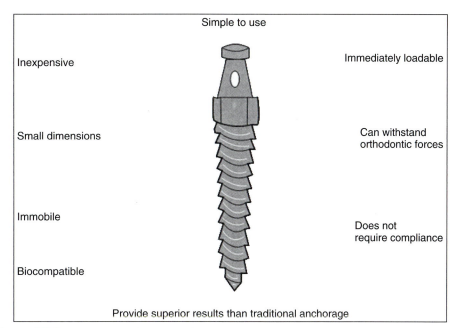

Figure 11-1
Ideal Characteristics of Microimplant.

screw, ortho–anchor pin, orthoscrew, pin, and transitional implant.

Although "micro" may mean one-millionth (10^{-6}); e.g., micrometer), this prefix is also widely used in medical and dental fields to emphasize small size (e.g., micrognathia, microdontia, microglossia). The term "implant" is used for any material retained more than 1 month in the body, according to EEC/MDD norms (MDD 93/42/EEC of June 1993 concerning medical device, Annex IX, 1.2). Therefore the author believes *microimplant* is the best term to use.

RESORBABLE SCREWS FOR ORTHODONTIC ANCHORAGE

The risks associated with metallic microfixation devices used in pediatric craniofacial surgery and the need for subsequent removal led to the development of biodegradable miniosteosynthesis devices. Devices made of polylactic acid and polyglycolic acid and their copolymers have been used in the internal fixation of fractures and osteotomies in orthopedic surgery since the 1980s after extensive experimental studies.[29] The biocompatibility of certain resorbable materials and the urgent need for alternative methods to metallic fixation led to a rapid transition to biodegradable fixation in nonloaded osteosyntheses in the pediatric neurocranium after 1995.

COMMON PROBLEMS ASSOCIATED WITH METALLIC FIXATION

Problems related to rigid (metallic) fixation in the growing skull include restriction of growth and passive translocation of metallic implants (device transposition). Metallic fixation devices may also cause a distinct cosmetic deformity, palpability, or wound dehiscence, especially if placed under a scarred, tight scalp, as well as allergic reactions, and may interfere with radiological investigations and other imaging (e.g., MRI).

Compared with other metals, titanium is considered highly biocompatible with a high degree of corrosion resistance.[30,31] Although titanium ions may stay bound to local tissue, they may also bind to protein moieties that are transported through the bloodstream and lymphatics to remote organs.[32] Hypersensitivity reactions to titanium have been reported.[33] Corrosion and wear have also been suspected to induce chemical carcinogenesis.[34] However, reports are sparse, and titanium is the best material for implantation in regard to cost/benefit ratio.

Common reasons for metallic rigid fixation removal include palpable or prominent fixtures (34.5% of patients needing implant removal), loosening of plates and screws (25.5%), pain (25.5%), infection (23.6%), wound dehiscence/exposure of hardware (20%), and removal at the time of secondary procedures (9.1%).[35]

MATERIAL

Polylactic acid (PLA) and *polyglycolic acid* (PGA) are derivatives of cyclic diesters of glycolic and lactic acid and are produced by ring-opening polymerization, resulting in poly-alpha-hydroxy derivatives of the original acids.[36] Polymers exhibit a glass transition temperature (Tg), below which the polymer is solid and stiff and above which it is soft.[37] PGA is a hard, brownish crystalline polymer that melts at about 224° to 228°C, with a Tg of 36° C.[38] PGA lacks a methyl group, which makes it hydrophilic and thus more susceptible to hydrolysis and faster degradation than polylactide. PLA is a pale semicrystalline polymer with a Tg of 57° C and a melting point of 174° to 184° C.[38-41]

The asymmetrical lactic acid molecule has two stereoisomeric forms, L-lactide and D-lactide.[42] In the human body the L isomer exists in carbohydrate metabolism, and the D isomer is found in acidic milk. If the polymer consists only of the L isomer, it is called *poly-L-lactic acid* (PLLA), which has been used most often in orthopedic implants.

Weakness of the materials was the major limiting factor in the manufacture of mini-implants in the 1980s. Bulky, highly crystalline PLLA implants caused foreign body reactions,[43] which made all biodegradable implants suspect. Remnants of pure-PLA implants have been identified up to 8 years after implantation,[44] raising the question whether PLA is too "biostable" to be used as a bioresorbable material.[45]

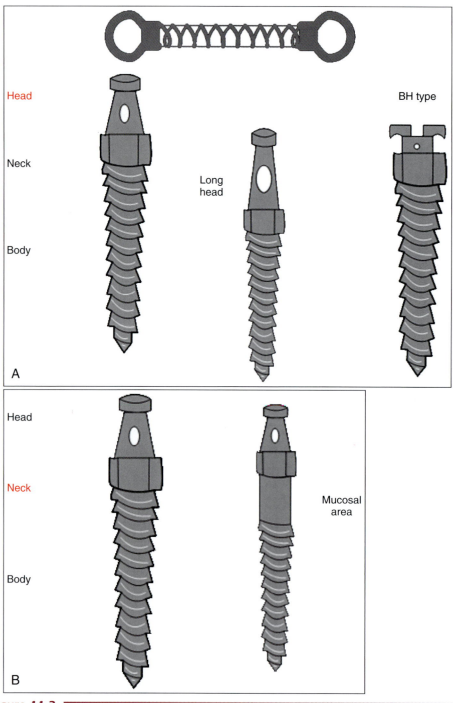

Figure 11-2

Three Parts of Microimplant. **A**, Head (*BH*, bracket head); **B**, neck; **C** and **D**, body.

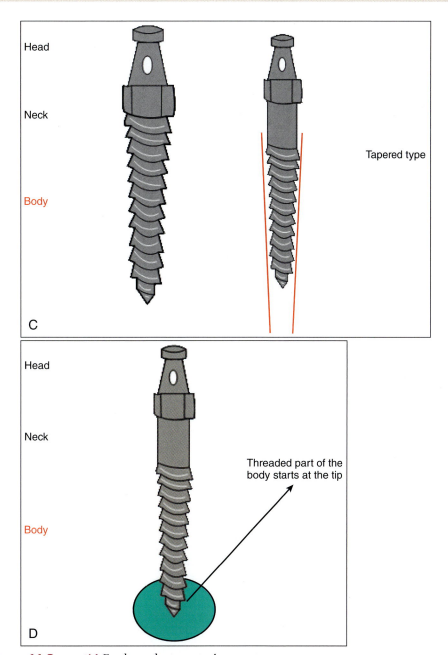

Figure 11-2, cont'd For legend see opposite page.

The *self-reinforcing technique* of Rokkanen and Törmälä enables the manufacture of extremely strong orthopedic *implants* and also thin but strong *mini-implants*.[29,46] The histological demonstration of *complete device resorption* without adverse local tissue effects is important before clinical application, because incomplete polymer elimination may eventually be associated with chronic inflammatory tissue changes.[47]

BIOCOMPATIBILITY

Bioabsorbable materials generally undergo a two-phase degradation process in the body. In the first, mainly physical phase, water molecules hydrolyze the chemical bonds of the polymer and cut long polymer chains to short chains. During this depolymerization process, the overall molecular weight and strength of the polymer are reduced, and the polymer is fragmented. The second phase involves phagocytosis of the fragments by macrophages, and the polymer mass rapidly disappears.[37] PGA is converted hydrolytically into glycolic acid and PLA into lactic acid, which is further metabolized in the citric acid cycle to carbon dioxide and water, and the final products are excreted through respiration or urine.

Hydrophilic *PGA*, although highly crystalline, becomes absorbed very quickly in the body, losing virtually all strength in 6 weeks[48] and all mass within 3 to 12 months.[39] Excellent biocompatibility and slow biodegradation of *PLA* have been documented in hundreds of reports; no inflammatory cell infiltration has been reported, and foreign body reactions have been limited to areas around the implanted material.[49-51]

Copolymers of PLA and PGA (PLGA) offer the capability of altering the degradation rate and mechanical properties of implants by changing the PLA/PGA ratio, which offers the potential to develop site-specific bone fixation and soft tissue anchoring devices.[14,52-54] Complete absorption of *PLGA 75/25* has been reported in 220 days, *PLGA 50/50* in 180 days,[42] and *PLGA 82/18* in 180 to 450 days.[53,55] No implant-related clinical foreign body reactions have been reported with PLGA implants.

An orthodontic implant anchor system consisting of an implant made of biodegradable polylactide (90/10) with a metal abutment was developed by Glatzmaier et al.[56,57] in 1995 and called BIOS (bioresorbable implant anchor for orthodontics system). Shear strength and maximum vertical strength were measured in biomechanical in vitro tests. The results suggest that BIOS can be used as an orthodontic anchoring system up to the time of degradation. However, ongoing clinical studies are evaluating practicability and biocompatibility of the BIOS implants.

CASE REPORT 11-1

Resorbable screws (1.6-mm diameter) made of the copolymer PLGA 75/25 were placed in the area of tooth #16. Two screws were placed because the distal screw was not well fixed, and it was decided to retain it and place another screw mesially (Figure 11-3, *A* and *B*).

The plan was to apply 120 g of force to distalize both premolars and canine until Class I was achieved. Because only 3 mm of distalization was needed, it was expected to move the teeth in place after 3 months of active force.

A plastic button was bonded with composite to the head of the screw (Figure 11-3, *C*). The button debonded 3 weeks later and was rebonded.

Three months later the upper premolars had distalized 3 mm, and some mobility of the screw was noticed. Eighty days after inserting the screws, the distal screw disappeared (Figure 11-3, *D*), and the same occurred for the other screw in 118 days (Figure 11-3, *E* and *F*).

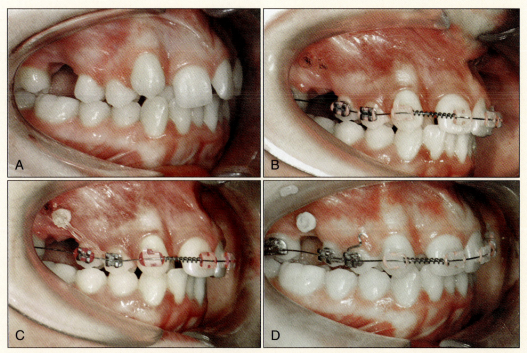

Figure 11-3 **A** and **B**, Two resorbable screws were placed to increase anchorage during premolar retraction. **C**, Plastic button was bonded to the head of the screw. **D**, Distal screw disappeared 80 days after insertion.

Continued

CASE REPORT 11-1—cont'd

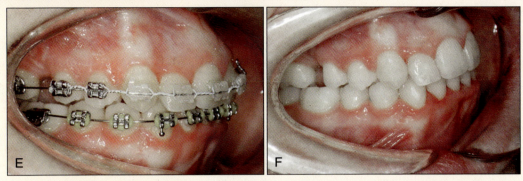

Figure 11-3, cont'd **E** and **F**, Mesial screw disappeared 118 days after insertion.

DISCUSSION

Absorbable screws are made of a resorbable copolymer, a polyester derivative of L-lactic and glycolic acids. Poly-L-lactic/polyglycolic acid copolymer degrades and resorbs in vivo by hydrolysis into L-lactic and glycolic acids, which are then metabolized by the body. The material is nontoxic, nonirritating, and 100% amorphous, metabolizing to CO_2 and H_2O.

The potential advantages of bioresorbable implants include less stress shielding of the bone that would be expected with metallic implants, less interference with modern imaging techniques, and elimination of the need for subsequent procedures to remove the implant. Recent improvements in the materials and design of bioresorbable plates and screws have addressed some of the problems with the first generation of resorbable implants. Bioresorbable fixation has been suggested as a means of overcoming drawbacks of miniplate fixation in the craniofacial complex while retaining the advantages.

SUMMARY

Microabsorbable screws can be applied with success for orthodontic purposes; however, the correct PLA/PGA ratio should be selected to obtain the maximum performance during treatment.[27,56-58] Further studies should involve the appropriate shape for orthodontics as well as root effect when tooth is moved against the screw.

BRACKET HEAD MICROIMPLANTS

Recently, different designs of microimplants became available for different purposes. Almost all have a hole in the head to attach accessories, and some have different types of slots or round heads.

The bracket head (BH) microimplant simplifies orthodontic treatment and offers many options for treatment without full fixed appliances.[25] The arch is fitted into the slot of the microimplant, which then works as a single tooth. The BH microimplant has two tie wings and one slot, which gives the same performance as a bracket and makes it easy to place the ligature. Two types of screw were developed for the BH implant, depending on the driving directions and according to the moment of force applied. Thus, the right-handed screw should turn clockwise and the left-handed screw should turn counterclockwise during driving.

For patients who need minor treatment or refuse to wear full fixed appliances, the BH implant is the best choice.

CASE REPORT 11-2

An adult female patient was referred by her dentist, who wanted to place an implant for #24. Because the space was too large (#24 and #25 missing), he wanted to close the space by 2 mm. It was decided to distalize #23 and correct the midline deviation with teeth drift. At the same time, #36 would be corrected.

A full fixed appliance was proposed to the patient, who refused. It was planned to place two BH microimplants and brackets on #23 and #36, and do the treatment with segmented wires. The estimated treatment time was 4 months.

A BH microimplant was placed mesial to #26 and another between #35 and #36. A segmented wire with a loop was inserted and attached to the BH to start distalization. At the same time another segmented wire was activated to upright #36 (Figure 11-4, *A-F*).

Four months later the space was closed 2 mm, and #36 was aligned (Figure 11-4, *G-I*). Microimplants were removed (Figure 11-4, *J-L*), and the patient was sent to the dentist to place the implant (Figure 11-4, *M-P*).

Continued

CASE REPORT 11-2—cont'd

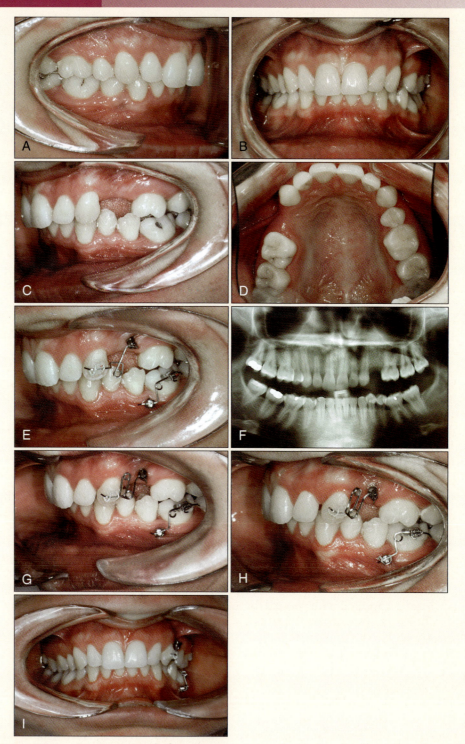

Figure 11-4 A to D, Patient before treatment. It was decided to distalize #23 and upright #36. E, Two bracket head microimplants were inserted, and segmented wires were placed to distalize upper canine and upright lower molar. F, Panoramic view. G to I, Progression of treatment. J to L, Both microimplants were removed and teeth aligned. M to O, Posttreatment intraoral photographs. P, Posttreatment panoramic radiograph.

CASE REPORT 11-2—cont'd

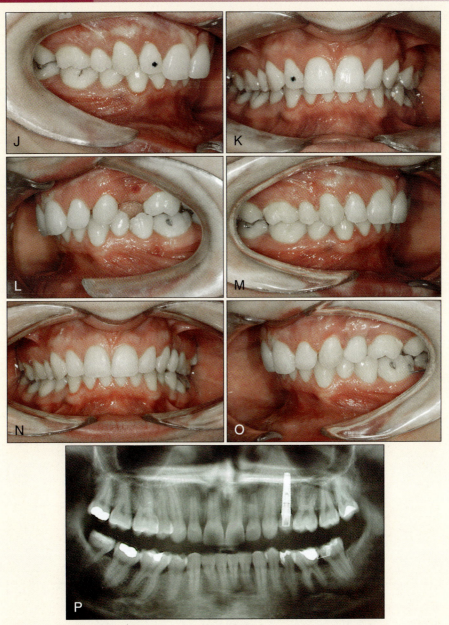

Figure 11-4, cont'd For legend see opposite page.

CASE REPORT 11-3

Orthodontic treatments based on intrusion of lower incisors require care during retention, especially if the patient has missing teeth. This case illustrates the advantage of the microimplants for lower-incisor intrusion as well as for retention after treatment.

An 18-year-old female patient presented with oligodontia (many teeth missing). A deep overbite and abnormal shape of some teeth were present (Figure 11-5, A-G). Tooth support was absent in the third quadrant, so it was decided to intrude lower incisors with the aid of two microimplants located in the area of #32 and #42 after leveling (Figure 11-5, H-J).

Sixteen months after treatment, the appliance was removed. Microimplants were removed, and two BH microimplants were placed in another position to allow a composite restoration of the missing lateral teeth (Figure 11-5, K-O).

The lower retainer was bonded to lower canines and also to the restorations (Figure 11-5, P-V). This is a unique approach to prevent relapse of the intrusion during treatment.

The patient was sent to the dentist, and both microimplants were replaced with prosthetic implants and crowns and were bonded to the retainer (Figure 11-5, W-BB).

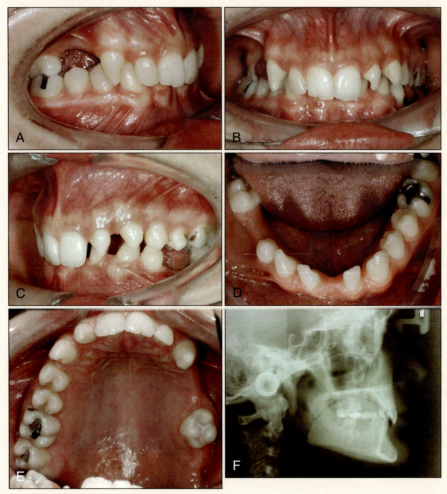

Figure 11-5 *A* to *G*, Patient with oligodontia and deep-bite malocclusion. *H* to *J*, Two microimplants were placed to help the intrusion of lower incisors. *K* to *O*, Both microimplants were removed and replaced by bracket head type in another position to allow a composite-buildup restoration. *P* to *V*, Retainer was bonded to the mandibular incisors, canines, and provisional restorations to avoid relapse after the intrusion, a "skeletal anchorage retainer."

CASE REPORT 11-3—cont'd

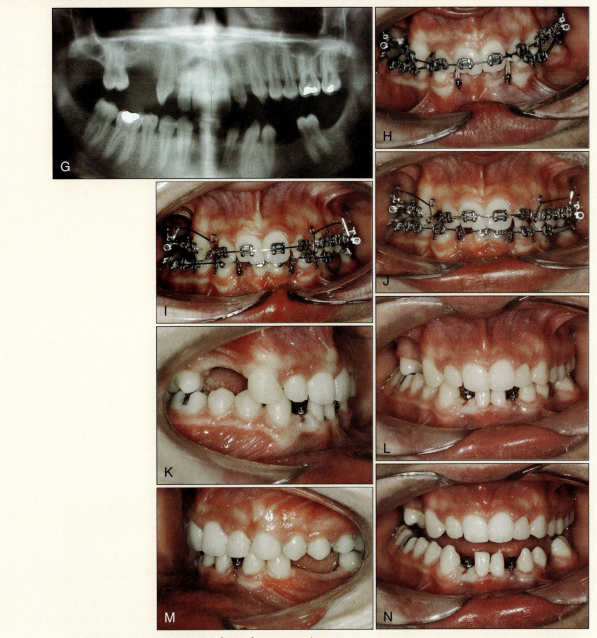

Figure 11-5, cont'd For legend see opposite page.

Continued

CASE REPORT 11-3—cont'd

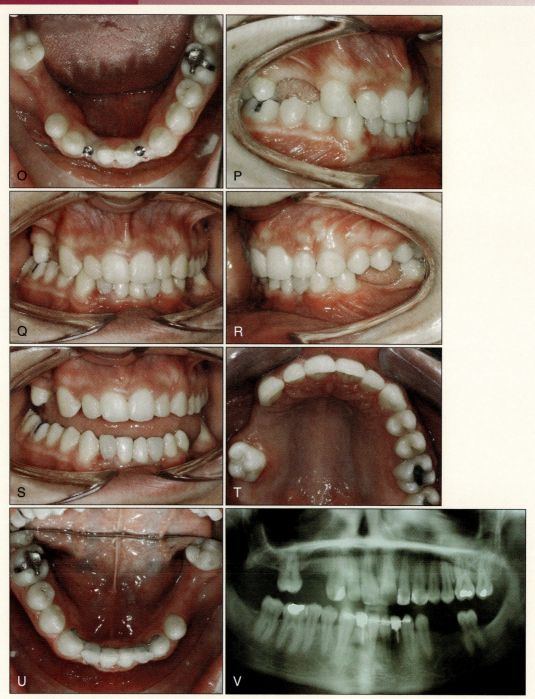

Figure 11-5, cont'd For legend see p. 246.

CASE REPORT 11-3—cont'd

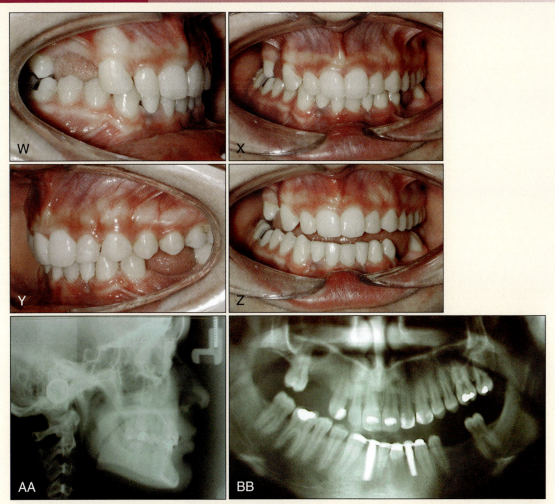

Figure 11-5, cont'd W to BB, Patient after treatment, with two prosthetic implants also bonded to the retainer.

Absolute anchorage is important for patients without enough tooth support to make movements such as intrusion. In this case, besides the anchorage for lower-incisor intrusion, the use of microimplants had the advantages of (1) absolute retention after treatment and (2) provisional restorations after debonding.

NONINVASIVE MINIPLATES

Titanium anchor plates have been used in orthodontics for correction of skeletal open bite and Class III malocclusions, increasing anchorage during treatment. Usually these plates are temporally fixed on the cortical plate of the mandible or maxilla with titanium monocortical miniscrews. Once the soft tissue surrounding the miniplate has healed, the anchor plate can be loaded.

Anchor plates can also be used in a way other than the traditional method (placed surgically on the cortical bone) in patients without posterior teeth and when a three-dimensional control will be necessary, as *noninvasive miniplates*.[27]

The anchor plate shape is selected according to the situation and adapted to the gingivae. It is inserted and tied to the microimplants. A bracket is then bonded in the desired position (angulation and vertical height). The shape of the plate can be changed with pliers to control the horizontal or sagittal direction.

CASE REPORT 11-4

A 30-year-old woman was referred by her dentist to have her upper front teeth aligned before prosthetic rehabilitation. She presented with moderate crowding, crossbite, and lack of space for #22 and canine crossbite on both sides. She had no posterior teeth on the upper jaw, and on the lower jaw #48 was to be extracted and #38 restored (Figure 11-6, A-E).

Because of the missing teeth, there was no support for orthodontic treatment. It was decided to treat the patient with TADs. A mini plate would be placed on the left side fixed with two microimplants, and one microimplant placed on the right side (Figure 11-6, F-H).

Two BH microimplants 1.5 mm in diameter and 7 and 8 mm in length were placed distal to #23. Another microimplant was placed distal to #13. They were left in place for 1 month to evaluate stability before starting with the fixed appliance. One month later the fixed appliance was bonded, and the miniplate was fixed into the slots of the BH microimplant. A bracket was bonded on the miniplate.

The miniplate was activated to increase the vestibular force on #23 to correct the crossbite (Figure 11-6, I-L). The treatment was done in 3 months (with fixed appliance bonded), and a retainer was made for nighttime use. The crossbite was corrected, and the teeth were aligned (Figure 11-6, M-P).

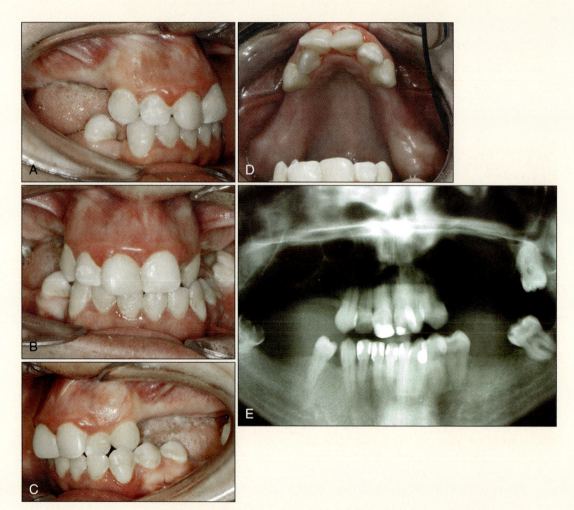

Figure 11-6 A to E, Patient before treatment without sufficient tooth support to align and correct crossbite on both sides. F to H, Miniplate was placed on the left side and fixed to the bracket head microimplant. A bracket was bonded on the miniplate. I, Miniplate activated. J to L, Anterior teeth alignment with a continuous wire. M to P, Patient after treatment, with all teeth aligned and crossbite corrected.

11 Skeletal Anchorage: Different Approaches

CASE REPORT 11-4—cont'd

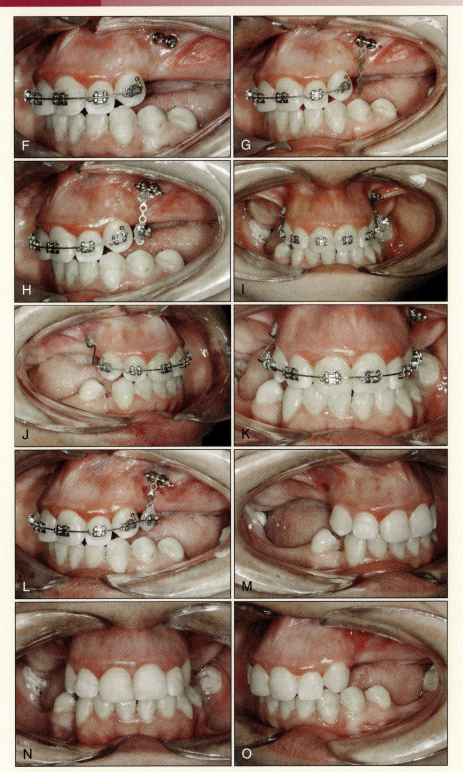

Figure 11-6, cont'd For legend see opposite page.

Continued

CASE REPORT 11-4—cont'd

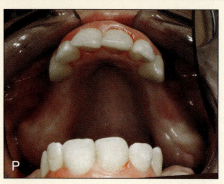

Figure 11-6, cont'd For legend see p. 250.

DISCUSSION

One of the advantages of skeletal anchorage is the possibility of treating patients without sufficient tooth support. Noninvasive miniplates are important in such cases because they can be activated during treatment in any direction. Because miniplates are fixed with more than one screw, the stability is greater than with only one microimplant.

Several miniplate designs were introduced to increase the potential of treatment with this approach (Figure 11-7, *A*). The main difference between these new plates (Dentos, Taegu, South Korea) and the regular plates is the area to be attached to the microimplants (Figure 11-7, *B*).

Another type of microimplant (Dentos) was introduced to facilitate fixation (Figure 11-8). This microimplant has the head with a screw to be inserted into the body. It can fix a regular plate (Figure 11-9, *A-G*) or a new plate (Figure 11-9, *H-J*).

RAPID CANINE DISTALIZATION AND SKELETAL ANCHORAGE

Tissue lengthening has been a long-desired goal of clinicians. In 1859, Wiscott described the use of two bars hooked to a telescopic third bar to achieve maxillary expansion. For long-bone lengthening, Codvila used intermittent traction on an osteotomized bone. However, the biological principles for bone lengthening were not described until the 1950s by a Russian orthopedic surgeon, Gravial Ilizarov, and only then could a surgical protocol be achieved.[59]

DISTRACTION OSTEOGENESIS

Since the studies of Ilizarov, the lengthening technique was widely used in orthopedics, but maxillofacial surgeons did not discover distraction until 1972. Using distraction for mandibular lengthening, Snyder[60] was the first to describe its use in the craniofacial skeleton of dogs. In 1992, McCarthy[61] reported using distraction osteogenesis to correct microsomia in four children. More recently the technique has been used in several other applications on the craniofacial skeleton.[62-72]

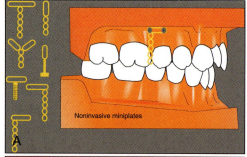
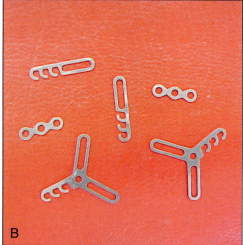

Figure 11-7

A, To overcome the drawback of the regular miniplates, several design changes were made. With these new miniplates, it is easier to adapt to the microimplants because of the significant space available for the fixation. *B*, Noninvasive miniplates.

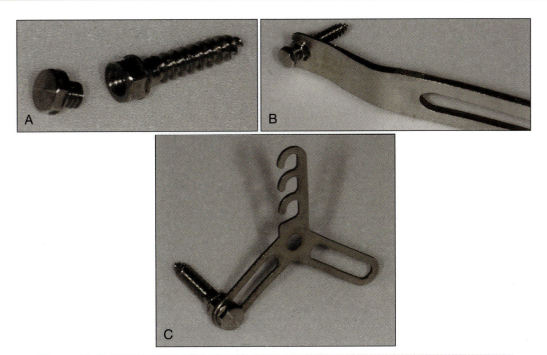

Figure 11-8
A, New type of microimplant for use with miniplates. B and C, New screw driver was made to allow the fixation without moving the microimplant after insertion.

The regular rate of tooth movement during canine retraction is about 1 mm per month. By orthodontically moving the tooth into the fibrous bone tissue created by distraction osteogenesis, however, the rate of orthodontic tooth movement could be as much as 1.2 mm per *week* in the mandible.[73]

The application of dental traction force to treat skeletal deficiencies has been reported since the eighteenth century. In 1876, Farrar reported his "positive system" to retract the canine into the space left after extraction of the first molar.[74,75] The distal movement was completed after 46 days. In 1887, Angle developed a retraction screw for the same purpose.[76]

Recent methods proposed to enhance the rate of tooth movement include Accelerated Osteogenic Orthodontics (Bill and Tom Wilcko),[77] Corticision (Young Guk Park), injection of biologically active peptides,[78] and rapid canine distraction.[79,80]

RAPID CANINE RETRACTION

Rapid canine retraction can be accomplished in several ways. In one technique the interdental distraction osteogenesis is followed by orthodontic tooth movement into the rapidly mineralizing bone regenerate. Osteotomies surrounding the canines are made to achieve rapid movement of the canines in the dentoalveolar segment, in compliance with the principles of distraction osteogenesis.[81]

Another rapid canine retraction technique consists of surgically undermining the interseptal bone distal to the canine, followed by rapid tooth movement into the previously extracted first premolar socket—"dental distraction." The rapid stretching of the periodontal ligament accelerates the periodontal cellular response without the initial delay seen during normal orthodontic tooth movement.[80]

Another procedure for rapid canine retraction involves bone decorticates (round cuts in internal and external cortical bone) together with alveolar bone removal distal to the canine.

The major drawbacks with these new approaches are the size and location of the distractors, which cause the patient discomfort, and some extrusion and tipping of the canine.

According to Farrar,[75] nonperceptible change in the position of the posterior teeth suggested that no anchorage loss occurred. This results from the lag period of minimal tooth movement that persists for approximately 2 to 3 weeks after applying a light or heavy orthodontic force.

ANCHORAGE WITH DISTRACTION

Skeletal anchorage can be applied in two different ways with dental distraction. When some problems occur during the distraction (e.g., distractor fracture, debonding, poor patient management with the screw), the lag period can pass, and the anchorage loss appears. In these cases a microimplant is placed distal to the distractor to stabilize it and to prevent this situation (Figure 11-10, *A-I*). The same microimplant can also be used

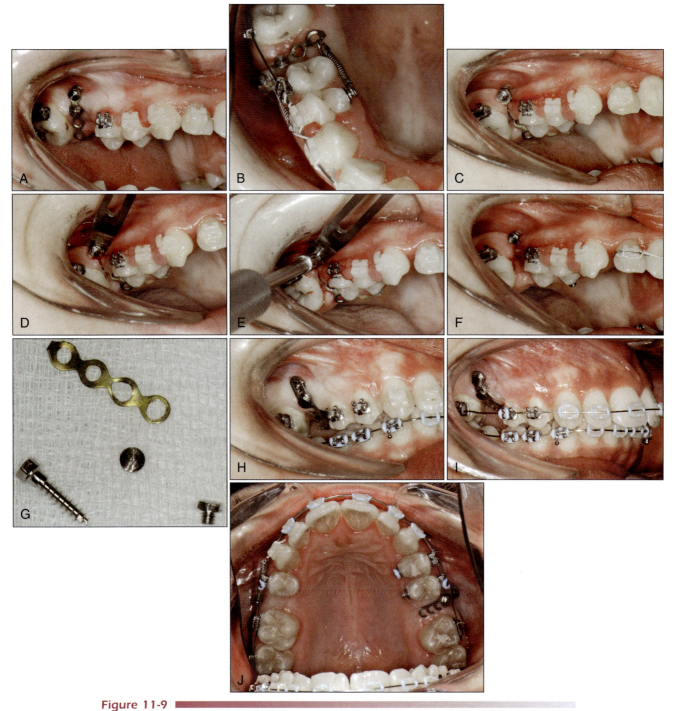

Figure 11-9
A and B, Regular miniplate attached with the new microimplant. C to G, Removal of miniplate using two screw drivers, one to fix the microimplant while the other removes the cap screw. H to J, New type of miniplate attached to new microimplant.

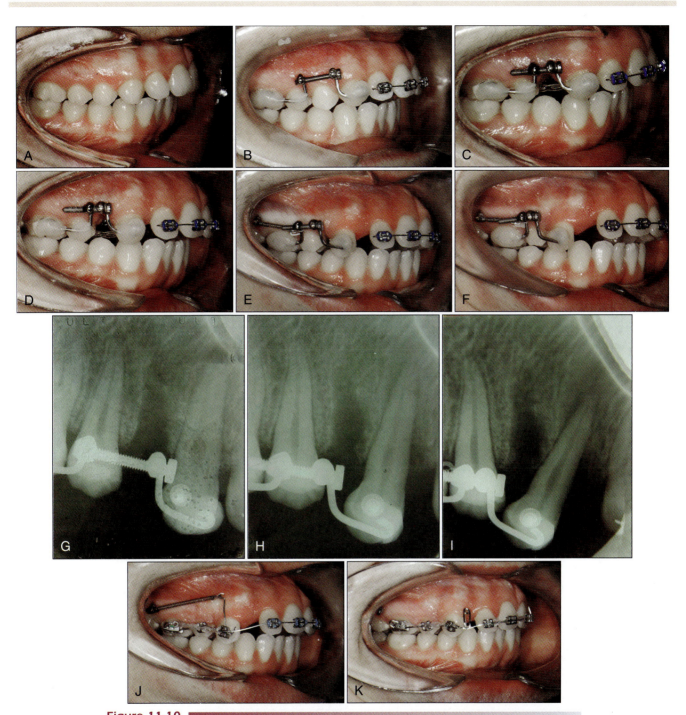

Figure 11-10

A and **B**, Distractor bonded, and patient ready for first premolar extraction. **C** and **D**, Five days and 10 days of distraction, respectively. Some problems occurred with the distractor, and it was rebounded. **E**, Thirty days after starting the activation, a microimplant was placed to stabilize the distractor. **F**, Forty days of distraction. **G**, **H**, and **I**, Periapical radiographs at 5 days, 30 days, and 40 days of distraction, respectively. **J** and **K**, Microimplant used to upright canine.

after distraction to upright the canine root and increase anchorage during retraction of incisors (Figure 11-10, J and K).

On the other hand, skeletal anchorage can be applied to stabilize the position of the distractor during dental distraction (Figure 11-11). This is particularly applicable when there are no braces or orthodontic wires to guide the canine during the distal movement, or when the distractor is not mounted in a telescopic arm, as usually done to avoid tipping caused by the space between the nut and the screw (Figure 11-12). After distractor removal, the microimplant can be used to increase anchorage during incisor retraction.

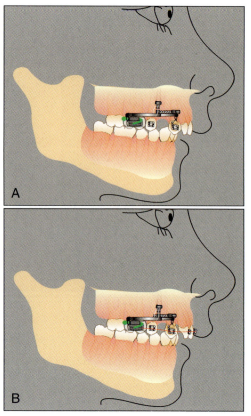

Figure 11-11
A, To maintain the distractor at the same level during distraction, a microimplant can be placed and attached to it. **B,** Braces and archwire as well as lingual buttons and elastic chain should be used to control the rotation.

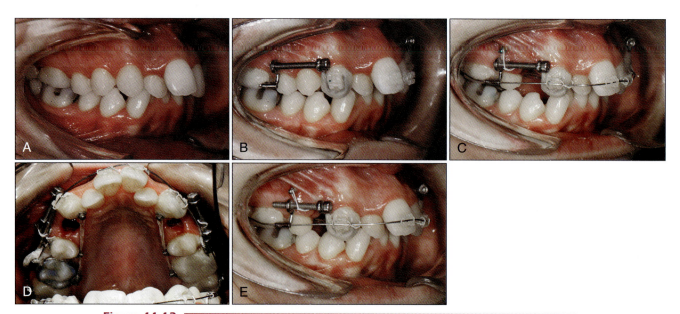

Figure 11-12
A to **L,** Sequence of distraction activation with images taken every 6 days, with 24 days of active distraction. The microimplant stabilized the dpistractor. **M,** Periapical radiograph at start of treatment. **N,** Panoramic radiograph after distraction.

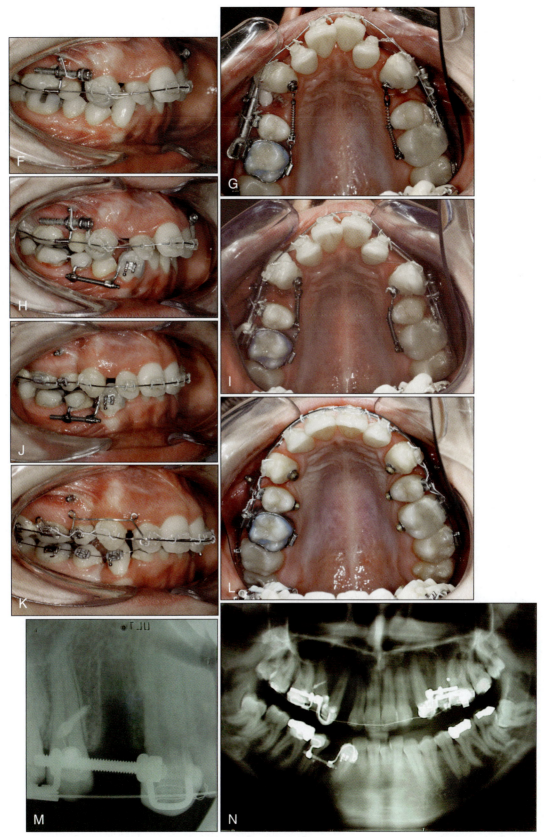

Figure 11-12, cont'd For legend see opposite page.

REFERENCES

1. Gainsforth BL: A study of orthodontic anchorage possibilities in basal bone, *Am J Orthod Oral Surg* 31:406-417, 1945.
2. Linkow LI: Implanto-orthodontics, *Clin J Orthod* 4:685-705, 1970.
3. Roberts WE, Helm FR, Marshall KJ, Gongloff RK: Rigid endosseous implants for orthodontic and orthopedic anchorage, *Angle Orthod* 59:247-255, 1989.
4. Sherman A: Bone reaction to orthodontic forces on vitreous carbon dental implants, *Am J Orthod* 74:79-87, 1978.
5. Block MS, Hoffman DR: A new device for absolute anchorage for orthodontics, *Am J Orthod* 107:251-258, 1995.
6. Melsen B, Petersen JK, Costa A: Zygoma ligatures: an alternative form of maxillary anchorage, *J Clin Orthod* 32:154-158, 1998.
7. Kokich VG, Shapiro PA, Oswald R, et al: Ankylosed teeth as abutments for maxillary protraction: a case report, *Am J Orthod* 88:303-307, 1985.
8. Wehrbein H, Glatzmaier J, Mundwiller U, Diedrich P: The orthosystem: a new implant system for orthodontic anchorage in the palate, *J Orofac Orthop* 57:143-153, 1996.
9. Umemori M, Sugawara J, Nagasaka H, Kawamura H: Skeletal anchorage system for open-bite correction, *Am J Orthop* 115:166-174, 1999.
10. Chung KR, Kim YS, Linton JL, Lee YJ: The miniplate with tube for skeletal anchorage, *J Clin Orthod* 36:407-412, 2002.
11. Schlegel KA, Schweizer C, Janson IR, Wiltfang J: A new anchorage concept for orthodontic treatment in the mandible, *World J Orthod* 3:353-357, 2002.
12. Clerck H, Geerinckx V, Siciliano S: The zygoma anchorage system, *J Clin Orthod* 36:455-459, 2002.
13. Kanomi R: Mini-implant for orthodontic anchorage, *J Clin Orthod* 31:763-767, 1997.
14. Costa A, Raffling M, Millstone B: Miniscrews as orthodontic anchorage: a preliminary report, *Int J Adult Orthod Orthog Surg* 13:201-209, 1998.
15. Bousquet F, Bousquet P, Mauran G, Parguel P: Use of an impacted post for anchorage, *J Clin Orthod* 30:261-265, 1996.
16. Park H, Bae S, Kyung H, Sung J: Micro-implant anchorage for treatment of skeletal Class I bialveolar protrusion, *J Clin Orthod* 35:417-422, 2001.
17. Lee JS, Park HS, Kyung HM: Micro-implant anchorage for lingual treatment of a skeletal Class II malocclusion, *J Clin Orthod* 35:643-647, 2001.
18. Bae SM, Park HS, Kyung HM, et al: Clinical application of micro-implant anchorage, *J Clin Orthod* 36:298-302, 2002.
19. Paik CH, Woo YJ, Kim J, Park JU: Use of miniscrews for intermaxillary fixation of lingual orthodontic surgical patients, *J Clin Orthod* 36:132-136, 2002.
20. Park HS, Kyung HM, Sung J: A simple method of molar uprighting with micro-implant anchorage, *J Clin Orthod* 36:592-596, 2002.
21. Maino BG, Bednar J, Pagin P, Mura P: The spider screw for skeletal anchorage, *J Clin Orthod* 37:90-97, 2003.
22. Ritto AK, Kyung HM: Solutions with micro implants, *Orthodontia J* 8:6-13, 2004.
23. Ritto AK: Micro implants in orthodontics, *Int J Orthod* 15(3):22-24, 2004.
24. Ritto AK: Easy movements with mini implants, *Orthod Soc Res Thailand* 4:1-6, 2004.
25. Ritto AK, Kyung HM: Bracket head micro implants, *Ortodontia J* 9:50-66, 2004.
26. Ritto AK: Micro implants in orthodontics: a useful tool to treat cases without teeth support, *Monografias Clinicas Ortodoncia* (in press).
27. Ritto AK: Skeletal anchorage: different solutions, *Int J Orthod* 16(4):39-48, 2005.
28. Ritto AK: The Ritto Appliance: an easy way to treat Class II malocclusions. In *Orthodontic treatment of the Class II noncompliant patient: current principles and techniques*, St Louis, 2006, Mosby-Elsevier, pp 67-91.
29. Rokkanen P, Böstman O, Vainionpää S, et al: Absorbable devices in the fixation of fractures, *J Trauma* 40:123-127, 1996.
30. Linder L, Albrektsson T, Branemark P, et al: Electron microscopic analysis of the bone-titanium interface, *Acta Orthop Scand* 54:45-52, 1983.
31. Carlsson L, Rostlund T, Branemark PI, et al: Osseointegration of titanium implants, *Acta Orthop Scand* 57:285-289, 1986.
32. Woodman JL, Jacobs JJ, Galante JO, Urban RM: Metal ion release from titanium-based prosthetic segmental replacements of long bones in baboons: a long-term study, *J Orthop Res* 1:421-430, 1984.
33. Lalor PA, Gray AB, Wright S, et al: Contact sensitivity to titanium in a hip prosthesis? *Contact Dermatitis* 23:193-194, 1990.
34. Sunderman FW Jr: Carcinogenicity of metal alloys in orthopedic prostheses: clinical and experimental studies, *Fundam Appl Toxicol* 13:205-216, 1989.
35. Orringer JS, Barcelona V, Buchman SR: Reasons for removal of rigid internal fixation devices in craniofacial surgery, *J Craniofac Surg* 9:40-44, 1998.
36. Gilding DK, Reed AM: Biodegradable polymers for use in surgery: poly(glycolic)/poly(lactic acid) homo and copolymers, *Polymer* 20:1459-1464, 1979.
37. Pietrzak WS, Sarver DR, Verstynen ML: Bioabsorbable polymer science for the practicing surgeon, *J Craniofac Surg* 8:87-91, 1997.
38. Törmälä P, Pohjonen T, Rokkanen P: Bioabsorbable polymers: materials technology and surgical applications. Proceedings of the Institution of Mechanical Engineers, Part H, *J Eng Med* 212:101-111, 1998.
39. Frazza EJ, Schmitt EE: A new absorbable suture, *J Biomed Mater Res* 5:43-58, 1971.
40. Vert M, Chabot F, Leray J, Christel P: Stereoregular bioresorbable polyesters for orthopaedic surgery, *Macromolec Chem Physics Suppl* 5:221-231, 1981.
41. Hollinger JO, Battistone GC: Biodegradable bone repair materials: synthetic polymers and ceramics, *Clin Orthop* 1:290-305, 1986.
42. Cutright DE, Perez B, Beasley JD, et al: Degradation rates of polymers and copolymers of 73 polylactic and polyglycolic acids, *Oral Surg Oral Med Oral Pathol* 37:142-152, 1974.
43. Bergsma EJ, Rozema FR, Bos RR, de Bruijn WC: Foreign body reactions to resorbable poly(L-lactide) bone plates and screws used for the fixation of unstable zygomatic fractures, *J Oral Maxillofac Surg* 51:666-670, 1993.
44. Matsusue Y, Hanafusa S, Yamamuro T, et al: Tissue reaction of bioabsorbable ultra-high strength poly (L-lactide) rod: a long-term study in rabbits, *Clin Orthop* 317:246-253, 1995.
45. Bostman OM: Current concepts review: absorbable implants for the fixation of fractures, *J Bone Joint Surg* 73A:148-153, 1991.
46. Törmälä P: Biodegradable self-reinforced composite materials: manufacturing structure and mechanical properties, *Clin Mater* 10:29-34, 1992.
47. Bergsma JE, de Bruijn WC, Rozema FR, et al: Late degradation tissue response to poly(L-lactide) bone plates and screws, *Biomaterials* 16:25-31, 1995.
48. Vasenius J, Vainionpää S, Vihtonen K, et al: Comparison of in vitro hydrolysis, subcutaneous and intramedullary implantation to evaluate the strength retention of absorbable osteosynthesis implants, *Biomaterials* 11:501-504, 1990.
49. Kulkarni RK, Pani KC, Neuman C, Leonard F: Polylactic acid for surgical implants, *Arch Surg* 93:839-843, 1966.
50. Cutright DE, Hunsuck EE: Tissue reaction to the biodegradable polylactic acid suture, *Oral Surg Oral Med Oral Pathol* 31:134-139, 1971.
51. Cutright DE, Hunsuck EE: The repair of fractures of the orbital floor using biodegradable polylactic acid, *Oral Surg Oral Med Oral Pathol* 33:28-34, 1972.

52. Miller RA, Brady JM, Cutright DE: Degradation rates of oral resorbable implants (polylactates and polyglycolates): rate modification with changes in PLA/PGA copolymer ratios, *J Biomed Mater Res* 11:711-719, 1977.
53. Eppley BL, Sadove AM: A comparison of resorbable and metallic fixation in healing of calvarial bone grafts, *Plast Reconstr Surg* 96:316-322, 1995.
54. Eppley BL, Sadove AM, Havlik RJ: Resorbable plate fixation in pediatric craniofacial surgery, *Plast Reconstr Surg* 100:1-7, 1997.
55. Eppley B, Reilly M: Degradation characteristics of PLLA-PGA bone fixation devices, *J Craniofac Surg* 8:116-120, 1997.
56. Glatzmaier J, Wehrbein H, Diedrich P: The development of a resorbable implant system for orthodontic anchorage. The BIOS implant system: bioresorbable implant anchor for orthodontic systems, *Fortschr Kieferorthop* 56:175-81, 1995.
57. Glatzmaier J, Wehrbein H, Diedrich P: Biodegradable implants for orthodontic anchorage: a preliminary biomechanical study, *Eur J Orthod* 18:456-459, 1996.
58. Ogawa K, Aoki T, Miyazawa K, Goto S: Absorbable implant used as orthodontic anchorage. 82nd General Session of the International Association for Dental Research, Honolulu, Hawaii, Poster 3326, 2004, School of Dentistry, Aichigakuin University, Nagoya, Japan.
59. Ilizarov GA: The tension-stress effect on the genesis and growth of tissues: the influence of the rate and frequency of the distraction, *Clin Orthop* 239:263-285, 1989.
60. Snyder CC, Levine GA, Swanson HM, Browne EZ: Mandibular lengthening by gradual distraction, *Plast Reconstr Surg* 51:506-508, 1973.
61. McCarthy JG, Schreiber J, Karp N, et al: Lengthening the human mandible by gradual distraction, *Plast Reconstr Surg* 35:1-10, 1992.
62. Bell WH, Gonzales M, Samchucov ML, Guerrero CA: Intraoral widening and lengthening of the mandible in baboons by distraction osteogenesis, *J Oral Maxillofac Surg* 57:548-562, 1999.
63. Guerrero CA et al: Mandibular widening by intraoral distraction osteogenesis, *Br J Oral Maxillofac Surg* 35:383-392, 1997.
64. Hoppenreijs TM, Freihofer HP, Stoelinga PJ, et al: Condylar remodeling and resorption after Le Fort I and bimaxillary osteotomies in patients with anterior open bite, *Int J Oral Maxillofac Surg* 27:81-91, 1998.
65. Hoppenreijs TM, Stoelinga PJ, Grace KL, Robben CM: Long-term evaluation of patients with progressive condylar resorption following orthognathic surgery, *Int J Oral Maxillofac Surg* 28:411-418, 1999.
66. Makarov MR, Harper RP, Cope JB, Samchucov ML: Evaluation of inferior alveolar nerve function during distraction osteogenesis in the dog, *J Oral Maxillofac Surg* 56:1417-1423, 1998.
67. Soares MM, Guerra F, Duarte PSS: Posterior edentulous mandible lengthening using distraction osteogenesis, *J Oral Maxillofac Surg* 60:S25, 2002.
68. Soares MM, Guerra F, Duarte PSS, Correa CA: Augmentation of the edentulous mandibular ridge by distraction osteogenesis, *Int J Oral Maxillofac Surg* 32:S9, 2003.
69. Soares MM, Marinho L, Duarte PSS, Correa CA: Maxillary advancement on cleft lip patients using distraction osteogenesis, *J Int Congr Maxillofac Craniofac Distract* 4:83-97, 2003.
70. Soares MM, Marinho L, Duarte PSS, Correa CA: Correction of deformity resultant from TMJ anquilosis by distraction osteogenesis, *J Int Congr Maxillofac Craniofac Distract* 4:163-167, 2003.
71. Soares MM, Guerra FB, Duarte PSS, Correa CA: Autogenous bone graft x distraction osteogenesis for anterior maxillary augmentation. *Transactions of the Second Asia Pacific Congress of Maxillofacial and Craniofacial Distraction*, Asia Association of Craniofacial Surgery, 2004, pp 192-197.
72. Wolford LM, Reiche-Fishel O, Mehra P: Changes in temporomandibular joint dysfunction after orthognathic surgery, *J Oral Maxillofac Surg* 61:655-601, 2003.
73. Cohen SR, Burstein FD, Stewart MB, Rathbun MA: Maxillary midface distraction in children with cleft lip and palate: a preliminary report, *Plast Reconstr Surg* 99:1421-1426, 1997.
74. Farrar JN: An inquiry into physiological and pathological changes in animal tissues in regulating teeth, *Dent Cosmos* 18:19, 1876.
75. Farrar JN: Regulation of teeth made easy. II. Rotation concluded: positive and probable systems, *Dent Cosmos* 20:18, 1878.
76. Angle EH: *Treatment of malocclusion of the teeth*, Philadelphia, 1907, White Dental Manufacturing.
77. Wilcko W, Ferguson DJ, Bouquot JE, Wilcko T: Rapid orthodontic decrowding with alveolar augmentation: case report, *World J Orthod* 4:197-205, 2003.
78. Penolazzi L, Lambertini E, Borgatti M, et al: Decoy oligodeoxynucleotides targeting NF-κB transcription factors: induction of apoptosis in human primary osteoclasts, *Biochem Pharmacol* 66:1189-1198, 2003.
79. Liou EJ, Polley JW, Figueroa AA: Distraction osteogenesis: the effects of orthodontic tooth movement on distracted mandibular bone, *J Craniofac Surg* 9:564, 1998.
80. Liou EJ, Huang CS: Rapid canine retraction through distraction of the periodontal ligament, *Am J Orthod Dentofacial Orthop* 114:372, 1998.
81. Iseri H, Kisnisci R, Bzizi N, Tuz H: Rapid canine retraction and orthodontic treatment with dentoalveolar distraction osteogenesis, *Am J Orthod Dentofacial Orthop* 127:533-541, 2005.

CHAPTER 12
Clinical Application of Microimplants

Hyo-Sang Park

Many attempts have been made in the past to create suitable anchorage appliances, one of the most important factors for successful orthodontic treatment. None of the intraoral orthodontic appliances has been shown to obtain "perfect" anchorage control, whereas extraoral appliances provide reliable and suitable anchorage only with compliant patients. Intraoral skeletal anchorage systems such as the dental implant,[1,2] miniplate,[3] and miniscrew or microscrew implant[4-11] provide absolute anchorage. Among skeletal anchorage devices, endosseous implants[1,2] failed to become popular because of anatomical limitations resulting from their bulky size and long waiting time for osseointegration.

The microscrew implants are most often used because of their tiny size, immediate loading, and low cost. The small size enables microimplants to be placed easily and closer to the dental arch, facilitating the delivery of the desired mechanics.

FEATURES OF MICROIMPLANT

Initially, surgical microscrews were placed into the bone and used as anchorage. A steel ligature wire was tied around the neck of the surgical microscrew and bent to form a hook,[6,7] to provide an attachment for elastic material. Drawbacks to using surgical microscrews as orthodontic anchorage include fracture of microscrews, peripheral screw inflammation, soft tissue impingement around canine eminence, and difficulty in making a hook for the screw head.

The microimplant was developed to enhance ease of use and improve efficiency.[12] The "ease of use" features include an attachment on the head for an elastic material or wire and a self-drilling screw with a cutting flute at the apex. The heads of the microimplant have several shapes, such as small head (SH), long head (LH), no head (NH), circle head (CH), bracket head (BH), and fixation head (FH) (Figure 12-1). The SH, LH, and FH types have a shank-shaped, tapered head that move elastics away from soft tissue to minimize soft tissue impingement. The microimplant was developed to provide easy placement by adding the cutting flute at the apex. In other words, self-drilling microimplants were developed to eliminate the need for pilot drilling.

The features that improve efficiency include changes in the thread shape and the diameter of the trunk (in the thread-bearing portion), which reduce the risk of fracture of the microimplant. The material was also changed from pure titanium to titanium alloy to minimize fracture. To increase the success rate, the trunk (threaded par) has minimal taper, 0.1-mm from neck to apex.

Each type of microimplant has various diameters, offering many options to clinicians. The diameters range from 1.3 to 1.8 mm at the neck and 1.2 to 1.7 mm at the apex. The 1.3-mm microimplant is most frequently used in the maxillary alveolar bone between the teeth, and the 1.3- to 1.4-mm diameter is most frequently used in the mandibular alveolar bone between the teeth and the retromolar area. The 1.4- to 1.5-mm diameter can be used for the midpalatal area. The length of microimplants ranges from 5 to 12 mm. The most common lengths of microimplants are as follows:

- 7 to 8 mm in maxillary buccal area
- 8 to 12 mm in maxillary palatal area
- 5 to 6 mm in mandibular retromolar, posterior teeth, and anterior teeth area
- 5 to 6 mm in maxillary anterior teeth area

The SH type is used most often. The LH type can be used to ensure the head is accessible in clinical situations involving thick, soft tissue or a deep vestibule. The NH type can be used when it is difficult to expose the head beyond the soft tissue; a ligature wire should be tied and extended through the soft tissue to provide a hook for force application. The CH type can be used to position the elastic material away from the soft tissue farther than the SH type. The FH type was developed to be used as an intermaxillary fixation screw when performing orthognathic surgery in lingual orthodontics. The BH type has a .018-inch slot on the head, and it is available in two types, right-handed and left-handed. The right-handed BH microimplant is tightened by turning it clockwise, and it can be used when a counterclockwise moment on the screw is expected.

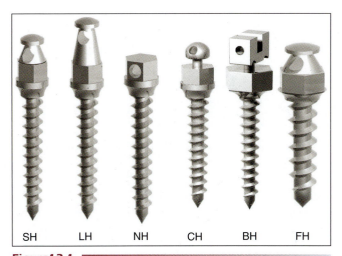

Figure 12-1

Types of microimplants. *Left to right*, Small head, long head, no head, circle head, bracket head, fixation head.

SURGICAL PLACEMENT OF MICROIMPLANT

The two surgical placement methods for microimplants are the drill (self-tapping) method and the drill-free (self-drilling) method. The drill method requires pre-drilling with a pilot drill before placement, whereas the microimplant can be placed without drilling using the drill-free method.

The bone density and thickness of the cortical bone are less in the maxilla than that in the mandible.[13-15] According to Lohr et al.,[16] a self-tapping screw is suitable for the dense, thick bone and a self-drilling screw for the thin cortical bone area.

Clinicians can inject one-third to one-fourth ampule of anesthetic solution into the mucosa (Figure 12-2, *A*). Injecting a small amount of anesthetic solution preserves sensation in the periodontal ligament. If a pilot drill or microimplant impinges into the periodontal ligament, the patient may experience pain. This indicates root contact and allows the clinician to change the direction of placement. An anesthetic patch also works well (Figure 12-2, *B*). After the soft tissue is dried, the patch adheres to the mucosa and after 10 minutes achieves sufficient anesthesia.

When placing the microimplant into the nonattached gingiva, a small incision is necessary to prevent the soft tissue from rolling up around the drill or microimplant (Figure 12-3, *A*). There is no need to suture because the incision is less than 4 mm. When placing the microimplant into the attached gingiva or palatal masticatory mucosa, an incision is unnecessary (Figure 12-3, *B*).

When placing the microimplant into the alveolar bone in the maxilla and anterior teeth area of the mandible, the self-drilling method can be used. The microimplant is placed at a 30- to 40-degree angle to the long axis of teeth; a narrow microimplant is used to reduce

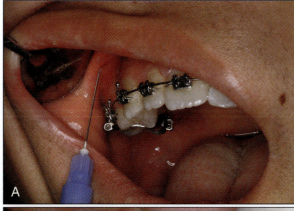
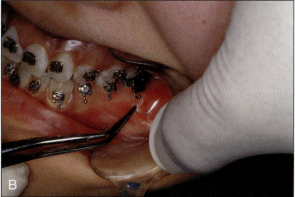

Figure 12-2

A, Injection of local anesthetic solution. **B**, Anesthetic patch for mucosal anesthesia.

the risk of root contact[7,8] (Figure 12-4, *A*). However, caution is required because introducing the microimplant 30 to 40 degrees to the bone surface causes slippage and surface damage. To prevent slippage and bulging of surface bone, a small pit with a round bur is needed. Another option is to introduce the microimplant 90 degrees to the bone surface until a hole in the cortical bone is completed (see Figure 12-3, *B*). After making the hole, withdraw and change the path of insertion to 30 to 40 degrees to the long axis of teeth (see Figure 12-4). This also prevents slippage and bulging damage of surface cortical bone. For an adult male patient or a patient with dense bone, it is better to make a hole with a pilot drill before placement of a microimplant, even in the maxilla. The drilling can be done only in the cortical bone. The microimplant can easily penetrate the cancellous bone with its sharp edge and surrounding threads. However, the palatal bone needs to have prior drilling before placement.

When placing the microimplant into the dense and thick bone (e.g., mandibular posterior teeth, retromolar area), a drilling method is appropriate (Figure 12-5, *A*). The drilling may lead to heat generation in the bone, a common cause of failure.[17] The drilling should be performed under copious irrigation with coolants. The diameter of the pilot drill should be smaller than that of the microimplant. I prefer a 0.9-mm pilot drill when

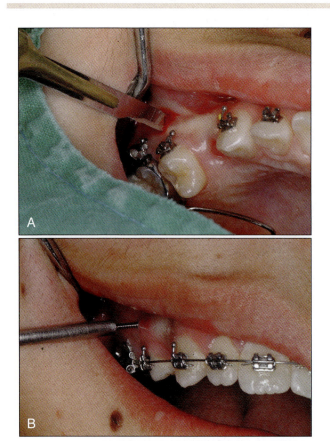

Figure 12-3
A, Small, vertical incision is used when placing the microimplant in oral mucosa. **B,** No incision is required when placing the microimplant in attached gingiva.

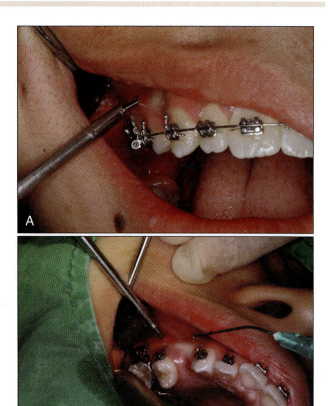

Figure 12-4
A, Placement of the microimplant with the drill-free method and no incision. Note that the angulation to the long axis of tooth is approximately 40 degrees. **B,** Placement of the microimplant with the drill-free method and incision.

placing a 1.3-mm-diameter microimplant. After making a hole with the pilot drill, the microimplant can be introduced into the hole and tightened with a screwdriver (Figure 12-5, *B*).

Microimplants are removed by simply unscrewing them, without local anesthesia.

CLINICAL APPLICATIONS OF MICROIMPLANT ANCHORAGE SLIDING MECHANICS

EXTRACTION TREATMENT

Microimplant anchorage (MIA) sliding mechanics can serve several purposes in treatment procedures for retracting anterior teeth with extraction of premolars (Box 12-1). The step-by-step procedures using MIA sliding mechanics in extraction treatment are listed next.

Maxillary Arch

1. Place a microscrew implant into the alveolar bone between a second premolar and a first molar on both sides.
2. Bond .022-inch, preadjusted appliances and a transpalatal bar to maintain archform and to control the torque of the posterior teeth (not for anchorage reinforcement) (Figure 12-6, *A*). A lingual sectional archwire between the first and second molars can be used to control the second molars (Figure 12-6, *B*).
3. Perform a partial canine retraction by tying back the canine to the microscrew implant to distalize the canine until the anterior teeth are in alignment.
4. Perform an en masse retraction of the six anterior teeth (Figure 12-6, *C*). Use a .016 × .022–inch stain-

> **BOX 12-1** Characteristics of Microimplant Anchorage (MIA) Sliding Mechanics in Extraction Treatment
>
> - MIA allows bodily retraction of the upper six anterior teeth by applying force closer to the center of resistance.
> - This procedure potentially induces the early changes in the facial profile because all six anterior teeth are retracted simultaneously.
> - Uprighting and slight intrusion of the lower molars induces the autorotation of the mandible, which helps in improving the facial profile.
> - Simultaneous retraction of the incisors with the canines reduces the treatment time.

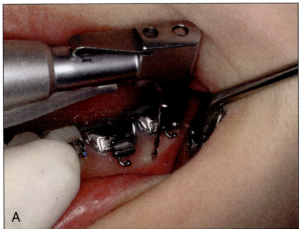

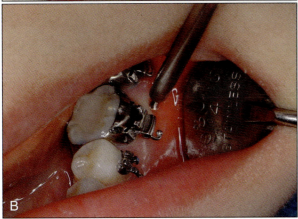

Figure 12-5
A, Predrilling with a pilot drill to make a hole. **B,** Introduction of the microimplant into a predrilled hole and tightening.

less steel archwire with anterior hooks between lateral incisors and canines. Use a nickel-titanium (Ni-Ti) closing-coil spring to connect the anterior hooks to the microscrew implants, and apply 150 g of force on each side.
5. To finish, provide occlusal settling with up-and-down elastics.

Mandibular Arch
1. Place a microscrew implant between the first and second molars on both sides.
2. Perform a partial canine retraction by tying back the canine to the second premolar.
3. Perform en masse retraction of the six anterior teeth using a .019 × .025–inch stainless steel archwire.
4. Apply an intrusion force to the lower molars by ligating an elastic thread from the microscrew implant to the lower archwire (Figure 12-6, *D*).
5. To finish, provide occlusal settling with up-and-down elastics.

The need to apply lingual root torque to prevent lingual tipping is reduced during anterior teeth retraction by using a force passing through or near the center of resistance of the anterior teeth segment in the upper arch (Figure 12-7; see Figure 12-6, *C*). In fact, a .016 × .022–inch archwire in a .022 bracket slot cannot exert lingual root torque on the anterior teeth because of the play between the bracket slot and the archwire. The anterior teeth, however, can be retracted bodily by using a force passing close to the center of resistance.[7,8,18,19] The play between the archwire and the bracket slots produces less friction in the posterior teeth segment. To minimize friction on the posterior teeth in the upper arch, the second molar may not be engaged in the main archwire. The second molars can be controlled by a sectional archwire between the first and second molars.

The factors controlling the mode of the anterior teeth retraction are the occlusogingival position of the microscrew implant, the height of anterior hooks, and the amount of torque-curve given on the archwire. The insertion site should be 8 to 10 mm gingival to the archwire when retracting the six anterior teeth.[7,18] This low position of the microimplant tends to produce minimal lingual tipping of the anterior teeth. On the other hand, the microscrew implants should be placed in a low position (~4 mm gingival to archwire when distalizing entire dentition in nonextraction).[9,20] The height of the anterior hooks should be 3 to 5 mm to obtain slight intrusion and bodily retraction of the anterior teeth. The force direction should be upward and backward. The force usually passes slightly below the center of resistance of the six anterior teeth.[21] The torque-curve incorporated into the archwire between the lateral incisors and canines and distal to the canines affects the mode of the incisor retraction. By moving the canine distally 1 or 2 mm before incisor retraction, clinicians can increase the lingual tipping of the upper incisors. When too much lingual tipping of the anterior teeth is evident, intrusion force from another microimplant placed between upper central incisors can effectively prevent lingual tipping of the upper incisors.

The mandibular microscrew implant is necessary when treating high-angle cases, may not be required in average-angle cases, and is not needed in low-angle cases. The mandibular microscrew implant can be used to apply an intrusive force to the posterior teeth. The tendency of buccoversion by the intruding force on the buccal side should be nullified by incorporating lingual crown torque in the archwire. In addition to intrusion of posterior teeth, the forward movement of the lower molars with an upright position moves the fulcrum forward and closes the mandibular plane angle (MPA), which results in an increase of the SNB (sella-nasion–point B) angle, a reduction of the ANB (point A-nasion–point B) angle, and resultant improvement of the facial profile[8,18,19] (see Figure 12-7). This is definitely true in a young, growing patient, but in an adult the change may be limited. As Klontz[22] advocated, the vertical control of posterior teeth with proper angulation of anterior teeth is important to improve facial harmony in high-angle cases. The intrusion of upper molars with the aid of microimplants closes the mandibular plane and produces profile changes.[23]

Text continued on p. 269

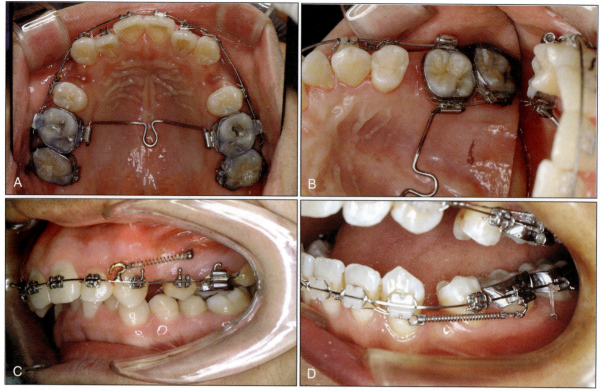

Figure 12-6

A, Transpalatal bar for maintaining archform. **B,** Lingual section of archwire to control an upper second molar. **C,** Upper microimplant was placed between the second premolar and first molar, with application of nickel-titanium (Ni-Ti) coil retraction force from the microimplant. **D,** Lower microimplant was placed between the first and second molars, with intrusive force applied from the microimplant to the archwire.

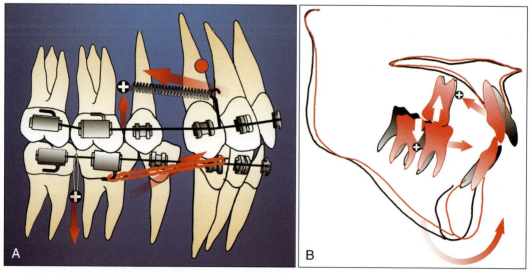

Figure 12-7

A, Upper retraction force passing near the center of resistance of the anterior teeth segment helps to control the torque of the upper anterior teeth. **B,** Intrusion of upper posterior teeth and lower posterior teeth, uprighting of lower posterior teeth, and mesial movement of lower posterior teeth can cause closure of the mandibular plane, improving the facial profile.

CASE REPORT 12-1

A 23-year-old female patient with a convex profile had a Class I skeletal pattern with bialveolar protrusion (Figure 12-8 and Table 12-1). She had a 4-degree ANB angle, a 36.5-degree angle from Frankfort horizontal (FH) to mandibular plane (MP), and a flat occlusal plane (FH to OP of 10 degrees). The overjet was 3.5 mm and the overbite 1 mm. Arch-length discrepancies in maxillary and mandibular arches were 0.5 mm and 2.5 mm, respectively. She had Class I canine and molar relationships. The treatment plan included the extraction of both upper and lower first premolars and maxillary microimplants for anchorage control.

Treatment Progress

After extraction of the four first premolars, straight wire appliances (.022 × .028 inch) were bonded and banded, and leveling was initiated. The maxillary microscrew implants (1.3 mm in diameter, 7 mm in length; AX12-107, Absoanchor, Dentos, Daegu, South Korea) were placed into the buccal alveolar bone between the maxillary second premolars and the first molars (Figure 12-9, A-C). Two weeks after placement, a ligature wire between the microscrew implants and maxillary canines was attached to maintain the canine anterior-posterior position during initial alignment. After 2 months of treatment, .016 × .022–inch stainless steel archwire with hooks was inserted, and 200 g of force by an Ni-Ti coil spring was applied to retract the maxillary anterior teeth on each side (Figure 12-9, D-I). A torque bend of approximately 5 degrees was provided on the archwire between the lateral incisors and the canines and distal to the canines.

Most of the profile changes occurred within 10 months of treatment (Figure 12-10). At 17 months of treatment, the patient had a harmonious facial profile and a functional occlusion with Class I dental relationships (Figure 12-11).

Treatment Results

The facial profile was improved with the retraction of upper and lower lips. The ANB angle was decreased by 1 degree (from 4 to 3 degrees). The MPA was decreased from 36.5 to 36 degrees in accordance with a decrease in anterior facial height (see Figure 12-11 and Table 12-1).

The panoramic radiograph revealed no obvious root resorption and adequate root parallelism (Figure 12-12, A and B). Cephalometric superimposition showed a controlled tipping movement of the upper anterior teeth with considerable amount of intrusion at the root apex (Figure 12-12, C). The mandibular molars and incisors were upright. The upper posterior teeth did not show discernible anchorage loss. By retracting the six anterior teeth together, the profile change was achieved early in the treatment.

TABLE 12-1 Cephalometric Measurements in Case Report 12-1

Measurements	Pretreatment (degrees)	Posttreatment (17 mo)
SNA	82.5	81.5
SNB	78.5	78.5
ANB	4	3
FMA	36.5	36.0
PFH/AFH	62	61.5
FH to OP	10.5	10.5
FH to UI	120	104
IMPA	91.5	77.5
Upper lip to E line	1 mm	−1 mm
Lower lip to E line	6 mm	0 mm

SNA, Sella-nasion–point A; *SNA*, sella-nasion–point B; *ANB*, point A-nasion–point B; *FMA*, Frankfort mandibular plane angle; *PFH/AFH*, posterior/anterior facial height; *FH*, Frankfort horizontal; *OP*, occlusal plane; *UI*, upper incisor; *IMPA*, lower incisor to mandibular plane angle.

Continued

CASE REPORT 12-1—cont'd

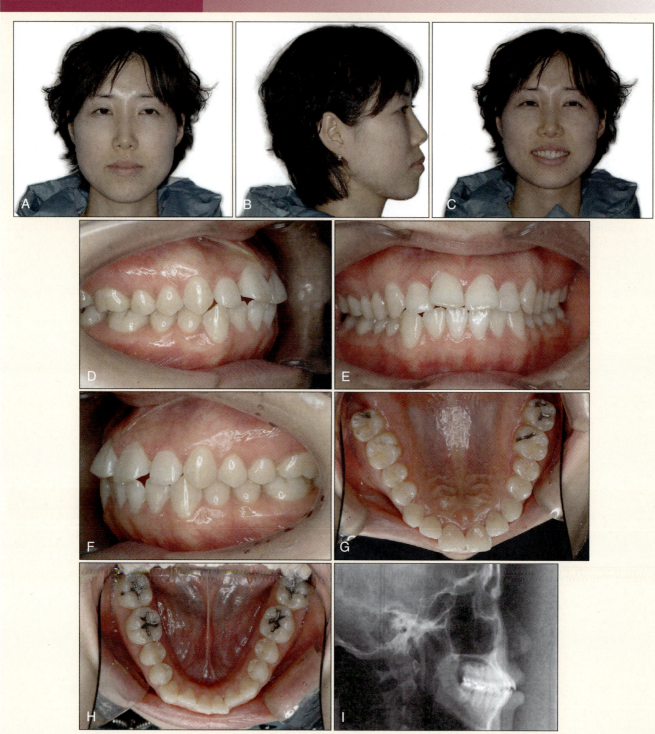

Figure 12-8 Pretreatment. **A** to **C**, Facial photographs. **D** to **H**, Intraoral photographs. **I**, Cephalometric radiograph (cephalograph).

CASE REPORT 12-1—cont'd

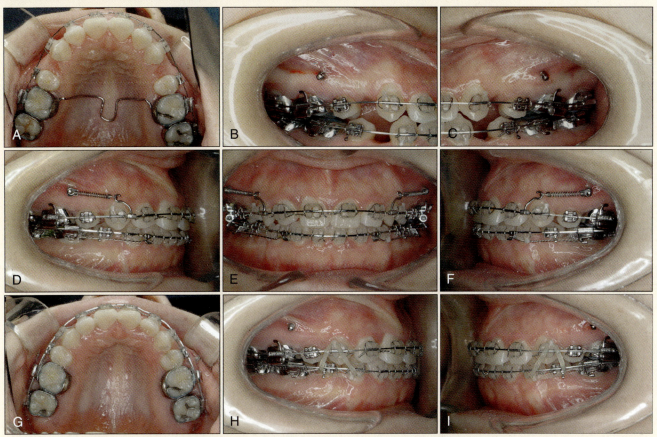

Figure 12-9 Treatment Progress. **A**, Transpalatal bar to prevent archform distortion. **B** and **C**, Upper microimplant placed into the alveolar bone between the second premolar and first molars. **D** to **F**, Ni-Ti coil retraction force was applied from the microimplants to hooks attached on the archwire. **G** to **I**, After removal of the transpalatal bar, triangular up-and-down elastics were used to settle down the occlusion.

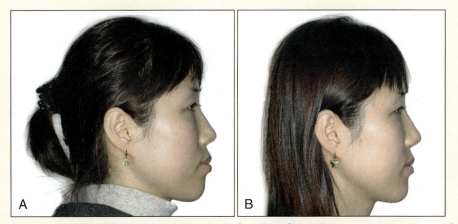

Figure 12-10 Profile Changes. Changes in facial profile with treatment at **A**, 6 months, and **B**, 10 months.

Continued

CASE REPORT 12-1—cont'd

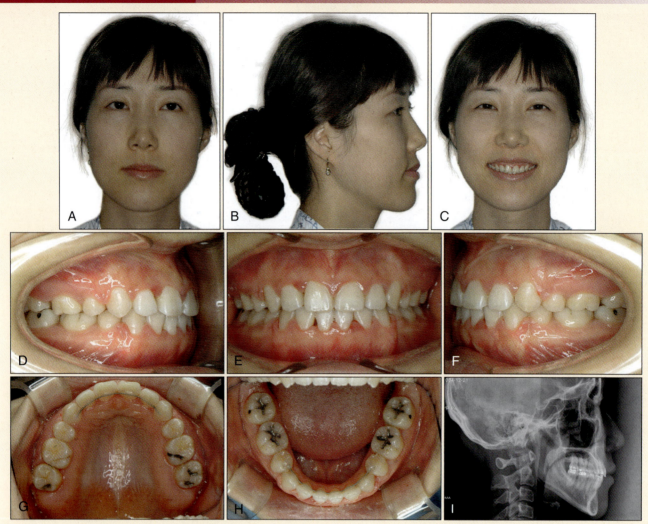

Figure 12-11 Posttreatment (17 months). **A** to **C**, Facial photographs. **D** to **H**, Intraoral photographs. **I**, Cephalograph.

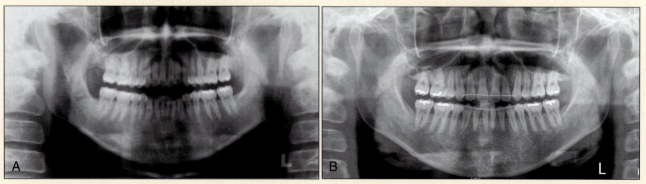

Figure 12-12 Treatment Results. Panoramic radiographs: **A**, pretreatment; **B**, posttreatment.

CASE REPORT 12-1—cont'd

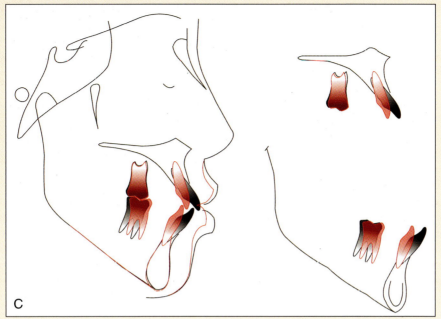

Figure 12-12, cont'd C, Cephalometric superimposition: pretreatment *(black line)* and posttreatment (17 months) *(red line)*.

NONEXTRACTION TREATMENT

In nonextraction treatment, all posterior teeth need to be retracted to resolve crowding in the anterior teeth.[9,20] To provide anchorage for distal movement of the posterior teeth, the maxillary microimplants can be placed into the buccal alveolar bone between the second premolar and first molar or into the palatal alveolar bone between the first and second molars. The occlusogingival position of the microimplant should be low and close to the attached gingiva to increase the horizontal component of force.[9] The mandibular microimplant can be placed between the first and second molar, distobuccal to the second molar or retromolar area. An anteriorly placed microimplant produces an intrusive force component that causes reduction of the Frankfort mandibular plane angle (FMA) during retraction of teeth. When dealing with a low-angle case, inclusion of the second molar into the main arch may result in an opening of the FMA (Box 12-2). If clinicians want to obtain lingual root movement of the upper anterior teeth during retraction of the entire maxillary arch, then an archwire with long anterior hooks can be used.[24]

After placement of microimplant, a distal force can be applied to the canine or first premolar to retract posterior teeth. This produces some space mesial to the canine or first premolar, and the space can be used to align the anterior teeth. After aligning the anterior teeth, all teeth including posterior teeth and anterior teeth can be distalized.

BOX 12-2 Characteristics of MIA Sliding Mechanics in Nonextraction Treatment

- With en masse movement of teeth, the treatment time is reduced.
- For each tooth, tooth movement is slow, but the total treatment time is reduced by moving the teeth together.
- Compared with molar-distalizing appliances, MIA sliding mechanics causes no round-tripping of the anterior teeth (flaring of incisors).
- Less rotation and less tipping movement are expected.

CASE REPORT 12-2

A 28-year-old female patient presented with a slightly convex profile and a Class I skeletal pattern with a high MPA (Figure 12-13 and Table 12-2). She had an ANB angle of 2.5 degrees and FMA of 37 degrees. The overbite and overjet were 3 mm, and the arch-length discrepancy was −1 mm and −5.5 mm in the maxillary and mandibular arches. She had Class I canine and molar relationships, and no third molar was present. The treatment plan included distalization of posterior teeth using MIA in both jaws.

Treatment Progress

After .022-inch straight wire brackets were bonded, initial leveling started with a .014 Ni-Ti wire. After 1 month of treatment, maxillary microimplants (SH1311-06, Absoanchor, Dentos) were placed into the alveolar bone between the second premolar and first molar. The mandibular microimplants (SH1311-08, Absoanchor) were placed between the first and second molars (Figure 12-14, A-E). Immediately after placement of the microimplant, distal force was applied to canines from microimplants by an Ni-Ti coil spring in the upper arch and an elastomeric thread in the lower arch. After alignment of anterior teeth, all teeth were retracted simultaneously against the microimplants (Figure 12-14, F-K).

At 20 months of treatment, the upper and lower anterior teeth were aligned with distal movement of the posterior teeth (Figure 12-15). Functional occlusion with Class I canine and molar relationships was obtained.

Treatment Results

The panoramic radiographs revealed no obvious root resorption (Figure 12-16). The facial profile was improved with retraction of anterior teeth as well as the posterior teeth. The MPA decreased by 1 degree. The upper and lower anterior teeth showed lingual tipping, and the posterior teeth were distalized bodily (see Figure 12-16, C).

TABLE 12-2 Cephalometric Measurements in Case Report 12-2

Measurements	Pretreatment (degrees)	Posttreatment (20 mo)
SNA	79	79
SNB	76.5	77
ANB	2.5	2
FMA	37	36
PFH/AFH	64	65
FH to OP	12.5	12.5
FH to UI	121.5	110.5
IMPA	84.5	79
Upper lip to E line	−2.5 mm	−4 mm
Lower lip to E line	0 mm	−2 mm

CASE REPORT 12-2—cont'd

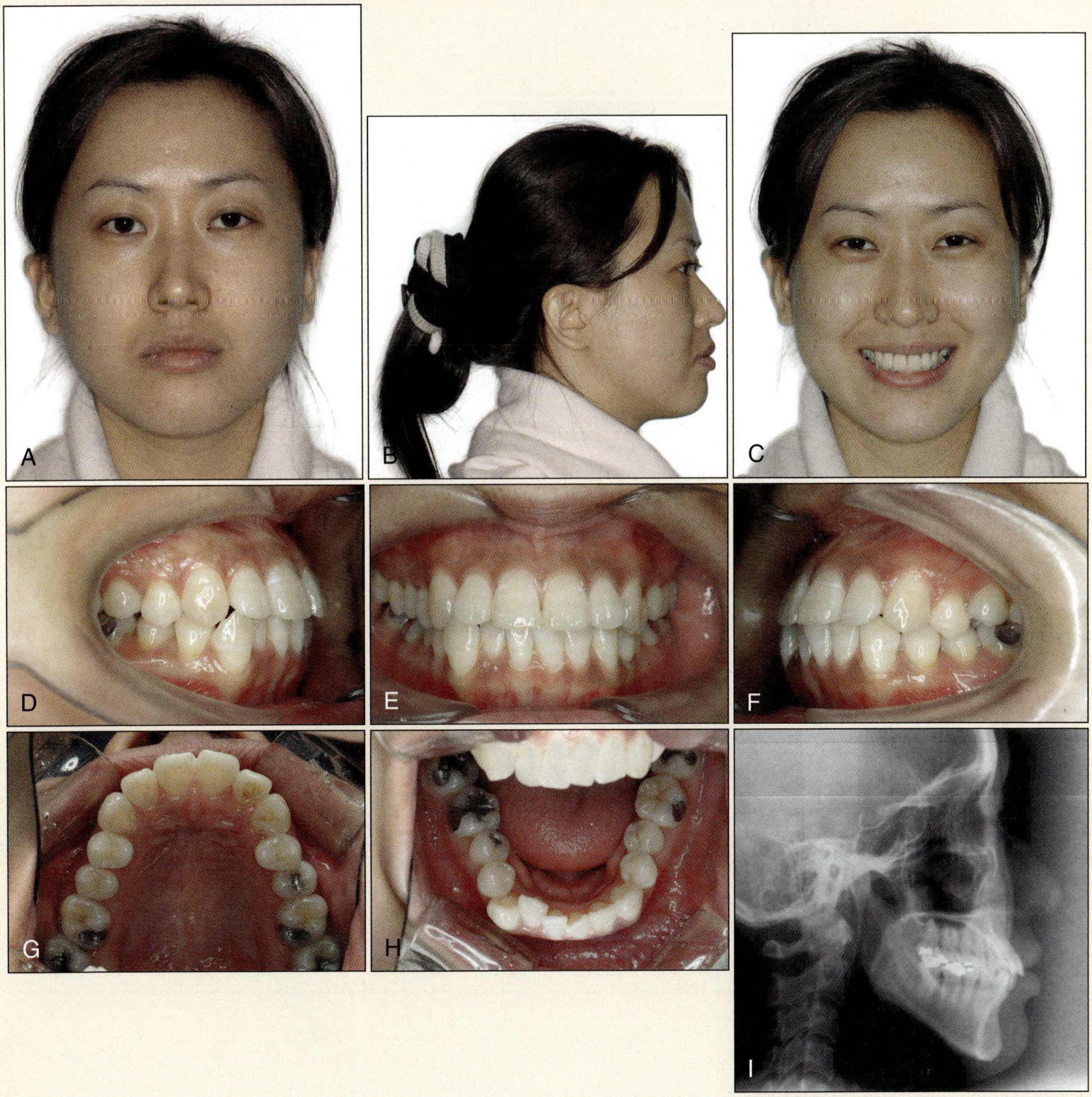

Figure 12-13 Pretreatment. **A** to **C**, Facial photographs. **D** to **H**, Intraoral photographs. **I**, Cephalograph.

Continued

CASE REPORT 12-2—cont'd

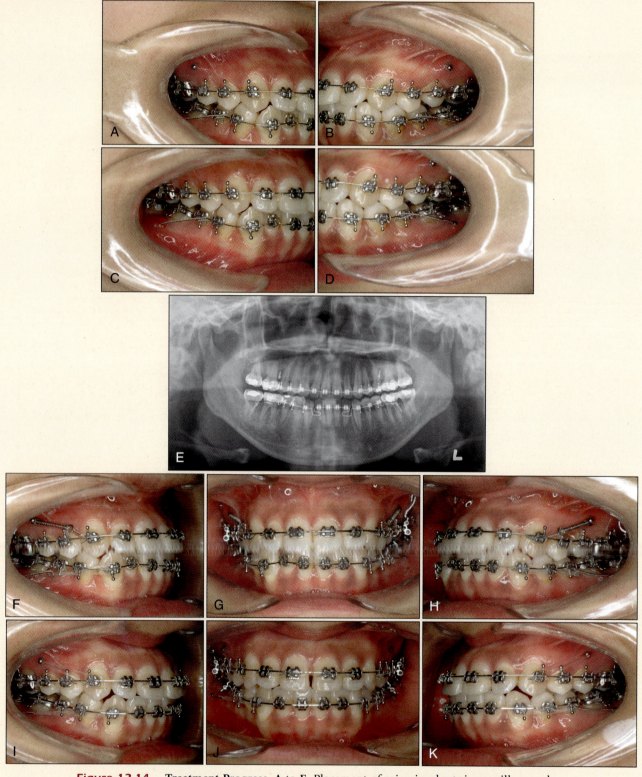

Figure 12-14 Treatment Progress. **A** to **E**, Placement of microimplants in maxillary and mandibular arches. **F** to **H**, Distal retraction of posterior teeth after 2 months of treatment. **I** to **K**, Retraction of whole arches after 6 months of treatment.

12 Clinical Application of Microimplants 273

CASE REPORT 12-2—cont'd

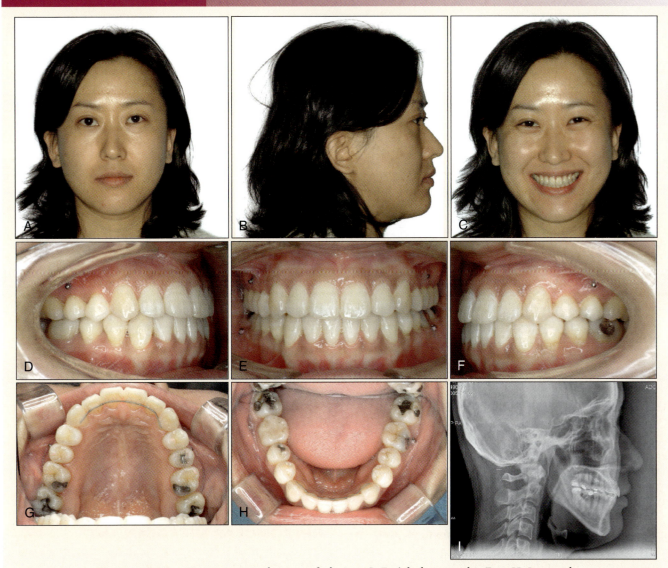

Figure 12-15 Posttreatment (20 months). A to C, Facial photographs. D to H, Intraoral photographs. I, Cephalograph.

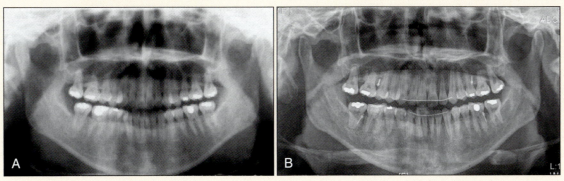

Figure 12-16 Treatment Results. Panoramic radiographs: A, pretreatment; B, posttreatment.

Continued

CASE REPORT 12-2—cont'd

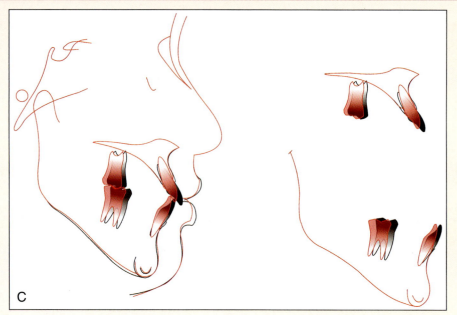

Figure 12-16, cont'd C, Cephalometric superimposition: pretreatment *(black line)* and posttreatment *(red line)*.

MICROIMPLANTS IN VARIOUS CLINICAL SITUATIONS

Clinical situations using microimplants include molar uprighting, molar intrusion, molar distalization, forced eruption of the teeth, anchorage for the periodontally compromised patient, and treatment of occlusal canting.

Microimplants can be a powerful tool for providing anchorage for whole-dentition treatment as well as movement of one or two teeth. The preprosthetic orthodontic treatment requires precise control of the moving teeth and absolutely no movement in the anchorage part. To minimize side effects, clinicians try to include as many teeth as possible into the anchorage unit. However, deterioration of occlusion in an anchorage unit is still a concern. The microimplants can eliminate the need for anchorage from the teeth.

MOLAR UPRIGHTING WITH ONE RETROMOLAR MICROIMPLANT

A mesially tipped lower molar can be uprighted distally with a microimplant placed into the retromolar area.[11]

CASE REPORT 12-3

A 14-year-old female patient had mesially tipped lower second molars and impacted third molars (Figure 12-17, *A* and *B*). To upright the second molars, the third molars were extracted, and a microimplant (SH12-06, Absoanchor) was placed into the right retromolar area (Figure 12-17, *C*). A ligature wire was tied around the head and extended toward the expected direction of the force application. After bonding a lingual button onto the distal surface of the lower-right second molar, which was exposed surgically, approximately 80 g of force was applied with elastomeric thread (Super thread, T-045, RMO, Denver) (Figure 12-17, *D*). At 3 months of treatment, the lower-right second molar was uprighted enough to expose the occlusal surface, the lingual button was bonded onto the occlusal surface of the crown, and a distal force was applied continuously (Figure 12-17, *E*). At 6 months of treatment, a minitube was bonded onto the exposed buccal surface of the crown (Figure 12-10, *F*), and the second molar was aligned with conventional mechanics. After 8 months of treatment, the mesially tipped lower-right second molar was uprighted (Figure 12-17, *G* and *H*).

Because the direction of force determines the mode of tooth movement, the position of the microimplants should be determined by considering the force direction three-dimensionally. Buccolingually, the microimplant needs to be placed slightly buccal to the center of the alveolar crest. Because the lower molars tend to tip ligually, disto-buccal force can upright the tipped molar distobuccally

CASE REPORT 12-3—cont'd

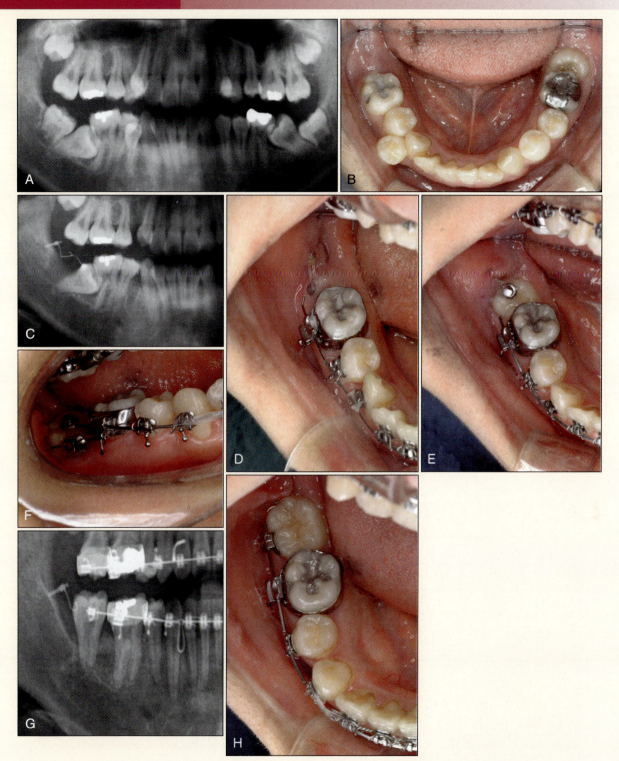

Figure 12-17 Initial panoramic radiograph (**A**) and intraoral photograph (**B**) showing mesially tipped lower second molars. **C,** Placement of microimplant into right retromolar area. Uprighting force application from microimplant: **D,** 1 month; **E,** 3 months; **F,** 6 months of treatment. **G** and **H,** At 8 months of treatment, mesially tipped lower-right second molar was uprighted.

Continued

CASE REPORT 12-3—cont'd

to obtain suitable occlusion.[11] Intrusion or extrusion of the uprighting molar can be controlled by the occlusogingival position of the head of the microimplant. The uprighting of a tipped molar tends to produce passive extrusion,[25] which may bring about *trauma from occlusion* (TFO). To prevent this, force in a downward and backward direction is needed. Therefore, a fundamental requirement involves checking the direction of the force three-dimensionally and predicting the response of the tooth to applied force.

MOLAR UPRIGHTING WITH TWO JOINED MICROIMPLANTS

The microimplant is weak on torsional force but strong in pulling or pushing force. Most of the application of force to the microimplant is a pulling force to retract or protract teeth and to intrude teeth.

To upright a molar with a two-tooth system, the anchorage part needs to withstand a very strong force. Because of its comparative weakness to torsional force,[26] a careful approach is needed to upright a molar with a bracket on one microimplant. The microimplant should be thick and long and should have remained unloaded for a long time before applying the torsional force. On the other hand, joining two microimplants can provide much more resistance to torsional force than one microimplant.[27] In addition, bonding a bracket on the head of two joined microimplants provides precise control of the tooth with conventional archwire mechanics.

CASE REPORT 12-4

A 44-year-old female patient was referred from the prosthetic department. She had an upright, mesially tipped lower-left second molar that needed uprighting. (Figure 12-18, A-C). A third molar was extracted to enhance uprighting. The two microimplants (SH1312-07, Absoanchor, Dentos) were placed into the edentulous ridge and tied together with a steel ligature wire. Core resin (Bisfil Core, Bisco, Schaumburg, Ill) was added on the heads, and a .018 standard bracket was bonded. After bonding another bracket on second molar, a sectional archwire formed with a .016 × .022–inch Titanium Molybdenum Alloy (TMA) archwire was used to apply force (Figure 12-18, D and E). To hold the upper posterior teeth vertically, a sectional archwire was bonded on the buccal surface of the first and second molars.

After 8 months of treatment, the molar was uprighted. After 4 months of retention, all brackets and microimplants were removed (Figure 12-18, F and G). The microimplants stayed firm throughout treatment and adequately withstood the torsional force. The removal torques measured were 12.29 and 16.49 Ncm, which are comparatively strong.

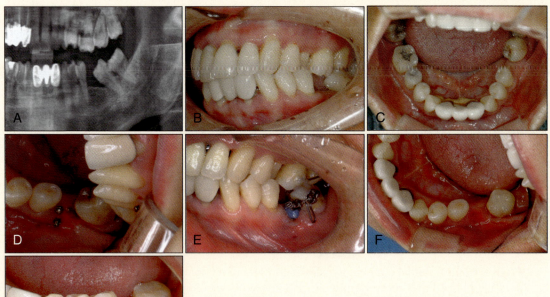

Figure 12-18 Initial panoramic radiograph (**A**) and intraoral photographs (**B** and **C**) showing mesial tipping of lower-left second molar. **D** and **E**, The two joined microimplants with a sectional wire to upright the second molar. **F** and **G**, Posttreatment intraoral photographs showing the uprighted lower second molar.

MOLAR INTRUSION

Molar intrusion is a frequently encountered problem that is difficult to treat with conventional orthodontic mechanics. To obtain pure intrusion of a molar or molars, the force should pass through the center of resistance; otherwise, the molar can be tipped. Several methods of molar intrusion using microimplants have been discussed in the literature.[7,28]

Upper Molar Intrusion with Buccal and Palatal Microimplants

To intrude two upper molars, the simple method is to apply intrusive force from both the buccal and the lingual side by placing one microimplant into the buccal side and another one into the palatal side.

Again, to obtain pure intrusion of molars, the applied force should pass through the center of resistance, buccolingually as well as mesiodistally.[29] Mesiodistally, adjacent teeth may act as anchorage to prevent tipping of molars, and the force applied to the center of the two molars should not produce tipping. In the buccolingual dimension, however, the force exerted from the microimplant is more vertical on the buccal side than the palatal side, and it may produce a palatal tipping movement. This should be prevented by placing the palatal microimplants toward the gingiva and leaving some length of the buccal microimplant to protrude from the bone and mucosal surface.

CASE REPORT 12-5

A 24-year-old female patient had the upper-left first and second molars extruded beyond the occlusal plane (Figure 12-19, A). Dental implants were placed into the lower arch. The intrusion of upper molars was planned to correct the occlusal plane and provide a better prosthesis.

The 8-mm-long microimplant (SH1312-08, Absoanchor) was placed between the first and second molars buccally, while the 10-mm-long microimplant (SH1312-10) was placed into the palatal alveolar bone between the first and second molars. Immediately after placement, an intrusive force of 70 g from both microimplants was applied to the brackets on teeth with an elastomeric thread (Super thread, T-045). The head of the microimplant in the palatal side was covered by bonding resin to minimize tongue irritation (Figure 12-19, B and C).

After 6 months of treatment, the molars were intruded approximately 2 mm (Figure 12-19, D and E). After delivering the lower prosthesis, the microimplants and brackets were removed (Figure 12-19, F and G). The debonding is delayed to prevent relapse.

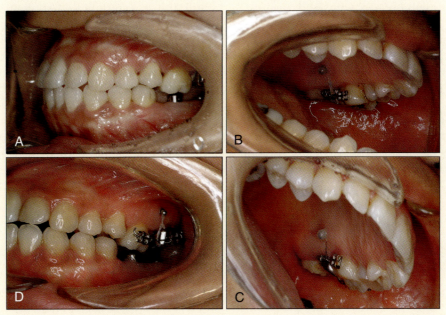

Figure 12-19 **A**, Initial intraoral photograph showing extrusion of upper first and second molars. **B** and **C**, Application of intrusion force from the buccal and palatal microimplants. **D** and **E**, Intraoral photographs showing intrusion of upper molars at 6 months of treatment.

CASE REPORT 12-5—cont'd

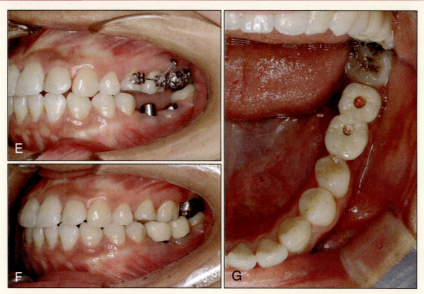

Figure 12-19, cont'd D and E, Intraoral photographs showing intrusion of upper molars at 6 months of treatment. F and G, Posttreatment intraoral photographs.

Molar Intrusion with Bracket Head Microimplant

The two types of BH microimplants are right-handed and left-handed. The right-handed BH microimplant is tightened by turning the microimplant clockwise.

Loading of force in a tightening direction may have a positive effect on stability. To withstand torsional force, however, the microimplant should be thick and long and should remain in the alveolar bone unloaded for at least 3 months to allow osseointegration. Force in the pulling direction with minimal torsional force can be loaded to a thick-diameter microimplant without adverse results.

The intrusion of one molar may produce tipping when one microimplant is used. To prevent tipping, four microimplants are required to align the force to pass through the center of resistance of the molar.[30] However, the transpalatal bar with a hinge joint on the molar in the opposite side and an ordinary soldered connection to the intrusion side can prevent a tipping movement, with one microimplant placed in the palatal or buccal alveolar bone on the side of molar intrusion. Still, this is a complicated appliance.

Using the BH microimplant can prove to be a simpler alternative for intrusion of one molar. The palatal cusp of the upper molar tends to extrude more than the buccal cusp when antagonists are missing. Therefore, it is rational to apply more force to the palatal cusp than to the buccal cusp to obtain a similar amount of intrusion. The palatally placed BH microimplant can provide intrusion force to the palatal cusp and buccal torque by twisting a sectional archwire as illustrated in the next case report.

CASE REPORT 12-6

A 32-year-old male patient presented with extruded upper-right second molars (Figure 12-20, A-C). The palatal cusp was extruded more than the buccal cusp. The 1.5-mm-diameter, 10-mm-long, right-handed BH microimplant (BH1514-10-R, Absoanchor) was placed into the palatal alveolar bone between the upper first and second molars (Figure 12-20, D-F). A .017 × .025 TMA archwire was engaged into the .018 bracket slot on the head. Intrusive force with buccal crown torque was applied to the bracket on the palatal surface of the molar from the microimplant. At 4 months of treatment, the palatal cusp was intruded with slight intrusion of the buccal cusp (Figure 12-20, G-I). The microimplant and bracket were removed after the patient received a prosthesis in the lower arch.

CASE REPORT 12-6—cont'd

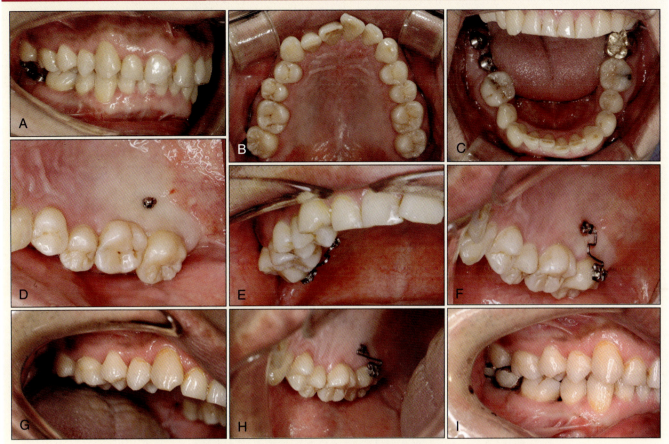

Figure 12-20 **A** to **C**, Initial intraoral photographs showing the extruded palatal cusp of the upper-right second molar. **D** to **F**, Bracket head–type microimplant and a sectional wire to intrude the second molar. **G** to **I**, Intraoral photographs after intrusion and after prosthetic treatment.

Molar Intrusion with Direct or Indirect Anchorage

The use of a microimplant as orthodontic anchorage can be divided into direct and indirect anchorage. Direct anchorage is used most often, but the movement of one or two teeth is difficult to control precisely,[31] because the only force that can be obtained from the microimplant is a pulling or pushing force. The indirect anchorage system is similar to typical orthodontic mechanics, except for the inclusion of the microimplant. The microimplant is connected to a tooth or a group of teeth, which can then be used to perform precise, three-dimensional control of the teeth with conventional archwire mechanics.

MOLAR DISTALIZATION

Many molar-distalizing appliances have been developed and their clinical application described.[32] Treatment effects of molar-distalizing appliances can be summarized by distal movement of the molars, anterior movement of the premolars, and flaring of the incisors. The anterior teeth are moved forward during distalization of molars and retracted during space closure. The resultant position of the upper molars after completion of treatment has been reported slightly anterior to its original position.[33] With microimplants, molars can be distalized effectively without reactive mechanics on anterior teeth.

CASE REPORT 12-7

A 55-year-old female patient had an extruded lower-left second molar that interfered with proper fabrication of a maxillary prosthesis (Figure 12-21, A and B).

To apply intrusive force through the center of resistance or to apply intrusion force from both the buccal and the lingual side or through the center of resistance, the microimplant should be placed into the buccal as well as lingual alveolar bone. The placement of microimplant into the lingual alveolar bone is difficult because of limited access. Therefore, indirect anchorage with the buccal microimplant was planned for this patient.

A microimplant (SH1312-07, Absoanchor) was placed between the first and second premolars and connected to the first premolar with a .016 × .022–inch stainless steel wire. The intrusive force was applied with a sectional TMA archwire from the buccal and lingual side (Figure 12-21, C and D). After 8 months of treatment, the second molar experienced 2 mm of intrusion (Figure 12-21, E-G) with no movement of the tooth in the anchorage part.

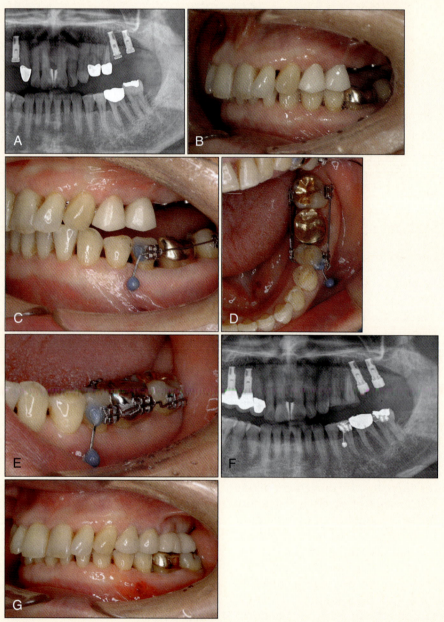

Figure 12-21 Initial panoramic radiograph (**A**) and intraoral photograph (**B**) showing the extruded lower-left second molar. **C** and **D**, Connection of microimplant to second premolar and use of premolar as anchorage for second-molar intrusion. **E**, Intraoral photograph, and **F**, panoramic radiograph, after intrusion. **G**, Intraoral photograph after final restorations.

CASE REPORT 12-8

A 9-year-old boy had a Class II molar relationship on both sides (Figure 12-22, A-C). The distal movement of upper posterior teeth was planned. After cementation of a modified transpalatal bar, microimplants (SH1312-08, Absoanchor) were placed into the palatal alveolar bone mesial to the first molars (Figure 12-22, D and E). Immediately after placement, an elastomeric thread was tied to apply a distalizing force. After 3 months of force application, a Class I molar relationship was achieved by the distal movement of the molars (Figure 12-22, F-H).

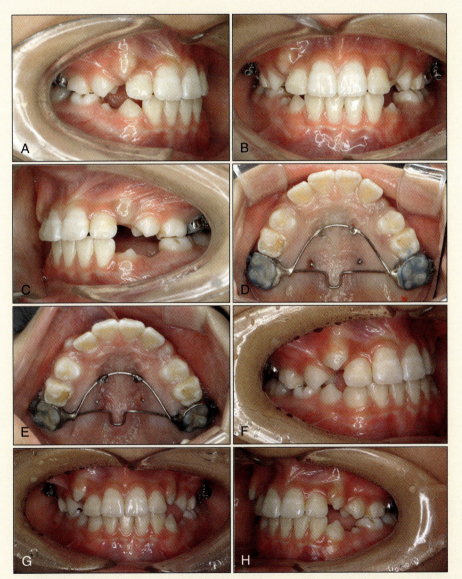

Figure 12-22 A to C, Intraoral photographs showing Class II molar relationship. D and E, Distal force application from the microimplants to a modified transpalatal bar. F to H, Class I molar relationship that was achieved by distal movement of the upper molars.

FORCED ERUPTION

When providing prosthetic treatment for a severely decayed tooth or a tooth with a fracture line below the alveolar crest, orthodontic forced eruption is an important treatment option. Forced eruption can be performed by using the adjacent teeth as anchorage, with negligible movement of the anchorage teeth because of the relatively low force level needed to extrude a tooth. However, forced eruption of a tooth whose adjacent teeth are missing is extremely difficult. A removable appliance is one option but then it depends greatly on patient compliance.

ANCHORAGE FOR PERIODONTALLY COMPROMISED PATIENT

When managing periodontally compromised teeth, the lack of bony support results in unsuitable anchorage. Connecting the microimplant to the anchor tooth (or teeth) can eliminate reciprocal reactive mechanics.

CASE REPORT 12-9

A 54-year-old female patient was referred from the prosthetic department to erupt the upper-right canine orthodontically (Figure 12-23, *A-C*). She had missing lateral incisors and decayed central incisors, which made it difficult to obtain anchorage with conventional mechanics. Two microimplants (SH1312-08, Absoanchor) were placed into the missing lateral incisor area (Figure 12-23, *D-G*). After tying them together with a ligature wire, core resin was added, and a bracket was bonded. A small hook was cemented into the root canal of the decayed upper-right canine. This hook was located close to the center of the canine so that it did not produce a tipping movement during extrusion (Figure 12-23, *H-J*). A sectional wire was bent to position its hook to the center of the canine. If needed, the wire could be adjusted to obtain mesial or distal tipping or buccal or lingual tipping. Immediately after placement of microimplants, 40 g of force was applied. For esthetic reasons, a temporary bridge was cemented.

After 4 months of treatment, the canine experienced 3 mm of extrusion. A steel ligature was tied with no force in order to provide retention for 2 months (Figure 12-23, *K-M*).

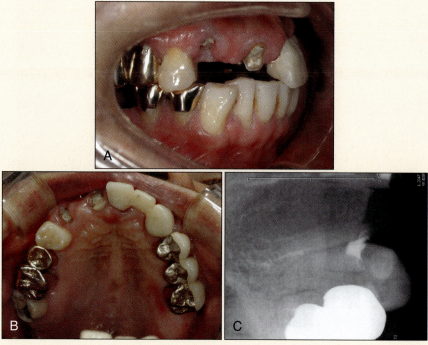

Figure 12-23 A to C, Intraoral photographs and periapical radiograph showing severely decayed upper left canine.

CASE REPORT 12-9—cont'd

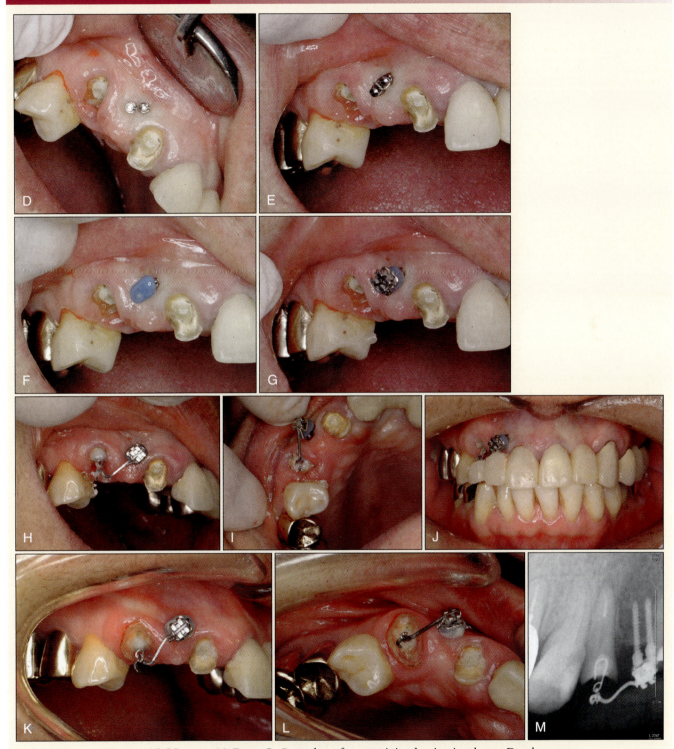

Figure 12-23, cont'd D to G, Procedure for two joined microimplants: D, placement of two microimplants; E, tying ligature wire; F, adding core resin; G, bonding a bracket. H to J, Sectional wire with a hook extended to the center of canine. K to M, Intraoral photographs and periapical radiograph after forced eruption.

CASE REPORT 12-10

A 45-year-old female patient was sent from the prosthetic department to close a space between the upper-right first premolar and the distally migrated second premolar (Figure 12-24, A and B). She had severely damaged periodontal support. Periodontal treatment and oral hygiene instruction were already completed. To eliminate the movement of the first premolar, a microimplant was planned.

After placement of the microimplant (SH1312-10, Absoanchor) into the palatal alveolar bone, a sectional archwire was bent and connected with a core resin from the microimplant to the palatal surface of the first premolar (Figure 12-24, C and D). After bonding brackets on the buccal and palatal side, less than 50 g of force was applied to protract the second premolar.

After 5 months of treatment, the space was closed by forward movement of the second premolar (Figure 12-24, E and F). A fixed retainer was bonded on the first and second premolars, and all braces (including the microimplant) were removed (Figure 12-24, G and H). There was no movement at the first premolar, which was connected to the microimplant. The second premolar moved forward.

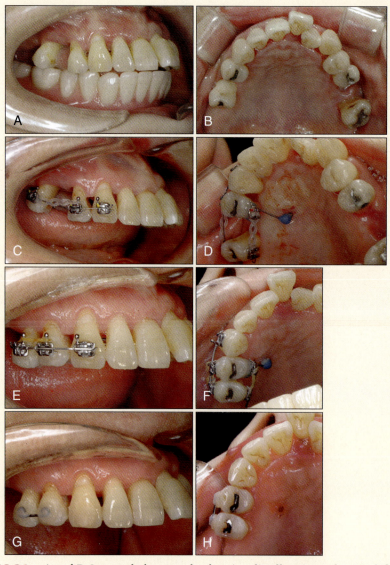

Figure 12-24 A and B, Intraoral photographs showing distally migrated upper-left second premolar. C and D, Connection of microimplant to first premolar for reinforcing anchorage. E and F, Intraoral photographs showing space closure at 5 months of treatment. G and H, Fixed bonded retainer and removal of the microimplant.

CORRECTION OF CANTED OCCLUSAL PLANE

Facial asymmetry is often associated with canting of the occlusal plane. The cant in the occlusal plane may compromise facial appearance and beauty, with concurrent canting of the lip line. The canted occlusal plane can be corrected with extrusion of teeth on the side with more superiorly positioned teeth, using vertical elastics. The intrusion of teeth in the extruded side, however, cannot be achieved with conventional orthodontic mechanics. The microimplant placed in the buccal alveolar bone can apply intruding force to posterior teeth and can be used to correct the canted occlusal plane. Correcting the canted occlusal plane can reduce the need for maxillary surgery in facial asymmetry treatment, combining two jaw procedures into one jaw surgery.[7] The precise control of the occlusal plane with orthodontic treatment can bring more predictable results.

CASE REPORT 12-11

A 16-year-old female patient had a canted occlusal plane (Figure 12-25, A). To correct the canting of the occlusal plane, intrusion of the upper teeth on the right side was planned. A microimplant (SH1312-07, Absoanchor) was placed into the buccal alveolar bone between the second premolar and first molar, and intrusion force was applied (Figure 12-25, B-D). To prevent buccal tipping of teeth during application of intrusion force on the buccal side, a transpalatal bar was installed. After 8 months of treatment, the canting of the occlusal plane was corrected (Figure 12-25, E). The steel ligature wire was tied to hold the teeth vertically afterward.

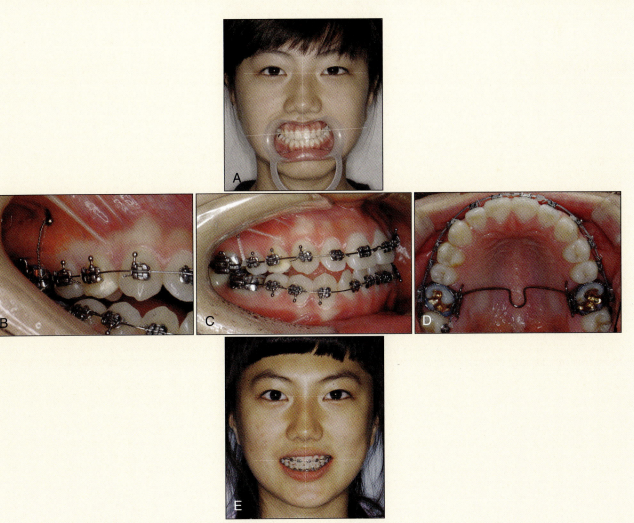

Figure 12-25 A, Initial extraoral photograph showing canting of the occlusal plane. B to D, Intrusion of upper-right posterior teeth and transpalatal bar to prevent buccal tipping of teeth. E, Extraoral photograph showing a corrected occlusal plane.

SUCCESS AND FAILURE OF MICROIMPLANT ORTHODONTICS

Success in microimplant orthodontics is defined as a microscrew with minimal mobility and inflammation and the ability to obtain full functional correction either through direct or indirect anchorage. In 1999, Park and Kim[34] reported a success rate of 82% after 5 months of observation. In 2003 a 93% success rate was reported during a 15.8-month observation period.[35] Other studies have shown a similar level of success.[36-38] Microimplant orthodontics has a learning curve; with more experience, the success rate increases.

Regarding the causes of microimplant failure, Miyawaki et al.[36] reported that small diameter of the screw (<1.0 mm), inflammation, and a high MPA are risk factors for the screws placed in the mandibular posterior teeth area. Cheng et al.[37] found that the mandibular posterior teeth area and nonkeratinized mucosa are also risk factors for miniscrew failure. Additionally, Park et al.[38] found that mobility, right side of the jaw, the mandible, and inflammation are among 17 clinical variables in microimplant failure.

CONCLUSION

Microimplants can provide absolute anchorage for the movement of whole dentition, as well as the movement of one or two teeth for prosthetic needs. It simplifies treatment mechanics by eliminating reactive mechanics.

REFERENCES

1. Shapiro PA, Kokich VG: Uses of implants in orthodontics, *Dent Clin North Am* 32:539-550, 1988.
2. Roberts WE, Nelsen CL, Goodacre CJ: Rigid implant anchorage to close a mandibular first molar extraction site, *J Clin Orthod* 28:693-704, 1994.
3. Umemori M, Sugawara J, Mitani H, et al: Skeletal anchorage system for open bite correction, *Am J Orthod Dentofac Orthop* 115:166-174, 1999.
4. Creekmore TD, Eklund MK: The possibility of skeletal anchorage, *J Clin Orthod* 17:266-269, 1983.
5. Kanomi R: Mini-implant for orthodontic anchorage, *J Clin Orthod* 31:763-777, 1997.
6. Park HS: The skeletal cortical anchorage using titanium microscrew implants, *Korean J Orthod* 29:699-706, 1999.
7. Park HS: *The use of micro-implant as orthodontic anchorage* Seoul, South Korea, 2001, Nare.
8. Park HS, Bae SM, Kyung HM, Sung JH: Micro-implant anchorage for treatment of skeletal Class I bialveolar protrusion, *J Clin Orthod* 35:417-422, 2001.
9. Park HS, Kwon DG, Sung JH: Nonextraction treatment with microscrew implant, *Angle Orthod* 74:539-549, 2004.
10. Lee JS, Park HS, Kyung HM: Micro-implant anchorage in lingual orthodontic treatment for a skeletal Class II malocclusion, *J Clin Orthod* 35:643-647, 2001.
11. Park HS, Kyung HM, Sung JH: A simple method of molar uprighting with micro-implant anchorage, *J Clin Orthod* 36:592-596, 2002.
12. Kyung HM, Park HS, Bae SM, et al: Development of orthodontic micro-implants for intraoral anchorage, *J Clin Orthod* 37:321-328, 2003.
13. Champy M, Pape H, Gerlach KL, Lodde JP: Mandibular fracture. In Kruger E, Schilli W, editors: *Oral and maxillofacial traumatology* vol 2, Chicago, 1986, Quintessence, pp 19-43.
14. Park HS: An anatomical study using CT images for the implantation of micro-implants, *Korean J Orthod* 32:435-441, 2002.
15. Park HS, Lee YJ, Jeoung SH, Kwon TG: Bone density of the alveolar and basal bone in the maxilla and the mandible, *Am J Orthod Dentofacial Orthop* 133:30-37, 2008.
16. Lohr J et al: Comparative in vitro studies of self-boring and self-tapping screws: histomorphological and physical-technical studies of bone layers, *Mund Kiefer Gesichtschir* 4:159-163, 2000.
17. Eriksson AR, Albrektsson T: Temperature threshold levels for heat-induced bone tissue injury: a vital-microscopic study in the rabbit, *J Prosthet Dent* 50:101-107, 1983.
18. Park HS, Kwon DG: Sliding mechanics with microscrew implant anchorage, *Angle Orthod* 74:703-710, 2004.
19. Park HS, Kwon OW, Sung JH: Microscrew implant anchorage sliding mechanics, *World J Orthod* 6:265-274, 2005.
20. Park HS, Lee SK, Kwon OW: Group distal movement of teeth with microscrew implants, *Angle Orthod* 75:510-517, 2005.
21. Melsen B, Fotis V, Burstone CJ: Vertical force considerations in differential space closure, *J Clin Orthod* 24:678-683, 1990.
22. Klontz HA: Facial balance and harmony: an attainable objective for the patient with a high mandibular plane angle, *Am J Orthod Dentofac Orthop* 114:176-188, 1998.
23. Park HS, Kwon OW: The treatment of openbite with microscrew implants, *Am J Orthod Dentofacial Orthop* 126:627-636, 2004.
24. Park HS, Bae SM, Kyung HM, Sung JH: Simultaneous incisor retraction and distal molar movement with microimplant anchorage, *World J Orthod* 5:164-171, 2004.
25. Roberts WW, Chacker FM, Burstone CJ: A segmental approach to mandibular molar uprighting, *Am J Orthod* 81:177-182, 1982.
26. Costa A, Raffini M, Melsen B: Miniscrew as orthodontic anchorage, *Int J Adult Orthod Orthogn Surg* 13:201-209, 1998.
27. Lee JS, Kim DH, Park YC, et al: The efficient use of midpalatal miniscrew implants, *Angle Orthod* 74:711-714, 2004.
28. Park HS, Jang BK, Kyung HM: Maxillary molar intrusion with micro-implant anchorage (MIA), *Aust Orthod J* 21:129-135, 2005.
29. Melsen B, Fiorelli G: Upper molar intrusion, *J Clin Orthod* 30:91-96, 1996.
30. Park YC, Lee SY, Kim DH, Jee SH: Intrusion of posterior teeth using mini-screw implants, *Am J Orthod Dentofacial Orthop* 123:690-694, 2003.
31. Yun SW, Lim WH, Chun YS: Molar control using indirect miniscrew anchorage, *J Clin Orthod* 39:661-664, 2005.
32. Bussick T, McNamara JA: Dentoalveolar and skeletal changes associated with the pendulum appliance, *Am J Orthod Dentofacial Orthop* 117:333-343, 2000.
33. Ngantung V, Nanda RS, Bowman SJ: Posttreatment evaluation of the distal jet appliance, *Am J Orthod Dentofacial Orthop* 120:178-185, 2001.
34. Park HS, Kim JB: The use of titanium microscrew implants as orthodontic anchorage, *Keimyung Med J* 18:509-515, 1999.
35. Park HS: Clinical study on success rate of microscrew implants for orthodontic anchorage, *Korean J Orthod* 33:151-156, 2003.
36. Miyawaki S, Koyama I, Inoue M, et al: Factors associated with the stability of titanium screws placed in the posterior region for orthodontic anchorage, *Am J Orthod Dentofacial Orthop* 124:373-378, 2003.
37. Cheng SJ, Tseng IY, Lee JJ, Kok SH: A prospective study of risk factors associated with failure of mini-implants used for orthodontic anchorage, *Int J Oral Maxillofac Implants* 19:100-106, 2004.
38. Park HS, Jeong SH, Kwon OH: Factors affecting the clinical success of mini- or microscrew implants used as orthodontic anchorage, *Am J Orthod Dentofacial Orthop* 130:18-25, 2006.

CHAPTER 13
Clinical Suitability of Titanium Microscrews for Orthodontic Anchorage

Ulrike B. Fritz and Peter R. Diedrich

The number of adult patients requiring orthodontic therapy has greatly increased in recent decades. However, adults frequently present with pathological findings such as periodontal and endodontic diseases and early loss of posterior teeth. Therefore the use of the native dentition for orthodontic anchorage is frequently limited, and extraoral appliances are rejected for esthetic reasons. However, osseointegrated implants have proved to be compliance-free, stable anchorage units in orthodontics (Figure 13-1).

Numerous histological and clinical studies have confirmed the value of osseointegrated titanium implants.[1,2] Even a longer application of orthodontic forces in all three dimensions results in no implant dislocation. Experimental animal studies have verified that orthodontic loading has a positive impact on the periimplant bone situation in terms of bone-remodeling rate and density. Continuous orthodontic loading resulted in osseous adaptation mechanisms and additional periimplant bone apposition, which lead to increased stability[1,2] (Figure 13-2). Conventional implants, most frequently inserted bicortically in the palate, offer "absolute anchorage" and 100% success rate. However, disadvantages include the following:

- Restricted indication
- Limited insertion sites
- Long osseointegration period (6 weeks)
- Complicated implantation and removal procedures
- Complex design and size
- High cost

In recent years the trend in medicine has been to favor atraumatic procedures. The dimensions of the fixtures have become smaller over time, with manufacturers developing titanium microscrew systems in various designs during the past 8 years.[3] These methods are derived from maxillofacial fixation techniques and rely on mechanical retention for anchorage. The diameters vary between 1 and 2 mm and the lengths between 4 and 14 mm. Clinical experiences and case reports are promising because small implants offer advantages to the orthodontist as well as the patient.[4-6] These advantages are as follows:

- More orthodontic treatment options
- Simple, atraumatic insertion and explantation
- Direct loading
- Increased patient comfort
- Favorable cost/benefit ratio

So far, however, minimal evidence is available concerning the failure rate of microscrews. We reported that in situ time varied from 17 days to more than 1 year.[7] Although promising case reports are available, studies with a high predictive potential on the clinical long-term behavior of microscrews are rare. A direct comparison of the failure rates in different studies is problematic

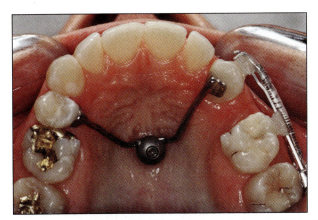

Figure 13-1
Skeletal Orthodontic Anchorage with Conventional Implant. Implant is bicortically inserted in the palate (Orthosystem, Straumann, Waldenburg, Switzerland). Treatment aim is mesialization of teeth #26 and #27 using a passive, stainless steel sectional arch and a superelastic coil. The upper-left canine is stabilized by an implant-supported palatal bar.

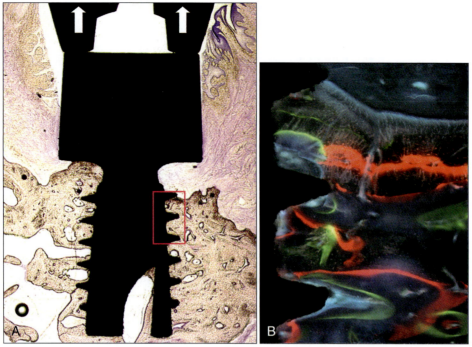

Figure 13-2

Vertically Loaded Fixture (Orthosystem) with Almost Complete Osseointegration (animal experiment). A, Polychrome sequential labeling technique underlines the periimplant bone deposition: close attachment and differentiation of the bone to lamellar maturity. **B,** Stain analysis documents retrospectively the pronounced osteodynamics: several apposition lines at the alveolar margin, as well as longitudinal and cross-sectional osteons in the periimplant bone.

because of differences in study designs, implant systems, and insertion techniques. A few clinical studies reported failure rates of 20% to 30%,[7-10] although the reasons or risk factors are still unclear.

SCREW DESIGN

The microimplant system Dual Top Anchor (Jeil Medical, Promedia, Germany) uses screws made of a titanium alloy (titanium-vanadium). Sterilization of the screws and the insertion kit must be performed in the dental office before clinical use.

Five different Dual Top screw types are available: JA, G1, G2, JB, and JD. The screws have four components: head, neck, platform, and screw body (Figure 13-3). The hexagonal head of Dual Top G2 has a .022 × .025 cross-slot for incorporation of a rectangular archwire. The head in the bracket design facilitates a stable three-dimensional connection of the microscrew and the appliance and easy archwire management.

The smooth platform surface enhances soft tissue wound healing and prevents the screw head from impairing labial and buccal mucosa. The conical screw body has a self-drilling and self-tapping design and a twisted cone point. The threads have a 105-degree upward angle and a 130-degree downward angle designed for

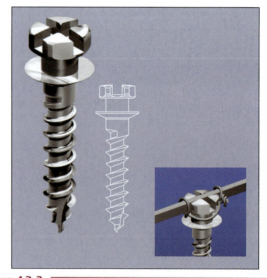

Figure 13-3

Self-Tapping Titanium Screw (Dual Top G2). Screw head has a cross-slot to hold a rectangular archwire.

orthopedic screw *osteosynthesis*, that is, maximum stability with minimum trabecular traumatization.

The Dual Top screws are available in three different diameters (1.4, 1.6, and 2 mm) and in lengths of 6, 8, and 10 mm (Table 13-1).

TABLE 13-1	Diameter and Length of Microscrews*
Diameter (mm)	Length of Thread (mm)
1.4	6 or 8
1.6	6, 8, or 10
2.0	6, 8, or 10

*Dual Top screw types JA, G1, G2, JB, and JD.

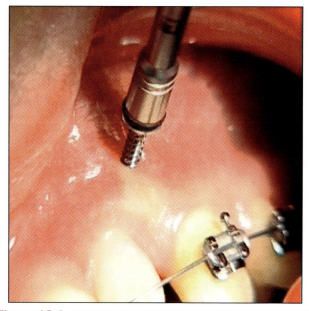

Figure 13-4
After local anaesthesia, Dual Top screw is inserted with manual screwdriver. No mucosal punching, incision/flap surgery, or pilot hole is used.

IMPLANT INSERTION

Choice of insertion site and screw type depends on the indication, with reference to radiographs (panoramic radiograph, lateral cephalograms, periapical radiographs where necessary) and clinical findings (bone supply, interradicular space, position of mental foramen, dimensions of maxillary sinus, soft tissue situation, e.g., attached gingiva, oral mucosa). In general, positioning of the microscrew head within attached gingiva is recommended. If inserting the device in mobile mucosa is unavoidable (e.g., spina nasalis anterior, fossa infrazygomatica, symphysis), the microscrew tends to "submerge"; inflammatory tissue proliferation results in coverage of the screw head.

Before microscrew insertion, patients are informed about the surgical procedure, risks, complications, and postoperative directives.

After infiltrative local anesthesia with epinephrine-free anesthetic, a pilot hole (2-mm depth) is drilled directly through the mucosa using a low-speed, water-cooled pilot drill (0.9-mm bur diameter) in cases with dense cortical bone in the mandible. Pilot holes are avoided in the maxilla and, where appropriate, in the mandible, because the holes may impair the essential primary stability of the screw. Neither punching of the mucosa nor incision/flap surgery is necessary. The screws are inserted slowly with a manual screwdriver (Figure 13-4) or with the help of a contra-angle, low-speed handpiece under adequate cooling with sterile sodium chloride (NaCl) solution. To achieve a close implant-bone contact, it is crucial to maintain the initial drilling direction.

Before surgery the patient rinses the mouth with a 0.1% chlorhexidine digluconate solution and is instructed to apply chlorhexidine gel on the screw head and the surrounding soft tissue daily. Antibiotic therapy is not performed.

Microscrews can be loaded directly after insertion. Generally, two loading alternatives are available. With *direct* screw loading the active forces are directly transferred to the screw (Figure 13-5, *A*). With *indirect* loading, the screw is connected to an adjacent tooth by a passive, segmented archwire, thus establishing a combined periodontal/implant-supported anchorage (Figure 13-5, *B*).

The implants are removed with the same manual screwdriver used for insertion. Local anesthesia is not necessary. The mucosa at the insertion site heals without complication within days.

IMPLANT SITES

Larger implants need a relatively extensive bone supply, which limits the number of insertion sites. Microscrews, however, offer a wider and more flexible range of applications, with typical insertion sites in the *maxilla* (upper jaw) as follows:
- Spina nasalis anterior
- Palate
- Crista infrazygomatica
- Alveolar process

If palatal implants are planned in growing patients, insertion at the midpalatal suture should be avoided. Sufficient bone support is likely about 1 mm from the suture (Figure 13-6).

Interradicular implantation depends on the width of the septum. A typical histological section of a human maxilla reveals the variability of adjacent interradicular sites. Whereas the bone volume is copious between canine and first premolar, the space between the premolars is an issue (Figure 13-7). In narrow-root topographies, an additional x-ray film using an individual positioning device can be recommended to allow targeted insertion of the screw. In general, optimal conditions for interradicular implant placement in the upper

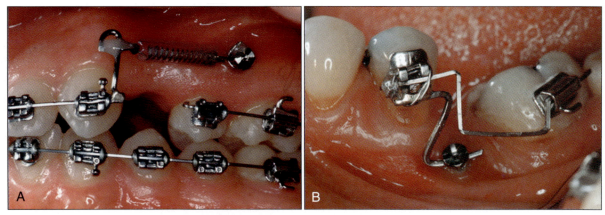

Figure 13-5

Microscrew Loading Alternatives. A, Direct screw loading. The reactive anchorage loading is transferred straight to the position-stable implant. En masse retraction of the upper incisors after premolar extraction, with stabilization of the posterior anchorage unit by an interradicularly positioned microscrew. The extension permits force application close to the center of resistance and results in translatory movement of the incisors. **B,** Indirect anchorage type. The screw is connected by a passive stabilization wire to the adjacent tooth. For uprighting of a tilted molar, a microscrew is inserted in the edentulous alveolar ridge in the region of tooth #36 and is connected to the premolar bracket by a passive, rectangular wire serving as anchorage for the interception of a counterclockwise moment. The uprighting spring consists of .016 × .022–inch Titanium Molybdenum Alloy (TMA) archwire.

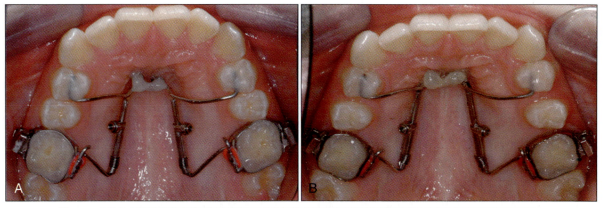

Figure 13-6

A, Microscrew-supported skeletonized Distal Jet appliance with occlusal rests bonded to the first premolars. Treatment objective is bilateral distalization of the first and second molars. Two microscrews serve as additional anchorage for the appliance. The screws were inserted 1 mm paramedian. **B,** Comparison of initial situation and findings after 4 months reveals the effective anchorage quality of the palatal microscrews.

and lower jaw are a broad septum, thick cortical bone, and dense bone marrow.

In the *mandible* (lower jaw) the typical sites for microscrew implantation are as follows:
- Retromolar region
- Alveolar process
- Symphysis

Cephalometric analysis provides valid information about the subapical bone supply for implantation in the symphysis.

The slender nature of the microscrews allows for the range of insertion sites and clinical applications such as molar anchorage, intrusion, mesialization, distalization, molar uprighting, en masse incisor retraction and

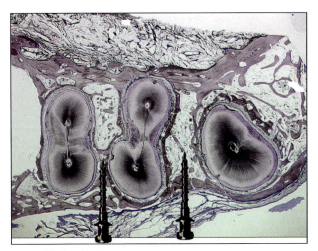

Figure 13-7
Histological section of a human specimen illustrates the variability of interradicular sites.

extrusion-intrusion, and preprosthetic premolar distalization for ridge augmentation.

COMPLICATIONS

INTRAOPERATIVE
- Trauma of vessel (palatine artery)
- Trauma of nerve (inferior alveolar, mental)
- Implantation in nasal or maxillary sinus
- Root contact
- Fracture of the screw

The practitioner should be familiar with anatomical structures, so intraoperative complications such as traumatic damage of adjacent roots, vessels, nerves, or the sinus are negligible. Screw fractures are rarely observed with implantation and explantation procedures (0%-3.5%).[11]

POSTOPERATIVE
- Periimplant inflammation
- Mucosal irritations, mainly in the mobile mucosa
- Mobility (see below)
- Failures

Even when correctly inserted, it is important to be aware that microscrews do not remain absolutely stationary.[11] When loaded over a period, the devices are displaced 1 to 1.5 mm in the direction of the applied force. Even though some displacement occurs, microscrews present enough stability to complete the treatment.

FAILURE RATE

We inserted 64 microimplants (Dual Top G2) in 41 patients (22 males, 19 females; mean age, 26 ± 13 years). Mean observation time was 151 ± 84 days (4.8 months), with at least 14 days, up to more than 400 days.

Eleven of 64 implants showed increased mobility but still served as anchorage. Thirteen failures occurred before the end of treatment, a failure rate of 20%. Because of the small number of implants, the study did not include statistical analysis. However, the following tendencies were observed:
- Implants with larger diameter were prognostically more favorable.
- Fewer failures occurred in the upper than in the lower jaw.
- Primary stability was crucial for the prognosis.
- Even mobile implants performed well as anchorage.

CASE REPORT 13-1

Diagnosis
A 51-year-old woman was advised by the department of prosthodontics to register at the department of orthodontics. Initial clinical findings included the following (Figure 13-8, A and B):
- Dentition with prosthetic rehabilitation
- 26-year-old fixed partial denture
- Teeth #11 and #13 with gingivitis
- Gingival recession of about 3 to 4 mm
- Exposed crown margins

The patient found the uneven gingival margin of teeth #11 and #13 esthetically displeasing, so planning focused on harmonization of the gingival margin before the prosthetic procedure.

Treatment Plan
- Instructions to the patient
- Removal of supragingival and subgingival plaque and calculus to eliminate marginal infection.
- Orthodontic extrusion of the abutment teeth #11 and #13 by an implant-supported, limited fixed appliance.
- Retention of treatment result for at least 3 months.
- Prosthetic procedure

A fixed appliance was designed to extrude the abutment teeth #11 and #13 with a light, continuous force. A microscrew (Dual Top, 2 × 8 mm) was inserted vestibularly into the edentulous alveolar bone in the region of tooth #12 under local anesthesia to anchor the appliance and to intercept the reactive intrusive force.

Continued

CASE REPORT 13-1—cont'd

The bridge to be extruded was not separated, and the crowns of #11 and #13 were bonded with ceramic brackets. The two brackets were connected with a passive .019 × .025–inch stainless steel archwire. Another segmented, .019 × .025 archwire was fixed into the slot of the screw head perpendicular to the archwire connecting the brackets. The two sectional wires were connected by a cross-tube, fixed with composite to the horizontal wire, so that only vertical movements were possible. The required extrusion force of 20 cN was generated by a superelastic open-coil spring, placed between the head of the screw and the cross-tube. The microscrew was loaded immediately after insertion (Figure 13-8, C and D). The palatal surfaces of the pontic and the crowns were continuously reduced to provide sufficient space for the eruption (Figure 13-8, E).

The patient did not feel impaired in eating or oral hygiene and did not find the esthetic disturbance severe. She adapted to the orthodontic appliance within a few days. During treatment the screw head was coated with composite to prevent pressure sores.

After a 10-week period of active eruption, a new, longer coil spring was inserted to reactivate the system. The 4-month active treatment period was followed by a 3-month retention phase (Figure 13-8, F and G).

After debonding and removal of the microscrew without local anesthesia, the prosthetic procedure was started. At its removal the microscrew was still firmly anchored in the alveolar bone. The gingival margin of the two central incisors had an almost uniform level; slight gingival recession had developed only at tooth #13, to be covered partly by a connective tissue graft before prosthetic treatment (Figure 13-8, H).

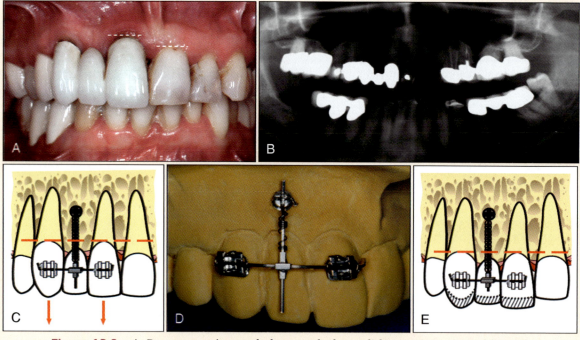

Figure 13-8 **A,** Pretreatment intraoral photograph shows disharmonious gingival line of the upper central incisors, 3 to 4 mm of gingival recession at abutment teeth #11 and #13, and exposed crown margins with inflammation of the marginal gingiva. **B,** Pretreatment panoramic radiograph reveals inadequate prosthetic reconstruction in the upper jaw. **C,** Design of the limited extrusion appliance: two brackets, sectional arches, and superelastic open coil. **D,** Rectangular stainless steel archwire is attached with brackets to the bridge and runs via a cross-tube along an additional vertical guiding archwire. The extrusive force is transmitted by an inserted superelastic coil. **E,** During extrusion the incisal edges of the crowns are continuously shortened, and the palatal surfaces of the bridge are grinded to gain space for eruption.

CASE REPORT 13-1—cont'd

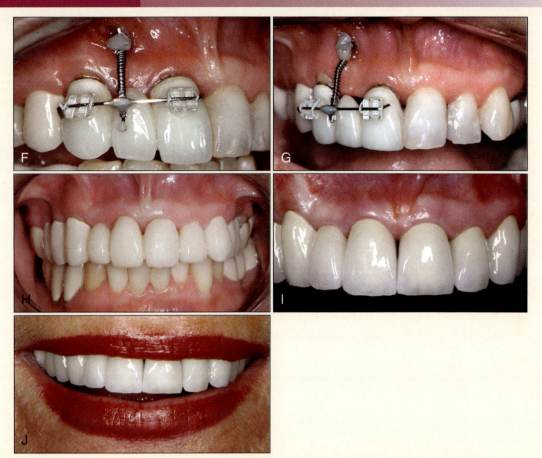

Figure 13-8, cont'd F, Inflammation-free gingiva 6 weeks after treatment. Bridge moves along the vertical guide archwire. G, Clinical finding on completion of 4-month extrusion period. Gingival margin of the first incisors have a uniform level, but not on the canine. H, After removal of appliance and temporary bridge on teeth #15 to #25. Recession at tooth #13 was partly covered by a connective tissue graft. I, Teeth on completion of prosthetic treatment. J, Patient's smile at the end of treatment.

On completion of prosthetic rehabilitation, the patient's improved smile was attractive and convincing (Figure 13-8, I and J).

Targeted eruption or intrusion of single teeth represents an excellent opportunity to harmonize the gingival margin of the incisors before the prosthetic procedure. In this case the application of a single microscrew permitted the extrusion of a three-unit fixed bridge without involving other teeth.

CONCLUSION

Microscrews are being increasingly used for anchorage in modern orthodontic settings. They represent a beneficial, non–compliance-bases alternative to conventional anchorage techniques. The slenderness and uncomplicated insertion of microscrews permit biomechanically creative solutions. Complex anchorage strategies are superfluous; the interception of reactive forces and moments becomes more manageable; and the size of the appliance can be minimized. Thus, microscrews open up new anchorage perspectives.

Although microscrews have many advantages, conventional implants are superior with respect to stability and success rate. Success depends on many factors, from loading protocols to screw characteristics and insertion sites. Future research should involve randomized clinical trials to assess individual patient risks (anatomical conditions, oral hygiene, smoker/nonsmoker, habits) and other risk factors for failure.

REFERENCES

1. Fritz U, Diedrich P, Kinzinger G, Al-Said M: The anchorage quality of mini-implants towards translatory and extrusive forces, *J Orofac Orthop* 64:293-304, 2003.
2. Wehrbein H, Yildirim M, Diedrich P: Osteodynamics around orthodontically loaded short maxillary implants, *J Orofac Orthop* 60:409-415, 1999.
3. Prabhu J, Cously RRJ: Current products and practice: bone anchorage devices in orthodontics, *J Orthod* 33:288-207, 2006.
4. Kim TW, Lee SJ: Correction of deep overbite and gummy smile by using a mini-implant with a segmented wire in a growing Class II Division 2 patient, *Am J Orthod Dentofacial Orthop* 130:676-685, 2006.
5. Kinzinger GSM, Diedrich PR, Bowman SJ: Upper molar distalisation with a miniscrew-supported Distal Jet, *J Clin Orthod*, 2006, pp 672-678.
6. Roth A, Yildirim M, Diedrich P: Forced eruption with microscrew anchorage for preprosthetic leveling of the gingival margin: case report, *J Orofac Orthop* 65:513-519, 2004.
7. Fritz U, Ehmer A, Diedrich P: Clinical suitability of titanium microscrews for orthodontic anchorage: preliminary experiences, *J Orofac Orthop* 65:410-418, 2004.
8. Berens A, Wiechmann D, Dempf R: Mini- and micro-screws for temporary skeletal anchorage in orthodontic therapy, *J Orofac Orthop* 67:450-458, 2006.
9. Miyawaki S, Koyama I, Inoue M, et al: Factors associated with the stability of titanium screws placed in the posterior region for orthodontic anchorage, *Am J Orthod Dentofacial Orthop* 124:373-378, 2003.
10. Park HS, Jeong SW, Kwon OW: Factors affecting the clinical success of screw implants used as orthodontic anchorage, *Am J Orthod Dentofacial Orthop* 130:18-25, 2006.
11. Liou EJ, Pai BC, Lin JC: Do miniscrews remain stationary under orthodontic forces? *Am J Orthod Dentofacial Orthop* 126:42-47, 2004.

CHAPTER 14

Treatment Planning with Endosseous Implants for Orthodontic Anchorage and Prosthodontic Restoration

Flavio Andres Uribe and Ravindra Nanda

The origins of temporary anchorage devices (TADs) for orthodontic tooth movement can be traced back to prosthetic alveolar ridge devices used for tooth replacement. In 1969, Linkow[1] used a mandibular endosseous blade implant in a Class II patient to retract the upper incisors. This implant was made of cobalt-chromium alloy (Vitallium) and was placed to restore mandibular missing teeth. In the 1960s, Brånemark pioneered the development of osseointegrated titanium endosseous implants for restoration of edentulous sites, which have shown remarkable long-term success rates.[2] In the 1980s, Roberts explored the possibility of loading these endosseous titanium implants for orthodontic tooth movement in animal models.[3] Later he applied the same methodology clinically, describing the use of skeletal anchorage with osseointegrated titanium implants in orthodontics in a series of case reports.[4]

Skeletal anchorage for orthodontic tooth movements has relied primarily on the biocompatibility and osseointegration attributes of titanium. Titanium devices attached to the jaws for absolute anchorage in orthodontics can be divided into two categories: temporary and permanent. Previous chapters describe the different types of TADs. If numerous edentulous spaces are available in the arch, however, conventional prosthetic dental implants should be considered. Although in some cases the permanent type of absolute anchorage lacks the mechanical efficiency and versatility of its temporary counterpart, it should remain a viable option. Placement of conventional implants offers a twofold benefit, as an adjunct for orthodontic anchorage and thereafter as a means of adequately restoring the necessary missing teeth.[5]

TREATMENT OPTIONS FOR EDENTULOUS PATIENTS

Patients missing numerous teeth usually present clinically with collapsed buccal occlusions that includes supraerupted molars and premolars. The malocclusion frequently extends to the anterior teeth because of loss of posterior support. Supraerupted incisors, impinging deep bites, extensive occlusal wear, flared upper incisors, and anterior spacing are common findings in these patients. Often, anterior spacing is the primary reason patients seek treatment (Figure 14-1). These patients need a comprehensive treatment plan, including replacing the missing teeth with prosthetic restorations. Before the permanent restorations can be placed, however, proper interdental spacing and inclination of the remnant teeth, as well as an adequate occlusal plane, need to be reestablished to obtain a predictable, long-lasting prosthetic rehabilitation.

Treatment alternatives for a patient with partial edentulism vary according to the location and extent of the edentulous sites. The prosthetic alternatives may consist of either fixed or removable partial dentures. Patients with a single edentulous space or one or two missing teeth may be treated with space closure using TADs, as described in other chapters.

COST AND IMPROVED OCCLUSION
Patients who require orthodontic treatment in addition to prosthetic restorations face certain financial burdens. Primarily motivated by a discontent regarding their anterior dental esthetics, patients seek orthodontic or prosthetic treatment to improve their smile. Often these same patients are apathetic or oblivious to the posterior segment, which is only a secondary concern.

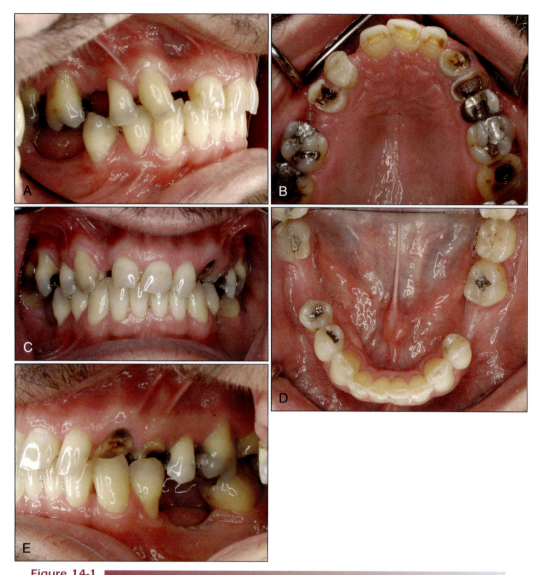

Figure 14-1

A to E, Intraoral photographs of 48-year-old man with a mutilated dentition referred from the prosthodontic division for preprosthetic orthodontic treatment. Patient was primarily concerned with the esthetics of the anterior region. Intraoral examination revealed multiple missing teeth, especially in the posterior segments; excessive wear of the anterior and posterior teeth; supraerupted molars; and multiple occlusal planes and tooth inclinations.

Nevertheless, it is imperative to implement orthodontic treatment for better tooth inclination and a functional occlusal plane. If molars are missing, TADs are a good option. As the treatment progresses, both esthetics and function are improved; the posterior teeth may be intruded and the spaces distributed to receive a less costly prosthetic solution, such as a removable partial denture. Ultimately, the patient will obtain the desired esthetics economically, but also an improved occlusion. The resulting occlusion should also be an excellent foundation for possible future placement of a fixed restoration, depending on the financial situation and motivation of the patient.

FIXED BRIDGES VERSUS IMPLANTS

Fixed bridges have been traditionally considered a better option to restore edentulous spaces than their removable counterparts.[6] This assertion is particularly applicable in patients with heavily restored teeth adjacent to the edentulous area. Orthodontics can also be used preprosthetically in these patients to reduce edentulous spaces through partial space closure and subsequent fabrication of a fixed bridge. TADs can also be used as adjuncts during the preprosthetic orthodontic treatment to achieve significant intrusion and anterior-posterior movement of the adjacent teeth to the edentulous site. However, patients with edentulous sites distal to the

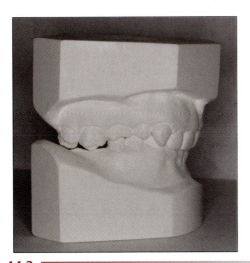

Figure 14-2
Diagnostic cast of patient missing the entire right mandibular buccal segment distal to the second premolar. The maxillary first and second molars have supraerupted to the edentulous area. Patient needs a conventional implant or a removable partial denture to restore occlusal function. Interocclusal space is needed for either option.

canine or premolars in any of the posterior segments, as well as patients dissatisfied with ridge-supported removable partial denture wear, will require conventional implants to restore adequate occlusion. Moreover, if teeth are present opposing the edentulous segment, the preferable means of establishing adequate occlusion will be achieved using conventional implants (Figure 14-2).

Current treatment planning in prosthetics has increasingly incorporated endosseous dental implants into removable as well as fixed devices. Integrating implants into the treatment plan is an excellent choice because data indicate their long-term survivability. Implants also provide a fixed restorative option without affecting the adjacent teeth.[7] For patients who need extensive preprosthetic work, the absolute anchorage provided by endosseous implants increases the range of orthodontic tooth movements. Significant space closure and molar intrusion can be attained with the direct or indirect anchorage provided by the implants.

Protraction and intrusion of molars are among the most difficult tooth movements in orthodontics.[8] The partially edentulous patient often requires both these orthodontic movements, which become exponentially more difficult with less teeth available for anchorage. Fortunately, absolute anchorage with TADs and conventional dental implants have made these orthodontic tooth movements predictably achievable.[9]

TEMPORARY ANCHORAGE VERSUS IMPLANTS

The clear challenge is the decision to use TADs or conventional dental implants, particularly for patients with one or more edentulous areas of approximately 10 to 15 mm. These patients usually are missing one molar (usually the first) along with one or two premolars. Often the second molars are present, and thus teeth delimit the edentulous site at both ends. One option is to use TADs to close the edentulous space and attain an acceptable occlusion. The other option is to place a conventional dental implant, with the advantage of absolute anchorage to correct the inclination of the adjacent teeth and distribute the edentulous spaces properly to restore permanently the dental implants. The latter option would entail partially closing, maintaining, or opening the edentulous space. This space management decision is made during the planning stage by an interdisciplinary team of clinicians.

The prosthodontist and the orthodontist should determine the ideal distribution of the edentulous spaces. They will decide which spaces will be closed (and to what extent) and which spaces will be maintained or opened. However, an important factor is cost efficiency. Placing conventional implants is more costly than closing an edentulous site using TADs, but efficiency of treatment clearly favors conventional implants; closing a molar space by translatory movement requires more than 18 months.[10] Ultimately, the patient must choose between implants to restore the edentulous sites, with more cost for the prosthesis, or fewer (or no) implants, with more time complying with orthodontic appliances.

A treatment plan with the least amount of absolute anchorage devices, including dental implants, delivered within a reasonable time would seem the most cost-effective alternative in these patients. This can be accomplished with conventional implants placed at the beginning (before orthodontic appliances) or in the middle of treatment. Thus, the implants usefulness is twofold: delivering the difficult, anchorage-dependent, orthodontic movements and thereafter acting as a prosthetic device to accomplish occlusal function.

INTERDISCIPLINARY TEAM

Treatment planning with conventional dental implants for orthodontic anchorage involves several important considerations. First, the orthodontist requires a multidisciplinary team in place with good communication. Each specialist has a specific role and timed intervention. The orthodontist spends the most time with the patient[11] and therefore may lead the team. Knowing the limitations of orthodontic movement, the orthodontist can maintain a realistic, comprehensive plan.[12]

Often the prosthodontist is involved in the treatment-planning phase and later, at the end of orthodontic treatment. Initially providing input on the final tooth positions for an optimal prosthodontic outcome, the prosthodontist later helps determine the amount of compensation in the crown inclinations that can be achieved once the teeth are prepared for the final restorations. These inclination modifications allow slight variation in some of the final tooth positions; orthodontic tooth movement is not as precisely predictive as a crown preparation or restoration.

The periodontist/oral surgeon then evaluates the implant site(s) already determined by the prosthodontic/orthodontic specialist, considering the following factors:
- Conformity of the bone at specific sites.
- Density of bone at feasible locations.
- Navigating any nerves that might interfere with implant placement.
- Locating and mapping the blood vessels.
- Anticipating any interference from anatomical structures.

Through a clinical and radiographic inspection, the periodontist/oral surgeon will determine if any additional procedures, such as bone grafting, are needed before the implant placement is finalized.

TREATMENT-PLANNING CONSIDERATIONS

An important consideration with conventional implants versus TADs is evident in the treatment-planning process; each implant requires a different margin of placement error. This factor has major implications in the planning. TADs are often shorter than conventional implants and are removed once their usefulness is depleted. However, it is important not to confuse impermanence with inaccuracy. The vital concern with TADs, especially mini-implants and miniscrews, is not to impinge on any major anatomical structure, such as the maxillary sinus, the mandibular nerve, the nasal floor, or a dental root.

On the other hand, permanent placement of conventional implants requires evaluation of not only anatomical structures but also the angulation and depth of placement. There is approximately a 1-mm range of error in the mesiodistal, buccolingual, and occlusogingival direction. Any deviation above this range results in compromised restorative work. For this reason, placement of dental implants in the upper anterior esthetic zone for orthodontic anchorage is not recommended. If the patient has a high smile line, even greater caution must be taken.

However, Figure 14-3 provides an exception to this planning advice. This patient was missing the entire maxillary anterior segment and wanted to stop wearing her removable partial denture. To reduce the anterior spacing and upper intercanine width, the patient had two block grafts and two implants placed in the maxillary central incisor region, which were later used for anchorage to move the adjacent teeth. Fortunately, this patient did not display the cervical portions of her maxillary incisors on smiling.

Patients with complete dentition are subject to broadly the same analytical outcome criteria as partially edentulous patients. The same esthetic and functional occlusal objectives are set.[13] The only difference is that by incorporating conventional implants in the edentulous spaces, it is possible to accomplish movements otherwise impossible with traditional orthodontic mechanotherapy. Briefly, the skeletofacial objectives are first defined, then the final incisor position in three dimensions, followed by the molar objectives in the three dimensions.

VISUALIZED TREATMENT OBJECTIVE AND DIAGNOSTIC WAX-UP

Formulating a sound, understandable treatment plan requires a three-dimensionally visualized treatment objective. This can be accomplished in a diagnostic wax-up mounted on an articulator (Figure 14-4, *A-E*). This wax-up is almost indispensable in complex multidisciplinary cases.[11,14] At the University of Connecticut, the *occlusogram* is considered an essential component in visualizing treatment objectives in the transverse and anterior-posterior (A-P) planes of space (Figure 14-4, *F-H*).[15] A *visualized treatment objective* (VTO) using the lateral cephalometric radiograph (cephalograph) depicts the objectives in the vertical and A-P planes (Figure 14-5). The information achieved from the occlusogram and VTO is then transferred to the diagnostic wax-up (Figure 14-6, *A-E*).

One caveat should be noted regarding the diagnostic wax-up. Although a useful tool in the treatment-planning process, the initial dental relationship is lost once the wax-up is completed. To avoid this complication and maintain the initial reference, it is important to obtain a copy of the original models. The most efficient method is to score the lingual or palatal side and the buccal or labial side of the original model.[12] The scored model is then replicated. The copy will become the *working model* on which the final wax-up will be established. The indentations serve as reference areas for the diagnostic model in relation to the working model (see Figure 14-4, *A* and *B*).

Silicon impression material is used to imprint the buccal surfaces of all the teeth and the indentations in the lingual or palatal side of the model. This silicon impression of the initial model is trimmed to remove the incisal edge of the teeth and then placed on the working model to view the magnitude and direction of the planned tooth movements (Figure 14-6, *F* and *G*). The wax-up is then compared to the occlusogram to ensure that the tooth movements are accurate (Figure 14-6, *H-M*). Additionally, the working model depicts the specific site where the conventional implant will be placed at the beginning of orthodontic treatment, later to be restored after appliances are removed (see Figure 14-6, *A* and *B*). This information is then transferred to the diagnostic model using the silicon impression mate-

14 Treatment Planning with Endosseous Implants for Orthodontic Anchorage

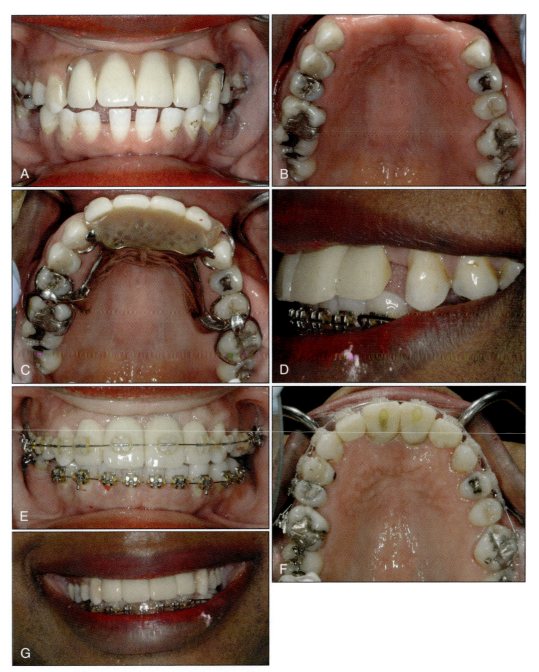

Figure 14-3
A, This 43-year-old woman presented to the prosthodontic division seeking to replace her removable partial denture with a fixed prosthesis. **B,** Patient had a large edentulous space from canine to canine, with reduced alveolar ridge height and width. Intercanine width needed to be reduced for adequate size of maxillary incisors. **C,** Two implants were placed on the sites of the central incisors after block-graft ridge augmentation. Two lateral incisors were cantilevered from the central incisors. **D to F,** The implants were used as anchorage to achieve proper mesiodistal width of the incisors by reducing the intercanine width and protracting the left maxillary buccal segment. **G,** Although placing implants in the anterior region for absolute anchorage is not recommended for esthetic reasons, this patient's smile did not display the cervical portion of the incisors.

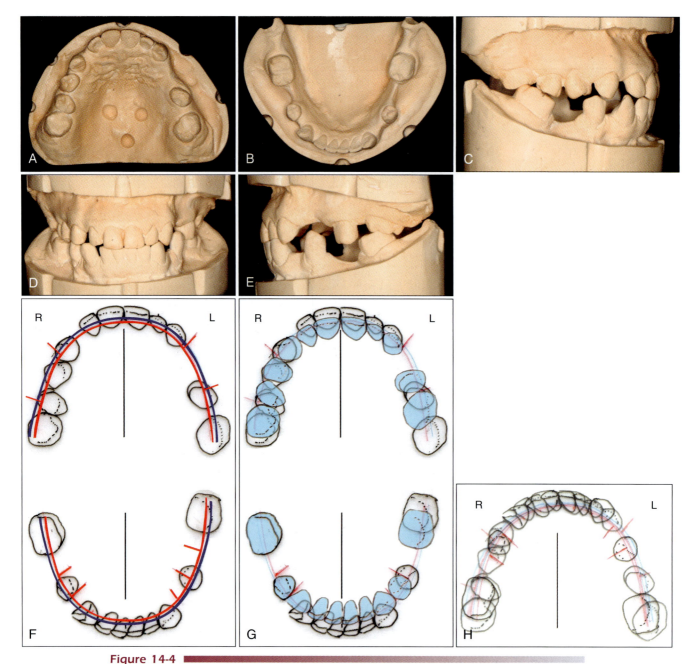

Figure 14-4
A to E, Diagnostic casts of a patient presenting for comprehensive orthodontic and prosthodontic care. F, After determining the treatment objectives, an occlusogram helps in visualizing the necessary tooth movements in the transverse and anterior-posterior dimension. The blue and red lines represent the final positions of the teeth. G, Occlusogram with the actual tooth movements. H, Occlusogram showing the final occlusal relationship.

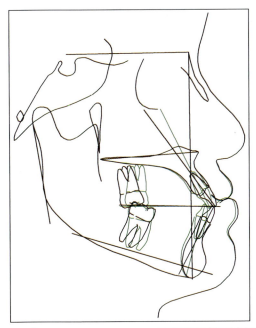

Figure 14-5

Visualized treatment objective (VTO) from a lateral view depicts the projected vertical and anterior-posterior (A-P) movements *(green line)*. These movements should match the magnitude of A-P movements in the occlusogram. The VTO and the occlusogram provide a 3D model of the treatment plan.

rial, to fabricate the surgical stent. The position of the conventional implant is now registered in the diagnostic model with an acrylic tooth in the proper buccolingual and mesiodistal position (Figure 14-6, *N-S*). Finally, the occlusogram is used to corroborate the proper position of the conventional implant. This is an important step because this model's essential purpose is to fabricate the surgical stent necessary for the proper placement of the endosseous implant.

INTEROCCLUSAL ANALYSIS FOR IMPLANT PLACEMENT

Implant sites are usually analyzed mesiodistally and buccolingually, whereas the occlusogingival dimension is often ignored or not evaluated as thoroughly. The relationship of the ridge to the occlusal plane must be carefully evaluated in the edentulous areas. The relationship of the edentulous area to the opposing teeth should also be appraised and the occlusal plane changes anticipated. Furthermore, if a tooth will be extracted for periodontal reasons or is deemed unrestorable, a change in the distance of the ridge to the occlusal plane should be anticipated, resulting in more interocclusal space. All these factors need to be considered in the diagnostic phase because the implants will be placed before initiat-

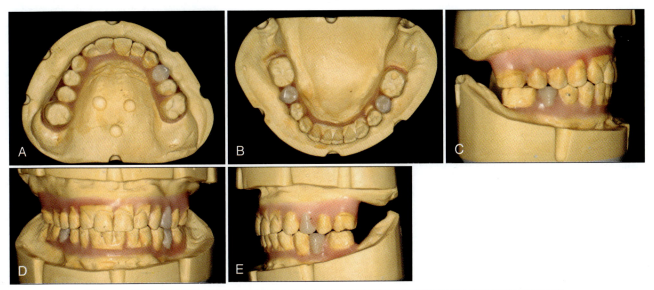

Figure 14-6

A to **E**, Diagnostic wax-up based on the occlusogram and visualized treatment objective (VTO). Note that the wax-up does not portray the magnitude or direction of the necessary tooth movements.

Continued

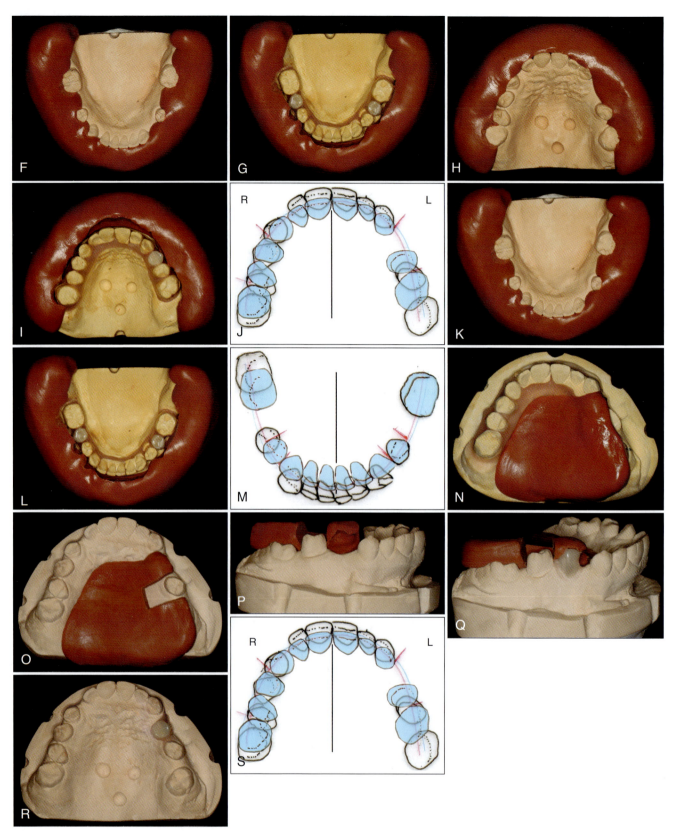

Figure 14-6, cont'd **F** and **G,** To evaluate magnitude and direction of tooth movements, the diagnostic model is duplicated with indentations scored in the model. The wax-up is finished in the working model, and silicon material is used to relate the initial (diagnostic model in red stone) to the final position of the teeth (working model in yellow stone). **H** to **M,** Magnitude and direction of tooth movements are compared to the occlusogram, ensuring that wax-up reflects planned final position of the teeth. **N** to **S,** Silicon material is used to transfer the final position of the implant from the working model (**N**) to the diagnostic model (**O-R**). If no occlusogingival changes are planned with treatment, the diagnostic model with the acrylic tooth can be replicated for fabrication of the surgical stent.

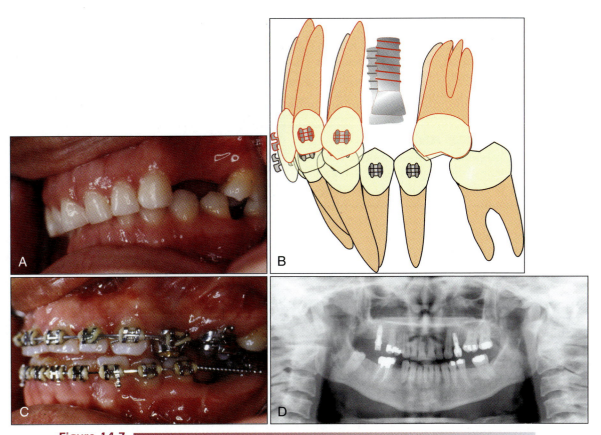

Figure 14-7
A, Intraoral photograph showing need for a significant change in the occlusal plane. **B,** Final occlusal plane inclination dictates the direction of implant placement before the initiation of orthodontic treatment. **C,** Significant maxillary incisor intrusion and occlusal plane rotation. **D,** Panoramic radiograph shows how the implant inclination of the left maxillary first premolar did not account for the occlusal plane change when placed at the beginning of orthodontic treatment.

ing the orthodontic movements in the majority of these patients.

As mentioned, interocclusal clearance is a critical factor at the site of placement. In most patients the occlusogingival position will be calculated in reference to the marginal ridges of the adjacent teeth. However, any change in occlusal plane inclination to be obtained with orthodontic treatment must be considered, because the marginal ridge position of the teeth adjacent to the implant will change vertically. Figure 14-7 shows a buccal segment that was differentially intruded. Absolute anchorage was used to rotate the occlual plane counterclockwise. The endosseous implant significantly intruded the teeth anteriorly and slightly intruded the mesial cusp of the first molar. Although the implant was adequately planned in mesiodistal and buccolingual dimensions, unfortunately the change in occlusal plane inclination was not considered before implant placement. A posttreatment panoramic radiograph shows how the longitudinal axis of the implant, parallel to the adjacent teeth at the beginning of treatment, was substantially off at the end of treatment (see Figure 14-7, *D*).

Esthetics and retention of the final restoration are also important factors to consider in relation to occlusogingival analysis in the treatment-planning phase. Not accounting for the final position of the occlusal plane with intrusion may result in a dental implant short in occlusogingival height and an unesthetic display of the implant fixture or abutment. Improper inclination also may lead to an abutment that needs to be placed at an angle to the longitudinal axis of the fixture. This remedial adjustment would be required to ensure a final restoration that coincides with the occlusal plane of the adjacent teeth.

The previous example highlights the importance of incorporating a VTO into the treatment plan; predicting the amount of occlusal change caused by orthodontic treatment is indispensable. Indeed, to plan properly for the correct occlusogingival position and mesiodistal longitudinal axis inclination of the implant, a VTO is critical. As described, the VTO is used to evaluate the occlusal change that will result from orthodontic treatment. The final vertical position of the incisors and buccal segments are clearly delineated, and this information is then transferred to the wax-up. The same procedure using the silicon impression material is used to transfer the information from the diagnostic model. Thus, the direction and magnitude of tooth movements in the vertical dimension from their initial position are evaluated on the final wax-up, and a thorough treatment plan is established.

ALVEOLAR BONE RIDGE ANALYSIS

After evaluating the mesiodistal, buccolingual, and occlusogingival dimensions, the surgical stent is ready to be fabricated. This is done by duplicating the diagnostic model containing the acrylic crowns representing the final position of the implants after orthodontic treatment. A vacuum-formed, clear sheet of the model is used to fabricate the surgical stent. The surgical stent is then tried on the patient's mouth, and the positions of the implant crowns are analyzed with respect to the edentulous ridge.

To evaluate the bone height at the implant site and its relationship to the final tooth restoration, a panoramic radiograph is taken, with a surgical stent duplicate representing the final implant crown positions. Radiopaque "bullets" (or metal wires or gutta-percha points) incorporated into this surgical stent duplicate indicate the proper location and longitudinal axis of the of the implant crowns[12] (Figure 14-8). Serious angulation problems in the position of the final implant can result if this step is not carefully followed (Figure 14-9).

Panoramic radiographs provide a two-dimensional relationship, with information on the height of the bone and surrounding structures, and help to determine the appropriate implant length. To achieve a three-dimensional (3D) analysis of the site, the ridge width needs to be evaluated. This is done most often through clinical inspection by sounding the ridge with a periodontal probe before surgery. In other cases the anatomy of the ridge is inspected at surgery after flap reflection. With the advent of cone-beam computed tomography (CBCT), the 3D analysis of the site can be obtained with the surgical stent in place. The quality and quantity of bone in the implant site and the relationship to the surrounding anatomical structures (e.g., maxillary sinus, mandibular canal, incisive canal, adjacent teeth) can be analyzed.[16,17] Figure 14-10 shows a patient who was to receive two implants on the mandibular left molar region. CBCT was used to visualize and evaluate the implant sites and ensure an ideal placement.

Evaluation of the bone at the determined implant site might reveal inadequacies in width, height, or both. To obtain the appropriate bone dimensions, a decision must be made and different options weighed. Bone can be generated by orthodontic movement of the adjacent teeth through the edentulous space, or bone grafts can be placed in the deficient area. Both approaches will

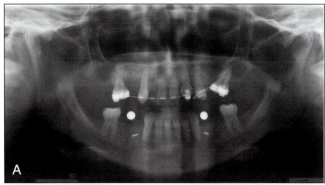
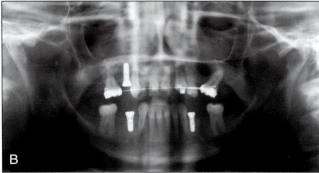

Figure 14-8
A, Panoramic radiograph showing radiopaque "bullets" used to evaluate the relationship of bone characteristics and surrounding anatomical structures to the selected site for implant placement. **B**, Panoramic radiograph reflecting the final position of implants.

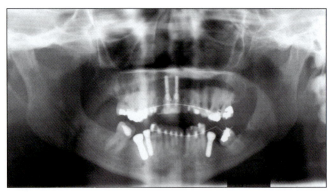

Figure 14-9
Panoramic radiograph showing implants with significant angulation problems. A restorative dentist will need to perform extensive compensation in the abutments and in the crown fabrication. Implant fixture replacement should be considered.

delay the possibility of using the planned implant for absolute anchorage. If the former approach is chosen and absolute anchorage is required before the implants are placed, TADs are ideal. Alternatively, the remnant teeth can be used as anchorage to generate bone at the

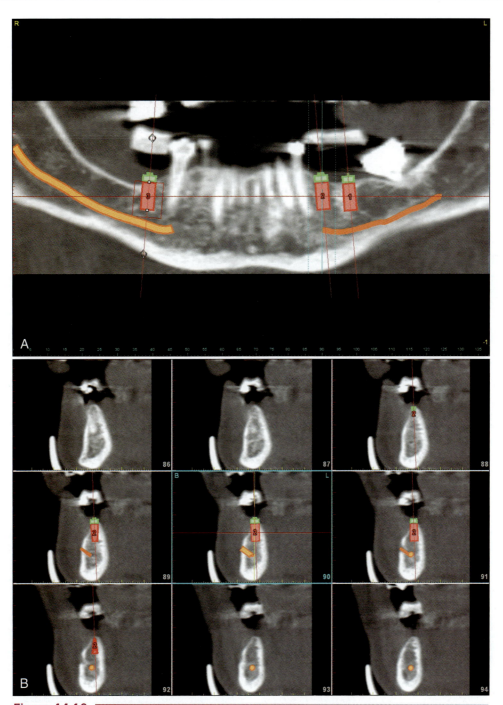

Figure 14-10

A and B, Cone-beam computed tomography (CBCT) used to evaluate bone characteristics of implant sites. This technology allows in-depth analysis of the alveolar ridge in quantity (height and width) as well as quality (density) of the bone in the selected implant site.

site. Once the implant is placed and osseointegration occurs, the side effects are controlled (Figure 14-11).

Grafting the area is another approach to a dimensionally deficient edentulous area. If the grafting area is small and the width deficient, the implant can be placed and particulate autogenous bone added as necessary to cover the implant. When the defect is more extensive, an autogenous block graft may be preferred. The graft usually provides both adequate height and adequate width (Figure 14-12). As a general rule, this graft is usually harvested from the symphysis, ramus buccal shelf, or the hip.[18]

In general, grafting procedures are more successful in gaining and maintaining width than height.[19] If an implant is not placed in the grafted area within a short period, the grafted bone may loose volume in both

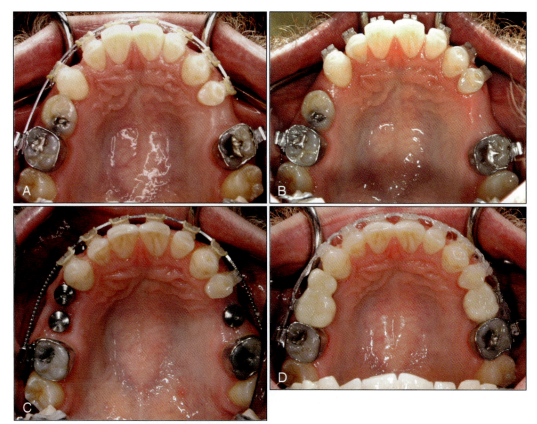

Figure 14-11

A to D, Intraoral photographs showing alveolar ridge development in the maxillary premolar region through reciprocal anchorage. Absolute anchorage was used after the ridge was developed to control the excessive distal movement of the left maxillary molar (side effect).

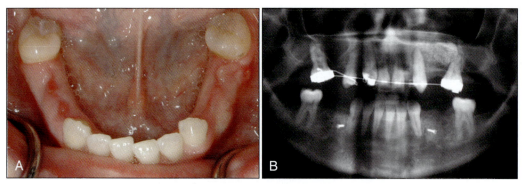

Figure 14-12

A, Lower arch with adequate bone height and width achieved after onlay grafts of autogenous bone were placed bilaterally in the premolar region. B, Panoramic radiograph shows the newly placed bone grafts with screws securing it in place.

height and width.[20] Block grafts often need a host bed prepared to receive the graft so that good coupling is achieved between the autogenous graft and the native bone. In some cases, when teeth are tipped into the implant site, orthodontic treatment must be started to achieve an adequate space for the graft. Figure 14-13 shows a lower-right molar tipped mesially and the space partially closed. The molar had to be uprighted before the area could be grafted and an implant placed. By grafting after the orthodontic movement, the quality and quantity of the bone site can be revaluated before implant placement in determining the type and extent of the bone graft needed.

Maxillary bone height deficiency in the buccal segments is usually related to a low maxillary sinus floor. Because esthetics may not be an issue in this area, two

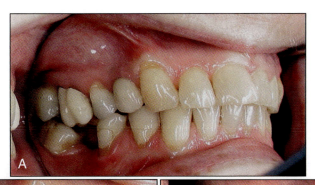
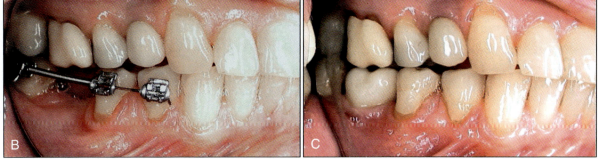

Figure 14-13
A, This patient was to receive a dental implant in the mandibular right first molar region. B, Inadequate ridge height and width precluded implant placement. Second molar needed to be uprighted to achieve adequate space for grafting and subsequent implant placement (C).

options are available when grafting is considered. First, a sinus lift can increase the bone height and house an implant. Sinus floor elevation by osteotome usually provides about a 3-mm gain in bone height.[21] The second option is a block graft to normalize the alveolar height, possibly resulting in a more esthetic restoration.

IMPLANT LOADING

One of the major drawbacks of using conventional implants as anchorage compared with TADs is the necessary delay in loading to achieve osseointegration. Waiting time before implant loading for a partially edentulous jaw is approximately 3 months, although new implant-surface characteristics may reduce this to 6 weeks.[22] Some of the current technological developments on the surface of the implants may further reduce this healing period. Straumann* has recently developed a new surface called "bioactive SLA" that may reduce the waiting period for loading to about 3 to 4 weeks. However, the implant loading time is usually extended 9 to 12 weeks if a graft was previously placed.[23]

Once the implant has osseointegrated, two methods are available to load it for orthodontic anchorage. The first is to place the abutment that matches the fixture with a temporary crown made of acrylic and cemented on top of the abutment. To fabricate this temporary tooth, the stent for the implant placement surgery is used as a template. Orthodontic appliances are then attached to the osseointegrated implants to provide skeletal anchorage. The method of attachment to the temporary tooth can be either bonding or banding. One notable advantage to banding is that it offers the possibility of placing an attachment on the lingual surface. This lingual attachment may be used to provide anchorage across the arch for movements such as molar protraction or root correction (Figure 14-14).

Fracture or breakage is always a risk when cementing to a temporary tooth. The weak link is found in two components of the system: the adhesion of the acrylic to the abutment and the band or bracket to the acrylic. A stronger system involves casting a temporary abutment on which a band can be cemented or a bracket can be bonded (Figure 14-15). This alternative method is not susceptible to the fragility of the crown-abutment interface and thus is less inclined to break. However, it is more unsightly, and the abutment needs to be untorqued and replaced when the restoration is cemented permanently at the end of treatment.

BIOMECHANICS WITH ENDOSSEOUS IMPLANTS

Conventional implants are placed in the alveolar ridge, so the mechanics depend mainly on direct anchorage. Molar protraction and anterior segment retraction are viable movements that can be achieved and incorporated to any orthodontic technique. The important con-

---
*Straumann USA LLC, 60 Minuteman Road, Andover, MA 01810.

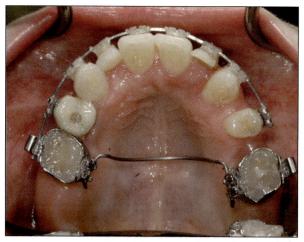

Figure 14-14

Transpalatal arch (TPA) can be used from an implant to correct excessive tooth inclinations in the contralateral side of the arch. In this patient the implant was used as indirect anchorage by splinting it to the maxillary right first molar and activating it to achieve mesial root correction of the contralateral first molar.

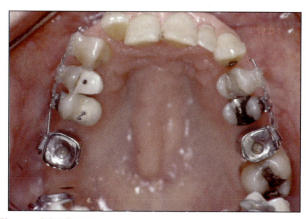

Figure 14-15

Custom-made bands cemented to fit the custom abutments placed on the maxillary first molars.

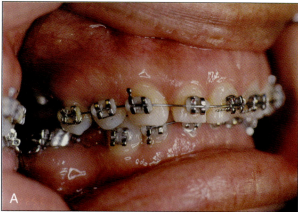

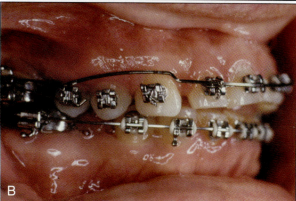

Figure 14-16

A and B, Two cantilever systems were extended from the maxillary right molar (endosseous implant) to intrude the maxillary incisors as well as the second premolar.

sideration when retracting anterior teeth with implant anchorage is that because the line of force is primarily applied buccal to the center of resistance of the implant, the moment of the force will tend to unscrew the abutment. This usually is not a problem with the abutments that are torqued permanently. In contrast, screw-retained abutments are more prone to loosen with these types of movements. Therefore, the clinician should check for abutment loosening when delivering these forces on all implants, but more critically on screw-retained abutments.

As mentioned, protraction and retraction are directional forces easily delivered by conventional implants. Vertical forces, however, are not included. Although conventional implants provide adequate anchorage in the A-P and transverse dimension, vertically their efficiency is limited because of their location in the alveolar ridge. Thus, this type of implant is limited in its ability to obtain significant intrusion in the buccal segments. This shortcoming is more apparent if the force application is done through a step bend in the main archwire. However, the use of cantilever systems can circumvent this flaw. When using a cantilever system extended from a conventional implant, the clinician can obtain adequate incisor intrusion and intrusion of the buccal segments, more specifically the premolars (Figure 14-16).

As an example, Figure 14-17 shows the significant incisor intrusion obtained by extending an intrusion arch, from two conventional endosseous dental implants placed in the posterior maxillary region. The patient had a significant amount of intrusion, well above the 2-mm range considered the maximum magnitude of movement in the envelope of discrepancy.[24] This magnitude of incisor intrusion resulted in a very good esthetic result, resembling the outcome of a surgical Le Fort I maxillary impaction. In terms of the buccal segment, a similar cantilever system can be used for intrusion. Figure 14-18 shows a patient with an excessive deep bite and supraeruption of the premolars, with power arms extending from the acrylic. These arms offer the possibility of directing a line of force to achieve the intrusion in the buccal segments.

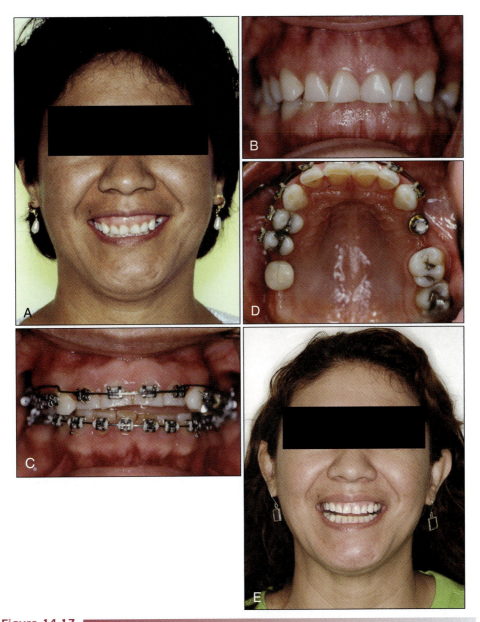

Figure 14-17

A and B, Pretreatment facial and intraoral photographs. C and D, Significant maxillary incisor intrusion was obtained by using a cantilever system extended from two endosseous implants in the right and left buccal segments. E, Smile image shows the significant improvement in gingival display with the extensive incisor intrusion.

As previously mentioned, if the lingual aspect of conventional implant is banded or bonded, other active applications used in direct anchorage may be available. In this configuration a force can be applied from the implant for protraction of a molar in the other side of the arch. A transpalatal arch (TPA) with a couple applied in the implant side will apply a mesial force in the lingual attachment of the contralateral tooth. Figure 14-19 shows an ankylosed primary tooth used as an-chorage to achieve the molar protraction of a contralateral mandibular molar, to close the edentulous area. The mesial force on the mandibular right second molar is delivered through a lingual arch from the ankylosed primary molar. The same force delivery system can be achieved to intrude a tooth or a group of teeth in the contralateral side of the arch. This can be accomplished by placing a third-order bend on the lingual attachment of the implant, generating an intrusive force on the tooth or teeth to which the palatal arch is attached (Figure 14-20). In both these active applications of palatal arches, the side that is generating either the protrusive or the intrusive force must not be tied in the bracket slot, to achieve a "pure" cantilever system.

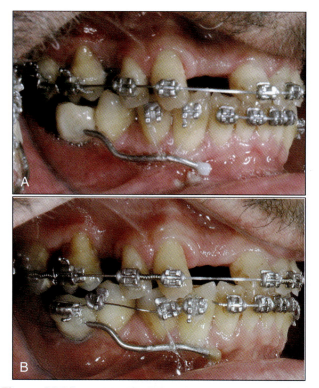

Figure 14-18
Power arm extended from an implant temporary acrylic crown in the mandibular molar can be used to intrude premolars.

Root correction can be accomplished in the same manner by applying a tip-back/tip-forward bend on the TPA. Figure 14-21 shows a molar that has significantly tipped mesially. A TPA was placed, anchoring the implant to the tipped molar. The TPA was made passive on the legs, and then both sides of the arch were activated to produce a mesial tip on the root. Because the movement is around the center of resistance, a small space may open mesial to the tipped molar. The same TPA with the activation previously described can be used to accomplish the molar protraction needed (Figure 14-22).

IMPLANTS TO ACHIEVE INTRAARCH AND INTEROCCLUSAL SPACE

Careful planning of multidisciplinary cases lays the foundation for intelligent use of a single implant to achieve multiple objectives. Figure 14-23 shows a patient who had an edentulous space on the mandibular right quadrant. The patient had a brachycephalic facial pattern with a significant deep bite. The maxillary second molar had supraerupted to the edentulous space. To restore the mandibular posterior-right edentulous area, the first choice might be to place a mini-implant to intrude the maxillary second molar, then two conventional implants to restore the edentulous area. In this patient, however, a conventional implant was used to intrude the maxillary molar, with opposing forces delivered by a magnet.

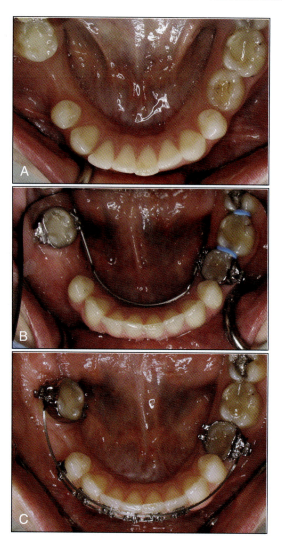

Figure 14-19
A, Ankylosed primary molar that biologically resembles an implant offers the possibility of absolute anchorage. **B** and **C,** Active lingual arch is used to deliver a protrusive force to a molar in the contralateral side to reduce the size of the edentulous space.

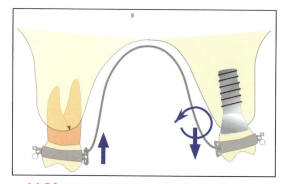

Figure 14-20
Intrusive force delivered from transpalatal arch (TPA) from an implant in the contralateral side in the molar area. TPA requires a point contact (not engaged in slot) on the molar tooth to achieve a pure intrusive force. The couple and the extrusive force generated on the molar implant will not be expressed.

14 Treatment Planning with Endosseous Implants for Orthodontic Anchorage

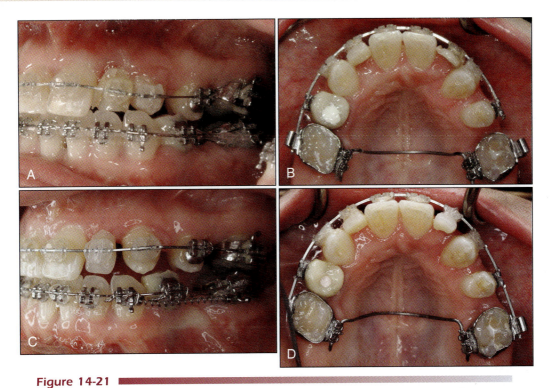

Figure 14-21

A to D, Implant in the maxillary right premolar used indirectly to deliver a mesial root correction moment on the tipped left maxillary molar.

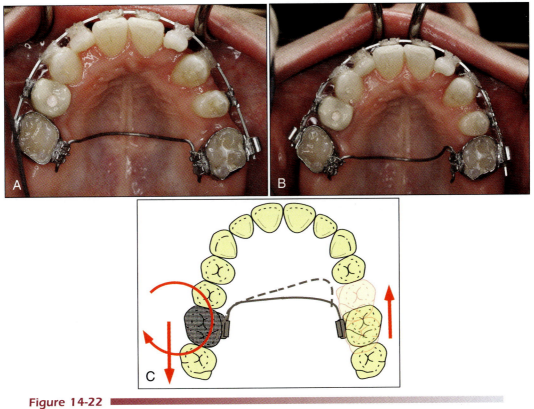

Figure 14-22

A to C, Transpalatal arch can also be used to provide a mesial force directly or indirectly from the implant to the contralateral molar.

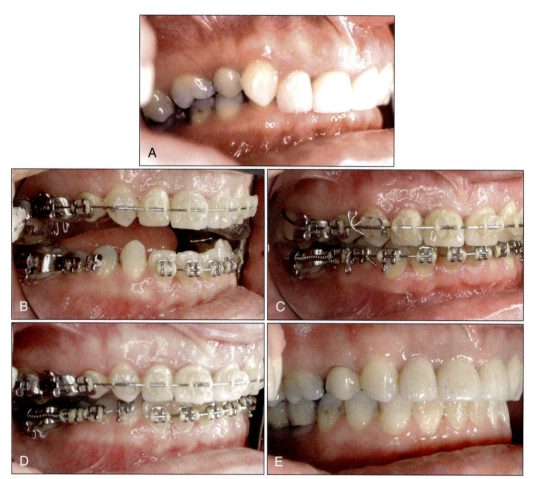

Figure 14-23
A, Patient missing intermaxillary space for the restoration of the edentulous area distal to the mandibular right second premolar. An implant was placed distal to the premolar and used as absolute anchorage to intrude the extruded maxillary second molar. **B,** Magnet was used to achieve this objective. **C** and **D,** This same implant was later used to protract the lower-right buccal segment and achieve a Class I canine occlusion. **E,** Second implant was placed mesial to the implant placed at the beginning of treatment to restore the right mandibular buccal segment.

After adequate intrusion of the maxillary molar was achieved, the implant was restored with a temporary tooth, with a bracket placed to protract the right mandibular buccal segment to achieve a Class I canine occlusion. Simultaneously, the alveolar ridge was developed for the placement of another implant.

CONCLUSION

Conventional implants offer similar possibilities for anchorage as temporary devices. However, conventional implants in this context have limited demand, required only by patients with edentulous spaces. Treatment planning for partially edentulous patients usually involves the integration of varied disciplines. Intricate mechanics often are required to achieve the desired movements, especially intrusion of the buccal segment or movement on the contralateral side of the arch. Planning must be precise, and consensus among team members is crucial.

Absolute anchorage is a fairly new concept in orthodontics, whether achieved by conventional implants or TADs, with great potential. Nevertheless, traditional dogma still prevails; the clinician's duty is to consider the most cost-effective treatment for the patient, keeping conventional implants as an option.

ACKNOWLEDGMENT

Special thanks to Dr. Ruben Mesia for his help in the laboratory and graphic work. We are also indebted to Dr. Zehra Pradhan and Dr. Brett Holliday for their contribution in the preparation of this manuscript.

REFERENCES

1. Linkow LI: The endosseous blade implant and its use in orthodontics, *Int J Orthod* 7(4):149-154, 1969.
2. Buser D et al: Long-term evaluation of non-submerged ITI implants. Part 1. 8-year life table analysis of a prospective multicenter study with 2359 implants, *Clin Oral Implants Res* 8(3):161-172, 1997.
3. Roberts WE et al: Osseous adaptation to continuous loading of rigid endosseous implants, *Am J Orthod* 86(2):95-111, 1984.
4. Roberts WE, Marshall KJ, Mozsary PG: Rigid endosseous implant utilized as anchorage to protract molars and close an atrophic extraction site, *Angle Orthod* 60(2):135-152, 1990.
5. Kokich VG: Managing complex orthodontic problems: the use of implants for anchorage, *Semin Orthod* 2(2):153-160, 1996.
6. Wostmann B et al: Indications for removable partial dentures: a literature review, *Int J Prosthodont* 18(2):139-145, 2005.
7. Adell R et al: Long-term follow-up study of osseointegrated implants in the treatment of totally edentulous jaws, *Int J Oral Maxillofac Implants* 5(4):347-359, 1990.
8. Sugawara J: A bioefficient skeletal anchorage system. In Nanda R, editor: *Biomechanics and esthetic strategies in clinical orthodontics*, St Louis, 2005, Mosby-Elsevier, pp 295-309.
9. Huang LH, Shotwell JL, Wang HL: Dental implants for orthodontic anchorage, *Am J Orthod Dentofacial Orthop* 127(6):713-722, 2005.
10. Roberts WE, Arbuckle GR, Analoui M: Rate of mesial translation of mandibular molars using implant-anchored mechanics, *Angle Orthod* 66(5):331-338, 1996.
11. Kokich VG, Spear FM: Guidelines for managing the orthodontic-restorative patient, *Semin Orthod* 3(1):3-20, 1997.
12. Smalley WM: Clinical and laboratory procedures for implant anchorage in partially edentulous dentitions. In Higuchi KW, editor: *Orthodontic applications of osseointegrated implants*, Chicago, 2000, Quintessence, pp 33-70.
13. Nanda R, Uribe F: Individualized orthodontic treatment planning. In Nanda R, editor: *Biomechanics and esthetic strategies in clinical orthodontics*, St Louis, 2005, Mosby-Elsevier, pp 74-93.
14. Willems G et al: Interdisciplinary treatment planning for orthodontic-prosthetic implant anchorage in a partially edentulous patient, *Clin Oral Implants Res* 10(4):331-337, 1999.
15. Faber RD: Occlusograms in orthodontic treatment planning, *J Clin Orthod* 26(7):396-401, 1992.
16. Sato S et al: Clinical application of a new cone-beam computerized tomography system to assess multiple two-dimensional images for the preoperative treatment planning of maxillary implants: case reports, *Quintessence Int* 35(7):525-528, 2004.
17. Almog DM et al: Cone beam computerized tomography–based dental imaging for implant planning and surgical guidance. Part 1. Single implant in the mandibular molar region, *J Oral Implantol* 32(2):77-81, 2006.
18. Petrungaro PS, Amar S: Localized ridge augmentation with allogenic block grafts prior to implant placement: case reports and histologic evaluations, *Implant Dent* 14(2):139-148, 2005.
19. Cordaro L, Amade DS, Cordaro M: Clinical results of alveolar ridge augmentation with mandibular block bone grafts in partially edentulous patients prior to implant placement, *Clin Oral Implants Res* 13(1):103-111, 2002.
20. Malchiodi L et al: Jaw reconstruction with grafted autologous bone: early insertion of osseointegrated implants and early prosthetic loading, *J Oral Maxillofac Surg* 64(8):1190-1198, 2006.
21. Li TF: Sinus floor elevation: a revised osteotome technique and its biological concept, *Compend Contin Educ Dent* 26(9):619-720 (quiz, 630, 669), 2005.
22. Cochran DL, Morton D, Weber HP: Consensus statements and recommended clinical procedures regarding loading protocols for endosseous dental implants, *Int J Oral Maxillofac Implants* 19(suppl):109-113, 2004.
23. Nelson K et al: Histomorphometric evaluation and clinical assessment of endosseous implants in iliac bone grafts with shortened healing periods, *Int J Oral Maxillofac Implants* 21(3):392-398, 2006.
24. Sarver DM, Proffit WR: Special considerations in diagnosis and treatment planning. In Graber TM, editor. *Orthodontics: current principles and techniques*, St Louis, 2005, Mosby-Elsevier, pp 3-70.

PART V

SKELETAL ANCHORAGE

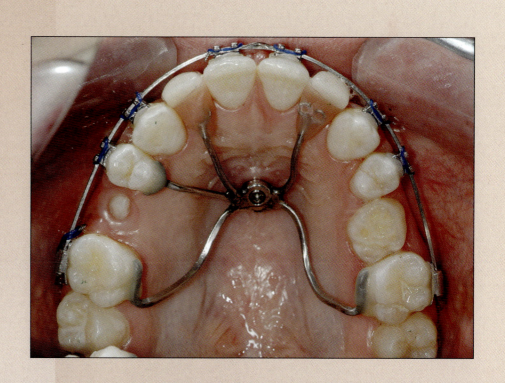

CHAPTER 15

Skeletal Anchorage System Using Orthodontic Miniplates

Junji Sugawara, Makoto Nishimura, Hiroshi Nagasaka, and Hiroshi Kawamura

INITIAL CASE FINDINGS

In 1992 we treated a 29-year-old woman who had a severe anterior crossbite.[1] The midline of her upper dentition had significantly shifted to the left because her upper-left canine and first premolar were missing (Figure 15-1, A-F). Cephalometric analysis revealed a near-average-size mandible, so jaw surgery was not an option. Correcting her anterior crossbite with traditional orthodontic mechanics seemed difficult, however, because she had no molars for anchorage in the lower dentition.

The patient's alveolar bone at the molar region was not thick enough to contain permanent implants at that time. Therefore an osteosynthesis miniplate and a miniscrew, components routinely used in patients requiring jaw surgery, were placed as temporary orthodontic anchorage devices in lieu of the missing teeth. A simple titanium miniscrew was inserted on one side and a titanium miniplate on the other (Figure 15-1, G). Interestingly, she had significant pain with the miniscrew, probably caused by the ligature wire through the mucosa, but no discomfort with the miniplate.

After debonding and prosthetic construction, the patient's profile was significantly improved, primarily due to backward and downward rotation of the mandible (Figure 15-1, H-M). Using an interdisciplinary approach, her occlusion improved dramatically. This motivated us to develop our skeletal anchorage system (SAS) because this first SAS-treated patient experienced no discomfort with the miniplate.

FEATURES OF ORTHODONTIC MINIPLATES AND SCREWS

Our SAS consists of orthodontic miniplates and monocortical fixation screws[2] (Figure 15-2, A). The plates and screws are made of commercially pure titanium that is biocompatible and suitable for osseointegration.

The miniplate has three parts: head, arm, and body (Figure 15-2, B). The *head* component has three continuous hooks for the application of various orthodontic force vectors. This component is exposed intraorally and positioned outside the dentition so as not to interfere with tooth movement. There are two different types of head components based on the direction of the hooks. The *arm* component is transmucosal and is available in three different lengths—short (6.5 mm), medium (9.5 mm), and long (12.5 mm)—to accommodate individual morphological differences. The *body* component is positioned subperiosteally and is available in three different configurations: T-plate, Y-plate, and I-plate (see Figure 15-2, B). The T-plates can be modified and used as "L-plates" by removing one of the circles at the body portion. The surface of the arm and the body in contact with the bone surface is sandblasted to facilitate osseointegration. Other parts are treated (anodic oxidation) to reduce infection at the transmucosal region.

The monocortical screws, 5.0 mm in total length and 2.0 mm in diameter, are inserted through the holes in the miniplate. The surgical site requires at least 2 mm of cortical bone thickness to fix the miniplate, and accordingly a 1.5-mm-diameter pilot hole is drilled before insertion of each screw. Each screw has an internal-tapered square head with self-tapping threaded body.

INDICATIONS FOR SKELTAL ANCHORAGE

Orthodontic treatment with SAS allows predictable three-dimensional tooth movement of the maxillary and mandibular molars without the need for patient compliance. Therefore, many indications exist for SAS treatment, as follows:

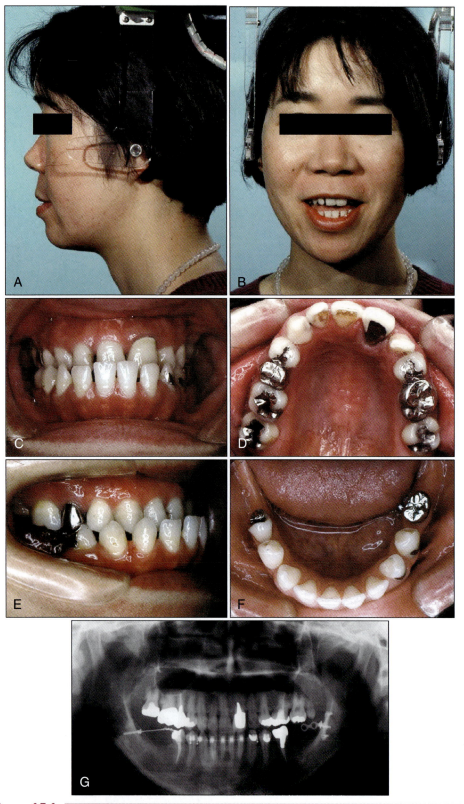

Figure 15-1

Severe Anterior Crossbite in 29-Year-Old Woman. Initial facial (**A** and **B**) and intraoral (**C-F**) photographs. **G,** Panoramic radiograph showing a miniscrew and a miniplate as temporary anchorage devices.

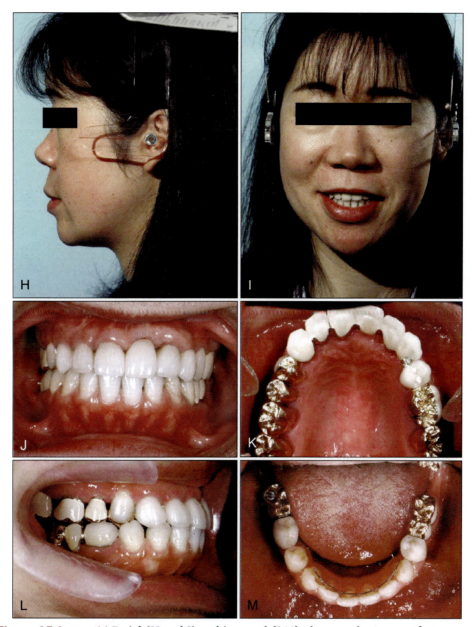

Figure 15-1, cont'd Facial (**H** and **I**) and intraoral (**J-M**) photographs 3 years after treatment. This is the first patient to receive treatment with the authors' skeletal anchorage system (SAS), from 1992.

- Nonsurgical camouflage treatment of skeletal malocclusions, such as Class II, Class III, open bite, deep bite, and facial asymmetry.
- Nonextraction treatment of various types of malocclusions characterized by incisor protrusion or anterior crowding.
- Traction of deeply impacted teeth.
- Second-phase treatment of growing patients who need molar movement.
- Presurgical and postsurgical orthodontic treatment of surgical cases.
- Re-treatment of failed cases with complex orthodontic problems.
- Interdisciplinary treatment for patients with occlusal collapse who have severe dental problem (e.g., periodontitis, missing teeth).

TIMING OF TREATMENT

The most significant use of SAS is molar distalization, in which the third molars are usually extracted before SAS treatment. This treatment should begin after the adolescent growth period, when a final decision regarding extraction of the third molars can be made. SAS is thus rarely applied to the first phase of treatment for growing patients, although the traction of deeply impacted teeth is an exception (Figure 15-3).

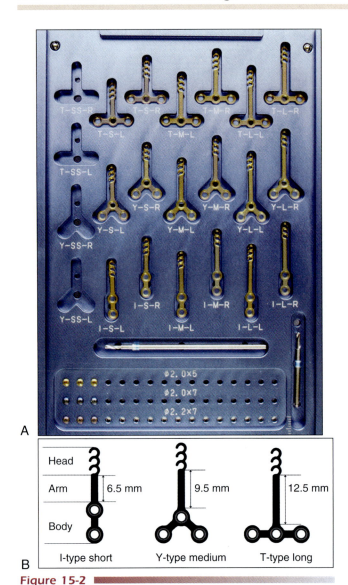

Figure 15-2

A, Orthodontic miniplates and screws. B, Three components and three configurations of orthodontic miniplates.

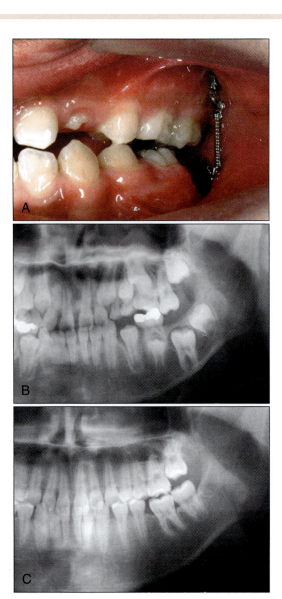

Figure 15-3

Deeply Impacted First Molar. A, Intraoral photograph, and B, panoramic radiograph, before traction. C, Panoramic radiograph after traction.

POSITIONING OF MINIPLATES

In general, the lateral wall of the maxilla is too thin to fix the miniplates with screws. The maxillary sites allowing screw fixation are limited to the zygomatic buttress and the piriform rim. These two sites are almost always thick enough to fix the plates on the bone with screws. At the zygomatic buttress, the Y-plate is usually implanted to intrude and distalize upper molars. At the piriform rim, the I-plate is usually placed for intrusion and protraction of upper molars.

In the mandible, it is possible to fix screws in most locations, except for sites adjacent to the mental foramen. The L-plate and T-plate are usually placed in the mandibular body to intrude, protract, or distalize lower molars, or at the anterior border of the ascending ramus to extrude impacted molars.

ORTHODONTIC MECHANICS WITH THE SAS

The most significant advantage of the SAS is that it allows predictable 3D molar movement: distalization, intrusion, protraction, extrusion, and buccolingual movement. However, because 92% of SAS application involves distalization, intrusion, and protraction of the maxillary and mandibular molars, these three representative movements are discussed.

DISTALIZATION OF MAXILLARY MOLARS

Distalization of molars has long been considered a difficult tooth movement even with headgear, especially in adult patients. However, by using SAS mechanics for

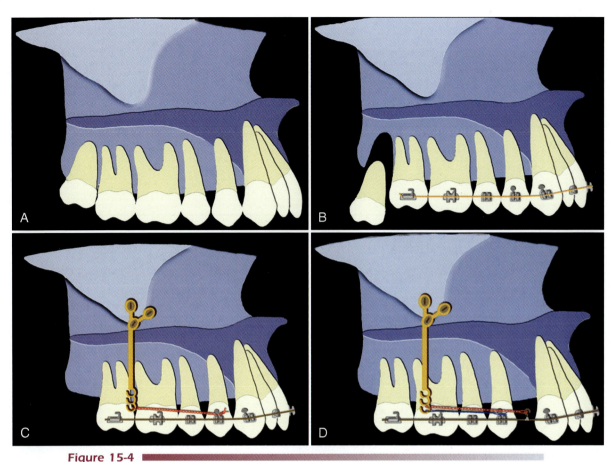

Figure 15-4
A to **D**, Biomechanics for distalization of maxillary molars. See text.

molar distalization, it is now possible to correct anterior crowding of the maxillary dentition, Class II denture bases, maxillary asymmetrical dentition, and proclined incisors in a Class III surgical case without bicuspid extraction.[3]

Figure 15-4 shows the procedures for the en masse distalization of the maxillary posterior teeth for correction of Class II malocclusion. Previously, single-molar distalization was the norm for correcting such malocclusions; however, with the development of SAS, en masse movement of the posterior molars became a common method, which reduced treatment time considerably.

- Before SAS treatment, extraction of the maxillary third molars is usually necessary to make space for molar distalization. In anterior crowding cases, leveling and aligning of the posterior segments should be done first (see Figure 15-4, *A* and *B*).
- Y-plates are implanted with monocortical screws at the zygomatic buttresses. A rigid, .018 × .025–inch, stainless steel archwire is then engaged. Orthodontic force using elastics or nickel-titanium (Ni-Ti) closed-coil springs for en masse distalization of the maxillary posteriors is added at the first bicuspids. The magnitude of orthodontic force can be up to 400 to 500 grams of force (gf) on each side (see Figure 15-4, *C*).
- After distalization of the maxillary posterior segment, canine retraction or en masse retraction of anterior segment through various mechanics is available (see Figure 15-4, *D*).

DISTALIZATION OF MANDIBULAR MOLARS

Distalization of the mandibular molars has long been considered to be much more difficult than that of the maxillary molars, because effective mechanics have not been available in traditional orthodontics. A headgear has not been an option for distalization of the mandibular molars. After development of SAS, if patients accept minor surgery for miniplate implantation, distalization of the mandibular molars is no longer a problem.[4]

Indications are cases with anterior crowding in the mandibular dentition, asymmetrical mandibular dentition, anterior crossbite with Class III denture,[5] and retroclined lower incisors in Class II surgical cases.

Figure 15-5 shows the procedures for distalization of the mandibular molars for correction of Class III

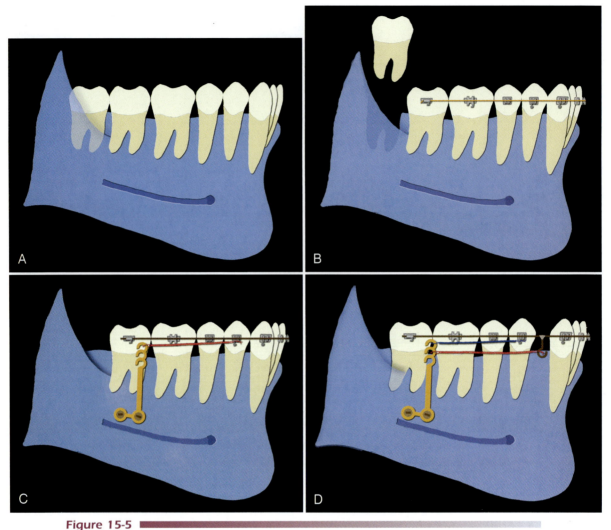

Figure 15-5
A to D, Biomechanics for distalization of mandibular molars. See text.

malocclusion. The basic mechanics are almost the same as for the distalization of the maxillary molars.

- Before SAS treatment, the mandibular third molars are extracted to create space for molar distalization (see Figure 15-5, A and B).
- After leveling and aligning the mandibular dentition, L-plates are implanted at the molar region of the mandibular body. Orthodontic force for en masse distalization of the posterior teeth is then applied. The magnitude of distalizing force can be up to 400 to 500 gf on each side (see Figure 15-5, C).
- After distalization of the posterior teeth, it is possible to achieve en masse movement of the anterior segment or canine retraction using various mechanics (see Figure 15-5, D).

INTRUSION OF MAXILLARY MOLARS

It has been extremely difficult to intrude the maxillary molars with traditional orthodontic mechanics. Therefore the patients who needed intrusion of the posterior dentition for open-bite correction had to undergo orthognathic surgery. However, orthodontic intrusion of the maxillary molars is now possible with the SAS.[6] The intrusion of maxillary molars causes clockwise rotation of the occlusal plane and counterclockwise rotation of the mandible. Such morphological changes improve anterior open bite with skeletal Class II relationship, as well as long face profiles. SAS treatment is indicated for patients with anterior open bite who have a large interlabial gap with excessive lower facial height, vertical maxillary excess, and skeletal Class I to moderate Class II jaw relationship.

Figure 15-6 shows the procedures undertaken in a typical example of open-bite correction by the intrusion of maxillary posterior teeth.

- A high percentage of patients with anterior open bite and vertical maxillary excess exhibit double maxillary occlusal planes. In such cases, leveling and aligning of the posterior segment should begin before leveling and aligning of the anterior dentition. If correction of the posterior segment is not begun first, the upper incisors will extrude more than expected, and conse-

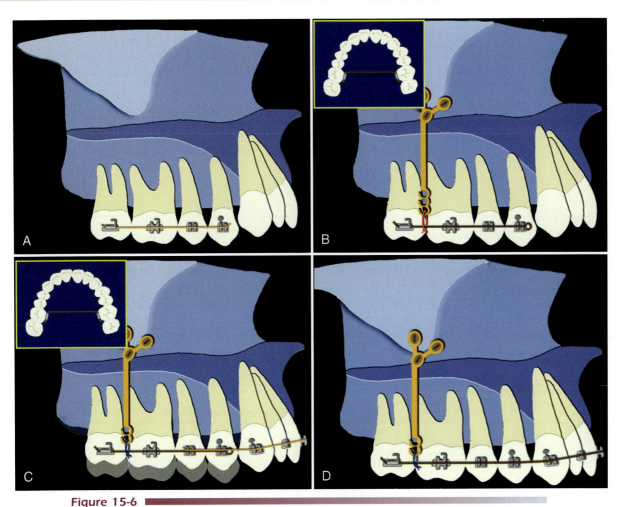

Figure 15-6
A to **D**, Biomechanics for intrusion of maxillary molars. See text.

quently, exposure of the maxillary incisors may be aggravated. In patients who exhibit a single occlusal plane, leveling and aligning should be done simultaneously (see Figure 15-6, *A*).

- After the engagement of rigid rectangular archwire in the buccal side and a transpalatal arch (TPA) in the lingual side, an elastic intrusive force will be provided from Y-plates placed at the zygomatic buttresses. The magnitude of the intrusive force can be up to 400 gf on each side. The purpose of the TPA is to prevent the buccal flaring of molars (see Figure 15-6, *B*).
- When the maxillary molars are intruded at the same level as anterior teeth, brackets are bonded on the anterior segment and aligned with a continuous archwire (see Figure 15-6, *C*).
- Simultaneously, the archwire is ligated to the miniplates to intrude molars and maintain their exact position for a few months (see Figure 15-6, *D*).

INTRUSION OF MANDIBULAR MOLARS

It has been much more difficult to intrude the mandibular molars than the maxillary molars with traditional mechanotherapies. Even with orthognathic surgery, it has been almost impossible to impact the mandibular molar region because of the risk of injuring the inferior alveolar nerve. SAS treatment is indicated for patients with anterior open-bite who have a large interlabial gap with excessive lower facial height, mandibular molar height excess, and skeletal Class I or mild Class III jaw relationship.[7-11]

Figure 15-7 shows the procedures undertaken in a typical example of open-bite correction by intrusion of the mandibular molars.

- Some patients with anterior open bite and lower molar height excess exhibit double mandibular occlusal planes (see Figure 15-7, *A*).
- Leveling should be carried out segmentally. Otherwise, the mandibular incisors will extrude more than expected. In patients with a single occlusal plane, leveling should be done with a continuous archwire (see Figure 15-7, *B*).
- After the engagement of a rigid rectangular archwire in the buccal side and a lingual arch in the lingual side, an elastic intrusive force of about 400 to 500 gf will be provided from L-plates placed at the molar region of the mandibular body. The lingual arch or lingual crown torque to a rectangular archwire

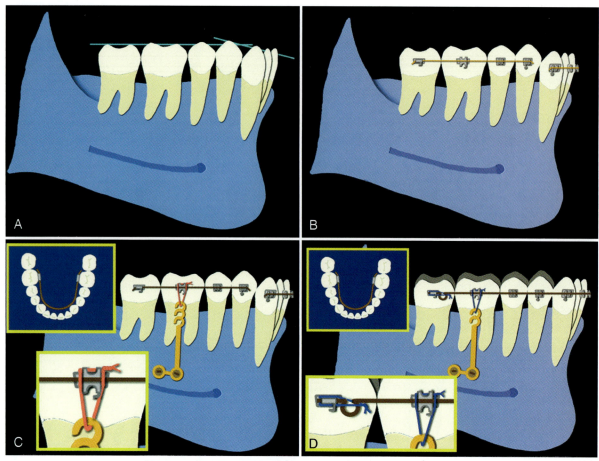

Figure 15-7
Biomechanics for intrusion of mandibular molars. See text.

must be set to prevent molar buccal flaring (see Figure 15-7, C).
- When the mandibular molars are intruded at the same level as the anterior teeth, brackets are bonded on the anterior segment and aligned with a continuous archwire. Simultaneously, the archwire is ligatured to the anchor plates to intrude the molars and maintain their exact position (see Figure 15-7, D).

PROTRACTION OF MAXILLARY MOLARS

Protraction of maxillary molars is occasionally needed. SAS treatment is indicated for patients who have an anterior crossbite caused by maxillary deficiency; congenital missing maxillary teeth, particularly lateral incisors or second bicuspids; asymmetrical maxillary dentition; and Class III jaw relationship.

Figure 15-8 shows the procedures to move maxillary molars mesially.
- Some patients present with anterior crossbite or asymmetrical maxillary dentition (see Figure 15-8, A).
- After leveling and aligning of maxillary dentition, an I-plate is implanted at the piriform rim, where the cortical bone is relatively thick. Orthodontic elastic force for protraction is then applied at the molars from the I-plate; about 400 gf can be applied unilaterally (see Figure 15-8, B).
- Entire maxillary dentition begins to move mesially (see Figure 15-8, C).
- The maxillary dentition would tend to show counterclockwise rotation if such mechanics were continued over time, because the line of force vector passes below the center of resistance (CR) of the maxillary dentition (see Figure 15-8, D).

PROTRACTION OF MANDIBULAR MOLARS

Protraction of mandibular molars is usually needed in patients who have a spaced mandibular dentition, congenital missing mandibular second bicuspids, asymmetrical maxillary dentition, decompensation of the mandibular incisors in presurgical orthodontics, and Class II molar relationship.

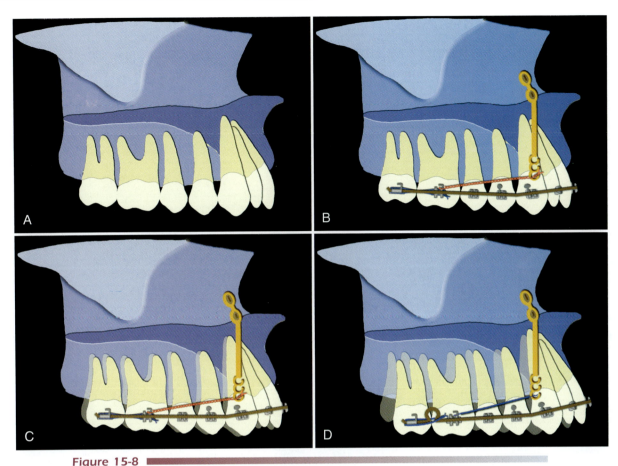

Figure 15-8

A to **D**, Biomechanics for protraction of maxillary molars. See text.

Figure 15-9 shows the procedures to protract mandibular molars, assuming decompensation of the mandibular incisors in presurgical orthodontics.

- In a patient with a spaced mandibular arch, protraction of the mandibular molars is indis-pensable to eliminate remaining space after proclination of the mandibular incisors (see Figure 15-9, *A*).
- After leveling and aligning of the maxillary dentition, L-plate is placed at the canine region of the mandibular body. Then, orthodontic elastic force for protraction is applied at the first molars from the first hook of L-plate. The magnitude of protractive orthodontic force can be as much as 200 gf unilaterally (see Figure 15-9, *B*).
- After completion of protraction of the first molar, protraction of the second molar begins (see Figure 15-9, *C*).
- The second molar is ligatured to the anchor plates to prevent relapse. In addition, the mandibular teeth tend to show mesial tipping because the line of force vector is above the CR of the mandibular dentition, and consequently the mandibular incisors are flared and intruded. To prevent such side effects, countermechanics are needed (see Figure 15-9, *D*).

SURGICAL PROCEDURES

IMPLANTATION OF MINIPLATES

Figures 15-10 and 15-11 show the surgical procedures for implantation of miniplates in the maxilla and the mandible, respectively. The procedure is performed under local anesthesia with intravenous (IV) sedation.

- Initially, a mucoperiosteal incision is made in the buccal vestibule (see Figures 15-10, *A*, and 15-11, *A*).
- A vertical incision is usually made in the maxilla and a horizontal incision in the mandible. The mucoperiosteal flap is elevated after the subperiosteal dissection to expose the bony cortex (see Figures 15-10, *B*, and 15-11, *B*).
- Based on the distance between the surgical site and the dentition on the pretreatment panoramic radiograph, the appropriate shape and length of the anchor plate is selected. The plate is contoured to the bone surface and placed in its final position. One of the holes is marked with crystal violet (see Figures 15-10, *C*, and 15-11, *C*).
- A pilot hole is drilled after removing the positioned plate (see Figures 15-10, *D*, and 15-11, *D*).

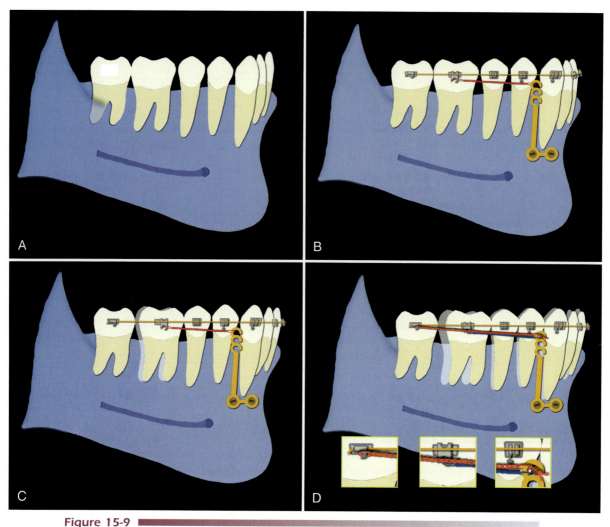

Figure 15-9
Biomechanics for protraction of mandibular molars. See text.

- A self-tapping monocortical screw is placed in the hole of the miniplate body (see Figures 15-10, *E*, and 15-11, *E*).
- The remaining holes are drilled and the remaining screws inserted to attach the anchor plate firmly to the bone surface (see Figures 15-10, *F* and *G*, and 15-11, *F* and *G*).
- The surgical site is closed with resorbable sutures (see Figures 15-10, *H*, and 15-11, *H*).

The implantation surgery takes approximately 10 to 15 minutes for each miniplate.

REMOVAL OF MINIPLATES

Immediately after orthodontic treatment, all miniplates are removed (Figures 15-12 and 15-13). As with implantation, the miniplates are removed under local anesthesia.

- Initially, a mucoperiosteal and subperiosteal dissection is performed to expose the miniplate (see Figures 15-12, *A* and *B*, and 15-13, *A* and *B*).
- Although the monocortical bone screws have been removed, the miniplate is still firmly attached to the bone surface because of the thin layer of newly deposited bone, frequently covering the miniplates (see Figures 15-12, *C*, and 15-13, *C*).
- After removing the miniplate, new bone formation is often observed surrounding the plate as well (see Figures 15-12, *C*, and 15-13, *C*).
- The surgical site is then closed with resorbable sutures (see Figures 15-12, *D*, and 15-13, *D*).

COMPLICATIONS AND COUNTERMEASURES

Most patients who have miniplates implanted undergo mild to moderate facial swelling for several days after surgery, as expected. The most common postsurgical complication is infection, with clinical evidence of pain, swelling, and pus production around the miniplate[12,13] (Figure 15-14). Such infection occurs in about 10% of patients. Mild infection can be controlled by careful brushing techniques and antiseptic mouthwash. In more severe cases, antibiotics are required. To prevent infection postsurgically, it is important to educate

Text continued on p. 331

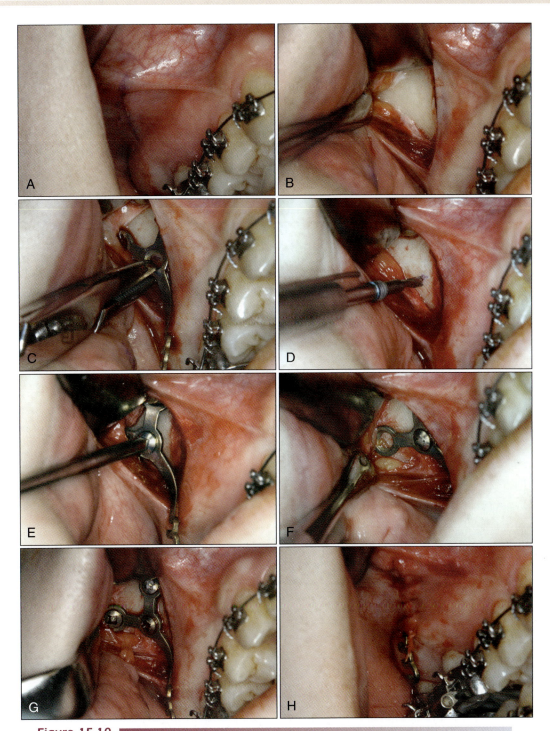

Figure 15-10
A to H, Procedure for implantation of miniplate in zygomatic buttress. See text.

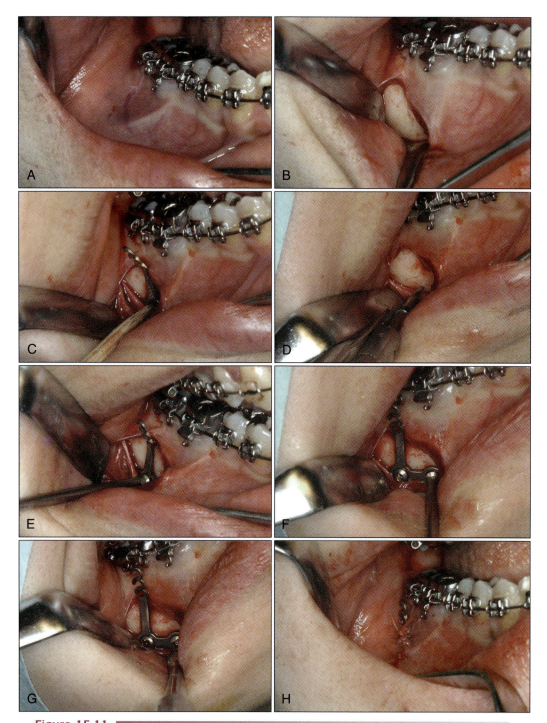

Figure 15-11
A to H, Procedure for implantation of miniplate in mandibular body. See text.

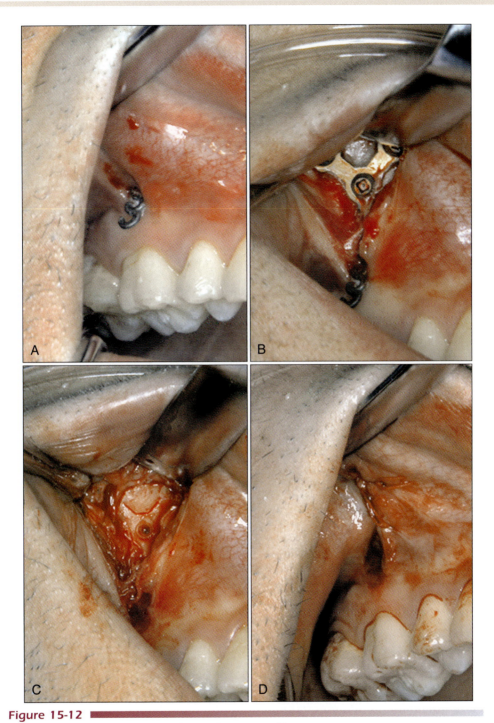

Figure 15-12
A to D, Procedure for removal of miniplate in maxilla. See text.

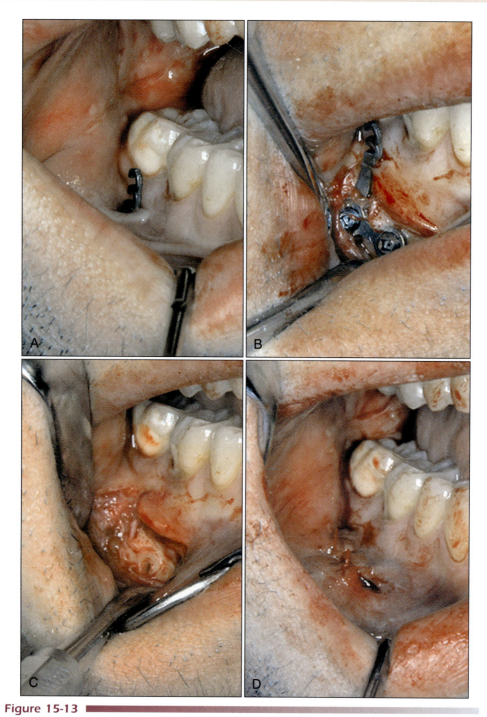

Figure 15-13
A to **D**, Procedure for removal of miniplate in mandible. See text.

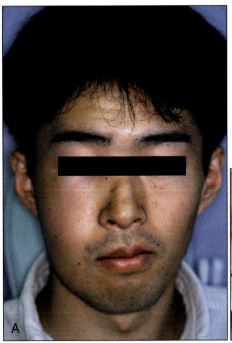
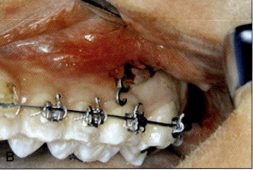

Figure 15-14
A, Facial swelling caused by infection. B, Pus production caused by infection.

patients in oral home care. Also, mechanically cleaning the exposed part of the miniplate at all routine orthodontic appointments greatly reduces postoperative infection.

Plate loosening occurred in only 1.7% of our cases. Other potential complications include plate fracture and mucosal dehiscence around the plate, neither of which has occurred during SAS treatment to date.

CASE REPORT 15-1

A 25-year-old Japanese woman presented with open bite, difficulty with incising, and temporomandibular disorder (TMD) (Figure 15-15). She underwent orthodontic treatment with multibracketed appliances for open-bite correction when she was 12 years old for about 2 years under a general practitioner (a part-time orthodontist took charge of her treatment). Her open bite recurred, and she had difficulty with incising. Interestingly, to maintain her incising function, composite resin had been applied at the incisal edges of her upper central incisors. After removing the composite resin, it was confirmed that her maxillary central incisors were intact.

Problem List
The patient had a complex list of orthodontic problems. The lateral cephalometric radiograph was taken in natural head position and centric relation with relaxed lip posture (Figure 15-16, A). The cephalometric template analysis indicated that her major skeletal and soft tissue problems were a large interlabial gap, deficient exposure of the upper incisors, excessive lower facial height, and Class II jaw relationship (Figure 15-16, B). She also had a severe anterior open bite, lower anterior crowding, a narrow upper dental arch, proclined incisors, and missing upper first bicuspids (Figure 15-17; see also Figure 15-15). We decided that almost all her orthodontic problems could be solved using SAS biomechanics.

Treatment Goals
In an open-bite case with skeletal Class II jaw relationship, dental problems as well as skeletal and soft tissue profile can be improved through three-dimensional movement of the maxillary and mandibular molars with the SAS mechanics.

According to the cephalometric prediction (Figure 15-18, A), the patient's treatment goal included intrusion of the maxillary and mandibular molars by 1.0 mm and 2.0 mm, respectively. This would generate counterclockwise rotation of the mandible, thus improving the excessive lower facial height, anterior open bite, and large interlabial gap. Simultaneously, Class II profile would be improved to Class I after counterclockwise mandibular rotation.

In addition to skeletal correction, some dental correction was needed to solve her orthodontic problems (Figure 15-18). At first, extrusion of the upper incisors by 1.5 mm was

Continued

CASE REPORT 15-1—cont'd

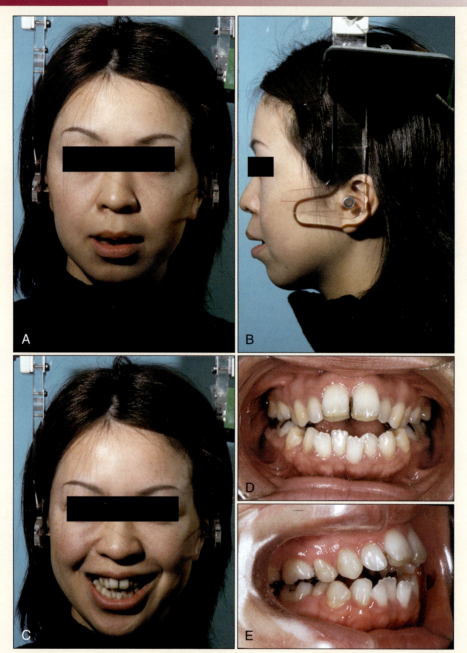

Figure 15-15 Pretreatment Evaluation. Facial (A-C) and intraoral (D-I) photographs at initial examination.

CASE REPORT 15-1—cont'd

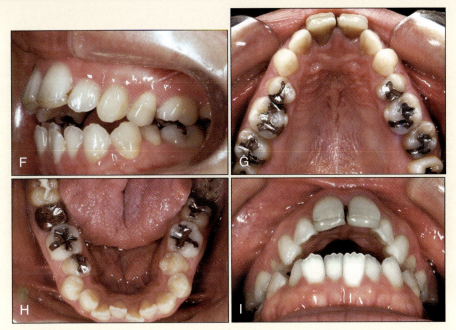

Figure 15-15, cont'd

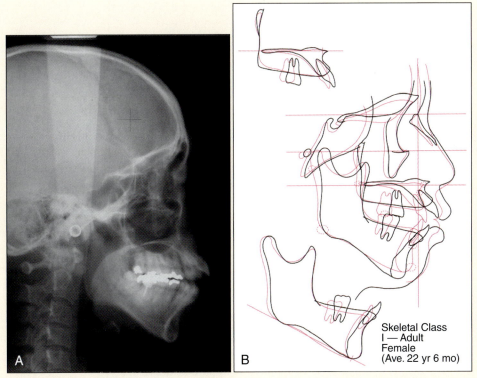

Figure 15-16 Cephalometric Evaluation. A, Cephalometric radiograph. B, Craniofacial Drawing Standards (CDS) analysis.

Continued

CASE REPORT 15-1—cont'd

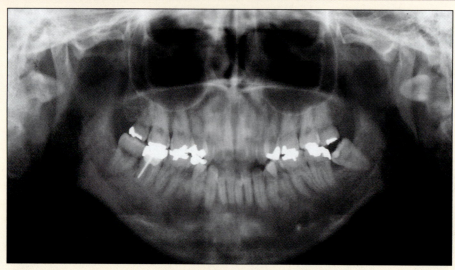

Figure 15-17 Panoramic Radiograph at Initial Examination.

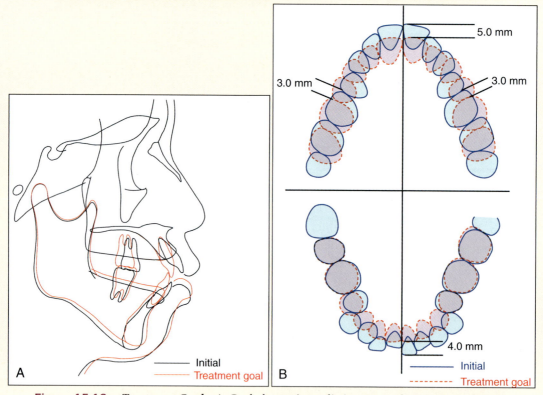

Figure 15-18 Treatment Goals. A, Cephalometric prediction. B, Occlusogram prediction.

required to improve her deficient exposure of the upper incisors in relaxed lip posture and smiling. Retroclination of the upper and lower incisors was also required, by 5.0 mm and 4.0 mm, respectively, to improve bidental protrusion. To ensure the incisal treatment goals, 3.0-mm distalization of the upper molars and extraction of the first bicuspids were needed bilaterally.

The final intercuspation was predicted with a diagnostic setup model based on the cephalometric and occlusogram treatment goals.

Treatment Plan

The following step-by-step plan was established to achieve the patient's treatment goals with the SAS mechanics:

CASE REPORT 15-1—cont'd

1. Extraction of #18, #28, #38, #48, #34, and #44.
2. Bonding brackets at the maxillary dentition and the mandibular posterior teeth.
3. Placement of a transpalatal arch (TPA) on #16 and #26.
4. Leveling and aligning of the maxillary dentition and the mandibular posterior segments.
5. Implantation of orthodontic miniplates at the zygomatic buttress and the mandibular body bilaterally.
6. Retraction of the lower canines with SAS.
7. Bonding brackets on the mandibular incisors; leveling and aligning of the mandibular dentition.
8. En masse retraction of the mandibular anterior teeth with SAS.
9. Intrusion and distalization of the maxillary posterior segments with SAS.
10. Intrusion of the mandibular posterior teeth with SAS.
11. Coordination of the maxillary and mandibular dentitions.
12. Detailing and finishing.
13. Debonding of all brackets and debanding.
14. Placement of a wraparound retainer on the maxillary dentition and a lingual-bonded retainer on the mandibular dentition.

Treatment Progress

In accordance with the patient's treatment plan, before orthodontic treatment, all the third molars and the mandibular first bicuspids were extracted. Subsequently, .022-inch preadjusted brackets were bonded and banded, leveling and aligning of the dentition were initiated with Ni-Ti wires (Figure 15-19, A-L).

A 0.032 × 0.032–inch TPA was placed on the maxillary first molars to prevent buccal flaring of the molars during intrusion with SAS. After engagement of rigid rectangular wires (0.018 × 0.022–inch stainless steel), orthodontic miniplates were fixed at the zygomatic buttress and the apical region of the mandibular molars, bilaterally (Figure 15-19, M-O).

Skeletal anchorage mechanics were applied approximately 3 weeks after implantation surgery. It was not necessary to wait for the osseointegration of the titanium screws and plates. Distalization and intrusion of maxillary posterior teeth and retraction of lower canines were initiated with elastic chain modules or Ni-Ti closed-coil springs. Magnitude of intrusive orthodontic forces for maxillary posterior teeth was about 500 gf. Subsequent to retraction of the mandibular canines, brackets were bonded at the mandibular anterior dentition. After leveling and aligning of the entire mandibular dentition, the patient's open bite was drastically reduced with the SAS.

At the detailing and finishing stage, occlusal equilibration was provided to maximize her intercuspation and to establish proper anterior guidance. Immediately after debonding, the patient was instructed to use a wraparound retainer with tongue cribs in the maxillary dentition, and a lingual-bonded retainer in the mandibular dentition was fixed. Tongue cribs were embedded in the retainer to make her aware of and stop her habitual tongue thrust (Figure 15-19, P and Q).

Posttreatment Evaluation

After debonding and as a result of SAS biomechanics for intrusion of the molars, the patient's orthodontic problems (large interlabial gap, open bite, excessive lower facial height) improved dramatically after counterclockwise rotation of the mandible (Figure 15-20, A-I). Although significant retroclination of the mandibular incisors was observed, the maxillary and mandibular dentitions were well aligned, and acceptable intercuspation and functional occlusion were established.

Her cephalometric superimpositions showed that her treatment goals were successfully achieved with the application of SAS biomechanics (Figure 15-20, J).

The stability of her occlusion has been favorably maintained during the 5-year follow-up after debonding (Figure 15-20, K-S). From her cephalometric superimpositions, her dentofacial change over 5 years clearly was minimal. The reason for her excellent dentofacial stability is elusive, but relapse of the intruded molars apparently was negligible. To assess the effectiveness of the retainer with tongue reminder, further investigation is needed.

Continued

CASE REPORT 15-1—cont'd

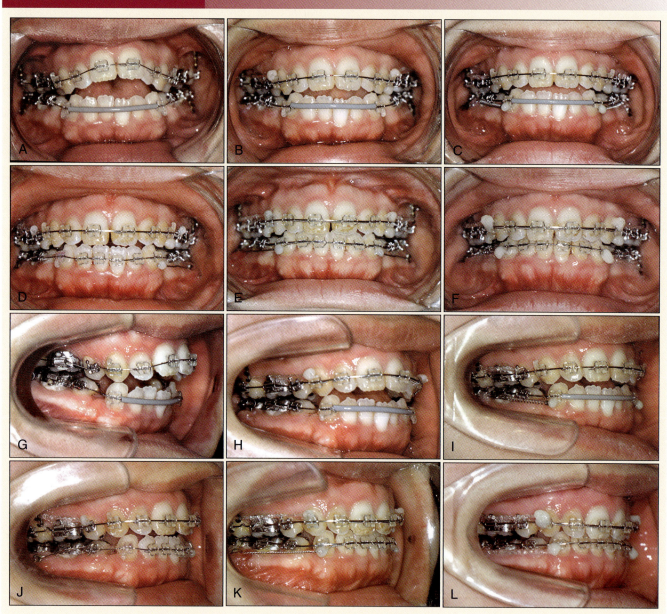

Figure 15-19 Treatment Progress. **A** to **F,** Intraoral photographs, frontal view. **G** to **L,** Intraoral photographs, lateral view.

CASE REPORT 15-1—cont'd

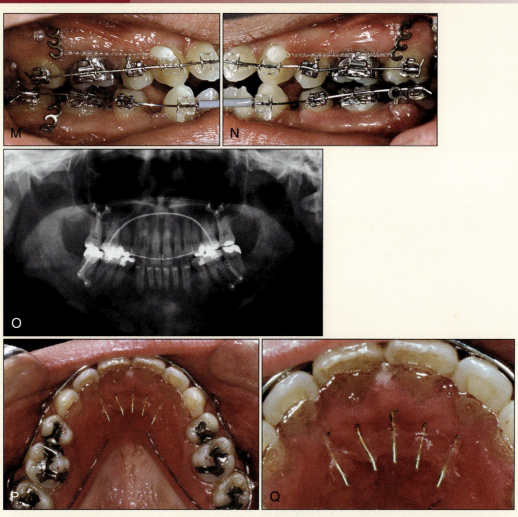

Figure 15-19, cont'd **M** to **O**, Intraoral photographs and panoramic radiograph showing implantation of miniplates. **P** and **Q**, Wraparound retainer with tongue crib.

Continued

CASE REPORT 15-1—cont'd

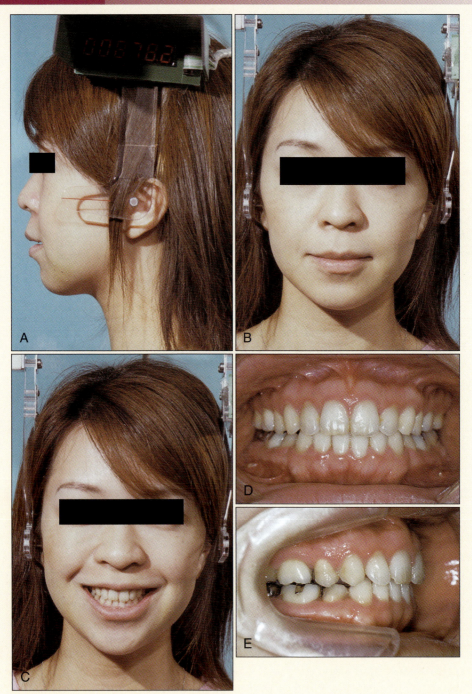

Figure 15-20 Posttreatment Evaluation. **A** to **C**, Facial photographs immediately after debonding. **D** to **I**, Intraoral photographs immediately after debonding. **J**, Pretreatment and posttreatment cephalometric superimposition.

CASE REPORT 15-1—cont'd

Figure 15-20, cont'd   For legend see apposite page.

Continued

CASE REPORT 15-1—cont'd

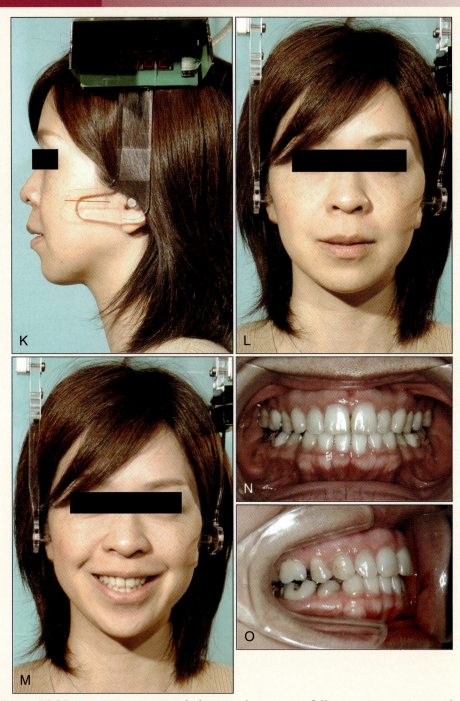

Figure 15-20, cont'd K to M, Facial photographs at 5-year follow-up. N to S, Intraoral photographs at 5-year follow-up.

CASE REPORT 15-1—cont'd

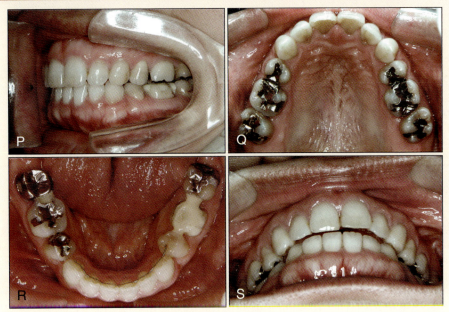

Figure 15-20, cont'd   For legend see opposite page.

SUMMARY

- Development of SAS has allowed three-dimensional movement of the molars with ease.
- Orthodontic miniplates do not disturb any type of tooth movement because these are placed outside the dental arches.
- Molars can be moved as easily as teeth in the anterior dentition.
- Patients no longer need to wear uncomfortable extra-oral appliances.
- Orthodontic therapy can proceed based on the individualized treatment goal and predictable outcome.
- Nonextraction cases can be significantly increased.
- Orthognathic surgical cases can be significantly decreased.

REFERENCES

1. Sugawara J: JCO interviews Dr. Junji Sugawara on the skeletal anchorage system, J Clin Orthod 33:689-696, 2000.
2. Sugawara J, Nishimura M: Minibone plates: the skeletal anchorage system, Semin Orthod 11:47-56, 2005.
3. Sugawara J, Kanzaki R, Takahashi I, et al: Distal movement of the maxillary molars in non-growing patients with the skeletal anchorage system, Am J Orthod Dentofacial Orthop 126:723-733, 2006.
4. Sugawara J, Daimaruya T, Umemori M, et al: Distalization of mandibular molars in adult patients with application of skeletal anchorage system, Am J Orthod Dentofacial Orthop 125:130-138, 2004.
5. Sugawara J, Umemori M, Mitani H, et al: Orthodontic treatment system for Class III malocclusion using a titanium miniplate as an anchorage, Orthod Waves 57:25-35, 1998.
6. Daimaruya T, Takahashi I, Nagasaka H, et al: Effects of maxillary molar intrusion on the nasal floor and tooth root using skeletal anchorage system in dogs, Angle Orthod 73:158-166, 2003.
7. Sugawara J, Baik UB, Umemori M, et al: Treatment and posttreatment dentoalveolar changes following intrusion of mandibular molars with application of skeletal anchorage system (SAS) for open bite correction, Int J Adult Orthod Orthognath Surg 17:243-253, 2002.
8. Umemori M, Sugawara J, Mitani H, et al: Skeletal anchorage system for open-bite correction, Am J Orthod Dentofacial Orthop 115:166-174, 1999.
9. Daimaruya T, Nagasaka H, Umemori M, et al: The influences of molar intrusion on the inferior alveolar neurovascular bundle and root resorption by using skeletal anchorage system in dogs, Angle Orthod 71:60-70, 2001.
10. Konno Y, Daimaruya T, Knazaki R, et al: The morphological and hemodynamical analysis in the dog dental pulp following molar intrusion using the skeletal anchorage system, Am J Orthod Dentofacial Orthop 132:199-207, 2007.
11. Kanzaki R, Daimaruya T, Takahashi I, et al: Remodeling of alveolar bone crest following molar intrusion with the skeletal anchorage system in dogs, Am J Orthod Dentofacial Orthop 131:343-351, 2007.
12. Nagasaka H, Sugawara J, Kawamura H, et al: A clinical evaluation on the efficacy of titanium miniplates as orthodontic anchorage, Orthod Waves 58:136-147, 1999.
13. Sato R, Sato T, Takahashi I, et al: Profiling of bacterial flora in crevices around titanium orthodontic anchor plates, Clin Oral Implant Res 18:21-26, 2007.

CHAPTER 16

Bone Anchorage: a New Concept in Orthodontics

Nejat Erverdi and Serdar Üşümez

Anchorage is perhaps one of the most important concepts in biomechanics of orthodontics. There are a number of methods to maintain and reinforce anchorage.[1,2] All these appliances and biomechanical procedures aim to achieve "maximum anchorage," which means favorably using 75% of the space. In some cases the maximum anchorage concept is insufficient, and the treatment goal requires the use of 100% of the space. "Stationary anchorage" can be used for such situations. The only way to achieve this in traditional orthodontics is through the use of extraoral appliances. Extraoral appliances are effective but have disadvantages; two major concerns are patient compliance[3-5] and possibly serious injuries.[6] Also, in many cases, only the orthodontic effect of extraoral fixation is required; unfortunately, orthodon-tic and orthopedic effects generally cannot be isolated from each other.

Recent developments in implantology now allow stationary anchorage without extraoral appliances or complex biomechanical procedures. Implants used for orthodontic anchorage are generally classified as *osseointegrated* or *nonosseointegrated* implants. Conventional dental implants and palatal implants are regarded as osseointegrated implants, and miniscrews, microscrews, and various surgical plates as nonosseointegrated implants. However, these two concepts are sometimes confused in orthodontics and need to be clarified.

Animal studies have shown that any contact between bone surface and titanium material results in osseointegration, which is required for the successful service of conventional dental implants and palatal implants.[7,8] The quality of osseointegration is based on the surface characteristics of the titanium implant and the quality of the bone.[9] Various treatment modalities are available for the implant surface to facilitate osseointegration.[10-13] Quality of the bone is related to the anatomical site where the implant is placed, age of the patient, and the general health conditions. On the other hand, screws that are used for fixation of the plates and the plates themselves are designed for temporary use only for fixation of two bony segments. In some cases, they are left permanently in place after healing to avoid another surgery, particularly in orthopedics. Ideally, however, it should be possible to remove them easily after the healing procedure. Therefore, their surfaces are finished smooth to avoid osseointegration. However, osseointegration still develops in these screws, but it is not strong enough to prevent the unscrewing process. An appropriate term for such interaction between bone and the screw can be *partial osseointegration*. However; the extent of osseointegration cannot be determined because it depends on the surface characteristics and the bone type where it is mounted. This term is appropriate for cases in which unscrewing is possible.

Orthodontic miniscrews have the same surface properties as the surgical fixation miniscrews because they are designed for temporary use only. Therefore, partial osseointegration is also valid for orthodontic miniscrews. However, as this amount of osseointegration is not clinically relevant we are going to use the term *nonosseointegrated implants* in this chapter to describe all anchorage attachments that are fixed to the bone in a temporary manner.

This chapter discusses clinical use of different orthodontic implants to correct different malocclusions. Although orthodontic implants can be used in any case, their use should be limited to cases in which treatment results will be improved, compared with conventional biomechanical procedures or radical surgery, which always carries a risk of morbidity. Otherwise, serious ethical concerns may arise. Therefore, the treatment methods presented in this chapter are compared with the conventional method, and the benefits of the implant method are clarified.

ZYGOMATIC ANCHORAGE WITH MULTIPURPOSE IMPLANT

Various methods for bone anchorage have been tested: cobalt-chromium (Vitallium) screws, vitreous carbon, Bioglass-coated aluminum oxide implants, stainless steel plates and screws,[14-22] Brånemark implants,[23,24] retromolar implants,[23] onplants,[25] zygomatic wires,[26] ankylosed teeth,[27] palatal implants,[28] miniplates,[29,30] and miniscrews.[18,22,31] Among these, zygomatic implants have particular importance as being widely used and tested in recent years.[17]

MULTIPURPOSE IMPLANT

The Multipurpose Implant (MPI) was designed by Erverdi and produced by Tasarim Med (Istanbul, Turkey). This implant has two parts: a miniplate with three holes for fixation and a round, straight extension 20 mm in length and 0.9 mm in diameter (Figure 16-1).

The extension is bendable, so that the point of force application can be carried to any location according to the biomechanical protocol. Screws 5 mm in length and 2.2 mm in diameter are advised for low-positioned holes to avoid perforation of the sinus mucosa. For the hole in a higher position, screws 7 or 9 mm in length can be used.

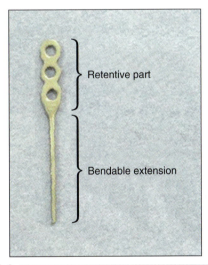

Figure 16-1
Multipurpose implant (MPI), with retentive part and bendable extension (Tasaraim Med, Istanbul, Turkey).

SITES FOR IMPLANT PLACEMENT

Two anatomical sites present enough bony thickness to fix an implant on the lateral wall of maxillary bone: nasal buttress and zygomatic buttress areas. The zygomatic buttress area is the site of choice for the specific purpose of intruding the maxillary posterior dentoalveolar segment (Figure 16-2).

As shown in case reports and investigations,[32,33] zygomatic implant–supported maxillary posterior intrusion is effective at the dentoalveolar level. Our cephalometric superimpositions demonstrated that the palatal plane was not affected by zygomatic implant–supported intrusion.[32] The center of resistance (CR) of the maxillary posterior segment to be intruded passes approximately through the mesial root of the first upper molar and zygomatic buttress area, when second molars are in occlusion (Figure 16-3, A). This makes the zygomatic buttress area an ideal point of force application to achieve parallel intrusion of this segment. In cases with first-premolar extraction, CR of the segment shifts slightly posterior about the distal root of the first molar (Figure 16-3, B). In this situation a slight distal step needs to be bent on the long extension of the implant, to adjust the point of force application to the same level as the CR of the intrusion segment.

SURGICAL METHOD FOR IMPLANT PLACEMENT

Incision is the most important part of the surgical procedure. The correct location of the incision is decided by digital palpation. By using the index finger, the zygomatic buttress is palpated, and the incision is made along the buttress in a vertical direction. The lower border of the incision is at the intersection of the attached and the mobile gingiva, and the total length is no longer than 1 cm. Care is taken to cut the periosteum completely during the incision, to prevent penetration of the buccal fat pad into the area. Mucoperiosteum is released and the area prepared for fixation of the implant

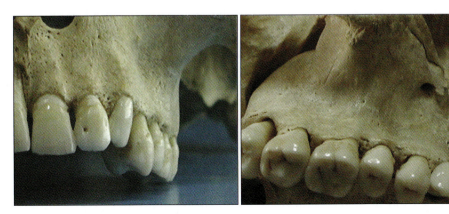

Figure 16-2
Zygomatic buttress is a curved bony area where the implants can be securely placed.

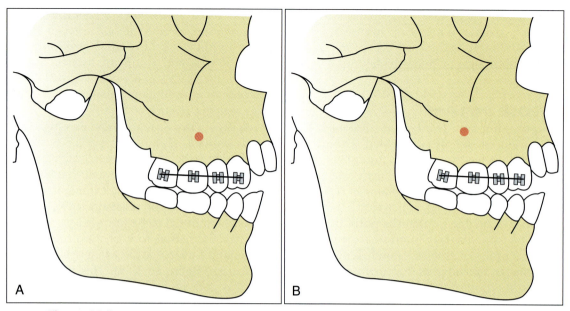

Figure 16-3
A, Center of resistance (CR) of the maxillary posterior segment to be intruded passes roughly through the mesial root of the first upper molar and zygomatic buttress area when second molars are in occlusion. **B,** In cases with first-premolar extraction, CR of the segment shifts slightly in the posterior direction, about the distal root of the first molar.

(Figure 16-4, *A* and *B*). The implant is first contoured according to the area to be fixed, and the free bendable end is cut in proper length and bent to form a hook to attach the orthodontic mechanic units (Figure 16-4, *C* and *D*). The implant is fixed to the bone with three screws, and the soft tissue is sutured (Figure 16-4, *E* and *F*).

The MPI is exposed into the oral cavity through the attached gingiva at the mucogingival junction. The location of the area where the implant is exposed is crucial to prevent inflammation. If the implant is exposed through the mobile gingiva, this will create a problem during treatment; the patient will have pain; and the result will be inflammation and loss of the implant.

COMPLICATIONS
Development of Inflammation
Inflammation may develop in any phase of treatment. In such a case, if the implant is not mobile, force application must be stopped and antibiotic treatment started, supported with bactericidal mouthwash. The healing period is about 15 days. Force application can be restarted when healing is complete, provided the implant is not mobile, which is unlikely.
Soft Tissue Impingement on Palate
If the palatal bars are not constructed far enough from the palate, they may impinge on the palatal mucosa during later stages of the dentoalveolar impaction. Bactericidal mouthwash may be used if the impaction is completed and the appliance is to be removed. If considerable impaction remains to be performed, the appliance should be replaced.

REMOVAL OF IMPLANTS
Removal of the implants is postponed until 1 month earlier than the completion of treatment. Removal is a simple procedure after accessing the implant site from, again, a short (1-cm) vertical incision. The screws are descrewed and the implant is removed. At this stage, growth of new bone chips may be observed over the implant and should be removed accordingly (Figure 16-5).

OPEN-BITE TREATMENT
One of the most difficult malocclusions to treat and maintain in orthodontics is the anterior open bite. Swinehart[34] defines open bite as the abnormal condition in which a group of teeth does not make occlusal contact because of a lack of vertical extension. Subtelny and Sakuda[35] defined open bite as a degree of openness available with lack of contact of the anterior teeth.

Etiological factors in open-bite malocclusion include heredity, functional disorders, bad habits, congenital malformations, trauma, and ankylosis. The statement by Sicher,[36] "Whenever there is a struggle between muscle and bone, bone yields," explains the close relationship between the developing open bite and functional disorders and bad habits. The incidence of open

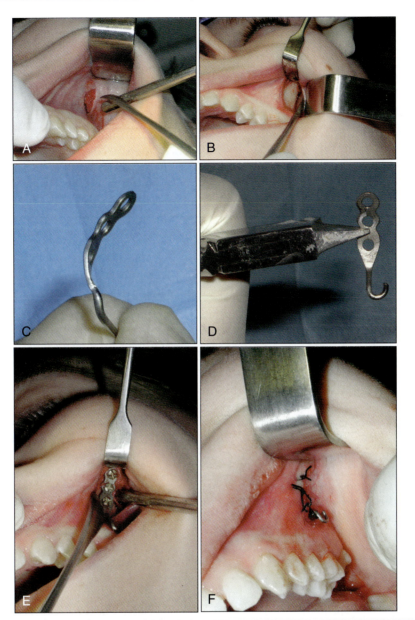

Figure 16-4

A and **B**, Incision of 1 cm is sufficient to access the zygomatic buttress area. Periosteum is elevated, and area is ready for implantation. **C** and **D**, Implant is contoured, and the free bendable end is bent into a hook to attach the orthodontic units. **E** and **F**, Screws 5 mm in length and 2.2 mm in diameter are recommended for low-positioned holes to avoid perforation of the sinus mucosa. For the hole in a higher position, screws 7 or 9 mm in length can be used.

bite is 4.2% at age 6 years and drops to 2.5% at age 14 years, perhaps because of the normalization of function during growth.[37]

Proffit[38] classified the anterior open bite into two groups, dental and skeletal. In *dental open bite* the problem is limited to dental changes. *Skeletal open bite* is especially important because it affects the skeletal structures, and treatment is challenging. This chapter discusses the treatment of this group. Morphological traits in skeletal open-bite malocclusion include excessive gonial, mandibular, and occlusal plane angles; decreased palatal plane angles; small mandibular body and ramus; increased lower anterior facial height; decreased upper anterior facial height; shorter nasion-basion distance; retrusive mandible; increased anterior and decreased posterior facial height; Class II tendency; divergent cephalometric planes; and steep anterior cranial base.[39]

Treatment of anterior open bite requires the following three steps:
1. Control of the etiological factor.
2. Correction of the morphogenetic pattern.
3. Customized retention protocol for the individual case.

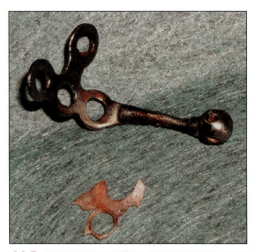

Figure 16-5
Explantation is as easy as placement. The area is exposed with the smallest incision possible.

Because of the many theories on cause, various treatment philosophies have been advocated for the correction of anterior open bite. These modalities include speech therapy; habit appliances; acrylic, magnetic, and spring-loaded bite plates; high-pull headgear; chin cap therapy; fixed appliances; implants; and different types of surgery.

The two most common morphological changes in open-bite malocclusion are overextruded maxillary posterior teeth and clockwise rotation of the mandible. Therefore, treatment of skeletal malocclusion requires the skeletal and dentoalveolar intrusion of the maxillary posterior dentoalveolar segment, to achieve anterior rotation of the mandible for correction of anterior open bite. True intrusion of maxillary posterior segment is possible only by orthognathic surgery. Besides complications and possible morbidity, patients who have orthognathic surgery undergo a long, painful postoperative healing period and loss of daily performance for at least 3 or 4 months. If maxillary posterior intrusion by bone anchorage solves these problems, this will be a new clinical method for the treatment of anterior open bite.

OPEN-BITE APPLIANCE

The open-bite appliance (OBA) was developed specifically for open-bite correction and has undergone various modifications with clinical experience.

FABRICATION
Wire Bending
The OBA has three palatal bars made of 1.5-mm, round stainless steel wire. Palatal bars are 4 mm apart from the palatal mucosa. Palatal arches are bent on two layers of wax to avoid impingement to palatal mucosa during intrusion (Figure 16-6, A).

Buccal bars are constructed using 0.8-mm, round stainless steel wire. They are adjusted to be parallel to the maxillary dental arch and are placed at least 5 mm buccal from the labial faces of the molars. Nickel-titanium (Ni-Ti) coil springs with required force magnitude are engaged on the buccal bars. Buccal bars extend from the second molar to the second premolar (Figure 16-6, B). In the coronal section, the angulation of the buccal bars needs to be made according to the width of the attached gingiva. In patients with insufficient gingival band width, the vertical height also is insufficient for activation of Ni-Ti coil springs. In these patients, buccal bars are angled downward to gain more vertical distance, which is necessary for activation of the coil springs (Figure 16-6, C).

Acrylic Cap
The intrusion appliance consists of two shallow, acrylic bite blocks connected with palatal arches and wire attachments on each buccal side, used for force application. An acrylic-cap splint is used for the retention of the appliance. It must cover whole occlusal surfaces of the posterior teeth and end at the level of the widest crown diameter. Occlusal thickness must be about 3 mm (Figure 16-7).

CLINICAL APPLICATION

After 7 to 10 days of wound healing and removal of the sutures, the OBA is first tried in the mouth to check for even occlusal contact bilaterally. The cusp tips of the appliance segments are trimmed flat to control bite opening during expansion and generation of eccentric and unilateral contact points. This step is especially important; occlusal interference is the main threat to the stability of the appliance.

The bonding material is glass-ionomer cement, which provides adequate appliance retention. After cleaning the residual adhesive material, coils are engaged to the implants and treatment begins. Two 9-mm Ni-Ti coil springs (Masel, Bristol, Pa) placed bilaterally between the tip of the implant and the outer wire create an intrusive force of 400 g (Figure 16-8).

Mode of Action
In OBA treatment the intrusive force has three components functioning in the same favorable way to intrude the maxillary dentoalveolar segment (Figure 16-9).

Coil Springs. Ni-Ti coil springs exerting bilateral intrusive force are the main intrusive component. The individual force is calculated for each case, as explained below. Because of the buccal bars, it is possible to exert a perpendicular force with this method. This means there will be no force loss.

Acrylic Cap. An acrylic cap with 3 mm of thickness is very effective in transferring forces from muscle tonus and occlusal function to the dentition as an intrusive vector.

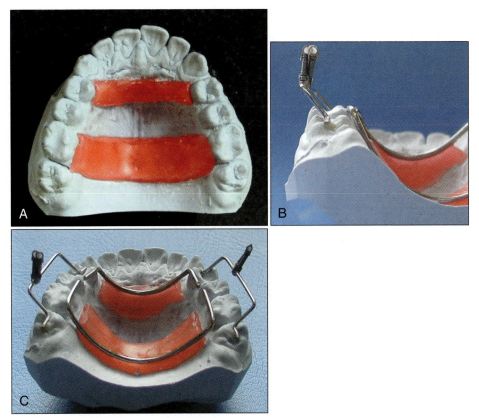

Figure 16-6
A, Palatal arches are bent on two layers of wax to avoid impingement to palatal mucosa during intrusion. B and C, Buccal bars house the Ni-Ti closed-coil spring and extend from second molar to second premolar. The angulation of this bar can be altered, as seen on C, to gain extra vertical distance to activate the coil springs.

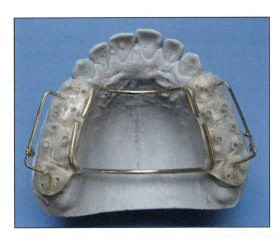

Figure 16-7
Acrylic cap covers the occlusal surfaces and extends about 1.5 to 2.0 mm away to the gingival margin. This amount of clearance between the acrylic and the gingiva ensures proper hygiene maintenance throughout the impaction period.

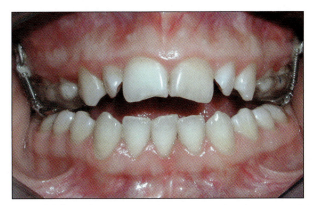

Figure 16-8
Intraoral application of open-bite appliance (OBA). At this stage, OBA should be checked for even occlusal contact bilaterally.

Palatal Bars. Palatal bars are in contact with the corpus of the tongue, transferring this intrusive force to the dentition.

Force Calculation

The chart developed by Ricketts for "bioprogressive therapy" is used for the calculation of the force magnitude. In this system, force is calculated according to the maximum cross section of the root area, using 100 and 150 g of force per square centimeter (cm^2) (Table 16-1).

CLINICAL EXPERIENCE

In the OBA treatment philosophy, upper third molars are extracted before the treatment. Patient selection is important, and patients with very good oral hygiene are good candidates for orthodontic implants. Patients must be instructed about the oral hygiene requirements and special care in cleaning the areas where the implant is exposed into the oral cavity.

Treatment is divided into two phases. In the first phase, open-bite correction is achieved with the OBA, taking approximately 5 months. The appliance is then removed, and the open bite is reduced by the autorotation of the mandible. Conventional orthodontic treatment of a Class I case resumes as the underlying malocclusion has been corrected with the OBA. In some patients the incisor position will not allow completion of the anterior rotation of mandible after removal of the OBA. In these patients, upper incisor leveling and proclination must be started during the intrusion phase of the OBA treatment. For this action, the acrylic in the buccal aspect of the premolar is removed and brackets are placed, including canine and incisors (Figure 16-10).

In the second phase of treatment, fixed appliances are placed completely, and the first molar is kept ligated to the implant until the end of treatment. In this way, vertical position of the posterior teeth is maintained.

Risk of Root Resorption

The only investigation on this subject reported in the literature found no clinically significant root resorption with OBA treatment.[40]

RETENTION

For the retention of OBA cases, canine-to-canine fixed lingual retainers are advised. It has been shown that muscle exercises are effective in increasing muscle tonus.[41] Natural chewing gums are suggested for patients to chew at least 3 or 4 hours daily in the first 3 months. These gums are hard, odorless, and tasteless (Figure 16-11). In the ensuing 3 months, chewing activity can be reduced to 1 or 2 hours daily.

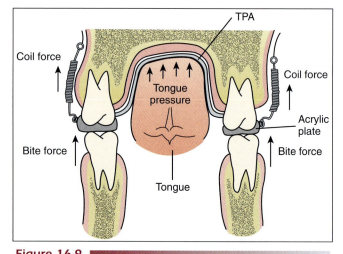

Figure 16-9
Combination of three intrusive force vectors are present with OBA. *TPA*, Transpalatal arch.

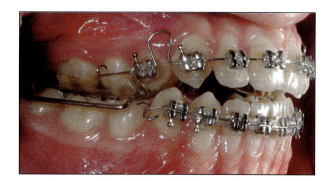

Figure 16-10
Leveling and aligning the anterior segment may be necessary to remove interferences and allow for proper autoclosure of the mandible. This is easily achieved by removing the acrylic in the buccal side of the premolar and placing brackets on the canine and incisors.

TABLE 16-1	Ricketts' Chart for Calculation of Force Magnitude						
Tooth	7	6	5	4	3	2	1
Root area (cm^2)	.70	.80	.30	.30	.45	.30	.40
150 g/cm^2	105.0	120	45	45	65	45	60
100 g/cm^2	70	80	30	30	45	30	40

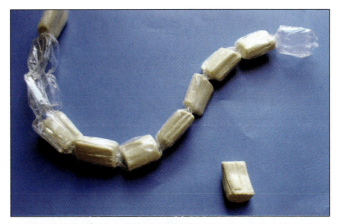

Figure 16-11
Natural chewing gums may be suggested in the first 3 months into retention to increase muscle tonus.

CASE REPORT 16-1

A 19-year-old female patient was referred with the chief complaint of anterior open bite. Her previous orthodontic treatment involved extraction of the two upper first bicuspids and the lower-right central incisor (Figure 16-12).

The growth pattern was vertical with lip tension. She was skeletally Class II with retrognathic maxilla and more retrognathic mandible. Clinical examination revealed that molar and canine relationships were Class II on both sides. She had a 3-mm anterior open bite and 10-mm overjet. The upper arch was constricted, and both arches showed crowding in the anterior region (see Figure 16-12, G and H). The smile line was high, posterior to the lateral teeth, and she had a posterior "gummy" smile with dark corners.

Treatment Objectives
1. Achieve correction of the maxillary posterior dentoalveolar vertical overgrowth.
2. Achieve correction of the anterior open bite and canine relationship with impaction of the maxillary posterior dentoalveolar segment.
3. Improve smile esthetics by eliminating the posterior gummy smile and dark corners.
4. Achieve expansion of the upper arch and alignment of the upper and lower arches.
5. Improve overall oral hygiene and periodontal health.

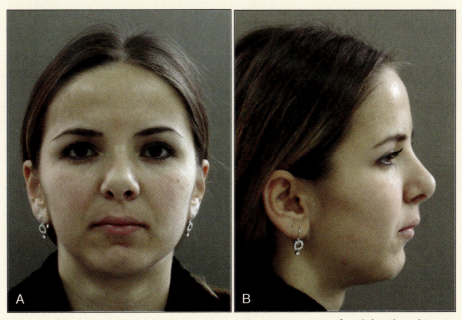

Figure 16-12 **Class II with Anterior Open Bite.** Pretreatment facial (A-C) and intraoral (D-H) photographs.

Continued

CASE REPORT 16-1—cont'd

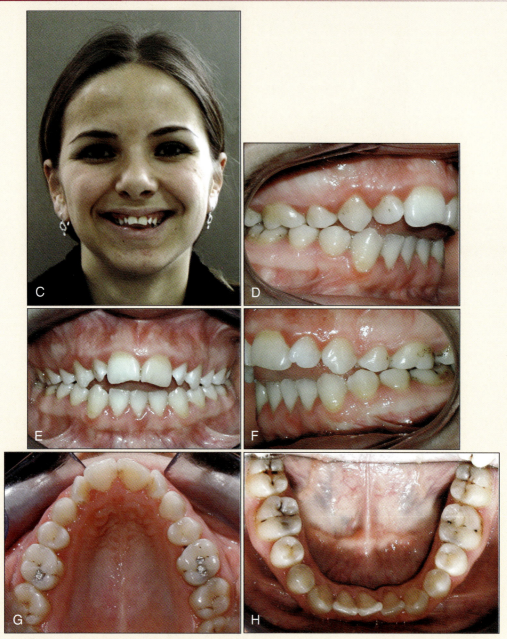

Figure 16-12, cont'd For legend see p. 349.

CASE REPORT 16-1—cont'd

Treatment Plan
Considering the excessively developed posterior maxillary dentoalveolar region, it was decided to impact the maxillary posterior dentoalveolar segment using zygomatic anchorage instead of a more invasive orthognathic surgery followed by fixed-appliance therapy.

Treatment Progress
After implant placement surgery and suture removal at day 7, the appliance was cemented and force application initiated. Two 9-mm Ni-Ti coil springs (Masel, Bristol, Pa) were placed bilaterally between the tip of the implant and the outer wire. This created an intrusive force of 400 g. The patient was seen at 4-week intervals and progress observed. No fixed appliances were placed until the completion of the posterior dentoalveolar intrusion in 7 months (Figure 16-13).

After completion of impaction, fixed orthodontic therapy was initiated, and the achieved impaction was maintained with wire ligation between the implant and the molar tubes throughout the treatment. This was followed by alignment of the arches and detailing of the occlusion with fixed mechanics. The incisal edges of the upper anterior teeth were recontoured for a better appearance. The teeth were retained by upper and lower 3-3 bonded retainers, and the patient was instructed to chew hard bubble gum 2 hours daily to strengthen the masticatory muscles and maintain physiological retention of the intrusion.

The anterior open bite is usually corrected in 5 to 6 months. Posterior segment intrusion is retained with wire ligation between molar tube and implant throughout treatment. The implants are removed about 1 month before debonding.

Results
At the end of treatment, a Class I canine and Class II molar relationship and correction of anterior open bite were

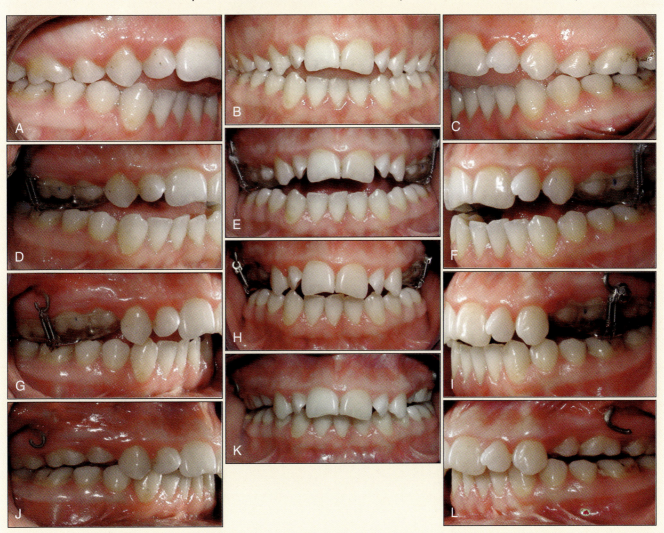

Figure 16-13 Treatment Progress with OBA. **A** to **L**, Intraoral photographs show dramatic deepening of the bite without extrusive mechanics on the incisors.

Continued

CASE REPORT 16-1—cont'd

achieved through the impaction of maxillary posterior dentoalveolar segment (Figure 16-14).

No particular extrusive mechanics was involved in the treatment. The molars were impacted by 3.6 mm and maintained throughout treatment. The posterior gummy smile was corrected, and the dark corners were eliminated. Figure 16-15 demonstrates the dramatic improvement in the smile.

Cephalometrically, the mandibular plane showed a counterclockwise autorotation of 4 degrees at the end of treatment. The overbite was improved by more than 5 mm; however, the overjet value was decreased to only 6.2 mm because of Bolton discrepancy originating from one missing lower incisor (Figure 16-16).

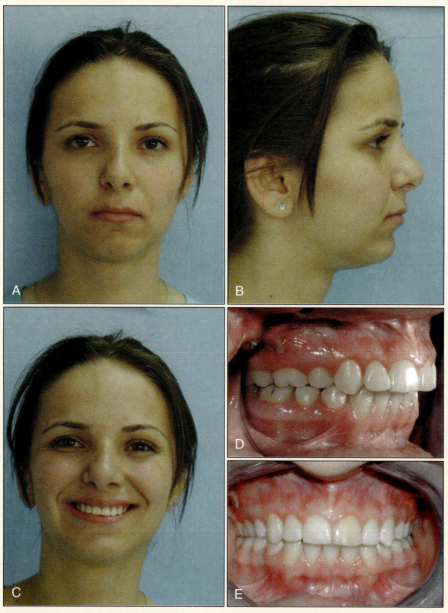

Figure 16-14 Treatment Results. Posttreatment facial (A-C) and intraoral (D-H) photographs.

CASE REPORT 16-1—cont'd

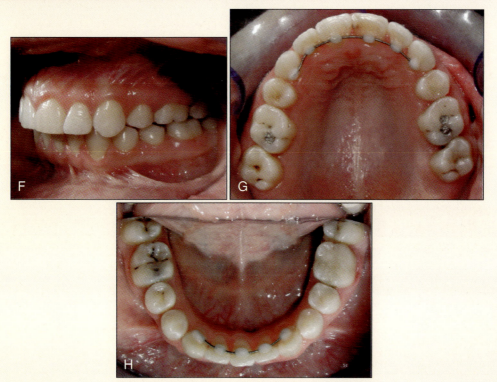

Figure 16-14, cont'd   For legend see opposite page.

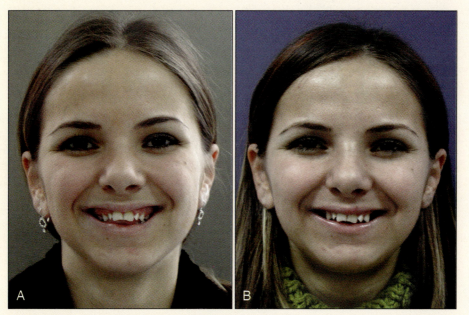

Figure 16-15   **Treatment Progress in Smile.** Pretreatment (**A**), treatment in progress (**B**), and posttreatment (**C**) photographs show dramatic improvement in the smile esthetics, with elimination of posterior gummy smile and dark corridors.

Continued

CASE REPORT 16-1—cont'd

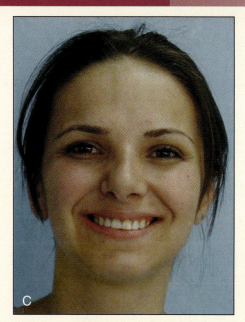

Figure 16-15, cont'd

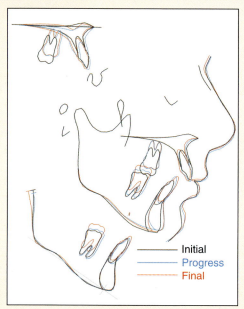

Figure 16-16 **Cephalometric Superimposition.** Significant autorotation of the mandible with molar intrusion is seen, despite that some of this rotation is counteracted during the fixed-appliance treatment period.

CASE REPORT 16-2

An 18-year-old female patient presented with a symmetrical frontal facial appearance, a gummy smile in the posterior region, and a slightly convex profile. Intraorally, she presented with a Class I molar and canine relationship, with a maxillary dentoalveolar constriction and 3 mm of anterior open bite (Figure 16-17).

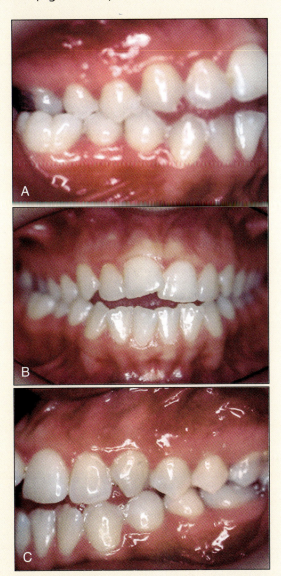

Figure 16-17 Class I with Anterior Open Bite. A to C, Pretreatment intraoral photographs.

Treatment Objectives
1. Achieve correction of the maxillary posterior dentoalveolar vertical overgrowth.
2. Achieve correction of the anterior open bite and canine relation with impaction of the maxillary posterior dentoalveolar segment.
3. Improve smile esthetics by eliminating the posterior gummy smile and dark corners.
4. Achieve expansion of the upper arch and alignment of the upper and lower arches.
5. Improve overall oral hygiene and periodontal health.

Treatment Plan
Taking into account the excessively developed posterior maxillary dentoalveolar region, it was decided to use skeletal anchorage for molar intrusion and fixed-appliance therapy.

Treatment Progress
After implant placement surgery and suture removal at the end of the first week, the appliance was cemented and force application initiated. The patient was seen at monthly intervals and progress observed.

Results
At the end of treatment, a Class I canine and molar relationship and 2 mm of positive overbite were achieved in 5 months. Because of the force application on the buccal side of the posterior segment, the dental posterior maxillary constriction was eliminated. After achieving good interdigitation, ideal overbite and overjet were achieved and the braces removed (Figure 16-18). On completion of treatment, the patient's smile and profile were significantly improved, and the posterior gummy smile was eliminated.

Cephalometry showed the improvement of the anterior open bite, clockwise occlusal plane rotation, and intrusion of the maxillary molars. Panoramic radiographs showed a flattening of the maxillary occlusal plane.

Posttreatment Evaluation
This patient was followed 5 years out of retention, and the occlusion and smile esthetics were totally stable (Figure 16-19).

Continued

CASE REPORT 16-2—cont'd

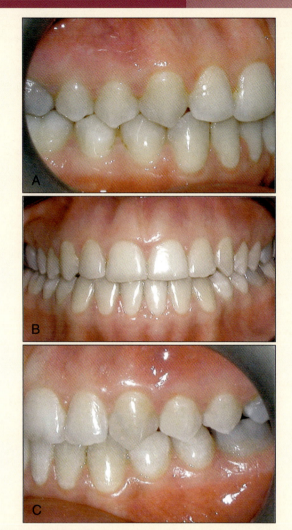

Figure 16-18 Treatment Results. A to C, Posttreatment intraoral photographs.

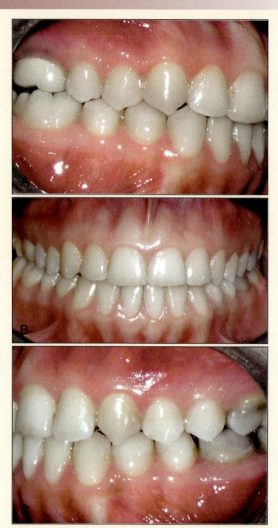

Figure 16-19 Five-Year Follow-Up. A to C, Intraoral photographs demonstrate the stability of achieved treatment goals.

ZYGOMATIC ANCHORAGE–SUPPORTED MOLAR DISTALIZATION

Nonextraction treatment is always the first option for clinicians. Extraoral appliances were used for many years for this purpose. Patient compliance problems and risk of injury reduced the use of extraoral appliances. In recent years, various intraoral molar-distalizing appliances have been developed.[42-51] The mode of activation is similar in these appliances and usually results in anchorage loss, as seen by the proclination of the incisors. The amount of anchorage loss ranges from 30% to 40%.[44,52-54] These appliances constitute an important part of clinician's armamentarium, although their use requires careful patient selection. Intraoral molar distalizers are very effective in cases in which crowding is present and upper incisor proclination is part of the treatment plan.

Implant-supported molar distalization has been performed with different designs by various investigators.[25,28,55-57] Palatal implants were used by many investigators, with successful results.[55,58-61] (Palatal anchorage uses osseointegrated implants and is discussed in Chapter 17.)

In this section we discuss our method for molar distalization with zygomatic anchorage. The surgical procedure is the same as described for open-bite treatment in the previous section.

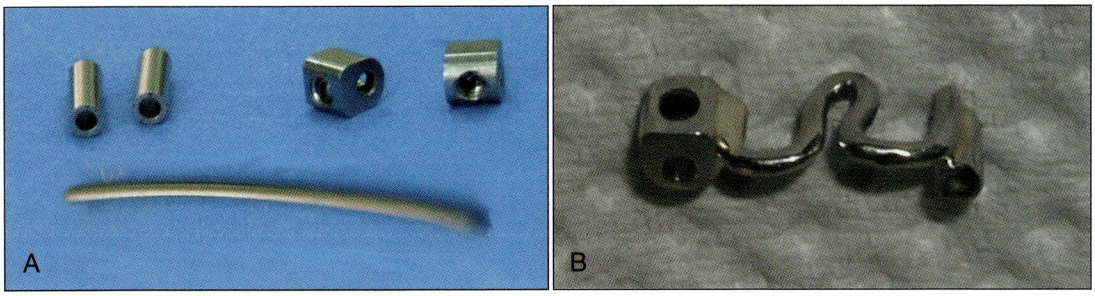

Figure 16-20
Easily accessible materials (A) are used to fabricate the orthodontic attachment (B) to carry the point of force application to the level of the archwire.

CONSTRUCTION OF MOLAR-DISTALIZING APPLIANCES

The MPI's retention plate is adjusted according to the curve of the zygomatic buttress area. The straight-bar extension exposed to the oral cavity is bent to form a lateral step. The length of the step must be at least 2 mm greater than the thickness of the soft tissue; this is important to maintain hygiene in this area. Later, the step bar must be bent toward the mesial direction (see Figure 16-1).

The next step is to carry the point of force application to the level of the archwire. A sliding lock with screw available commercially, a segmental tube with 0.5-mm inner diameter and 4 to 5 mm of length, and a segment of 0.8-mm-thick, round stainless steel wire is required for this purpose. A horizontal U bend is placed on the wire, which is soldered to the sliding lock on one end and to the tube from the other end. The U bend must be in the middle. The length of the wire segment is adjusted to carry the point of force application to the level of the archwire (Figure 16-20).

First molars are banded and first premolars and canines bracketed. A .016 × .022–inch, rectangular stainless steel wire is bent to extend from first molar to canine. A length of Ni-Ti open-coil spring is passed over the rectangular wire, and the wire is inserted into the molar tube. Later, the segmental tube on the lower end of the sliding-bar extension is passed over the rectangular wire, and the sliding lock is engaged on the mesial extension of the implant after compression of the open-coil spring. Sufficient activation to distalize the molars is provided by the compressed coil spring (Figure 16-21).

CLINICAL EXPERIENCE

In all patients requiring molar distalization, the maxillary third molars are extracted before treatment. The average distalization speed is approximately 1 mm per month. The system needs to be reactivated every 2 months. This can be done easily by shifting the sliding lock toward the distal direction or by adding a longer section of open-coil spring. After distalization of molars,

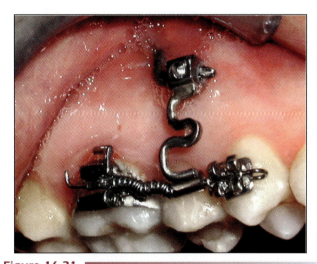

Figure 16-21
Compressed coil spring between the molar tube and the extension retained with the zygomatic implant provides required activation for the distalization of the molar.

second premolars move in the same direction by the action of the transseptal fibers. It is advisable to wait an additional 3 months after completion of the molar distalization to allow transseptal fibers to complete their action.

The unfavorable side effects seen during distalization are the distopalatal rotation and distal crown tipping of the molars. In some cases, distopalatal molar rotation requires an extra treatment procedure to be corrected. Including the second molars in the treatment mechanics is recommended to overcome this side effect. Distal molar crown tipping is negligible, about 3 to 4 degrees, and can be corrected in the later stages of treatment.

After the molar distalization is completed, the coil spring is removed, and the sliding lock is shifted toward the distal direction to achieve tight contact with the molar tube and lock in this position. In this way the molar position is maintained throughout treatment.

CASE REPORT 16-3

A 21-year-old female patient was referred with the chief complaint of dental crowding. Clinical examination revealed unilateral Class II molar relationship on the right side. The upper arch was constricted, and both arches showed slight crowding in the anterior region. The smile line was high, and she had gummy smile with dark corners (Figure 16-22).

Treatment Objectives
1. Achieve correction of the unilateral Class II molar and canine relationship.
2. Improve smile esthetics by eliminating the posterior gummy smile and dark corners.
3. Achieve expansion of the upper arch and alignment of the upper and lower arches.

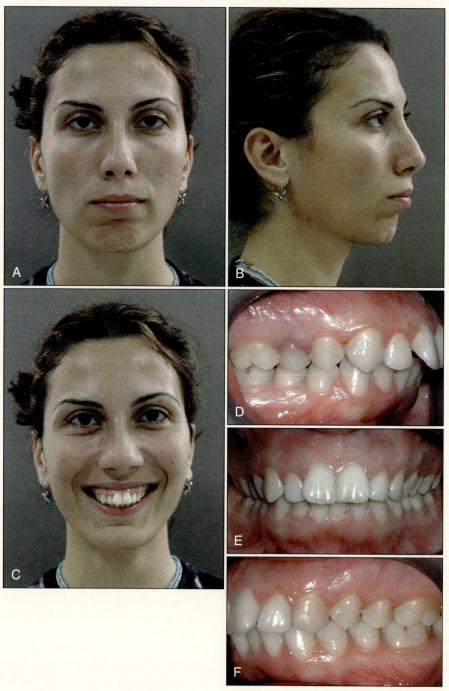

Figure 16-22 Molar Distalization. Pretreatment facial (**A-C**) and intraoral (**D-F**) photographs.

CASE REPORT 16-3—cont'd

Treatment Plan
It was decided to distalize tooth #16 using zygomatic anchorage, followed by fixed-appliance therapy.

Treatment Progress
After implant placement surgery and suture removal at day 7, tooth #16 was banded, #14 was bonded, and the force application was initiated. The patient was seen at 4-week intervals and progress observed. Distalization was completed in 5 months (Figure 16-23).

After completion of distalization, fixed orthodontic therapy was initiated, and the achieved distalization was maintained with wire ligation between the implant and the molar tubes throughout treatment. This was followed by alignment of the arches and detailing of the occlusion with fixed mechanics.

Results
At the end of treatment, a Class I canine and molar relationship and proper overjet and overbite were achieved (Figure 16-24). The maxillary arch was slightly expanded, improving the smile esthetics.

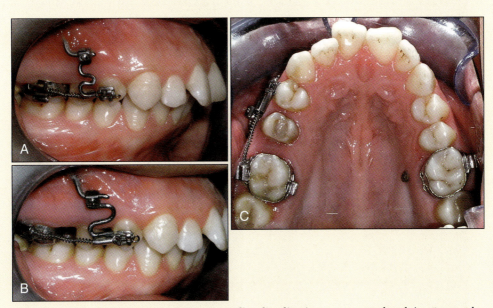

Figure 16-23 Treatment Progress. Molar distalization was completed in 5 months. A, Initial molar position. B and C, Final molar positions.

Continued

CASE REPORT 16-3—cont'd

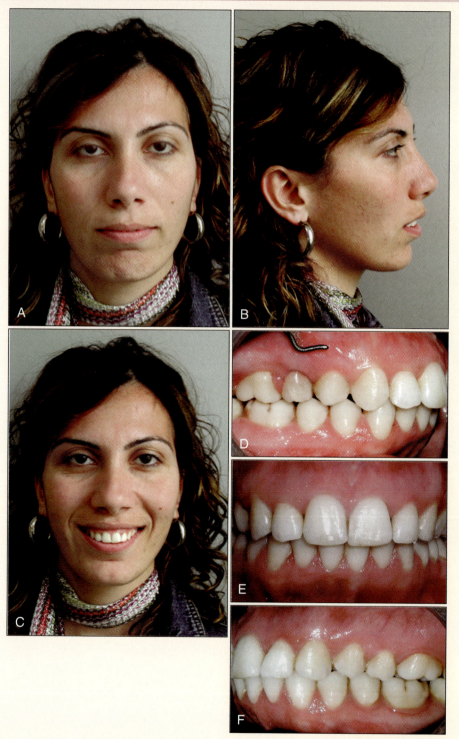

Figure 16-24 Posttreatment Evaluation. Facial (A-C) and intraoral (D-F) photographs after fixed-appliance therapy show symmetrical Class I molar relationship with improved functional and esthetic status.

ZYGOMATIC ANCHORAGE–SUPPORTED EN MASSE RETRACTION

In the treatment of Class II, Division 1 malocclusion characterized by maxillary excess, upper premolar extraction with incisor retraction is a common clinical procedure. In conventional edgewise mechanics, the first step is the canine distalization, followed by incisor retraction. The advantage of this clinical procedure is that because the canines are distalized first, anchorage is not forced excessively, and anchorage maintenance is simple. The disadvantage is that because the procedure has two steps, it takes longer.

Always of interest to some investigators,[62] en masse retraction has the advantage of a shorter treatment time because the canines are not distalized separately. The disadvantage is the difficulty in maintaining anchorage. Despite some anchorage bends and appliances, it is not easy to obtain maximum anchorage in en masse retraction biomechanics. As discussed previously, anchorage implants allow clinicians to obtain stationary anchorage.

IMPLANTS USED

Ball-ended plates developed by Surgi-Tech (Brugge, Belgium) are used (Figure 16-25). These implants contain a horizontal tube in the ball-end area that can be used for wire insertion. The surgical method is the same as for the zygomatic implant procedures previously discussed. Implants are loaded 10 days after the procedure, to allow healing of soft tissue.

MODE OF ACTION

The CR of the anterior segment, including six anterior teeth, was located 3.5 to 4 mm from the apex, as measured from the palatal side of the alveolar bone[63] (Figure 16-26).

The horizontal line drawn parallel to the occlusal plane passing through the tube in the center of the ball end is almost in the CR level; sliding mechanic is planned for use there. Archwire bent from .017 × 0.025–inch stainless steel wire is shaped to connect the six anterior teeth. Arch is bent toward the upper direction from the level of the distal edge of the canine bracket. At the level of the tube in the ball end of the implant, a horizontal bent is made again, and after the horizontal bend a helix facing toward the occlusal plane is placed. During placement of the helix, an Ni-Ti coil spring is placed in the helix. After helix placement, the archwire extends toward the distal direction and ends passing through the tube, with 2 mm of extension. The coil spring is activated between the wire extension and the coil (Figure 16-27).

This biomechanical procedure applies continuous retraction force passing through CR of the anterior segment. Its aim is to obtain parallel retraction of the anterior segment.

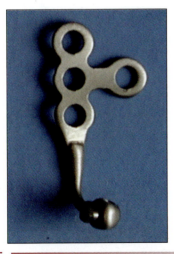

Figure 16-25
Zygoma implant (Surgi-Tech) used for en masse retraction.

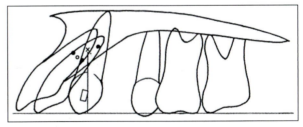

Figure 16-26
The center of resistance of anterior segment before en masse retraction.

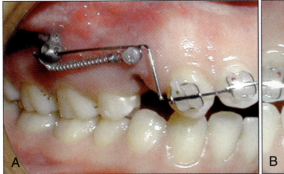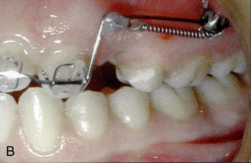

Figure 16-27
A and **B**, Intraoral mechanics for the en masse retraction of the upper incisors.

CASE REPORT 16-4

A 24-year-old female patient presented with a Class II, Division 1 malocclusion. Her chief complaints were an unesthetic facial appearance and a gummy smile. Her anamnesis showed no contraindication to orthodontic treatment. The patient was characterized by an excessively convex facial profile. Her facial appearance was characterized by a short mandibular corpus length, excessive lip strain in the closed-lip position, and an insufficient chin prominence. She had a gummy smile, with an excessive gingival margin showing in both anterior and posterior dentition, and a slight open bite with an associated tongue thrust. Clinical evaluation revealed a Class II molar and canine relationship on both sides, with a 12-mm overjet and 2-mm anterior open bite. The patient also had a maxillary midline diastema and undersized upper lateral incisors (Figure 16-28).

Treatment Objectives

The treatment plan consisted of extraction of the upper first premolars and retraction of the six anterior teeth to correct the excessive overjet. Because the patient refused to wear

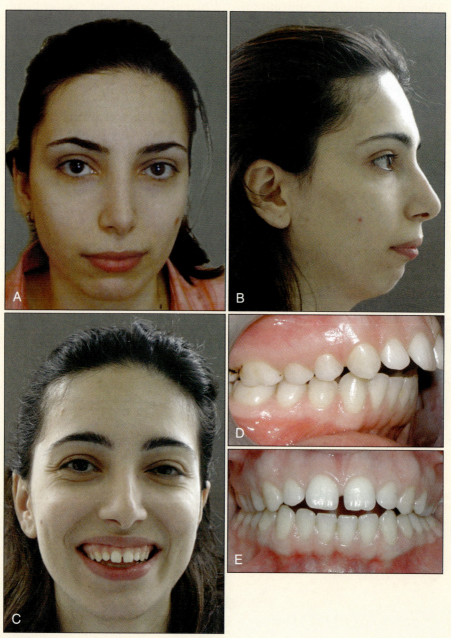

Figure 16-28 **Molar En Masse Retraction.** Pretreatment facial **(A-C)** and intraoral **(D-H)** photographs.

CASE REPORT 16-4—cont'd

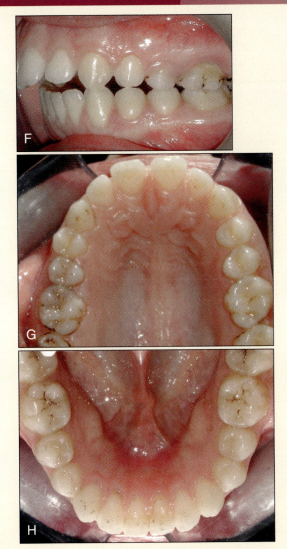

Figure 16-28, cont'd   For legend see opposite page.

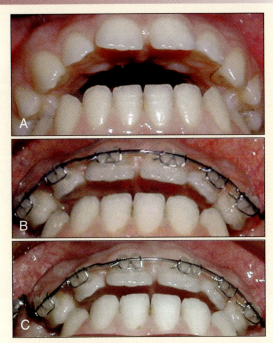

Figure 16-29 Treatment Progress of Overjet Reduction. **A,** Initial position. **B,** Position in fourth month. **C,** Position in sixth month.

headgear during treatment, en masse retraction had to be performed with the anchorage provided by the zygomaticomaxillary buttress.

Treatment Progress

The maxillary first premolars were extracted as part of the orthodontic treatment plan. Roth prescription brackets (.018 inch) were bonded to the upper six anterior teeth. Because there was only a slight misalignment in the incisor region, leveling was postponed until the end of en masse retraction. A .017 × .25–inch stainless steel archwire with slight steps, insets, and offsets was placed passive in the upper bracket slots. The archwire was bent vertically in the apical direction after the canine bracket on each side and after the formation of a helix, bent distally at the same vertical level as the tube on the ball end. The archwire was adjusted to pass through the tubes in the ball ends, and 2-mm wire extensions were left distal to the ball ends. The archwire was engaged in the brackets and tubes and ligated tightly. Ni-Ti closed-coil springs exerting 150 g of force were attached bilaterally to the helices on the archwire. Activation was completed by engaging the free ends of the coil springs to the extensions of the archwire distal to the tubes on both sides. To prevent soft tissue impingement, the helices and the ends of the coil springs were covered with adhesive material (see Figure 16-27).

The patient was requested to return to the clinic each month for control visits. No activation of the coil springs was necessary during these visits. Wire extensions distal to the tubes were shortened at each visit.

Figure 16-29 demonstrates the improvement in the overjet correction at 4 and 6 months compared with the pretreatment overjet. After correction of the overjet, molar bands and premolar brackets were applied and a round, .016-inch, Ni-Ti archwire engaged for leveling, followed by rectangular stainless steel archwires for finishing. No orthodontic treatment was performed in the lower arch. At debonding, slight diastema were left mesial and distal to the undersized upper lateral incisors, which were filled later. A canine-to-canine fixed lingual retainer was placed in the upper arch for retention.

Continued

CASE REPORT 16-4—cont'd

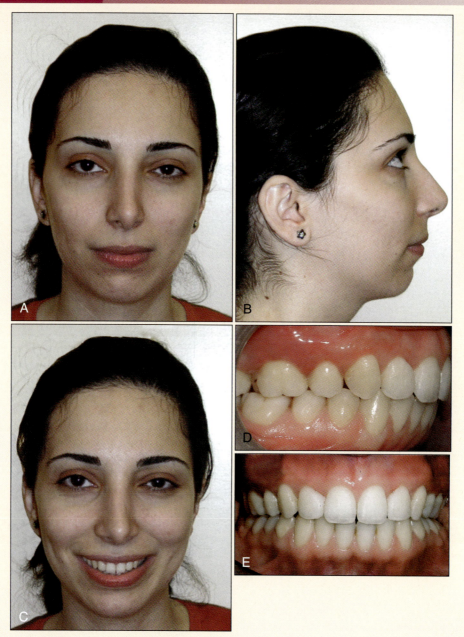

Figure 16-30 Treatment Results. Posttreatment facial (A-C) and intraoral (D-H) photographs.

CASE REPORT 16-4—cont'd

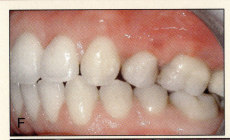
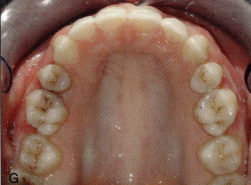
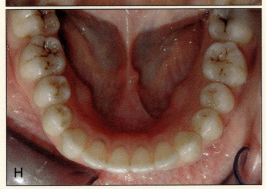

Figure 16-30, cont'd   For legend see opposite page.

Results

The overjet was reduced to normal limits in 6 months (Figure 16-30), and the overall treatment lasted 17 months. No movement in the molar area was observed.

Cephalometric superimposition showed that the incisor movement was controlled tipping rather than the bodily movement originally planned (Figure 16-31). A side effect observed during treatment was palatal tipping of the canines.

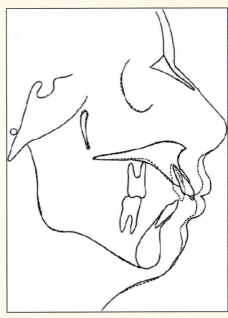

Figure 16-31   **Cephalometric Superimposition.** Incisor movement was controlled tipping rather than planned bodily movement.

CLASS II FUNCTIONAL TREATMENT WITH BONE ANCHORAGE

Class II malocclusion, one of the most popular subjects in orthodontics, affects about 25% of the general population.[64,65] It can originate from maxillary excess, retrognathic mandible, or a combination of both. The variable morphological pattern has led to different treatment approaches.

The prevalence of mandibular retrognathia in the total Class II population is about 60%. Fixed appliances, extraoral appliances, removable fixed appliances, fixed functional appliances, and orthognathic surgery are used to treat mandibular retrognathia. Fixed functional appliances are used most often (e.g., Herbst, Jasper Jumper, Twin Force Bite Corrector). Investigations showed that 30% of Class II correction from fixed functional appliances is attributed to skeletal response and 70% to dentoalveolar response.[66] Uncontrolled labial tipping of mandibular incisors is the common side effect of these appliances. The fixed-functional-appliance correction of Class II malocclusion requires about 6 months, with rapid labial tipping of the lower incisors limiting the time needed to obtain more skeletal response.

Application of mandibular prognathic force directly through the mandibular corpus can prevent the uncontrolled tipping of the mandibular incisors and allows enough time for skeletal growth, a key factor in the correction of mandibular retrognathia.

This section discusses the clinical effects of anteriorly directed force application through the bone on mandible.

IMPLANTS USED

Special implants were developed for this procedure, with different designs for left and right sides and with three parts. The first part is the *retentive plate*, which has three holes for fixation. For the right implant, the plate includes a triangular extension in the mesial side, designed to prevent the mesial rotation of the plate. The left plate is the same, except the triangular extension is in the reverse position. The second part of the implant is the *bar extension*, which has a thickness of 2 mm. Its function is to carry the point of force application to the lower canine area. The bar extends in the same direction with the retentive plate for 8 mm, and with a 30-degree angle, it uprights. Total bar length is 16 mm. This bar is also bendable, and slight adjustments can be made. The third part of the implant is the *ball end*, including a round tube 1 mm in diameter. The ball part is used for the attachment of the fixed functional appliance (Figure 16-32).

SURGICAL METHOD

A horizontal incision is made, connecting the distal level of canines along the intersection of attached and mobile gingiva. Vertical incisions are extended about 1 cm for both sides. Mucoperiosteum is released. The incision is very important; implants can be exposed into the oral cavity from the corner of the incisors on both sides. Implants need to be adjusted and placed accurately. The ball end must be in the middle level of mandibular canines and slightly in distal position. The bar must be 4 mm from the soft tissue, and the ball end must be 2 mm from the canine, for hygiene in this area. The angulation of the tube is also important and must be checked carefully (Figure 16-33).

CLINICAL PROCEDURE

After allowing 7 to 10 days for the healing of the soft tissue, the implant is ready for loading. The first step is to select Jasper Jumpers (JJ) of the right size. Distance between the distal edge of the extraoral tube and the mesial edge of the ball end is measured. To this distance, 12 mm is added: 4 mm for activation, 4 mm for the extension after molar tube, and 4 mm for the extension after ball end, for the free movement of JJ (Figure 16-34).

After placement of JJ, the patient is instructed about oral hygiene requirements. In every session, stability of the implants and oral hygiene are controlled.

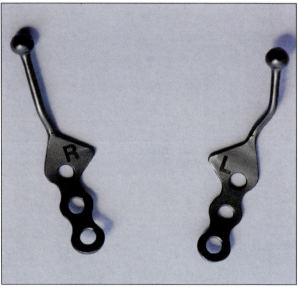

Figure 16-32
Left and right implants for bone anchorage are symmetrical and encompass three fixation holes. The triangular extension above the first hole provides support to overcome the stresses attempting to rotate the implant.

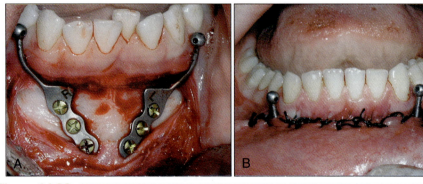

Figure 16-33
A, Two implants from Figure 16-32 are placed on either side of the symphysis in Class II malocclusion. **B,** Ball ends are exposed to the oral cavity from the canine region at the mucogingival junction.

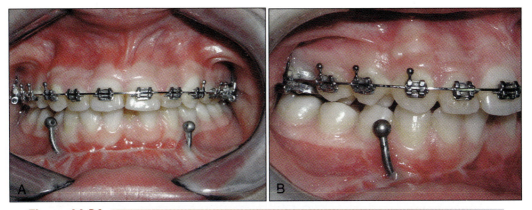

Figure 16-34

A and B, Same case as Figure 16-33. Healing is generally very good in about 10 days, and the implants are now ready to be loaded.

CASE REPORT 16-5

A 14-year-old female patient presented with a Class II, Division 1 malocclusion. Her chief complaint was crowding in the anterior region. The patient was characterized by a slightly convex facial profile resulting from a retrognathic mandible. She presented with a Class II molar and canine relationship on both sides, along with a 6-mm overjet. The maxilla was constricted, and the two upper laterals were trapped palatally. She also presented a slight amount of crowding in the lower anterior region (Figure 16-35).

Treatment Objectives

The treatment plan consisted of expansion and leveling of the upper arch, followed by fixed-functional-appliance therapy to eliminate the overjet and to correct the molar and canine relationships. The mandibular anchorage was to be provided by implants.

Treatment Progress

After rapid maxillary expansion, the upper arch was leveled and aligned. The lateral incisor positions were also corrected (Figure 16-36, A-H). At this stage, the two implants were fixed under local anesthesia, and force application was initiated with JJ (Figure 16-36, I-K).

Results

The overjet was reduced to normal limits in 5 months, and the overall treatment lasted 17 months (Figure 16-37).

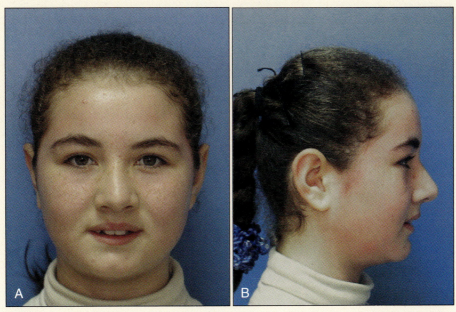

Figure 16-35 Bone Anchorage for Class II Treatment. Pretreatment facial (A-C) and intraoral (D-H) photographs.

Continued

CASE REPORT 16-5—cont'd

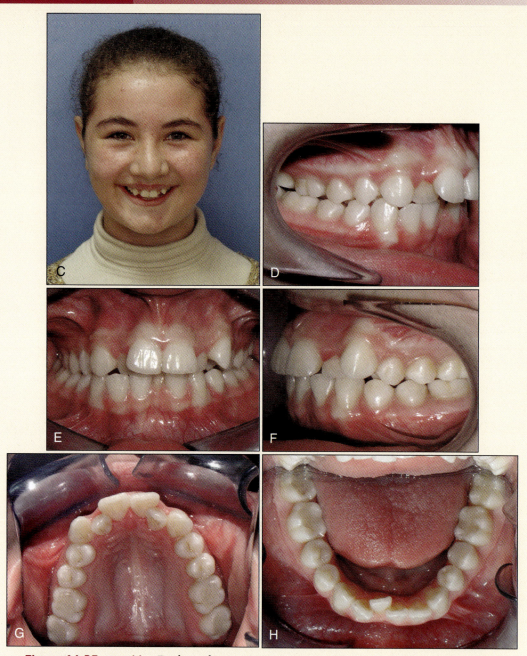

Figure 16-35, cont'd For legend see p. 367.

CASE REPORT 16-5—cont'd

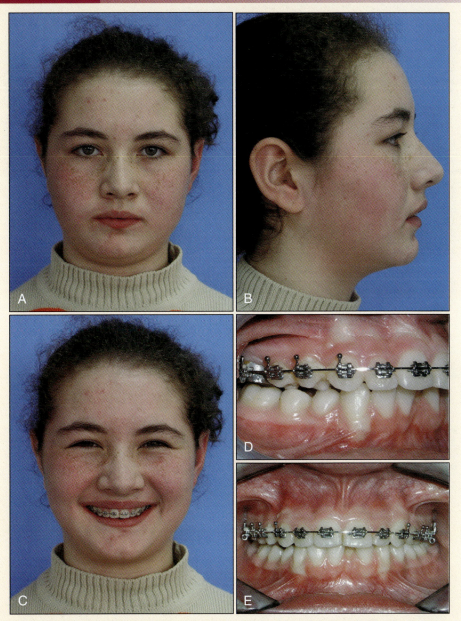

Figure 16-36 First Phase of Treatment. Facial **(A-C)** and intraoral **(D-H)** photographs show rapid maxillary expansion followed by leveling and aligning with the fixed appliance. **I** to **K,** Clinical application of Jasper Jumpers on mandibular implants. Ball end of the implants is designed so that the Jaspers can be easily fixed here.

Continued

CASE REPORT 16-5—cont'd

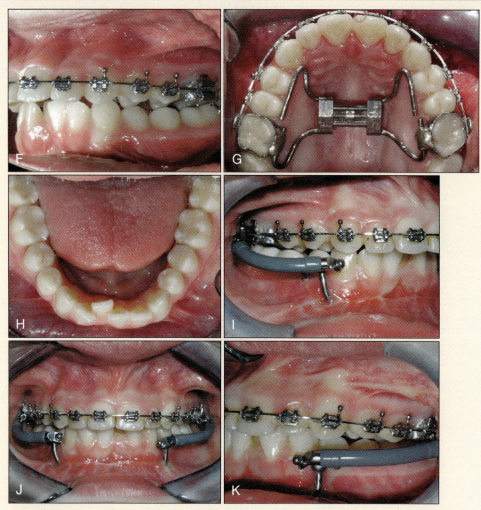

Figure 16-36, cont'd   For legend see p. 369.

CASE REPORT 16-5—cont'd

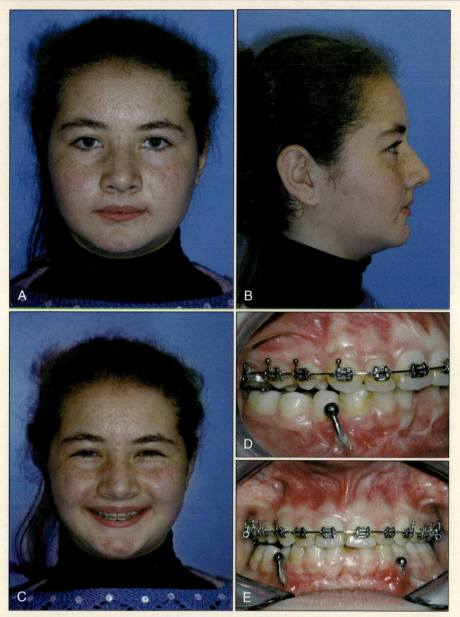

Figure 16-37 Treatment Results. Posttreatment facial (A-C) and intraoral (D-H) photographs show that the overjet was eliminated and that molar and canine relationships were corrected in 5 months, without adverse effects on the lower dental arch.

Continued

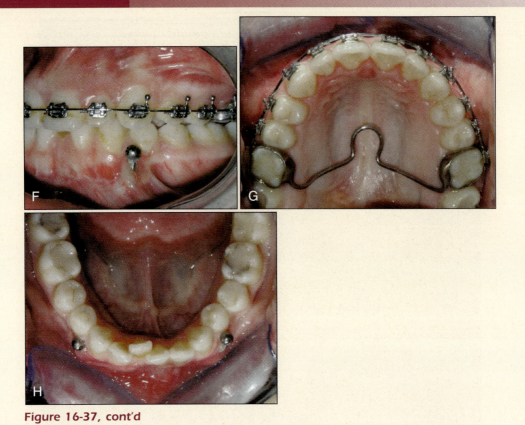

Figure 16-37, cont'd

CONCLUSION

Implants in the zygomatic buttress area are easy to place and remove under local anesthesia. Treatment generally progresses as expected, provided the implant is exposed into the oral cavity properly (from a stable gingival location) and the patient follows optimal oral hygiene protocol throughout treatment. Zygomatic anchorage implants can be used in various clinical scenarios where absolute anchorage is required, without depending on patient compliance. This type of an anchorage also enables the clinician to treat certain open-bite cases (e.g., overeruption of maxillary posterior dentoalveolar segment) that would otherwise require surgery. Zygomatic implants provide the orthodontist with new treatment possibilities, provided that careful case selection and proper surgical and clinical application are used.

REFERENCES

1. Higley LB: Anchorage in orthodontics, *Am J Orthod* 46:456-465, 1960.
2. Gray JB, Steen ME, King GJ, Clark AE: Studies on the efficacy of implants as orthodontic anchorage, *Am J Orthod* 83:311-317, 1983.
3. Egolf RJ, Begole EA, Upshaw HS: Factors associated with orthodontic patient compliance with intraoral elastic and headgear wear, *Am J Orthod* 97:336-348, 1990.
4. American Association of Orthodontists: Special bulletin on extraoral appliance care, *Am J Orthod* 75:457, 1975.
5. American Association of Orthodontists: Bulletin. Preliminary results of head gear survey, 1:2, 1982.
6. Samuels RH: A review of orthodontic face-bow injuries and safety equipment, *Am J Orthod Dentofacial Orthop* 110:269-272, 1996.
7. Creekmore TA, Eklund MK: The possibility of skeletal anchorage, *J Clin Orthod* 17:266-269, 1983.
8. Linder-Aronson S, Nordenram A, Anneroth G: Titanium implant anchorage in orthodontic treatment: an experimental investigation in monkeys, *Eur J Orthod* 12:414-419, 1990.
9. Albrektsson T, Branemark PI, Hansson HA, Lindstrom J: Osseointegrated titanium implants: requirements for ensuring a long-lasting, direct bone-to-implant anchorage in man, *Acta Orthop Scand* 52:155-170, 1981.
10. Javier Gil F, Planell JA, Padros A, Aparicio C: The effect of shot blasting and heat treatment on the fatigue behavior of titanium for dental implant applications, *Dent Mater* 11, 2006.
11. Nakagawa M, Zhang L, Udoh K, et al: Effects of hydrothermal treatment with CaCl(2) solution on surface property and cell response of titanium implants, *J Mater Sci Mater Med* 16:985-991, 2005.
12. Takemoto M, Fujibayashi S, Neo M, et al: Mechanical properties and osteoconductivity of porous bioactive titanium biomaterials, *Biomaterials* 26:6014-6023, 2005.
13. Wennerberg A, Albrektsson T, Andersson B: Design and surface characteristics of 13 commercially available oral implant systems, *Int J Oral Maxillofac Implants* 8:622-633, 1993.
14. Gainsforth BL: A study of orthodontic anchorage possibilities in basal bone, *Am J Orthod Oral Surg* 31:406-417, 1945.

15. Linkow LI: Implanto-orthodontics, *Clin J Orthod* 4:685-705, 1970.
16. Schlegel KA, Schweizer C, Janson IR, Wiltfang J: A new anchorage concept for orthodontic treatment in the mandible, *World J Orthod* 3:353-357, 2002.
17. Clerck H, Geerinckx V, Siciliano S: The zygoma anchorage system, *J Clin Orthod* 36:455-459, 2002.
18. Kanomi R: Mini-implant for orthodontic anchorage, *J Clin Orthod* 31:763-767, 1997.
19. Costa A, Raffling M, Millstone B: Miniscrews as orthodontic anchorage: a preliminary report, *Int J Adult Orthod Orthogn Surg* 13:201-209, 1998.
20. Bousquet F, Bousquet P, Mauran G, Parguel P: Use of an impacted post for anchorage, *J Clin Orthod* 30:261-265, 1996.
21. Park H, Bae S, Kyung H, Sung J: Micro-implant anchorage for treatment of skeletal Class I bialveolar protrusion, *J Clin Orthod* 35:417-422, 2001.
22. Lee JS, Park HS, Kyung HM: Micro-implant anchorage for lingual treatment of a skeletal Class II malocclusion, *J Clin Orthod* 35:643-647, 2001.
23. Roberts WE, Helm FR, Marshall KJ, Gongloff RK: Rigid endosseous implants for orthodontic and orthopedic anchorage, *Angle Orthod* 59:247-255, 1989.
24. Sherman A: Bone reaction to orthodontic forces on vitreous carbon dental implants, *Am J Orthod* 74:79-87, 1978.
25. Block MS, Hoffman DR: A new device for absolute anchorage for orthodontics, *Am J Orthod* 107:251-258, 1995.
26. Melsen B, Petersen JK, Costa A: Zygoma ligatures: an alternative form of maxillary anchorage, *J Clin Orthod* 32:154-158, 1998.
27. Kokich VG, Shapiro PA, Oswald R, et al: Ankylosed teeth as abutments for maxillary protraction: a case report, *Am J Orthod* 88:303-307, 1985.
28. Wehrbein H, Glatzmaier J, Mundwiller U, Diedrich P: The Orthosystem: a new implant system for orthodontic anchorage in the palate, *J Orofac Orthop* 57:143-153, 1996.
29. Umemori M, Sugawara J, Nagasaka H, Kawamura H: Skeletal anchorage system for open-bite correction, *Am J Orthop* 115:166-174, 1999.
30. Chung KR, Kim YS, Linton JL, Lee YJ: The miniplate with tube for skeletal anchorage, *J Clin Orthod* 36:407-412, 2002.
31. Maino BG, Bednar J, Pagin P, Mura P: The spider screw for skeletal anchorage, *J Clin Orthod* 37:90-97, 2003.
32. Erverdi N, Keles A, Nanda R: The use of skeletal anchorage in open bite treatment: a cephalometric evaluation, *Angle Orthod* 74:381-390, 2004.
33. Erverdi N, Üşümez S, Solak A: New generation open-bite treatment with zygomatic anchorage, *Angle Orthod* 76:519-526, 2006.
34. Swinehart EW: A clinical study of open-bite, *Am J Orthod Oral Surg* 28:18-34, 1942.
35. Subtelny JD, Sakuda M: Open bite diagnosis and treatment, *Am J Orthod* 50:337-358, 1964.
36. Sicher H, Weinmann JP: Bone growth and physiologic tooth movement, *Am J Orthod Oral Surg* 30:109, 1944.
37. Kelley JE, Harvey CR: An assessment of the occlusion of the teeth of youths 12-17 years, US Department of Health, Education and Welfare Pub No HRA 77-1644, 1977; *Vital Health Stat Series* 11:1-65, 1977.
38. Proffit WR: In Proffit WR, Fields HW, editors: *Contemporary orthodontics*, St Louis, 1986, Mosby.
39. Lopez-Gavito G, Wallen TR, Little RM, Joondeph DR: Anterior open-bite malocclusion: a longitudinal 10-year postretention evaluation of orthodontically treated patients, *Am J Orthod* 87:175-186, 1985.
40. Ari-Demirkaya A, Al Masry M, Erverdi N: Apical root resorption of maxillary first molars after intrusion with zygomatic skeletal anchorage, *Angle Orthod* 75:761-767, 2005.
41. Lowe AA: Correlations between orofacial muscle activity and craniofacial morphology in a sample of control and anterior open-bite subjects, *Am J Orthod* 78:89-92, 1980.
42. Cetlin NM, Ten Hoeve A: Nonextraction treatment, *J Clin Orthod* 17:396-413, 1983.
43. Wilson RC, Wilson WL: *Enhanced orthodontics. 1. Concept, treatment and case histories*, Denver, 1988, Rocky Mountain Orthodontics.
44. Gianelly AA, Vaitas AS, Thomas WM: The use of magnets to move molars distally, *Am J Orthod Dentofacial Orthop* 96:161-167, 1989.
45. Bondemark L, Kurol J: Distalization of maxillary first and second molars simultaneously with repelling magnets, *Eur J Orthod* 14:264-272, 1992.
46. Ten Hoeve A: Palatal bar and lip bumper in nonextraction treatment, *J Clin Orthod* 19:272-291, 1985.
47. Jeckel N, Rakosi T: Molar distalization by intra-oral force application, *Eur J Orthod* 13:43-46, 1991.
48. Pancherz H, Anehus-Pancherz M: The headgear effect of the Herbst appliance: a cephalometric long-term study, *Am J Orthod Dentofacial Orthop* 103:510-520, 1993.
49. Erverdi N, Koyuturk O, Kucukkeles N: Nickel-titanium coil springs and repelling magnets: a comparison of two different intra-oral molar distalization techniques, *Br J Orthod* 24:47-53, 1997.
50. Karaman AI, Basciftci FA, Polat O: Unilateral distal molar movement with an implant-supported Distal Jet appliance, *Angle Orthod* 72:167-174, 2002.
51. Gelgor IE, Buyukyilmaz T, Karaman AI, et al: Intraosseous screw-supported upper molar distalization, *Angle Orthod* 74:838-850, 2004.
52. Gianelly AA, Vaitas AS, Thomas WM: Distalization of molars with repelling magnets, *Clin Orthod* 22:40-44, 1988.
53. Joseph AA, Butchart CJ: An evaluation of the pendulum distalizing appliance, *Semin Orthod* 6:129-135, 2000.
54. Muse DS, Fillman MJ, Emmerson WJ, et al: Molar and incisor changes with Wilson rapid molar distalization, *Am J Orthod Dentofacial Orthop* 104:556-565, 1993.
55. Keles A, Erverdi N, Sezen S: Bodily distalization of molars with absolute anchorage, *Angle Orthod* 73:471-482, 2003.
56. Karcher H, Byloff FK, Clar E: The Graz implant supported pendulum, a technical note, *J Craniomaxillofac Surg* 30:87-90, 2002.
57. Wehrbein H, Feifel H, Diedrich P: Palatal implant anchorage reinforcement of posterior teeth: a prospective study, *Am J Orthod Dentofacial Orthop* 116:678-686, 1999.
58. De Clerck H, Geerinckx V, Siciliano S: The zygoma anchorage system, *J Clin Orthod* 36:455-459, 2002.
59. Wehrbein H, Hovel P, Kinzinger G, Stefan B: Load-deflection behavior of transpalatal bars supported on orthodontic palatal implants: an in vitro study, *J Orofac Orthop* 65:312-320, 2004.
60. Majumdar A, Tinsley D, O'Dwyer J, et al: The "Chesterfield stent": an aid to the placement of midpalatal implants, *Br J Oral Maxillofac Surg* 43:36-39, 2005.
61. Crismani AG, Bernhart T, Bantleon HP, Kucher G: An innovative adhesive procedure for connecting transpalatal arches with palatal implants, *Eur J Orthod* 27:226-230, 2005.
62. Guray E, Orhan M: "En masse" retraction of maxillary anterior teeth with anterior headgear, *Am J Orthod Dentofacial Orthop* 112:473-479, 1997.
63. Erverdi N, Acar A: Zygomatic anchorage for en masse retraction in the treatment of severe Class II division 1, *Angle Orthod* 75:483-490, 2005.
64. Abu Alhaija ES, Al-Khateeb SN, Al-Nimri KS: Prevalence of malocclusion in 13-15 year-old North Jordanian school children, *Community Dent Health* 22:266-271, 2005.
65. Soh J, Sandham A, Chan YH: Occlusal status in Asian male adults: prevalence and ethnic variation, *Angle Orthod* 75:814-820, 2005.
66. Cozza P, De Toffol L, Iacopini L: An analysis of the corrective contribution in activator treatment, *Angle Orthod* 74:741-748, 2004.

CHAPTER 17

Palatal Anchorage

Nejat Erverdi and Ahu Acar

OSSEOINTEGRATED IMPLANTS IN THE HARD PALATE

After the concept of osseointegration was introduced in implantology, orthodontists began to search for possible orthodontic applications of implants.[1-6] An osseointegrated implant is the functional equivalent of an ankylosed tooth, so it would be expected to serve well as a stationary anchorage unit. The term *stationary anchorage* means that the anchorage unit does not move in reaction to the applied orthodontic forces and moments.[7] When stationary anchorage is available, 100% of the extraction space can be closed with the movement of the anterior or posterior teeth, depending on the aim of the treatment. Experimental biomechanical studies,[8,9] studies on animal models,[9-14] and clinical investigations[15-17] have shown that dental implants placed in the alveolar bone were resistant to orthodontic force application. Because orthodontic patients generally have a complete dentition without any alveolar space available for implant placement, the retromolar area[4,18] and the median sagittal region of the hard palate[19-24] were suggested as suitable locations for implant placement.

The hard palate has long been used as an anchorage site in conventional orthodontics. The Nance button, a common anchorage appliance used in the hard palate, is a suitable choice in moderate anchorage situations, but it is not sufficient for maximum anchorage requirements. The hard palate is readily accessible to the surgeon and offers excellent periimplant conditions because of abundant attached mucosa. Osseointegrated implants placed in the hard palate can be used for anchorage reinforcement in many demanding orthodontic applications.[25-27]

ANATOMICAL CONSIDERATIONS IN PALATAL IMPLANT PLACEMENT

BONE THICKNESS

The midpalatal suture, the area adjacent to the midpalatal suture, and the incisor region are the areas with maximal bone height in the hard palate. In a computed tomography (CT) study, Gahleitner et al.[28] found that the overall mean palatal bone height was 5.01 mm, ranging from 0 to 16.9 mm. The maximum palatal height was 6.17 mm, measured 6 mm dorsally from the incisive canal. Henriksen et al.[29] reported that the actual bone available for midsagittal implants was 4.3 ± 1.6 mm. These findings indicate that sufficient bone exists for complete osseointegration of 4-mm implants; 6-mm implants should be used with caution.

It is widely accepted that diagnostic CT scans are the most reliable tools for detection of bone height in the hard palate area. On the other hand, because of factors such as cost-effectiveness, concerns about patient protection from excessive radiation, and clinical practicality, the lateral cephalograms are still frequently used for identification of palatal bone height (Box 17-1). Crismani et al.[30] reported that on lateral cephalograms, the palatal complex averaged 0.8 mm below the actual anatomical size. Wehrbein et al.[24] showed in dry skulls that at least 2 mm of extra bone depth was present in the sagittal area of the palate than indicated on a lateral cephalogram. This result should be regarded with caution, however, because presence of extra bone depth must not be taken into consideration in the calculation of actual bone thickness for implant placement. It should be reserved as a "safety distance" in preventing nasal perforation during implant placement.

INCISIVE CANAL PERFORATION

Implants placed in an anterior location along the midpalatal suture area can create incisive nerve injury. Using CT scans from 22 patients, Bernhart et al.[31] reported that to prevent perforation of the incisive canal, implants must be placed 6 to 9 mm distal to it.

ROOT INJURIES

Palatal implants placed in the anterior slope of the hard palate can cause incisor root injuries. In some cases the implant and the incisor root may not be in contact but may be in proximity, and thus it is important to consider both pretreatment and posttreatment incisor posi-

> **BOX 17-1 Guidelines for Palatal Implant Placement**
>
> 1. Lateral cephalograms are useful in detection of palatal bone height and optimal implant location.
> 2. A paramedian placement of the implants is recommended, and a slight lateral orientation is preferable, to find sufficient bone material.
> 3. To prevent incisive canal injury, implants should be placed 6 mm posterior to the incisive canal.
> 4. Posttreatment incisor position must be considered at the diagnostic stage.

tions. Root injury can easily occur during retraction of the incisors unless the implant is placed in the proper location. The levels of the upper first and second premolars provide the most appropriate anteroposterior (AP) site for implant entry.

MEDIAN OR PARAMEDIAN IMPLANT PLACEMENT

Melsen[32] concluded that ossification in the midpalatal suture was variable and was completed after age 27 years in men and even later in women. More recently, Schlegel et al.[33] reported in a cadaver study that complete ossification of the suture was rare before age 23 years. Also, because the anterior part of the midpalatal suture was often less ossified than the posterior region, a bone bed more favorable for osseointegration might be found posterior to the interconnecting line of the first premolars.

Both median[21,22] and paramedian[23,26,27] placement of palatal implants have been reported. In subjects with complete suture ossification, a median location would not create a problem. In the subjects with unossified sutures, however, the implant would be in contact with the fibrous tissue in the suture, and therefore the chances of total osseointegration would be less than for the implants with paramedian location. On the other hand, Schlegel et al.[33] reported that the connective tissue band in the midpalatal suture area was only 0.03 cm. Considering that the palatal implant has a diameter of 3.3 mm in the Orthosystem (Institute Straumann, Waldenburg, Switzerland) and 4.5 mm in the Frialit system (Friadent GmbH, Mannheim, Germany), only a very small portion of the implant would be in contact with the connective tissue when placed in the midpalatal suture area, minimizing the concerns about poor osseointegration.

Another critical issue is the possible effect of an implant placed in the midpalatal suture on transverse growth of the maxilla. Growth in the midpalatal suture increases the width of the palate and is considered to be more important than appositional remodeling of the alveolar processes in the development of maxillary width.[34] Björk and Skieller[35] found an average increase in maxillary width of 3 mm between ages 10 and 18 years, as measured between posterior implants on the radiographs of nine boys. Asscherickx et al.[36] evaluated the influence of orthodontic anchorage implants on transverse maxillary growth when inserted in the median palatal suture of growing dogs and reported restricted transverse growth of hard palate in the canine region. Because of ethical considerations, such investigations can be performed only in animals. In light of these findings, paramedian placement of palatal implants may be recommended in growing individuals.

ARTERIAL DAMAGE AND BLEEDING

There is always a risk of causing arterial damage during removal of the palatal soft tissue with a punch drill. To prevent bleeding during the procedure, an anesthetic with a vasoconstrictor agent should be infused around the area of implant placement. In cases with aggressive bleeding, the artery can be sutured.

RADIOGRAPHIC EVALUATION OF BONE HEIGHT AT IMPLANT SITE

An acrylic resin template that covers the occlusal surfaces of the maxillary teeth is constructed on a stone model of the maxilla. A spherical metal marker is embedded in the acrylic resin template at the highest point of the palate in the midline (Figure 17-1). The metal marker is placed to calculate the magnification of the radiograph when assessing the exact bony dimensions of the implant site and to create a reference point in the sagittal direction for identifying the drilling site.

A lateral cephalogram of the patient is obtained with the acrylic resin template in the mouth (Figure 17-2). Bone height at the implant site is measured in relation to the metal marker, which has a diameter of 5 mm. Patients who have at least 4 mm of bone height are accepted as suitable for palatal implant placement. Those without enough bone thickness are candidates for onplant placement.

SURGICAL TEMPLATE FOR POSITIONING IMPLANT

To construct a three-dimensional (3D) surgical template for accurate implant orientation, the following procedure is suggested.

The stone model used for template preparation is cut along the midpalatal line, passing through the mesial aspect of the central incisor. On the lateral cephalogram the maxilla and central incisor are traced on a tracing paper and then cut along the pencil line and superimposed on the paramedian section of the stone model. A drill insertion hole is prepared in the acrylic resin template, using a 2.5-mm-diameter stainless steel bur. A

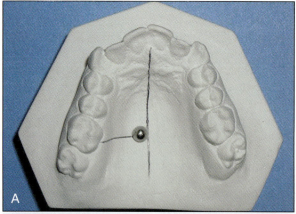

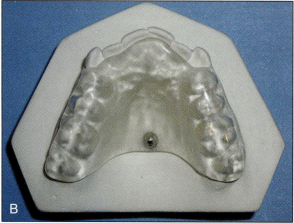

Figure 17-1
A, Spherical marker 5 mm in length is placed on the stone model at the highest point of the hard palate. **B,** Spherical marker is embedded in the acrylic template.

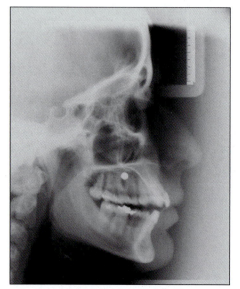

Figure 17-2
Lateral cephalogram of the patient is obtained with the template inserted in the patient's mouth. The spherical marker will be useful in measuring the actual bone height at the implant site.

cylindrical metal housing, 7 mm in length and 2.1 mm in diameter, with a pilot drill in it, is placed in the drill insertion hole. The implant drill is adjusted to emerge 8 mm out of the metal housing. In the sagittal plane the desired implant inclination in relation to the incisor roots and the nasal cavity is established. The implant axis is adjusted between 45 and 60 degrees to the occlusal plane. The implant should be oriented at least 3 to 4 mm above the apices of the incisor roots. The metal housing is then fixed to the acrylic template by cold-curing acrylic. In the transverse plane the metal housing should have a lateral orientation with 2 mm of distance from the midpalatal suture (Figure 17-3).

SURGICAL METHOD

Before the surgical procedure, the patient is asked to rinse the mouth with 0.2% chlorhexidine gluconate for 1 minute. After this rinsing, the palatal region is locally anesthetized with a vasoconstrictor agent. The surgical template is placed in the mouth to mark the implant position. A pilot drill is applied through the metal housing in the template. Mucosa is then removed using a punch drill, and the standard surgical protocol for placing the chosen implant system is followed. Drilling is carried out at 1000 rpm under internal and external sterile saline cooling. Drills with 8-mm-long stoppers are used in the following order: pilot drill of 2-mm diameter, twist drill of 3-mm diameter, and spade drill of 4.5-mm diameter (Figure 17-4).

Palatal implant (Friadent) is placed transmucosally so that a 4-mm length of the implant will stay in the bone and 4 mm will stay in the palatal mucosa and serve as an extension to reach the oral cavity. Transmucosal placement of the implant will be an advantage to avoid secondary surgery. To avoid postoperative pain, an analgesic agent is recommended, and the patient is instructed to use an antiseptic mouthwash twice daily for 2 weeks. The osseointegration of the palatal implants takes about 3 months, during which the implant should not be loaded.

After waiting 3 months for osseointegration, a "gingiva former" of proper size is screwed onto the implant. One week is usually sufficient for shaping of the palatal mucosa (Figure 17-5).

EVALUATION OF IMPLANT PLACEMENT METHOD

The accuracy of the implant placement method may be tested by superimposition of the presurgical and postsurgical lateral cephalograms taken with template in the mouth (Figure 17-6).

The acrylic resin template, described previously, serves only as a guide for the pilot drill. The following drills are applied through the initial hole created by the pilot drill. The operator should be extremely careful to

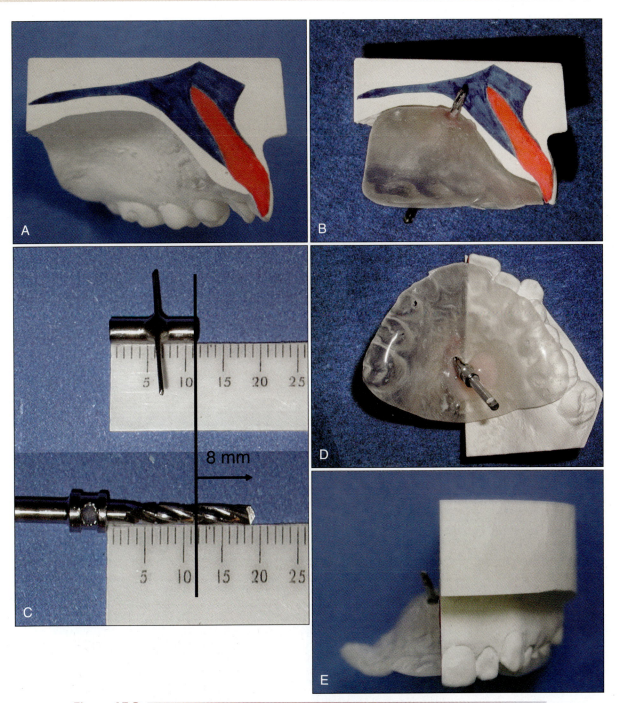

Figure 17-3
A, Maxillary tracing is superimposed on the model. B, Pilot drill should be oriented between 45 and 60 degrees to the occlusal plane. The drill axis should pass at least 3 to 4 mm above the apices of the incisors. C, Pilot drill is adjusted to emerge 8 mm out of the metal housing. D, Metal housing is fixed to the template with cold-curing acrylic. E, In the frontal plane, pilot drill should be about 2 mm laterally oriented from the median line.

maintain the orientation of the implant bed. Any significant deviation in the angulation of the handpiece relative to the initial path of the pilot drill can result in the destruction of the cortical bone shoulder surrounding the implant cavity. This permanent damage of the surrounding bone will reduce the primary stability of the implant.

Recently, an alternative method for surgical stent fabrication, which also involves combined cephalometric and model planning, has been described by Cousley and Parberry.[37] In this method the planned implant position is transferred to a mounted model using a premolar vertical reference plane constructed on the lateral cephalogram. The surgical stent described by the

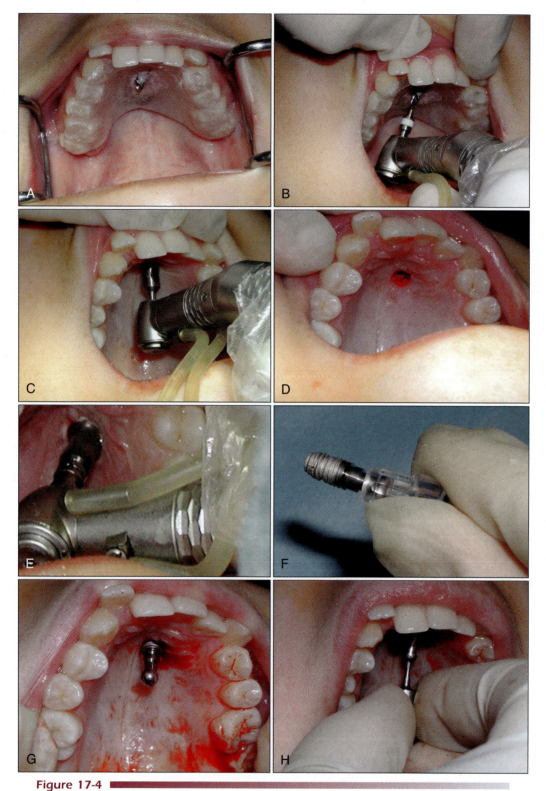

Figure 17-4

A, Paramedian and lateral orientation of the metal housing in the surgical template. B, Pilot drill application through the metal housing in the template. C, Template is removed from the mouth, and a punch drill is applied to the implant site to remove the mucosa. D, Implant site after removal of the mucosa. E, Preparation of the implant bed. F and G, Placement of the palatal implant. H, Removal of the implant carrier.

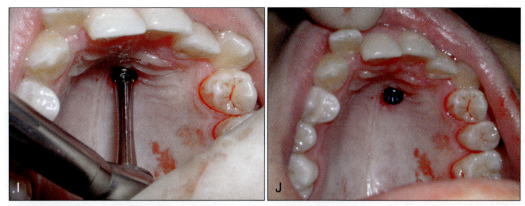

Figure 17-4, cont'd **I** and **J**, Screwing of the implant.

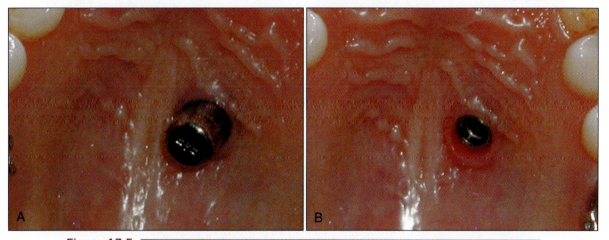

Figure 17-5

A, Gingiva former applied after 3 months. **B**, Shaping of the palatal mucosa by the gingiva former.

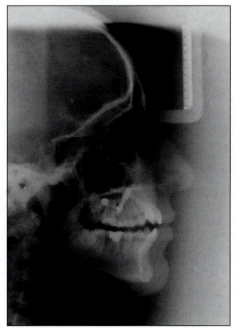

Figure 17-6

Superimposition of the presurgical and postsurgical lateral cephalograms taken with the template in the mouth. The implant is located on the same axis as the metal housing, indicating the accuracy of the implant positioning.

authors includes a guide channel for the orientation of all the drills used during implant bed preparation.

The surgical procedure for palatal implant placement proved to be successful and practical, with only a few complications (e.g., slight bleeding) that can easily be controlled. The surgical procedure lasts no longer than 10 to 15 minutes, and patient comfort during and after the procedure is excellent. The only risk is the possibility of the implant carrier being swallowed by the patient while it is being removed. In the standard surgical protocols of almost all implant systems, the implant carrier is removed after the initial placement of the implant in the cavity before screwing. The location of the implant and the possible vomiting reflex during implant carrier removal are the two factors creating the risk of swallowing the implant carrier. To avoid this risk, it is recommended to remove the implant carrier outside the mouth and to carry the implant to the cavity while it is seated on the screwing instrument. Care must be taken to hold the implant from the polished band, which is designed for gingival attachment. The implant carrier is removed while the implant is being held by a Weingart plier, and the implant is seated on the screwing instrument. The implant is then carried to the cavity using the screwing instrument and screwed directly (Figure 17-7).

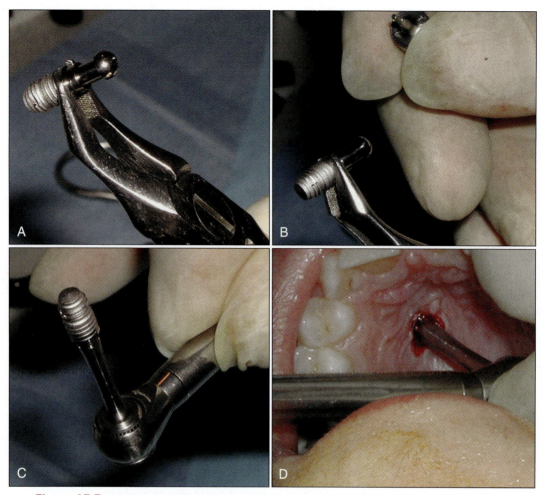

Figure 17-7
Safe Method for Removal of Implant Carrier. **A,** Implant is held from its polished neck section with Weingart pliers. **B,** Implant carrier being removed. **C,** Implant seated on screwing instrument. **D,** Implant is carried to its cavity with the screwing instrument.

CONSTRUCTION OF STATIONARY ANCHORAGE APPLIANCE

After removal of the gingiva former, a transfer kit is screwed onto the implant and a plastic cap mounted. The molar bands and the impression post are transferred to the stone model by a conventional impression technique. If necessary, premolar bands are transferred as well. An orthodontic abutment (Friadent) is fixed to the implant analog on the stone model (Figure 17-8).

On the stone model, a transpalatal arch (TPA) made of 1.2-mm-thick stainless steel wire is adjusted to connect the anchor teeth to the orthodontic abutment and then soldered to the bands (Figure 17-9). Care should be taken not to overheat the wire and create "dead wire," which can possibly cause anchorage loss. Anchorage effect of palatal implants is closely related to the rigidity of the TPA. A small mesial movement of premolars has been reported with TPAs made of .032 × .032–inch wire[21] and 1-mm-diameter round wire.[27] The TPA should tightly fit in the slot of the orthodontic abutment and should be rigid enough to withstand any deformation and rotational movement.

ORTHODONTIC MECHANICS WITH PALATAL IMPLANTS

Using the stationary anchorage provided by the palatal implant, orthodontic applications such as en masse retraction of six anterior teeth, molar distalization, and molar mesialization can be carried out without significant anchorage loss. For molar distalization with buccal mechanics, orthodontic abutment of the palatal implant can be connected to the first premolars (Figure 17-10). Molars can also be distalized using palatal mechanics supported by palatal anchorage. A representative case (case report 17-1) is presented.

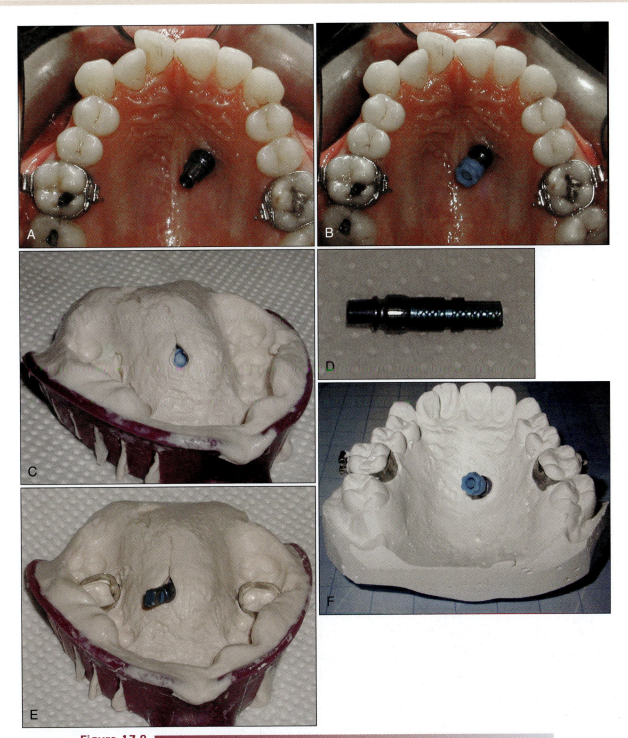

Figure 17-8

Impression Procedure. A, Transfer kit screwed onto the implant. **B,** Plastic cap mounted on transfer kit. **C,** Impression with plastic cap in it. **D,** Implant analog. **E,** Implant analog, plastic cap, and molar bands transferred to the impression. **F,** Stone model obtained with the implant analog, with molar bands.

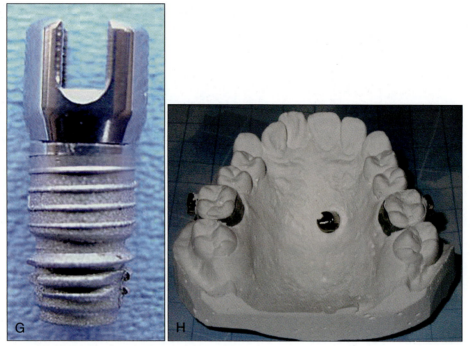

Figure 17-8, cont'd G, Orthodontic abutment. H, Orthodontic abutment is fixed to the implant analog.

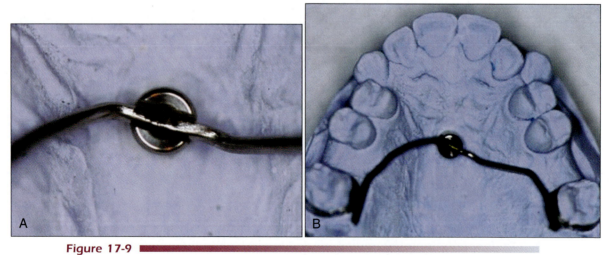

Figure 17-9

Stationary Anchorage. A, Transpalatal bar constructed of 1.2-mm-thick stainless steel wire is adjusted to fit into the slot of the orthodontic abutment. **B** and **C,** Transpalatal bar for reinforcement of molar anchorage. **D,** Transpalatal bar for reinforcement of premolar anchorage.

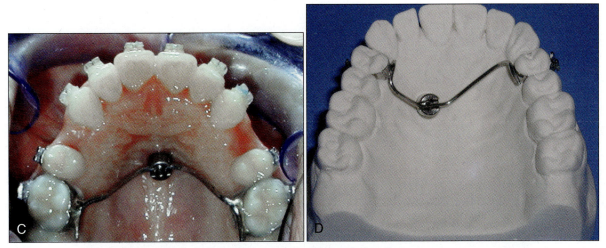

Figure 17-9, cont'd   For legend see opposite page.

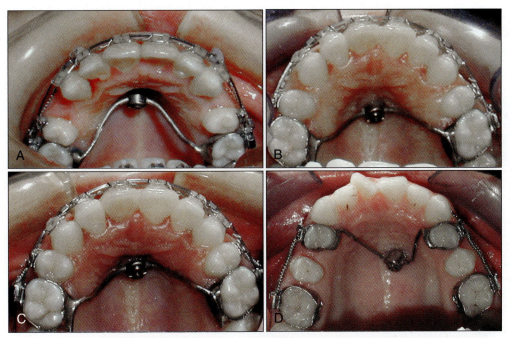

Figure 17-10

A to C, En masse retraction of six anterior teeth with palatal implant support. D to F, Molar distalization with buccally applied Ni-Ti open-coil springs. G, Once molar distalization is completed, the transpalatal arch (TPA) interconnecting the first premolars is removed, and a new TPA is constructed to reinforce molar anchorage during the remaining treatment. H, Retained second deciduous molars and missing second premolars in the upper arch. I to K, Mesialization of the permanent molars to close the spaces of the deciduous molars.

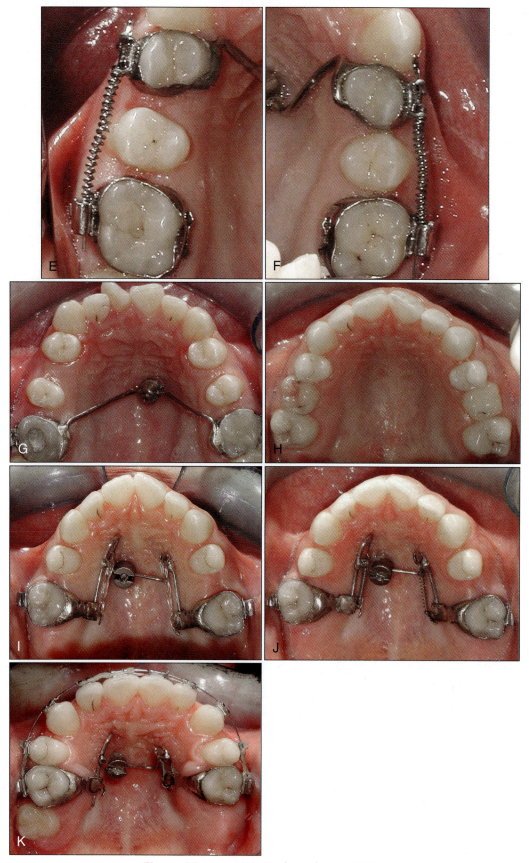

Figure 17-10, cont'd For legend see p. 383.

CASE REPORT 17-1: MOLAR DISTALIZATION WITH PALATAL MECHANICS

A 17-year-old patient presented with a chief complaint of crowding of her upper anterior teeth. She had a symmetrical face and a balanced profile. Intraoral examination showed Class II molar and canine relationship and severe crowding of the upper anterior teeth. Both upper canines were buccally positioned, with the left canine totally out of the arch. Both upper lateral incisors were in crossbite. The upper dental midline was on level with the facial midline, but there was about 1.5-mm midline discrepancy between the upper and lower arches. Overbite was 1 mm and overjet, 1.5 mm. There was slight constriction in the upper arch at the premolar region. Cephalometric evaluation showed that the patient had a skeletal Class I relationship and normal vertical dimensions of the face (Figure 17-11).

Treatment Goals
1. Elimination of the upper-arch crowding.
2. Bringing the teeth to normal overbite and overjet relationship.
3. Establishment of Class I molar and canine relationship.

Treatment Planning
A nonextraction treatment plan was adopted, which involved distalization of the upper molars with palatal implant support. The option of extraction treatment was rejected so as not to compromise the profile balance of the patient. Palatal implant anchorage was needed to prevent anchorage loss during molar distalization, which usually manifests as labial flaring of the upper anterior teeth.

Treatment Progress
After waiting 3 months for osseointegration of the palatal implant, molar distalization was initiated using mini-expansion screws (Hyrax II Expansion Screw 602-806-10, Dentaurum, Germay) against implant anchorage. The patient was instructed to turn the screws twice a week (half turn), and activation was continued until "super" Class I molar relationship was achieved on both sides. The distalization screws were kept in position for approximately 3 months for retention. During this period, distal drift of the premolars and some spontaneous eruption of the infrapositioned canines were observed. Just before initiation of the alignment of the teeth, the distalization screws were replaced by a TPA, again connected to the palatal implant (Figure 17-12).

Results
Molar distalization lasted about 6 months, and the overall treatment time was 20 months. Upper-right first molar was distalized 4.5 mm and left first molar, 5.1 mm. Some tipping of the molars was also observed. Dental alignment and Class I molar and canine relationship were achieved without significant alteration in facial profile (Figure 17-13). Upper and lower fixed lingual retainers were placed after removal of the brackets.

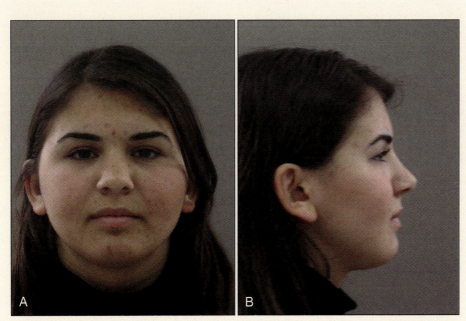

Figure 17-11 **Molar Distalization with Palatal Implants.** Pretreatment facial **(A-C)** and intraoral **(D-H)** photographs.

CASE REPORT 17-1: MOLAR DISTALIZATION WITH PALATAL MECHANICS—cont'd

Figure 17-11, cont'd

CASE REPORT 17-1: MOLAR DISTALIZATION WITH PALATAL MECHANICS—cont'd

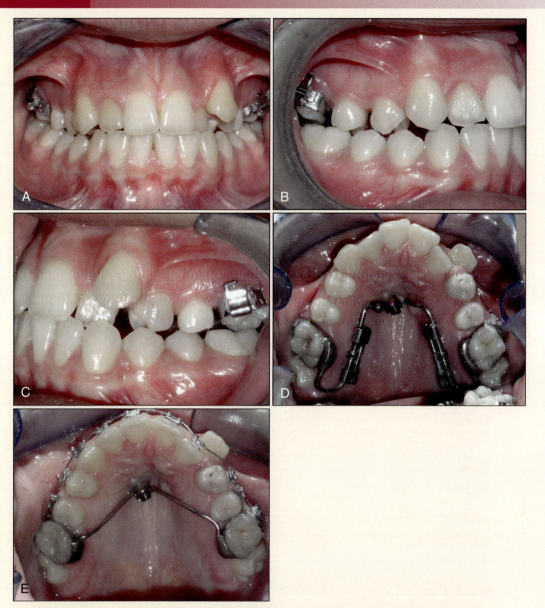

Figure 17-12 Treatment Progress. A to **D,** Intraoral photographs obtained toward end of the molar distalization phase. **E,** After removal of the distalization screws, TPA connected to the palatal implant was constructed to maintain the position of the first molars and to reinforce anchorage during the remaining treatment.

Continued

CASE REPORT 17-1: MOLAR DISTALIZATION WITH PALATAL MECHANICS—cont'd

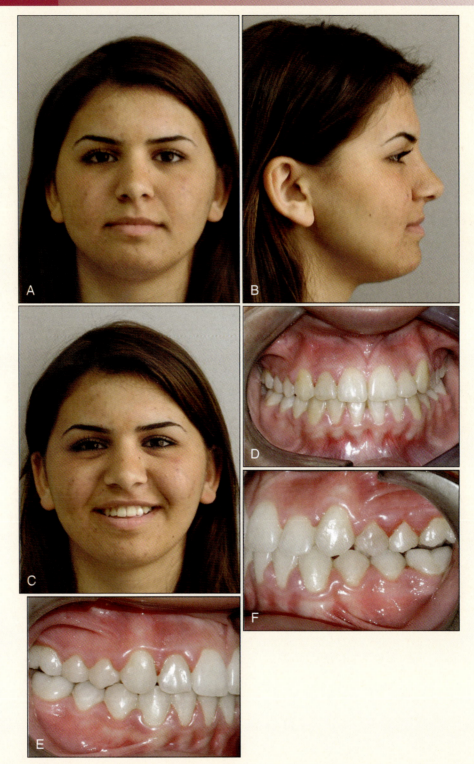

Figure 17-13 Treatment Results. Posttreatment facial (A-C) and intraoral (D-H) photographs.

| CASE REPORT 17-1: | MOLAR DISTALIZATION WITH PALATAL MECHANICS—cont'd |

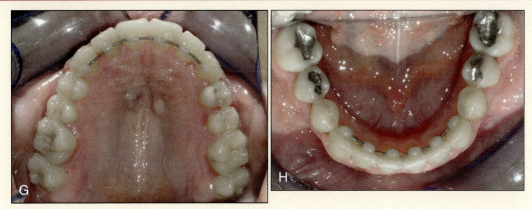

Figure 17-13, cont'd For legend see opposite page.

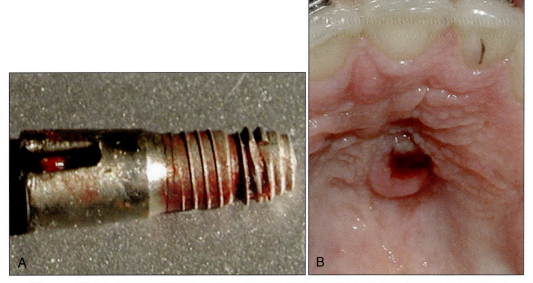

Figure 17-14
A, Palatal implant removed. B, Appearance of the implant site immediately after removal of the implant. Healing occurs rapidly, with no complications.

EXPLANTATION OF PALATAL IMPLANTS

The palatal implant is removed easily by unscrewing it counterclockwise. If a resistance is felt during unscrewing, a hollow drill may be used to loosen the implant first. The implant site heals rapidly, usually within 5 days (Figure 17-14).

FACTORS AFFECTING SUCCESS RATE OF PALATAL IMPLANTS

The success rate of palatal implants placed with the method previously described is about 82%. Zhao et al.[38] reported their success rate as 84.2%. Compared with the success rates given for dental implants,[39-42] the success rate of palatal implants seems to be lower. Two crucial factors affecting the success of palatal implants are *surgical method* (open vs. closed surgery) and *bone quality*.

Some investigators advocate the use of *open surgery* for palatal implant placement.[31,43] In this approach, when mucoperiosteum is released, the implant site becomes completely exposed. In this position, drilling would be safer, and the cortical bone shoulder surrounding the implant cavity would be protected. A well-maintained cortical bone shoulder enhances the primary stability of the implant, and the success rate may be higher. The disadvantages of open surgery are the severity of the procedure and the postoperative pain and discomfort.

In *closed surgery*, changes in the angulation of hand instrument may result in destruction of the cortical bone shoulder surrounding the implant, with a subsequent decrease in primary stability. The use of a surgical template for proper drill orientation becomes indispensable in closed surgery.

In implantology, bone is classified as type I, II, III, and IV. Type I bone is very rich in cortical bone but has limited vascularity. Type II bone is the best for osseointegration of implants, providing sufficient cortical anchorage for primary stability and having better vascularity than type I bone. Type IV bone is the least dense of all the bone types, and it requires the longest time for integration with an implant. The bone found in the hard palate is mostly type III or IV, meaning that it is rich in spongious bone with thinner layers of cortical bone than in type I and II bone. Cortical bone thickness usually does not exceed 2 mm in the entire hard palate; thus it is of utmost importance to maintain this thickness as much as possible during the surgical procedure.

CONCLUSION

Osseointegrated palatal implants provide an excellent solution in critical anchorage situations. These implants do not show clinically significant movement in reaction to orthodontic forces and eliminate the need for patient compliance during anchorage maintenance. The surgical procedure for palatal implant placement is relatively simple and does not cause major discomfort to the patient. Patient acceptance rate of palatal implants is satisfactory as well.[44]

ACKNOWLEDGMENT

With great appreciation to Drs. Serdar Sezen, Mustafa Ateş, and Musa Beceti for their valuable assistance with this chapter.

REFERENCES

1. Ödman J, Lekholm U, Branemark P-I, et al: Osseointegrated titanium implants: a new approach in orthodontic treatment, *Eur J Orthod* 10:98-105, 1988.
2. Roberts WE, Smith R, Zilberman Y, et al: Osseous adaptation to continuous loading of rigid endosseous implants, *Am J Orthod* 86:95-111, 1984.
3. Roberts WE, Helm FR, Marshall KJ, Gonglof RK: Rigid endosseous implants for orthodontic and orthopedic anchorage, *Angle Orthod* 59:247-256, 1989.
4. Roberts WE, Marshall KJ, Mozsary PG: Rigid endosseous implant utilized as anchorage to protract molars and close an atrophic extraction site, *Angle Orthod* 60:135-152, 1990.
5. Turley PK, Kean C, Sehur J, et al: Orthodontic force application to titanium endosseous implants, *Angle Orthod* 58:151-162, 1988.
6. Van Roekel NB: The use of Branemark system implants for orthodontic anchorage: report of a case, *Int J Oral Maxillofac Implants* 4:341-344, 1989.
7. Diedrich P: Different orthodontic anchorage systems: a critical examination, *Fortschr Kieferorthop* 54:156-171, 1993.
8. Chen J, Chen K, Garetto LP, Roberts WE: Mechanical response to functional and therapeutic loading of a retromolar endosseous implant used for orthodontic anchorage to mesially translate mandibular molars, *Implant Dent* 4:246-258, 1995.
9. Melsen B, Lang NP: Biological reactions of alveolar bone to orthodontic loading of oral implants, *Clin Oral Implants Res* 12:144-152, 2001.
10. Linder-Aronson S, Nordenram A, Anneroth G: Titanium implant anchorage in orthodontic treatment: an experimental investigation in monkeys, *Eur J Orthod* 12:414-419, 1990.
11. Ödman J, Grondahl K, Lekholm U, Thilander B: The effect of osseointegrated implants on the dento-alveolar development: a clinical and radiographic study in growing pigs, *Eur J Orthod* 13:279-286, 1991.
12. Sennerby L, Ödman J, Lekholm U, Thilander B: Tissue reactions towards titanium implants inserted in growing jaws: a histological study in the pig, *Clin Oral Implants Res* 4:65-75, 1993.
13. Smalley WM, Shapiro PA, Branemark P-I, et al: Osseointegrated titanium implants for maxillofacial protraction in monkeys, *Am J Orthod Dentofacial Orthop* 94:285-295, 1988.
14. Thilander B, Ödman J, Grondahl K, Lekholm U: Aspects on osseointegrated implants inserted in growing jaws: a biometric and radiographic study in the young pig, *Eur J Orthod* 14:99-109, 1992.
15. Haanaes HR, Stenvik A, Beyer Olsen ES, et al: The efficacy of two-stage titanium implants as orthodontic anchorage in the preprosthodontic correction of third molars in adults: a report of three cases, *Eur J Orthod* 13:287-292, 1991.
16. Ödman J, Lekholm U, Jemt T, Thilander B: Osseointegrated implants as orthodontic anchorage in the treatment of partially edentulous adult patients, *Eur J Orthod* 16:187-201, 1994.
17. Thilander B, Ödman J, Grondahl K, Friberg B: Osseointegrated implants in adolescents: an alternative in replacing missing teeth? *Eur J Orthod* 16:84-95, 1994.
18. Higuchi KW, Slack JM: The use of titanium fixtures for intraoral anchorage to facilitate orthodontic tooth movement, *Int J Oral Maxillofac Implants* 6:338-344, 1991.
19. Triaca A, Antonini M, Wintermantel E: Ein neues Titan-Flachschrauben-Implantat zur orthodonstischen Verankerung am anterioren Gaumen, *Inf Orthod Kieferorthop* 24:251-257, 1992.
20. Block MS, Hoffman DR: A new device for absolute anchorage for orthodontics, *Am J Orthod Dentofacial Orthop* 107:251-258, 1995.
21. Wehrbein H, Merz BR, Diedrich P, Glatzmaier J: The use of palatal implants for orthodontic anchorage: design and clinical application of the Orthosystem, *Clin Oral Implants Res* 7:410-416, 1996.
22. Wehrbein H, Glatzmaier J, Mundwiller U, Diedrich P: The Orthosystem: a new implant system for orthodontic anchorage in the palate, *J Orofac Orthop* 57:142-153, 1996.
23. Wehrbein H, Glatzmaier J, Yildirim M: Orthodontic anchorage capacity of short titanium screw implants in the maxilla: an experimental study in the dog, *Clin Oral Implants Res* 8:131-141, 1997.
24. Wehrbein H, Merz BR, Diedrich P: Palatal bone support for orthodontic implant anchorage: a clinical and radiological study, *Eur J Orthod* 21:65-70, 1999.
25. Wehrbein H, Feifel H, Diedrich P: Palatal implant anchorage reinforcement of posterior teeth: a prospective study, *Am J Orthod Dentofacial Orthop* 116:678-686, 1999.
26. Bantleon H, Bernhart T, Crismani AG, Zachrisson U: Stable orthodontic anchorage with palatal osseointegrated implants, *World J Orthod* 3:109-116, 2002.
27. Keles A, Erverdi N, Sezen S: Bodily molar distalization with absolute anchorage, *Angle Orthod* 73:471-482, 2003.

28. Gahleitner A, Podesser B, Schick S, et al: Dental CT and orthodontic implants: imaging technique and assessment of available bone volume in the hard palate, *Eur J Radiol* 51:257-262, 2004.
29. Henriksen B, Bavitz B, Kelly B, Harn SD: Evaluation of bone thickness in the anterior hard palate relative to midsagittal orthodontic implants, *Int J Oral Maxillofac Implants* 18:578-581, 2003.
30. Crismani AG, Bernhart T, Tangl S, et al: Nasal cavity perforation by palatal implants: false-positive records on the lateral cephalogram, *Int J Oral Maxillofac Implants* 20:267-273, 2005.
31. Bernhart T, Vollgruber A, Gahleitner A, et al: Alternative to median region of the palate for placement of an orthodontic implant, *Clin Oral Implants Res* 11:595-601, 2000.
32. Melsen B: Palatal growth studied on human autopsy material, *Am J Orthod* 68:42-54, 1975.
33. Schlegel KA, Kinner F, Schlegel KD: The anatomic basis for palatal implants in orthodontics, *Int J Adult Orthod Orthognath Surg* 17:133-139, 2002.
34. Björk A, Skieller V: Postnatal growth and development of the maxillary complex. In McNamara JA Jr, editor: *Factors affecting the growth of the midface*. Monograph 6. *Craniofacial growth series*, Ann Arbor, Mich, 1976, Center for Human Growth and Development, University of Michigan, pp 61-69.
35. Björk A, Skieller V: Growth of the maxilla in three dimensions as revealed radiographically by the implant method, *Br J Orthod* 4:53-64, 1977.
36. Asscherickx K, Hanssens JL, Wehrbein H, Sabzevar MM: Orthodontic anchorage implants inserted in the median palatal suture and normal transverse growth in growing dogs: a biometric and radiographic study, *Angle Orthod* 75:826-831, 2005.
37. Cousley RRJ, Parberry DJ: Combined cephalometric and stent planning for palatal implants, *J Orthod* 32:20-25, 2005.
38. Zhao Y, Su YC, Jiang XY, Du J: Clinical study on the stability of palatal implant anchorage, *Zhonghua Kou Qiang Yi Xue Za Zhi* 40:463-467, 2005 (abstract in English).
39. Bornstein MM, Schmid B, Belser UC, et al: Early loading of non-submerged titanium implants with a sandblasted and acid-etched surface: 5-year results of a prospective study in partially edentulous patients, *Clin Oral Implants Res* 16:631-638, 2005.
40. Fischer K, Stenberg T: Three-year data from a randomized, controlled study of early loading of single-stage dental implants supporting maxillary full-arch prostheses, *Int J Oral Maxillofac Implants* 2:245-252, 2006.
41. Telleman G, Meijer HJ, Raghoebar GM: Long-term evaluation of hollow screw and hollow cylinder dental implants: clinical and radiographic results after 10 years, *J Periodontol* 77:203-210, 2006.
42. Artzi Z, Carmeli G, Kozlovsky A: A distinguishable observation between survival and success rate outcome of hydroxyapatite-coated implants in 5-10 years in function, *Clin Oral Implants Res* 17:85-93, 2006.
43. Bernhart T, Freudenthaler J, Dortbudak O, et al: Short epithetic implants for orthodontic anchorage in the paramedian region of the palate: a clinical study, *Clin Oral Implants Res* 12:624-631, 2001.
44. Gunduz E, Schneider-Del Savio TT, Kucher G, et al: Acceptance rate of palatal implants: a questionnaire study, *Am J Orthod Dentofacial Orthop* 126:623-626, 2004.

CHAPTER 18

Skeletal Anchorage in Orthodontics Using Palatal Implants

Heiner Wehrbein, Britta A. Jung, Martin Kunkel, and Peter Göellner

Control of anchorage for orthodontic tooth movements represents a fundamental problem in the treatment of dental and skeletal dysgnathia. Available anchorage potential,[1,2] as well as that required for each anchoring task, must be taken into consideration so that undesired tooth movements and anchorage loss can be avoided. To prevent uncontrolled tooth movements, the existing anchorage potential of the natural teeth needs to be balanced with the required anchorage task. This may pose a clinical challenge when strict positional stability and maximal anchorage are needed.

According to these general rules, a reduced number of anchor teeth, advanced loss of periodontal attachment, or unfavorable distribution of teeth represents the typical clinical situation in which skeletal anchorage can be considered.[3] When traditional anchorage concepts such as the Nance button appliance, lingual arch, or even extraoral (headgear or Delaire face mask) devices are applied in such situations, they often produce unpredictable reactive forces and moments.[4,5] Specifically, these appliances often lead to protrusion of the incisors, cause extrusion and tipping of the anchoring teeth, and interfere with the alignment of the occlusal plane.

When extraoral devices are considered, compliance is a critical issue that may affect the outcome with these treatment options. Moreover, adolescent patients are often very reluctant to wear extraoral appliances.

For these reasons, temporary orthodontic anchorage implants were developed for the maxilla in the early 1990s. Since then, extensive clinical and experimental data have verified remarkable reliability and a sound clinical success rate for these implants.[4,6-12]

This chapter discusses some common skeletal orthodontic anchorage devices and their clinical use and potential benefits, focusing primarily on the use of palatal implants for orthodontic treatment tasks.

IMPLANTS FOR ORTHODONTIC ANCHORAGE

It is clinically relevant to know whether implants would be used as orthodontic anchoring elements to correct malocclusion and subsequently as abutments to support a fixed prosthetic appliance—orthodontic-prosthetic implant anchorage (OPIA)—or whether they are to function temporarily and exclusively as orthodontic anchorage elements (OIA). These principal requirements determine the overall concept of orthodontic anchorage, including factors such as insertion site, implant type, and dimension.

ORTHODONTIC-PROSTHETIC IMPLANT ANCHORAGE

In the OPIA setting the insertion site is determined fundamentally by subsequent use of the implant as a prosthetic abutment. For this reason, conventional prosthetic implants are inserted into the alveolar bone of the mandible or the maxilla. The position of orthodontic-prosthetic anchoring implants is determined by the patient's final occlusion, which should satisfy the individual restorative or prosthodontic requirements. Therefore, a preliminary implant setup may be reasonable.

To implement the OPIA concept, an orthodontic attachment (e.g., bracket, molar band) is fixed at the provisional crown or a prefabricated bonding base. The orthodontic force system acts at the superstructure of the implant. The reactive moments and forces are transmitted directly to the implant and its surrounding bone. Both direct and indirect anchorage can be established with this type of implant.

Indications
The OPIA technique may be indicated in patients with the following:

- Malpositioned anterior teeth and either unilateral or bilateral shortened dental arch.
- Malpositioned anterior or posterior teeth in association with edentulous spaces (gaps of two or more missing teeth), most frequently in the posterior mandible or maxilla.

Advantages

The combination of OPIA and the segmented-arch technique enables a stepwise expansion of the orthodontic device and allows for spearing parts of the dentition within the treatment process. First, only the neighboring teeth are bonded. When the alignment of these teeth has been accomplished, other parts of the dentition are included.

Because of the nature of OPIA, the implants remain in situ after completion of the orthodontic treatment. If necessary, this may be used for long-term retention.

Limitations

Implants for occlusal rehabilitation should not be inserted before completion of growth, because they may impair the development of the alveolar bone and, more important, will not keep up with the growth of the surrounding bone.[13,14] In clinical terms, early implant placement will unavoidably lead to infraocclusion of the implant with development of an open bite.

ORTHODONTIC IMPLANT ANCHORAGE

With respect to the insertion site, implant dimensions, scale, and direction of applied forces and duration of use, fundamental differences exist between OPIA and exclusively OIA. In contrast to the masticatory stresses of prosthetic implants, orthodontic loading exerts continuous, nonaxial forces at a comparatively lower level. Moreover, orthodontic implants are removed when malocclusion has been corrected, thus rendering long-term performance according to common success criteria (e.g., <0.1 mm of marginal bone loss/year) irrelevant.

Insertion Sites

In full-dentition patients, insertion of additional standard-dimension dental implants would be counterintuitive and, more important, would endanger the integrity of the radices. Thus, length-reduced and diameter-reduced implants (e.g., length <6 mm; diameter <2 mm), as well as bone plates with a transmucosal appendix, have been developed to take advantage of alternative bone sources. Specifically, the following regions have been used for orthodontic anchorage purposes:

- Interradicular septum[15,16]
- Supraapical and infrazygomatic area[16,17]
- Retromolar area in mandible[18,19]
- Palate (midline)[4,6,8-10]
- Paramedian anterior palate[20-22]

The anterior palate was recognized early as a promising source of bone for orthodontic anchorage purposes. Because of the palate's limited vertical bone dimension, short implants originally designed for epithetic use were the first devices transferred to an orthodontic setting (titanium flat screw[6]). Further conceptual approaches included resorbable anchors (BIOS Implant System[10]) and the palatal "onplant."[23]

In this context, palatal implants developed by Wehrbein et al.[8,9] have been extensively investigated experimentally and clinically and thus can be regarded as a benchmark for current orthodontic skeletal anchorage systems. Palatal implants are described later in detail.

Biomechanical Aspects

Apart from the basic destination of the implant itself, two fundamental anchorage concepts need to be distinguished for systematic reasons: direct and indirect anchorage. Direct orthodontic implant anchorage (DOIA) implies a force system acting immediately between the teeth to be moved and the implant.

The advantages and disadvantages of these concepts are discussed later. As a general rule, direct anchorage requires less technical effort but has limitations with respect to direction and dimension of tooth movements. On the other hand, indirect anchorage offers a range of treatment options but requires higher technical expenditure. The most convenient technical solution for establishing indirect orthodontic anchorage is a transpalatal arch, soldered or welded to a palatal implant abutment, which is bonded to the teeth or connected to molar bands. This technique provides a stable anchorage unit for various types and directions of tooth movement in treatment.

Osseointegration

The concept of osseointegration originated with the anatomist Brånemark (1977), who defined it as a "direct structural and functional connection between organized, living bone and the surface of the loaded implant."[24] Therefore, osseointegration is a fundamental prerequisite for implant therapy. In general, a complete covering of the implant surface with bone tissue is desirable. However, because orthodontic loading forces differ significantly from functional loading during mastication, a complete bone-to-implant contact is not required to achieve sufficient implant stability under orthodontic loading conditions.[20,25,26]

The typical bone-to-implant contact rates reported for orthodontic implants range from 34% to 93%.[4,7,8] In fact, it remains unconfirmed how much bone-to-implant contact would be sufficient to establish and maintain osseointegration, but extensive clinical evidence indicates that osseointegrated implants remain positionally stable under orthodontic and even orthopedic loading conditions.[7,11,18,27-31]

PALATAL IMPLANTS

The first generation of palatal implant (Orthosystem, Straumann, Basel, Switzerland) was a pure-titanium,

TABLE 18-1 Dimensions of Palatal Implants*

Dimension	Orthosystem	Palatal Implant
Endosteal diameter (mm)	3.3 and 4.0	4.1 and 4.8
Endosteal length (mm)	4.0 and 6.0	4.2
Neck height (mm)	2.5 and 4.5	1.8
Abutment (mm)	2.0	1.5
Material	Titanium	Titanium
Surface	SLA	SLA

*Straumann, Basel, Switzerland.
SLA, Sandblasted, large grit, acid etched.

one-piece endosseous implant specifically designed for orthodontic use. It is manufactured with a sandblasted, large-grit, acid-etched (SLA) surface and a self-tapping thread. The implant is connected to the orthodontic appliance by a steel abutment coping, onto which orthodontic arches are fixed in position by laser welding or soldering.

Since 2004 a second generation of this implant (Palatal Implant, Straumann) has been available. Compared with the first generation, the diameter of the second-generation implant has been slightly enlarged, from 3.3 to 4.1 mm, and the emerging profile modified from a 90-degree shoulder to a slightly concave, conical design (Table 18-1).

INDICATIONS

Palatal implants are most suitable for the following treatment objectives:

- Preparation of a positionally stable, posterior anchoring unit to retract, torque, or intrude front teeth in a controlled manner.
- Preparation of a stable anterior anchoring unit to mesialize or distalize side teeth and close or open spaces.
- Transverse expansion in adult patients having unilateral or bilateral crossbite.
- Stabilization of teeth (e.g., canines) in treatment with vertical elastics (e.g., Class II or Class III elastics)
- Expanding the superconstruction to a temporary denture in cases of aplasia or traumatic loss of front teeth during and after orthopedic treatment of growing patients.

Figure 18-1 provides some examples of common indications and superstructures.

IMPLANT INSERTION

As a general rule, a lateral cephalogram and an orthopantomogram should be taken before surgery. Except for severe deformities, neither computed tomography (CT) nor digital volume tomography (DVT) is required for preoperative assessment. The individual site of implant insertion is determined using a lateral cephalogram, which allows an estimation of the bone available in the anterior part of the maxilla. The distance between the incisors' edge and the preferred position of the implant can be directly transferred from the lateral cephalogram to the clinical setting (Figure 18-2).

Procedure

In most cases the implant will be inserted in the midsagittal plane or slightly paramedian at the level of the first premolars.

The surgical procedure is performed under local anesthesia. Briefly, after a mouth rinse with chlorhexidine digluconate, the palatal mucosa is removed at the prospective site of implant placement with a rotating mucosal trephine (Figure 18-3, A and B). Using a round bur, a slight bony groove is created in the middle of the exposed bone. The implant site is then prepared using ascending sizes of twist drills up to a diameter of 3.5 mm (Figure 18-3, C). All drilling procedures must be performed under copious irrigation with sterile physiological saline. A template allows for precise adjustment of the insertion depth according to the mucosal reference (Figure 18-3, D and E). Finally, the implant is inserted using an appropriate ratchet, and the healing cap is screwed on top (Figure 18-3, F and G).

The issue of preoperative antibiotics has not yet been systematically analyzed in the context of palatal implants. At the authors' institution, however, a single oral dose of a second-generation cephalosporin is administered 1 hour before surgery.

IMPLANT REMOVAL

Because of the high torque resistance of the Orthosystem implant, this device cannot simply be screwed out, but must be removed with a minor surgical procedure. Under local anesthesia, a guiding cylinder is screwed to the internal thread, and the implant is harvested by an appropriate trephine bur (Figure 18-4). The extraction site is left for secondary healing, which will take approximately 2 weeks to complete. Figure 18-5 shows histological sections of a palatal implant after removal.

LABORATORY PHASE

After a healing period of approximately 12 weeks, impressions for the laboratory phase can be taken with alginate and prefabricated transfer caps to obtain a working plaster model. Depending on the type of malocclusion and on biomechanical requirements, a custom palatal superstructure is fabricated on the working model (Figure 18-6). At our institution, the preferred concept for indirect orthodontic implant anchorage (IOIA) is the transpalatal arch (TPA). It provides a rigid connection between the desmodontal anchorage unit and the implant. The ends of the TPA can be bonded to one or several teeth using an adhesive technique (see Figure 18-1, A and B) or by connecting to molar

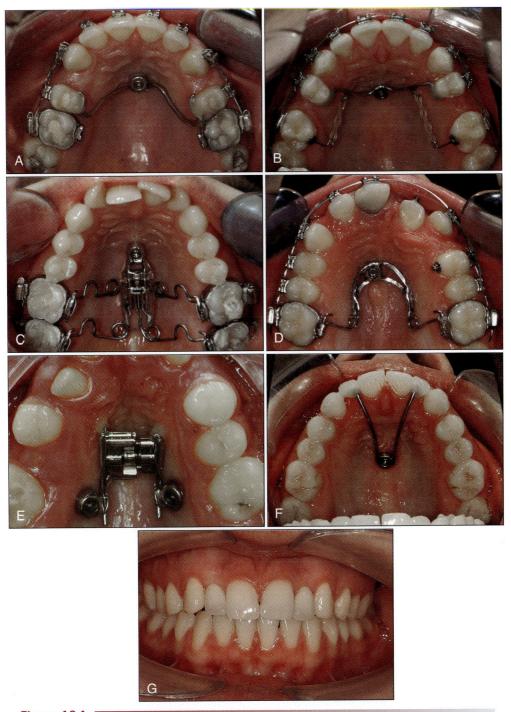

Figure 18-1
Examples of Implant-Borne Superstructures. Transpalatal arch (TPA) for preparation of a positionally stable posterior anchoring unit. **A,** to retract anterior teeth, and **B,** to mesialize #16 and #26. **C,** Implant-borne pendulum appliance for distalization of the posterior teeth. **D,** Modified TPA is inserted after active distalization. The ends of the TPA are connected to molar bands. **E,** Implant-supported rapid maxillary expansion (RME) for transversal expansion. **F,** and **G,** Implant-supported temporary prosthetic rehabilitation of teeth #12 and #22 in a growing patient. It was designed to hold the empty space open to prevent movement of the adjunct teeth and for esthetic reasons.

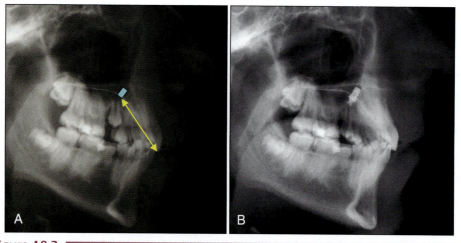

Figure 18-2
Lateral cephalogram used for preoperative assessment of the available bone. **A,** Distance between the incisor's edge and preferred site of the implant *(arrow)* can be transferred 1:1 to the clinical setting. **B,** Postoperative radiograph confirming the placement of the implant within the appropriate region of the anterior palate. Note the position of the implant at the level of the first premolars.

bands (see Figure 18-1, *C* and *D*). However, the direct implant-loading technique (DOIA), in the form of implant-supported pendulum appliances (see Figure 18-1, *C*) or implant-supported rapid maxillary expansion (RME) appliance (see Figure 18-1, *E*), are also used.

PALATAL IMPLANTS IN ADULTS AND GROWING PATIENTS

The use of palatal implants in adult patients has been reported by various authors.[1,2,6,8,9] Based on the original concept for treatment of the mature facial skeleton, a palatal implant is traditionally placed in the median region of the palate. In this anatomical region, two fundamental problems may be associated with implant placement in the growing facial skeleton. First, there is still a much larger proportion of connective tissue in the area of the suture than in an adult. There is also poorer interdigitation of the palatal plates; thus, lower primary stability is expected with palatal implants in the growing facial skeleton. Second, median implant placement may interfere with residual maxillary growth. In growing patients, placement of palatal implants in the paramedian region has therefore been recommended to prevent interactions with potential residual intermaxillary suture growth changes. Experimental data obtained from growing beagle dogs provided initial evidence of a minor transverse growth inhibition when palatal implants were placed in the midsagittal region.[32] Clinical data addressing potential long-term effects of endosseous palatal implants are not available at present.

Most interestingly, the predominant growth potential of the maxillary base is directed vertically during adolescence. Initial findings with palatal implants placed in the paramedian region in adolescent patients suggest that, in contrast to conventional alveolar bone prosthetic implants, there is caudal migration of these implants together with the maxillary complex. A partial submersion, as often seen in prosthetic implants inserted in the alveolar process, was not detected. With regard to midfacial growth, so-called growth-conditioned displacement causes anterior-caudal displacement of the nasomaxillary complex.[33] Specifically, the maxilla in particular moves caudally because of apposition processes in the oral and resorption in the nasal cortex. Within this process, the alveolar process and teeth are first passively shifted and then drift through apposition and resorption.[33,34] Pronounced growth inhibition is therefore to be expected in the adjacent alveolar bone tissue, approximately 0.8 mm per year, or about 5 mm total, when an implant is inserted in the alveolar process after age 12 years to adulthood.[22,34] On the other hand, in the region of the median palatine suture area, there is comparably less vertical growth because of remodeling processes, on an average of only 0.2 mm per year.[34,35]

Thus, with regard to residual vertical growth, significant growth inhibition is highly unlikely. The effect on transverse and sagittal growth of the maxilla has not yet been systematically analyzed in humans. In our institution, palatal implants are used from age 12 years if maximum anchorage is required and other anchorage aids are not indicated or are rejected (compliance, visibility, side effects).

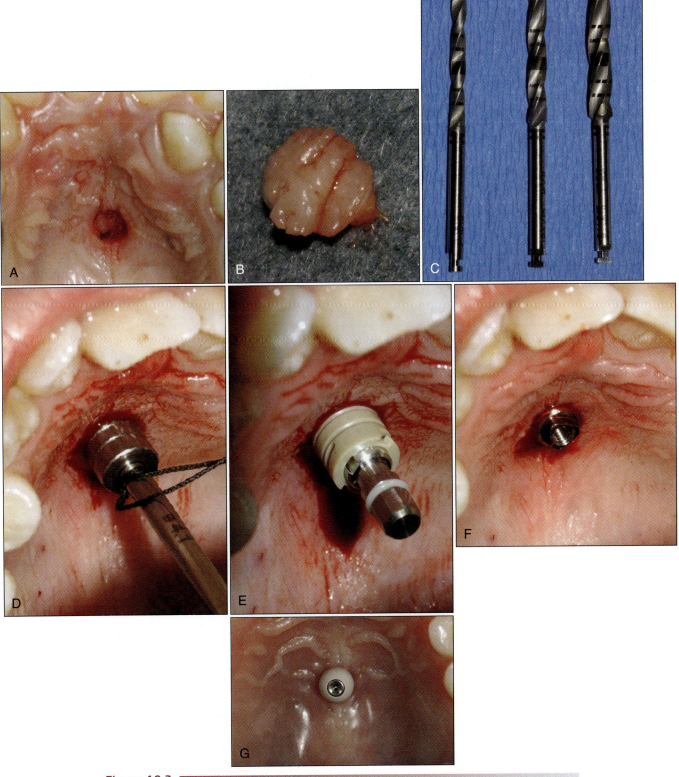

Figure 18-3

Surgical Treatment Steps. *Phase I*: **A,** Clinical aspect of hard palate after removal of palatal mucosa; **B,** mucosal patch as harvested by mucosal trephine. *Phase II*: **C,** Ascending sizes of twist drills as used for preparation of implant site; laser markings on each drill indicate the depth of drilling during the surgical phase. *Phase III*: **D,** After the final drilling procedure, a template is used to determine the insertion depth; **E,** identical markings at the template and the implant carriers allow for insertion to the planned submersion depth. *Phase IV*: **F,** Palatal implant after insertion and before placing the healing cap; **G,** palatal implant with healing cap.

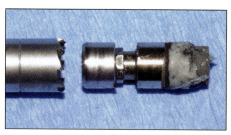

Figure 18-4
Implant Removal. Using a guiding cylinder, a trephine bur *(left)* is used for minimal invasive retrieval of the implant *(right)*.

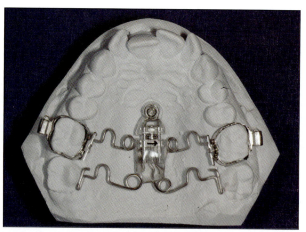

Figure 18-6
Laboratory Phase. Plaster working model with implant-supported pendulum appliance.

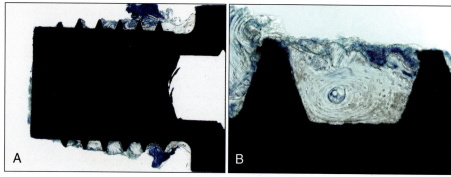

Figure 18-5
Histological Sections of Palatal Implant. A, After completion of active orthodontic treatment and implant removal (cutting and grinding technique according to Donath and Breuner, stained with toluidine blue). Because of trephine harvesting, the bone-to-implant contact zone is preserved to a depth of about 3 mm (original magnification, 25×). **B,** At higher magnification (200×), osseointegration of the SLA surface is confirmed.

CASE REPORT 18-1

This female patient was first evaluated at age 51 for orthodontic treatment, seeking esthetic improvement and maintenance for her teeth. Her family history revealed no remarkable problems. Intraoral examination revealed a conservative and prosthetically treated dentition.

Problem List
The patient's orthodontic problems at the initial examination were protrusion and elongation of maxillary front teeth (Figure 18-7, A and B), deep bite, a palatal position of the erupted canine (#13) with extraaxial load and severe periodontal destruction. In addition, physiological masticatory forces had led to jiggling of the teeth with increased mobility. Radiographic examination demonstrated advanced periodontal destruction with generalized horizontal bone and attachment loss of up to 80% in both arches, with vertical bone loss in the upper and lower front teeth (Figure 18-7, C). Further clinical findings revealed mild crowding of the lower and upper incisors, deep bite, and midline deviation. There was a Class I molar relationship on both sides with a Class II canine relationship of half premolar width on the right side and a Class I canine relationship on the left side (see Figure 18-7, A and B).

Treatment Concept and Treatment Progress
The interdisciplinary treatment concept provided the following treatment procedures:
- Preorthodontic periodontal therapy to treat marginal inflammation.
- Surgical insertion of a Brånemark-implant in the median region of the palate for preparation of a stationary posterior anchorage unit (Figure 18-7, D).
- Orthodontic treatment with IOIA for intrusion and buccal movement of tooth #13 and for intrusion of the upper

CASE REPORT 18-1—cont'd

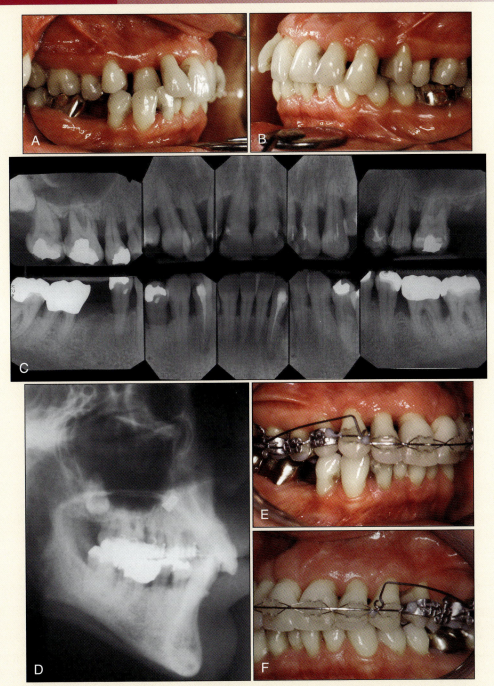

Figure 18-7 **A** and **B,** Initial clinical findings include periodontally compromised dentition, palatal eruption of #13, elongation of frontal teeth, and frontal crowding. **C,** Periapical radiographs of the dentition show severe periodontal bone loss. **D,** Cephalogram after insertion of extraoral Brånemark implant in the anterior palate. **E** and **F,** Clinical findings after intrusion of anterior teeth (segmented-arch technique). Posterior teeth were supported by an implant-borne TPA to avoid extrusion.

Continued

CASE REPORT 18-1—cont'd

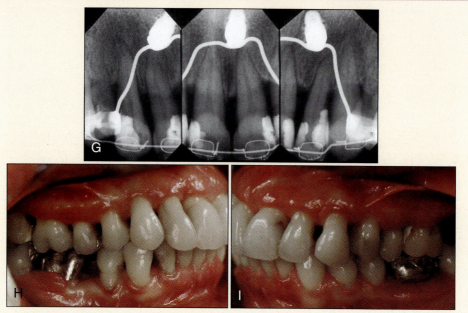

Figure 18-7, cont'd G, Periapical radiographs after intrusion. Implant-borne TPA was fastened to the first premolars to compensate for the clockwise moment and extrusion of posterior teeth during intrusion of anterior teeth. Only slight resorption occurred after intrusion of anterior teeth. **H** and **I,** Clinical findings after treatment (12 months).

front teeth against the implant-reinforced posterior teeth to avoid reactive tooth extrusion.
- Postorthodontic period with permanent retention and periodontal recall.

After a 3-month waiting period for implant healing, an impression was taken and a TPA inserted. With the implant-reinforced posterior teeth and segmented-arch technique, the intrusion and retraction of the anterior teeth, especially the correction of #13, were accomplished with no reactive extrusion of posterior teeth. Figure 18-7, E and F, shows clinical findings 9 months into orthodontic treatment. The radiographs in Figure 18-7, G, demonstrate the situation after intrusion of the canines and front teeth.

Treatment Outcome
Figure 18-7, H and I, shows the intraoral photographs taken immediately after treatment (12 months). Reactive extrusion forces of the periodontally compromised posterior teeth were compensated with an implant-borne TPA. The deep bite was corrected, and #13 was brought into proper position in the dental arch. After debonding, lingual bonded retainers from canine to canine were placed in the upper and lower arches.

CASE REPORT 18-2

A 14-year-old female patient presented to the authors' clinic with a family history of no apparent problems and a fixed appliance previously placed in a private practice (Figure 18-8, A and B).

Problem List
Her problem list at the initial examination was an impacted and buccally displaced premolar, #15. Radiographic examination demonstrated hypodontia associated with aplasia of teeth #12, #22, #25, #35, #25, and #41 (Figure 18-8, C). Hypodontia and apical root resorption led to an anchorage problem for further orthodontic treatment, especially for the elongation of the impacted and displaced #15. In particular, stationary anchorage was needed for the required space opening and later insertion of prosthetic implants in region #12 and #22 after completion of growth. Cephalometric analysis showed the tendency to Class III relationship. Clinical findings revealed a Class I molar and canine relationship. Figure 18-8, D, shows an intraoral maxillary photograph of the upper jaw at the initial examination.

Temporary Treatment Concept and Treatment Progress
The treatment concept provided the following procedures:
- Surgical insertion of a palatal implant (4.1 mm in diameter, 4.2 mm in length; Palatal Implant, Straumann; Figure 18-8, E).

CASE REPORT 18-2—cont'd

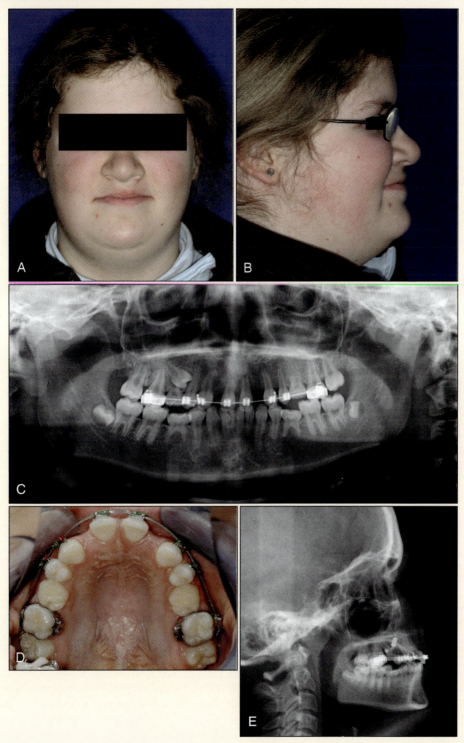

Figure 18-8 **A** and **B**, En face photograph and profile of 14-year-old patient. **C**, Panoramic radiograph after start of orthodontic treatment. **D**, Palatal view of maxillary dentition after start of orthodontic treatment elsewhere. **E**, Cephalogram after insertion of palatal implant (4.1 mm in diameter and 4.2 mm in length) into the anterior palate.

Continued

CASE REPORT 18-2—cont'd

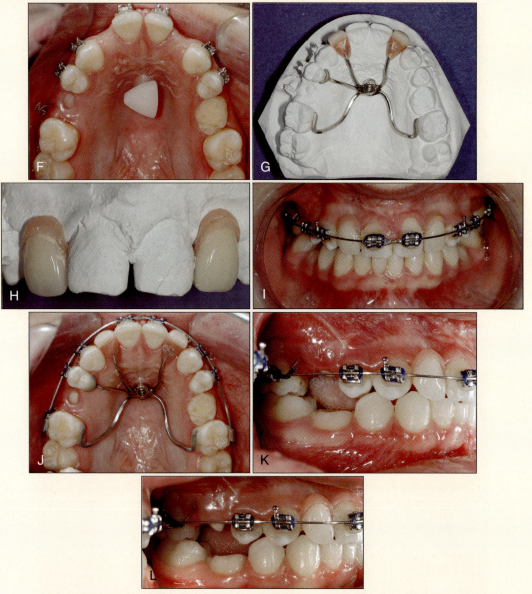

Figure 18-8, cont'd **F,** Situation before impression taking to fabricate the implant-borne superstructure. **G,** Model cast after fabrication of the anchorage unit. Note that only one palatal implant was used for multifunctional anchorage tasks: three-dimensional anchorage of three posterior teeth and temporary prosthetic replacement of teeth #12 and #22. **H,** Model cast with replaced incisors. **I,** Clinical finding with palatal implant-borne lateral incisors during orthodontic treatment. **J,** Palatal view after insertion of implant-borne superstructure. **K,** First, an elastic chain was used to elongate tooth #15. The chain was attached to the implant-borne first molar, thus avoiding intrusion forces to the molar. **L,** Lateral view at end of premolar elongation showing no open-bite development.

CASE REPORT 18-2—cont'd

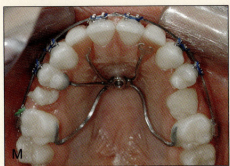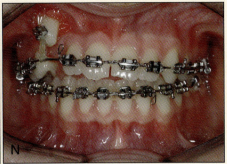

Figure 18-8, cont'd M, Palatal view after premolar movement. N, Potential side effect (bite opening) during canine elongation, if intraarch anchorage without skeletal anchorage is performed.

- Orthodontic treatment and temporary prosthetic replacement of #12 and #22 after a implant healing period of 12 weeks.
- Orthodontic correction of displaced #15 and malocclusion.
- Insertion of conventional prosthetic tooth implants in region #12 and #22 after completion of alveolar bone growth.

After an implant healing period of 12 weeks and conventional molding (Figure 18-8, F), a modified TPA (laser-welded stainless steel, 1.2 mm in diameter) was fabricated (Figure 18-8, G). The superstructure was expanded and connected to two resin-bonded prosthetic teeth by means of wire extensions (laser-welded stainless steel, 1.2 mm in diameter) to fill the gap left by the missing lateral incisors #12 and #22 as space maintainer (Figure 18-8, H and I). The TPA was then inserted and bonded on #16, #26, and #14 for preparation of an implant-supported anchorage unit. The premolar was then moved into position with light forces from elastics and nickel-titanium (Ni-Ti) overlay archwires (.014 and 0.016 inch). Figure 18-8, J to M, shows the treatment sequence during orthodontic tooth movement of #15 to its proper position.

The use of an implant-based TPA led to the elimination of undesired reactive forces and moments (intrusion of anchorage teeth). In this way the occurrence of an iatrogenic lateral open bite and, because of the load on the anchorage unit, additional root resorption could be avoided in this patient case. The existing canine and molar relationship was maintained during treatment. Figure 18-8, N, shows a potential side effect (bite opening) during canine elongation if intraarch anchorage without skeletal anchorage is performed.

As a result, one palatal implant served as prosthetic provisional solution to replace teeth #12 and #22 during orthodontic treatment (esthetic improvement) and fulfilled such functions as maintenance of the sagittal and vertical dimension (multifunctional anchorage task by using one implant).

CASE REPORT 18-3

A 23-year-old male patient was referred for orthodontic treatment with the chief complaint of unesthetic appearance of his teeth (Figure 18-9, A). His medical history was unremarkable. The patient demonstrated protruded lips and an unesthetic smile.

Problem List
Clinical examination and radiological evaluation revealed a mild skeletal Class II malocclusion caused by mandibular retrognathism (Figure 18-9, B). Further intraoral examination revealed a conservatively treated set of teeth, severe anterior maxillary crowding with slight proclination of upper and lower anterior teeth, an overjet of 9 mm, and an overbite of 4 mm. There was a full cusp angle Class II malocclusion on both sides (Figure 18-9, C and D). The lower arch had ideal alignment (Figure 18-9, E). The patient wanted to be treated short term with the least conspicuous appliance possible. He refused extraoral appliances in the form of headgear or orthognathic surgery with dental decompensation and surgical mandibular advancement.

Treatment Concept and Treatment Progress
In consideration of the patient's wishes, the treatment plan provided the following treatment procedures:
- Midpalatal insertion of palatal implant (3.3 × 6 mm; Orthosystem, Straumann; Figure 18-9, F), for stationary anchorage of the posterior segment.
- Extraction of #14 and #24.

Continued

CASE REPORT 18-3—cont'd

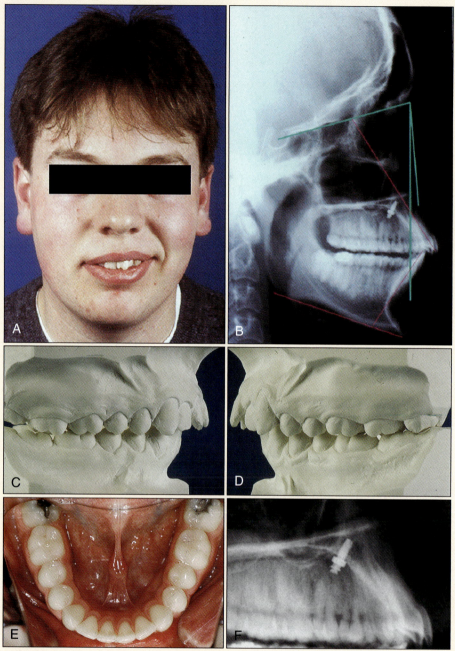

Figure 18-9 **A,** En face photograph of 23-year-old male shows an unesthetic smile. **B,** Cephalogram revealed mild skeletal Class II malocclusion. **C** and **D,** Pretreatment casts with full cusp angle Class II malocclusion, severe maxillary anterior crowding, and 9-mm overjet; view from right *(C)* and from left *(D)*. **E,** Intraoral photograph of lower arch. **F,** Cephalogram after palatal implant insertion (Orthosystem). **G,** Start of orthodontic treatment after extraction of upper first premolars and insertion of TPA at start of orthodontic treatment. **H** and **I,** Intraoral photograph (view from left) after partial canine retraction to resolve anterior crowding *(H)* and after completion of en masse retraction of anterior teeth *(I)*. **J,** Cephalometric superimpositions show the movement of anterior teeth and implant-supported premolars. **K** to **M,** Intraoral findings at end of treatment show Class II molar relationship was maintained at molars and Class I relationship obtained at canines. **N,** Extraoral findings at end of orthodontic treatment.

CASE REPORT 18-3—cont'd

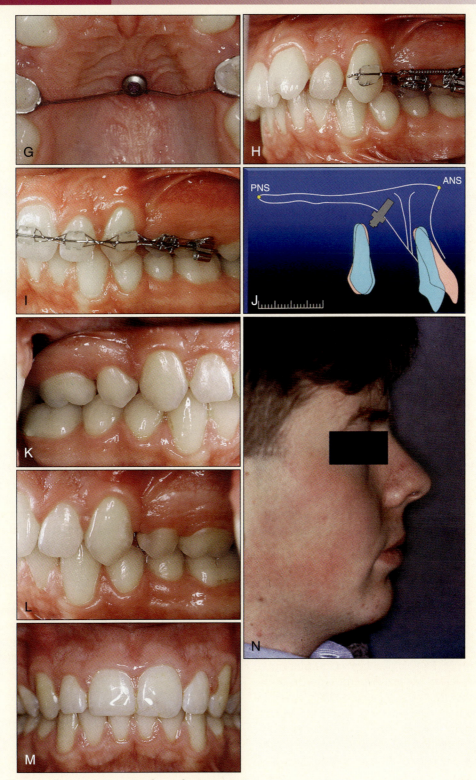

Figure 18-9, cont'd For legend see opposite page.

Continued

CASE REPORT 18-3—cont'd

- Orthodontic treatment with IOIA of posterior teeth for retraction of the canines, en masse retraction of anterior teeth, and palatal root torque for the incisors.
- Postorthodontic phase with permanent retention.

Approximately 10 weeks after implant insertion, the first premolars were extracted. About 2 weeks later, the second premolars bands were fitted, an impression was taken, and an individually configured TPA was produced in the laboratory. The TPA was inserted and active orthodontic treatment started in the same session. First, bilateral sectional arches were inserted for retraction of the canines, using Sentalloy traction springs with a continuous force of 1.5 N per side (Figure 18-9, G). When the canines were partially distalized (Figure 18-9, H and I), en masse retraction of the entire anterior segment against the implant-supported anchorage teeth was accomplished with a continuous force of 2 N per side. After 9 months of treatment, clinical examination revealed no anchorage loss of the anchored teeth in relation to the untreated mandibular dentition (see Figure 18-9, E). Palatal root torque was then applied to the incisors.

Treatment Outcome

The lateral cephalograms after implantation and toward the end of active treatment were overlaid on anterior nasal spine (ANS) and posterior nasal spine (PNS) to analyze the changes in the position of the relevant structures. The evaluation revealed no change in position of the TPA, mesial movement of the premolars by approximately 0.5 mm (uncontrolled tipping), and retraction of the incisors and canines by approximately 8 mm, in terms of an overall controlled tipping (Figure 18-9, J).

After 11 months of treatment, the Class II relationship was maintained, a Class I canine relationship was achieved, and the overjet was corrected (Figure 18-9, K-M). The extraction sites were closed exclusively from retraction of the anterior teeth. Additionally, a lingual bonded retainer from canine to canine was placed in the upper arch for long-term retention. Figure 18-9, N, shows the dentofacial esthetics after completion of active treatment.

CASE REPORT 18-4

A 24-year-old male patient presented for esthetic improvement of an existing malocclusion (Figure 18-10, A). The patient had already received orthodontic treatment in childhood, with extraction of four premolars. Moreover, the patient's mandibular second molar (#37) was extracted because caries and the extraction space were still present (Figure 18-10, B-E).

Problem List

Intraoral examination demonstrated that the midline had deviated 2 mm to the right in the maxilla, with 4 mm of anterior open bite and mild frontal crowding. An approximate Class I molar relationship existed on both sides (see Figure 18-10, C and D). Radiological evaluation (see Figure 18-10, F and G) revealed skeletal hyperdivergence of the jaw base relationship (NSL-ML, 37 degrees) with open-bite anomaly and maxillary retrognathism (SNA, 75 degrees; ANB, −1 degree). Proclination of the upper incisors (IS/NL, 122 degrees) and reclination of the lower incisors (li/ML, 87 degrees) had also occurred. In addition, the panoramic radiograph demonstrated generalized apical root resorptions (see Figure 18-10, F), especially of the upper anterior teeth, probably as a result of extensive use of intermaxillary elastics during early orthodontic treatment for bite closure. Symptoms of temporomandibular disorder (TMD), such as jaw clicking on both sides, were also present.

Treatment Concept and Treatment Progress

The patient refused orthognathic surgery but accepted orthodontic treatment, with the understanding that the treatment result could be compromised. In accordance with an attempt at dental compensation of the open-bite anomaly and space closure in the region of #37, the treatment concept provided the following treatment procedures:

- Surgical insertion of a palatal implant (3.3 × 6 mm; Orthosystem, Straumann).
- Orthodontic treatment after an unloaded implant healing phase of 12 weeks, with correction of the molar position by derotation and intrusion, as well as simultaneous correction of the jaw base relationship by autorotation of the mandible.
- Postorthodontic retention period.

The intrusion of the upper molars was achieved by DOIA (Figure 18-10, H and I). A TPA with a distal hook on both sides (laser-welded stainless steel, 1.2 mm in diameter) was bonded to #16 and #26 using adhesive technique. Two power chains, each from the distal hook of the molars to the applied attachments of the implant's fixation cap, were used for force transfer. For the planned intrusion, a vertical force of approximately 200 g per molar was applied for 18 months (Figure 18-10, J and K).

CASE REPORT 18-4—cont'd

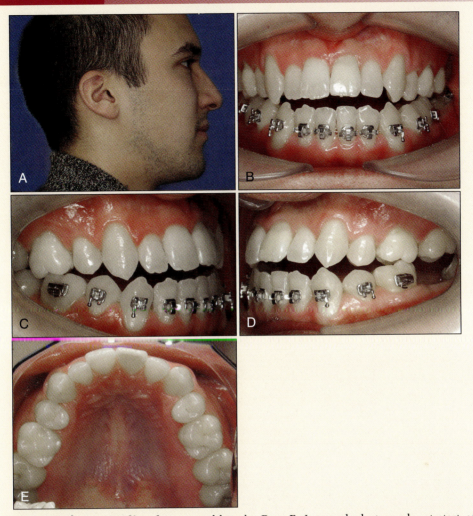

Figure 18-10 A, Profile of 24-year-old male. B to E, Intraoral photographs at start of treatment. Findings after orthodontic treatment in childhood with open bite.

Continued

CASE REPORT 18-4—cont'd

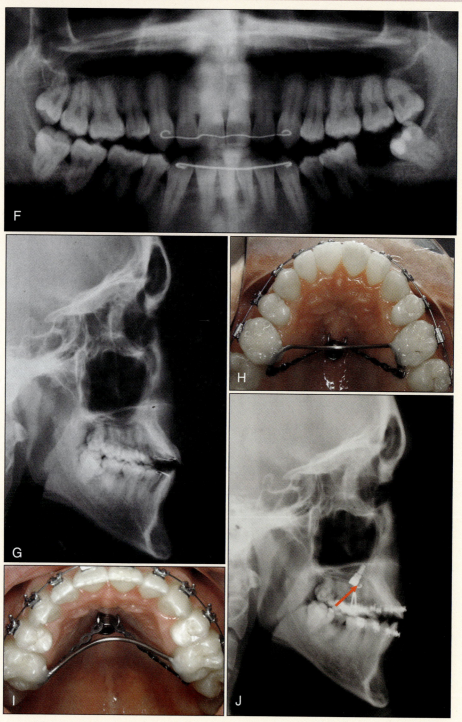

Figure 18-10, cont'd **F** and **G**, Pretreatment panoramic and lateral radiographs at the beginning of present treatment. **H** and **I**, Palatal views after implant insertion and application of a passive TPA to maintain the transverse dimension during molar intrusion. **J** and **K**, Lateral cephalograms with inserted TPA before *(J)* and after *(K)* the intrusion of the molars. Arrow demonstrates the applied attachments of the implant's fixation cap. For the intrusion, a vertical force of approximately 200 g per molar was applied. **L** and **M**, Final profile and profile with superimposed tracing of lateral cephalogram. **N**, Lateral cephalogram after molar intrusion, anterior rotation of mandible, and implant removal. The open bite was closed.

18 Skeletal Anchorage in Orthodontics Using Palatal Implants

CASE REPORT 18-4—cont'd

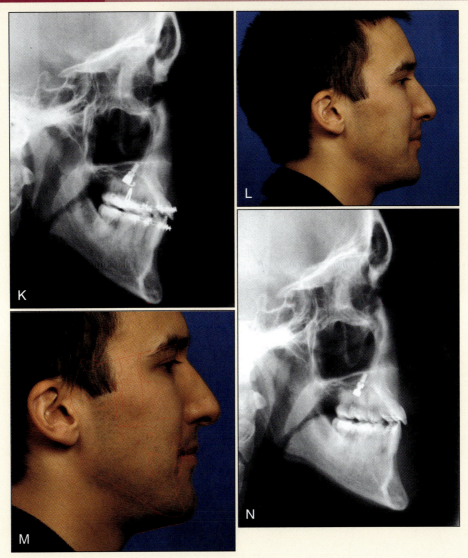

Figure 18-10, cont'd For legend see opposite page.

Continued

CASE REPORT 18-4—cont'd

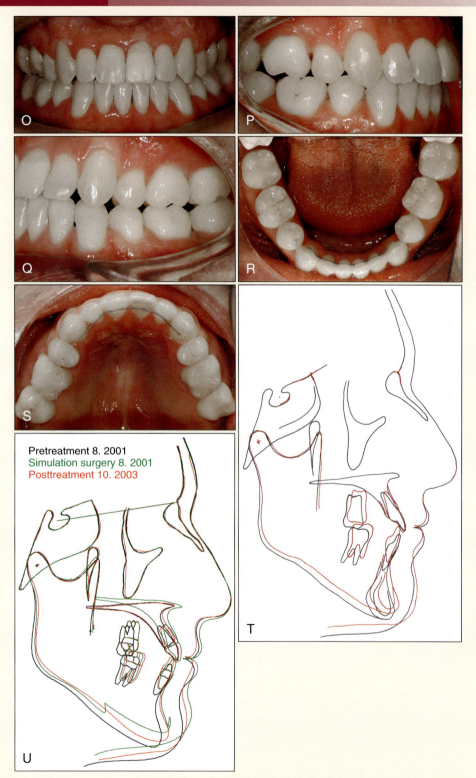

Figure 18-10, cont'd O to S, Intraoral photographs at end of treatment. T, Superimposition of lateral cephalograms before *(black)* and after *(red)* implant-based orthodontic treatment: intrusion and mesialization of maxillary molars as well as autorotation of mandible. U, Superimposition of dental and skeletal structures during orthodontic treatment compared with a surgical simulation.

CASE REPORT 18-4—cont'd

Treatment Outcome

After 28 months of active treatment, the fixed orthodontic appliance was removed. The anterior open bite was entirely corrected, and a dental Class I molar relationship on the right and a slight Class II molar relationship from space closure in region #37 were established (Figure 18-10, L-S). Anterior rotation of the mandible, with a 2-degree decrease in the NS-ML angle, was observed.

Superimpositions of lateral cephalograms before and after treatment show the dental and skeletal changes achieved by implant-based orthodontic treatment (Figure 18-10, T) as well as the movement of the incisors and molars during orthodontic treatment compared with a surgical simulation (Figure 18-10, U).

The question of whether this treatment outcome proves to be stable over a long period of time, and thus whether palatal implants might be used in the future for intentional "therapeutic" inhibition of unfavorable growth tendencies in growing patients, cannot yet be definitively answered. Currently, however, this treatment outcome seems to be stable, at 3 years and 2 months after debonding.

CONCLUSION

Skeletal orthodontic anchorage with palatal implants has expanded the orthodontic treatment spectrum and allowed up-to-date treatment, even in demanding anchorage conditions. One of the most important prerequisites for the successful application of skeletal anchorage with palatal implants is close interdisciplinary cooperation and knowledge in the fields of implantology, periodontology, and orthodontics/dentofacial orthopedics.

REFERENCES

1. Bernhart T, Dortbudak H, Wehrbein H, et al: Das Gaumenimplantat, *Inf Orthod Kieferorthop* 32:209-229, 2000.
2. Bernhart T, Vollgruber A, Gahleitner A, et al: Alternative to the median region of the palate for placement of an orthodontic implant, *Clin Oral Implants Res* 11:595-601, 2000.
3. Diedrich P: A critical consideration of various orthodontic anchorage systems, *J Orofac Orthop* 54:156-171, 1993.
4. Wehrbein H, Merz BR, Hämmerle CHF, Lang NP: Bone-to-implant contact of orthodontic implants in humans subjected to horizontal loading, *Clin Oral Implants Res* 9:348-353, 1998.
5. Wehrbein H: Implants used for anchorage in orthodontic therapy. In Lindhe J, Karring T, Lang NP, editors: *Clinical periodontology and implant dentistry* ed 4, Munksgaard, 2003, Blackwell, pp 1004-1013.
6. Triaca A, Antonini M, Wintermantel E: Ein neues Titan-Flachschrauben-Implantat zur orthodontischen Verankerung am anterioren Gaumen, *Inf Orthod Kieferorthop* 24:251-257, 1992.
7. Wehrbein H, Diedrich P: Endosseous titanium implants during and after orthodontic load: an experimental study in dog, *Clin Oral Implants Res* 4:76-82, 1993.
8. Wehrbein H, Merz BR, Diedrich P, Glatzmaier J: The use of palatal implants for orthodontic anchorage: design and clinical application of the Orthosystem, *Clin Oral Implants Res* 7:410-416, 1996.
9. Wehrbein H, Glatzmaier J, Mundwiller U, Diederich P: The Orthosystem: a new implant system for orthodontic anchorage in the palate, *J Orofac Orthop* 57:142-153, 1996.
10. Glatzmaier J, Wehrbein H, Diedrich P: Biodegradable implants for orthodontic anchorage: a preliminary biomechanical study, *Eur J Orthod* 18:465-469, 1996.
11. De Pauw GAM, Dermaut L, de Bruyn H, Johansson C: Stability of implants as anchorage for orthopedic traction, *Angle Orthod* 69:401-407, 1999.
12. Melsen B, Lang NP: Biological reactions of alveolar bone to orthodontic loading of oral implants, *Clin Oral Implants Res* 12:144-152, 2001.
13. Ödman J, Gröndahl K, Lekholm B: The effect of osseointegrated implants on the dento-alveolar development: a clinical and radiological study in growing pigs, *Eur J Orthod* 13:279-286, 1991.
14. Thilander B, Ödman J, Gröndahl K, Lekholm U: Osseointegrated implants in adolescents: an alternative in replacing missing teeth? *Eur J Orthod* 16:84-95, 1994.
15. Bousquet F, Bousquet P, Mauran G, Parquel P: Use of an impacted post for anchorage, *J Clin Orthod* 5:261-265, 1996.
16. Kanomi R: Mini-implants for orthodontic anchorage, *J Clin Orthod* 11:763-767, 1997.
17. Costa A, Raffini M, Melsen B: Miniscrews as orthodontic anchorage: a preliminary report, *Int J Adult Orthod Orthognath Surg* 13:201-209, 1998.
18. Roberts WE, Marshall KJ, Mozsary PG: Rigid endosseous implant utilized as anchorage to protract molars and close an atrophic extraction site, *Angle Orthod* 60:135-152, 1990.
19. Higuchi KW, Slack JM: The use of titanium fixtures for intraoral anchorage to facilitate orthodontic tooth movement, *Int J Oral Maxillofac Implants* 6:338-344, 1991.
20. Aldikacti M, Açikgöz G, Türk T, Trisi P: Long-term evaluation of sandblasted and acid-etched implants used as orthodontic anchors in dogs, *Am J Orthod Dentofacial Orthop* 125:139-147, 2004.
21. Bernhart T, Freudenthaler J, Dortbudak O, et al: Short epithetic implant for orthodontic anchorage in the paramedian region of the palate: a clinical study, *Clin Oral Implants Res* 12:624-631, 2001.
22. Wehrbein H: Orthodontische Implantatverankerung, *Kieferorthop* 18:117-124, 2004.
23. Block MS, Hoffmann DR: A new device for absolute anchorage in orthodontics, *Am J Orthod Dentofacial Orthop* 3:251-258, 1995.
24. Brånemark P-I, Hansson BO, Adell R, et al: Osseointegrated implants in the treatment of the edentulous jaw, *Scand J Plast Reconstr Surg* 11:1-7, 1977.
25. Ohmae M, Saito S, Morohashi T, et al: A clinical and histological evaluation of titanium mini-implants as anchors for orthodontic intrusion in the beagle dog, *Am J Orthod Dentofacial Orthop* 119:489-497, 2001.
26. Roberts WE, Helm FR, Marshal KJ, Gongloff RK: Rigid endosseous implants for orthodontic and orthopedic anchorage, *Angle Orthod* 59:247-256, 1989.
27. Roberts WE, Smith RK, Silbermann Y, et al: Osseous adaptation to continuous loading of rigid endosseous implants, *Am J Orthod* 86:95-111, 1984.

28. Shapiro PA, Kokich VG: Use of implants in orthodontics, *Dent Clin North Am* 32:539-550, 1988.
29. Van Roeckel NB: The use of Brånemark system implants for orthodontic anchorage: report of a case, *Int J Oral Maxillofac Implants* 4:341-344, 1989.
30. Haanaes HR, Slack JM: The efficacy of two-stage titanium implants as orthodontic anchorage in the preprosthodontic correction of third molars in adults: a report of three cases, *Eur J Orthod* 13:287-296, 1991.
31. Majzoub Z, Finotti M, Miotti F, et al: Bone response to orthodontic loading of endosseous implants in the rabbit calvaria: early continuous distalizing forces, *Eur J Orthod* 21:223-230, 1999.
32. Asscherickx K, Hanssens JL, Wehrbein H, Sabzevar M: Orthodontic anchorage implants inserted in the median palatal suture and normal transverse maxillary growth in growing dogs: a biometric and radiographic study, *Angle Orthod* 75:826-831, 2005.
33. Enlow DH: *Handbook of facial growth*, ed 2, Philadelphia, 1982, Saunders.
34. Björk A: Growth of the maxilla in three dimensions as revealed radiographically by the implant method, *Br J Orthod* 4:53-64, 1977.
35. Baumrind S, Korn EL, Ben-Bassat Y: Quantitation of maxillary remodelling, *Am J Orthod Dentofacial Orthop* 91:29-41, 1987.

Index

Page number followed by t indicates table; f, figure; b, box.
Terms in **bold** type are used in literature under the larger heading of *temporary anchorage devices*, 238-239

A

Aarhus (Denmark), University of, 84-86
Aarhus Anchorage System, 17, 74b, 84-85, 85f
   failure study of, 78, 84-88
   insertion procedure for, 85-86, 86f
   references on, 88-89
Absoanchor microscrew(s), 260-286
   Aarhus study of, 84-88
   anterior retraction and intrusion using, case report, 265f-269f
   canted occlusal plane correction using, case report, 285f
   en masse anterior retraction and intrusion using, case report, 270f-274f
   forced eruption using, case report, 282f-283f
   molar distalization using, case report, 281f
   molar intrusion using
     with bracket head, case report, 278f-279f
     with buccal and palatal implantation, case report, 277f-278f
     with direct or indirect anchorage, 279f-280f
   molar uprighting using
     with one microimplant, case report, 274f-276f
     with two joined microimplants, case report, 276f
Accelerated Osteogenic Orthodontics (Wilcko), 253
Acrylic cap, of Open Bite Appliance, 346, 347f
Acrylic coping, with extension arm, on miniscrew, 158, 159f, 160f
Acrylic resin template guide, 375-376, 376f, 377f
Adverse reactive forces, 76, 78f-79f, 80f
   causing extrusion, prevention of, 156-157, 157f
   device placement and avoidance of, 146. *See also* Appliance mechanics.
   in over-retraction, 174, 176f
Agenesis, dental, 223
Alveolar bone, 6-7, 8f
   biology of, 6-7, 8f
     osteogenic, 252-253, 304-305, 306f
     in tooth movement, 173-174
   bone grafting in, 305-307, 306f
   devitalization of, 8f, 10
   evaluation of, 104, 104f, 108, 253, 304-307
     in brachyfacial patient, 43, 44f-47f
     in dolicofacial patient, 32f-43f
   implant stability in, 8, 10, 10f, 88, 104, 104f. *See also* Stability.
   miniscrew penetration of, 100, 103f, 261, 262f
   stress modeling of, 25-26, 27f, 28t
Alveolar bone traces tooth movement, 173, 174

Anchor implant, 238
Anchor plate, 249, 250f-252f, 252. *See also* Miniplate(s).
Anchor screw, 238. *See also* Miniscrew(s)/microscrew(s).
Anchorage, 3, 342, 393
   direct or indirect, 146, 151-159, 198-199, 199f, 393. *See also specific orthodontic process or appliance.*
   mechanically retained, 15, 73, 74b
   nonosseointegrated, 342
   osseointegrated, 3, 6, 15-16, 73, 74b, 295, 342
Anchorage classification, and miniscrew position, 108f-110f
   Type A, 108, 109f
   Type B, 108, 109f, 110
   Type C, 110, 110f
Anchorage component, 3
Anesthesia, local, 99, 172, 261, 261f, 289, 289f
   with intravenous sedation, 325
Angle of insertion, of miniscrew, 101, 101f
Animal studies, of temporary anchorage devices
   applicability of, 73-74
   and primary stability, 76, 78
   references on, 47
   stress analysis in beagle dogs, 26, 28
     results of, 28, 31f, 32
Ankylosed teeth, 238, 343
Anodontia, 223
Anterior open bite, 126f, 344-346
   appliance mechanics in, 151-154, 175f-176f, 177, 184t, 188, 190-191
   direct and indirect anchorage, 154-157, 155f, 157f
   using miniplate skeletal anchorage, 317-341. *See also under* Miniplate(s).
     case report, 331f-341f
   using miniscrews, case report, 136f-143f
   using Open Bite Appliance, 344-349
   three-dimensional, case report, 218f-221f. *See also* Occlusal plane correction.
   using zygomatic anchorage of miniplate, case reports, 349f-356f
   with Class I relationship, and dentoalveolar protrusion
     treatment with miniscrews, case report, 190-191, 192f-193f
     treatment with Multipurpose Implant, case report, 355f-356f
   with Class II malocclusion

Anterior open bite—cont'd
    and high mandibular plane angle, 188, 190, 191f
    and retrognathic mandible and maxilla
        treatment with Multipurpose Implant, case report, 349f-354f
        treatment with miniplates and fixation screws, case report, 331f-341f
    with Class III malocclusion, and mandibular dentoalveolar protrusion, 177, 188, 189f-190f
    common morphological changes in, 346
    over-retraction in, osseous response in, 174, 176f
    relapse of intrusion in, 176f, 193, 195
Anterior-posterior movement, 154-157
    direct and indirect anchorage in, 154-157, 155f, 157f
    equivalent force systems in, 146, 147f, 148
    extrusion side effect in, preventing, 156-157, 157f
    in molar protraction, 134-135, 134f, 135f, 146, 147f, 148f
    in space closure, 75f-76f
Anterior retraction, and intrusion, 145, 151-154, 155f, 177
    alveolar osseous reaction in, 174, 176f, 193, 195
    appliance mechanics in, 108-120, 120f, 154-157, 177, 184f-188f, 184t
        using ball-ended miniplates, 361f-365f
        direct and indirect anchorage, 108f-110f, 154-157
        insertion site and sequence, 108, 109f-110f, 110
        line of force, 157, 157f
        in mandibular arch, 119, 120f
            case report, 269f-274f
        occlusal plane rotation in lateral plane, 263, 264f
        using palatal implant, 120f, 380, 383f, 398f-400f
        with resorbable microimplants, case report, 242f-243f
        sliding, 116-120, 262-274
        in vertical occlusal plane, 116, 116f, 117f, 118
        using zygomatic buttress anchorage, 361-365
    boundaries of tooth movement in, 173-174
    en masse, 108-120, 136, 156-157, 177, 188, 190-191, 269, 380. *See also* Occlusal plane correction; Whole arch movement/rotation.
    in anterior open bite, case report, 136f-143f
    in Class I bimaxillary dentoalveolar protrusion, case report, 177, 178f-179f
    in Class I malocclusion with overbite, 269f-274f
    in Class II, Division I malocclusion, case report, 361f-365f
    in Class II bimaxillary dentoalveolar protrusion, case report, 177, 180f-181f
    in Class II malocclusion, case report, 403f-406f
    in Class III mandibular dentoalveolar protrusion, case report, 177, 182f-183f
    extrusion side effects in, preventing, 156-157, 157f
    friction side effects in, preventing, 156-157, 157f
    in limited skeletal anchorage, 307-308, 309f

Anterior retraction, and intrusion—cont'd
    with bracket-head microimplants, case report, 246f-249f
    in edentulous patients, 296-297
    with mini-implant and transpalatal arch, 76, 77f-78f
    with surgical wire through infrazygomatic crest, 75, 75f-76f
    occlusal plane changes in, 116-118. *See also* Occlusal plane correction.
Anterior spacing, 295, 296f
Appliance design. *See* Appliance mechanics.
Appliance mechanics, 93-144, 145-163
    clinical application of
        in anterior open bite, 151-154, 175f-176f, 177, 184t, 188, 190-191. *See also* Anterior open bite.
        in anterior-posterior movement, 134-135, 146-148, 154-156, 177. *See also* Anterior-posterior movement.
        in anterior retraction, and intrusion, 108-120, 151-157, 177, 188, 190-191. *See also* Anterior retraction, and intrusion.
        in buccal segment intrusion, 151-154. *See also* Buccal segment intrusion.
        and conventional orthodontic mechanics, 116-118
        in crossbite correction, 145, 157, 214. *See also* Transverse occlusal plane correction.
        in forced eruption, 282f-283f
        for impacted molar, 132f-133f
        in less-than-ideal situations, alternatives and solutions, 161-162, 161f, 162f
        in limited anchorage, 284f, 307-312. *See also* Bone density; Edentulous space closure; Missing teeth; Site assessment.
        in malocclusions, 149-151, 154, 155f, 198-222. *See also* Occlusal plane correction.
        using miniplate skeletal anchorage, 317-341. *See also* Miniplate(s).
        in molar distalization, 126-128, 154-156, 199-201, 270f-274f, 281f. *See also* Molar distalization.
        in molar extrusion, 128-130, 148-149, 274, 276, 291f-293f. *See also* Molar extrusion (uprighting).
        in molar intrusion, 121-126, 148-151, 174, 177, 184f, 184t, 212-214. *See also* Molar intrusion.
        in molar mesialization, 78f-79f, 80f, 156, 223-225. *See also* Molar mesialization.
        in molar protraction, 134-135, 146-148. *See also* Molar protraction.
        in occlusal plane changes, 116-118
    references on, 143-144, 162-163
    and selection of appliance or system
        factors considered in, 148-149

Appliance mechanics—cont'd
  selection of appliance or system in, 148-162
  sliding
    versus loop mechanics, 116, 116f, 117f, 156-157
    in space closure, 75f-76f, 134-135, 149-157, 226-237, 249-252. *See also* Edentulous space closure.
    in whole arch movement/rotation, 136, 136f-143f, 198-222. *See also* Whole arch movement/rotation.
  sliding, 262-264
Archwires, stainless steel, 177
  attached to Quattro screw, 170f
  without first order curvature, 116
Asymmetric dentition, orthodontics in, 76
  and forward displacement of lower arch, 81f-82f
  using miniplates, 317-341. *See also* Miniplate(s).

B

Bands, custom-made, 307, 308f
BH. *See* Bracket head (BH) miniscrew(s).
Bilateral expansion appliances, 214, 216f
Bioabsorbable materials, 239-241
  degradation of, 241-242
Bioactive SLA surface, 307
Biofilm formation, 15, 15t
Bioglass-coated implants, 238
Bioglass implants, 14
Biological boundary, of orthodontic tooth movement, 167
Biological response, 14-21. *See also* Healing process.
  inflammatory, 15-16, 15t, 49, 150, 151f
    in labial frenulum, 105, 105f, 154
  to mechanically retained anchorage devices, 6-11, 15t, 16
  to osseointegrated anchorage devices, 15-16, 15t
Biomechanics. *See* Appliance mechanics.
Bioprogressive therapy, 348
BIOS (bioresorbable implant anchor for orthodontics system), 242, 393
Bisphosphonates, 18-19
Blade implants, 5, 6, 295
Bleeding
  and numbness, management of, 108
  in palate, during implant placement, 375
Block grafts, autogenous, 305-307, 306f
BMD (bone mineral density), 16
Bodily translation, in upper arch, 108. *See also* Anterior retraction, and intrusion; Whole arch movement/rotation.
Bone, alveolar, 6-7, 8f
  anchorage in. *See* Anchorage.
  biology of, 6-7, 8f. *See also* Bone remodeling; Cortical bone; Osteogenesis.
    osteogenic, 252-253, 304-305, 306f
    tooth movement and, 173-174

Bone, alveolar—cont'd
  bone grafting in, 304, 305-307, 306f
  classification of, 390
  devitalization of, 8f, 10
  evaluation of, 104, 104f, 108, 253, 304-307
    in brachyfacial patient, 43, 44f-47f
    in dolicofacial patient, 32f-43f
  implant stability in, 8, 10, 10f, 88, 104, 104f. *See also* Stability.
  miniscrew penetration of, 100, 103f, 261, 262f
  stress modeling of, 25-26, 27f, 28t
Bone crushing, advantages and disadvantages of, 10
Bone density (hardness), 16. *See also* Cortical bone.
  in brachyfacial patient, 43, 44f-47f
  determination of, 169-170, 170t
  in dolicofacial patient, case study, 32, 34f, 36f, 39f, 41f, 43f
  miniscrew insertion based on, 169-172, 170t, 171f, 261
Bone grafts, 304, 305-307, 306f
Bone height evaluation, of palate, 374, 375, 375b
Bone lengthening, 252
Bone mineral density (BMD), 16
Bone plates, 14, 15
  modified, 3
Bone remodeling. *See also* Osteogenesis.
  after implantation, 11, 11f, 15t, 16, 88
  and delayed failure of miniscrew implant, 104
  during incisor retraction, 174, 175f, 176f
  and migration of implant, 167-168
  during molar intrusion, 174
Bone traces tooth movement, 173, 174
Boundaries, of orthodontic tooth movement, 173-174, 176f
Brachyfacial patient
  bone study of, 43, 44f-47f
  implant orthodontics in, 154, 155f
Bracket addition, to miniscrew, 158-159, 159f
Bracket head (BH) miniscrew(s), 240f, 243, 249, 260, 261f
  Aarhus, 85f
  Absoanchor, in molar intrusion, case report, 278, 278f-279f
  proper ligature using, 87f, 88
  for tooth movement in edentulous spaces, case reports, 243f-245f, 246f-249f
Brånemark, biological concept of implantation, 5-6, 393
Brånemark implants, 4, 49, 238, 295, 342
Buccal segment intrusion, 151-154, 152f. *See also* Dentoalveolar protrusion.
  direct and indirect anchorage for, 151-154, 152f, 153f, 154f
  level or canted, appliance design, 151, 153, 153f, 154f
  plate system versus miniscrews in, 151

Buccal segment intrusion—cont'd
  pure translatory, appliance design, 151, 153f
  tipping prevention in, 153, 154f
Buccal tipping, 116, 116f

C

Canine distalization, rapid, using anchorage and distraction, 252-253, 255f, 256, 256f-257f
Canted occlusal plane(s), 214, 215f
Canted occlusal plane correction
  Absoanchor microimplants in, case report, 285f
  molar extrusion in, appliance design, 211, 211f
  molar intrusion in, appliance design, 151, 153f, 154f, 212-214, 212f, 213f
Cantilever system
  for anterior retraction, whole segment, 154, 157, 157f
  coupling of, with noninvasive miniplate, 159-160
  forces applied in, 158, 158f, 308
    direction of, 158-159, 159f
    magnitude of, 160, 160f
  for incisor intrusion, 154
  one couple, 158, 158f, 159f, 160f
  for retraction and intrusion in limited anchorage, 308, 308f, 309f
  second-order coupling of, with miniscrew, 158-159, 159f
  technical aspects of, 158
CB CT scanners. *See* Cone-beam computed tomography.
CB MercuRay, 25
Cephalogram, for palatal bone height evaluation, 375, 375b, 376f
Chewing gum, natural, 348, 349f
Circle head (CH) microimplant, 260, 261f
Cobalt-chromium alloy (Vitallium)
  blade implants, 5, 295
  screws, 14, 238
Coil spring(s)
  compressed, in molar distalization with Multipurpose Implant, 357, 357f
  in molar extrusion, attached to miniscrew head, 128-129, 130f
  nickel-titanium, 170f, 177, 346, 347f
  Sentalloy, on Aarhus mini-implant, 85f
    asymmetric tooth movement using, 81f-82f
    molar mesialization using, 78f-79f, 80f
Coil spring-arm, push-open, 224, 225-226, 226f
Compensating curve, 116, 116f
Compliance factor, in orthodontic process, 73-74
Complications
  of miniplate implantation, 326, 331, 344
  of miniscrew insertion, 105-108, 291
    abscess, 105
    bleeding and numbness, 108
    miniscrew fracture, 105, 108, 291
    pain, 108

Complications—cont'd
  root damage, 105, 107f
  soft tissue coverage, 105, 105f
  soft tissue inflammation and ulceration, 105, 105f
Cone-beam computed tomography (CB CT), 25. *See also specific case report.*
  in alveolar bone ridge analysis, 304, 305f
  of brachyfacial patient, 43f-47f
  in cortical bone thickness assessment, 8, 8f-9f
  of dolicofacial patient, 32f-43f
  references on, 47
Congenitally missing teeth, 223, 226
  case reports of orthodontic treatment, 226f-237f
Connecticut, University of, 298
Constriction, 149
Contra-angle handled screwdriver, 97, 98f
Controlled tipping, 118, 119f, 149
Conventional anchorage, in orthodontics, 73
Cope, J.B., 15, 15f
Core resin, 276f
Cortical bone, 6-7, 8f
  blood flow through, 8f
  devitalization of, 8f, 10
  hardness of, 170t
  insufficient, for miniscrew anchorage, 103, 104, 104f, 253
  miniscrew insertion in, 169-170, 171f, 261-262, 263f
  postoperative implant integration in, 8, 10, 10f
  in upper and lower posterior segment, 108
Corticision (Young Guk Park), 253
COSMOS/M, finite element modeling with, 25-26
Cost effectiveness, 145
Cost efficiency, 145-146
COX inhibitors. *See* Cyclooxygenase-2 (COX-2) inhibitors.
Crossbite, 214, 317, 318f. *See also* Transverse occlusal plane correction.
  severe anterior, skeletal anchorage system for, 317, 318f-319f. *See also* Skeletal anchorage.
Curve of Spee, compensating/reverse, 116, 116f
Cyclooxygenase-2 (COX-2) inhibitors, 18
Cyst, in area of upper bicuspid, case report, 233f-236f

D

Deep bite
  Class II, Division 1
    with maxillary midline deviation, case report, 227f-229f
    with missing mandibular bicuspids, case report, 227f-229f
  Class II, Division 1, relapsed, in brachycephalic woman, 5f
  Class II, Division 2, case report, 110f-115f
  and limited skeletal anchorage, case report, 246f-249f

Dental implants, 3, 15f, 73, 74b. *See also* Osseointegrated anchorage devices.
Dental open bite, 345
Dental trauma, incidence of, 223
Dentoalveolar dysplasia, K-1 System orthodontics in, 58f-72f
   assessment photography and cephalometric analysis, 58, 59f-60f
   insertion of implant, 58, 61f
   orthodontic treatment before second surgery, 58, 60, 62f
   posttreatment results, 62
      photography/radiography/cephalometric analysis, 62, 67f, 68f-69f
      two year, photography/radiography/cephalometric analysis, 64, 71f, 72f
   second surgery locating and engaging implants, 60, 62, 63f
   treatment progression, 60, 62, 64f, 65f, 66f
   stent preparation for surgery, 58, 61f
   third surgery for implant removal, 63-64, 70f
Dentoalveolar protrusion, 177
   appliance mechanics in, 177, 184t
   Class I, case reports, 190-191, 192f-193f, 265f-269f
   Class I bimaxillary, appliance mechanics, 177, 178f-179f
   Class II bimaxillary, appliance mechanics, 177, 180f-181f
   Class III mandibular, appliance mechanics, 177, 182f-183f
   miniplate orthodontics in, 317-341. *See also* Miniplate(s).
Dentos microimplants, 252, 253f, 254f. *See also* Absoanchor microscrew(s).
   and miniplates, 252, 252f
   stress analysis of, 76
Design, appliance. *See* Appliance mechanics, *or specific appliance or system.*
Devitalization, tissue, around miniscrew, 8, 8f, 10. *See also* Biological response.
Diagnostic wax-up, 298, 300f, 301, 301f-302f
Diameter, of miniscrews, 95, 96f, 260. *See also* Stability.
   and implant stability, 76, 84f, 169
      modeling, 26, 28f, 29f, 30f, 31t, 96f
   and length, 95, 95f
Differential moment concept, 73
Direct anchorage, 146, 151-159, 198-199, 199f. *See also specific orthodontic process or appliance.*
Distal Jet appliance, microscrew supported, 289, 290f
Distalization
   of mandibular teeth, boundaries of tooth movement, 173-174
   of maxillary teeth, boundaries of tooth movement, 173-174
   of molars, anchorage devices for, 145. *See also* Molar distalization.

Distalization—cont'd
   rapid canine, using anchorage and distraction, 252-253, 255f, 256, 256f-257f
Distraction, skeletal anchorage with, 253, 255f, 256, 256f-257f
Distraction osteogenesis, 252-253
Distractor, maintaining level of, 256, 256f
Dolicofacial patient, bone study of, case report, 32f-43f
   distal canine alveolar bone, 32, 35f, 36f
   lower anterior alveolar bone, 32, 38f, 39f
   lower molar alveolar bone, 34, 42f, 43f
   lower premolar alveolar bone, 32, 34, 40f, 41f
   molar site selection, 32, 37f
   three-dimensional skull reconstruction, 32, 32f
   upper anterior alveolar bone, 32, 33f, 34f
Driver assembly(ies), 98f
   with miniscrew in place, 98f
Driver tip(s), short and long, 97, 98f
Dual Top Anchor microscrew(s), 288-289
   design of, 288-289, 288f
   diameter of, 288, 289t
   extrusion mechanics using, case report, 291f-293f
   failure rate of, 291
   insertion procedure for, 289, 289f
   loading protocols for, 289, 290f
   removal procedure for, 289
   site assessment for, 289-291, 290f

E

Edentulous patients, treatment options for, 295-296. *See also* Prosthodontic restoration.
Edentulous space closure
   using bracket-head microimplants, case report, 243f-245f
   using direct and indirect anchorage, 156-157, 157f
   in mandibular anterior retraction, case report, 246f-249f
   in molar intrusion, 149
   in molar mesialization, 223-224
   in molar protraction, 134-135, 134f, 135f
   in patients with congenitally missing teeth, 226
      missing lateral incisors, upper and lower, case report, 229, 230f-232f
      missing mandibular bicuspids, case report, 226f-229f
      missing upper bicuspid, 233f-236f
   in periodontally compromised patient, 284f
   using resorbable screws, case report, 242f-243f
   in whole arch movement, 224-226
Edgewise system, compatibility with, 169
Elastic chain(s), linear force applied by, 93, 94f, 126f. *See also* Coil spring(s).
Elastomeric thread, 274f, 275f
   in mandibular arch during whole arch movement, 270, 272f

En masse movement of teeth. *See* Anterior retraction, and intrusion; Buccal segment intrusion; Whole arch movement/rotation.
Endosseous implants, 238, 295. *See also* Endosseous miniscrew(s).
 in orthodontic treatment and prosthetics, 295-313
  alveolar bone ridge analysis, 304-307
  anterior spacing as indication, 295, 296f
  financial considerations, 295-296
  fixed bridges or implants, 296-297
  loading implants, 307
  mechanics, 307-312
  occlusal plane analysis for implant placement, 301, 303-304
  occlusion improvement, 295-296, 310, 312
  placement planning, 298, 299f
  temporary anchorage or dental implant, 297
  three-dimensional visualization, 298, 300f, 301, 301f-302f
  treatment planning, 297-298
 references on, 313
 in removable and fixed devices, 297
 in restoring space, 310, 312, 312f
Endosseous miniscrew(s), 3-13
 biologic response to, 6-7, 10-11
 clinical questions about, 6
 development of, 3, 4-6
 failure rate of, 10
 healing and integration of, 8, 10-11
 importance of, 6
 laboratory testing of, 3-4
 manufacturing improvements of, 4, 10
 references on, 11-13
 self-drilling, 10
 site assessment for, 7-8
 stability of, 4, 11, 11f
Equipment, for miniscrew insertion, 97, 98f, 99. *See also specific implant.*
Equivalent force system(s), 118-119, 119f-120f, 146, 147f, 148
Eruption. *See* Forced eruption.
Expansion, 149
 appliances for bilateral and unilateral, 157, 158f, 214, 216f, 217f
 fixed appliances for, 214, 216f, 395f, 396
Extended arm(s), 177, 199-200, 200f
 and acrylic coping, on miniscrew, 158, 159f, 160f
 from implanted acrylic crown, 309, 310f
Extrusion mechanics, 148-149
 using Dual Top Anchor microscrews, case report, 291f-293f
 in forced canine eruption, 282
  case report, 282f-283f
 for impacted molar, case report, 132f-133f
 of molars. *See* Molar extrusion.
 side effects of, preventing, 156-157, 157f
 and skeletal anchorage, 317, 319, 320f

F

Failure, of miniscrew anchorage, 10, 78, 104, 172-173, 286
 Aarhus study of, 78, 84-88
 appliance design in, 85f, 86
 delayed, 104
 dentist/procedure-related, and solutions, 86, 88
 device-related, and solutions, 86
 Dual Top microscrews, 291
 immediate, 103, 104, 104f
 incorrect ligature placement in, 86, 87f, 88
 mechanical strength in, 76
 Orlus miniscrew system, 104
 osseointegration in, 10-11
 patient-related, and solutions, 88
 predictors of, 78, 84
 primary stability and, 76, 78, 86
 screwdriver positioning in, 86, 87f
 studies of, 76, 78, 84-88, 287-288. *See also* Finite element modeling (FEM) analysis.
Fibro-osseous integration, 49
Finite element modeling (FEM) analysis, 25-32, 76, 95-96. *See also* Stability.
 with COSMOS/M, 25-26
 references on, 47
 strain versus miniscrew diameter, 26, 28f, 29f, 30f, 31t, 95, 96f
 stress on miniscrew and bone, 25-26, 27f, 28t, 29f, 30f, 95, 95f
  stress distribution table, 31t
  tractional loading models, 28f
 surgical steel screws and titanium screws, 76
Fixation head (FH) microimplant, 260, 261f
Fixation screw(s), 3, 15, 15f, 342
 first report of, 6
 monocortical, 317, 320f
Fixation wires, 15f
Fixed bridges, advantages of, 296-297
Fixed expansion appliances, 214, 216f, 395f, 396
Force system(s), 17, 18t, 93-94, 94f, 146-148
 for anterior-posterior movement. *See* Anterior-posterior movement.
 for anterior retraction. *See* Anterior open bite; Anterior retraction, and intrusion.
 for buccal segment intrusion. *See* Buccal segment intrusion.
 for crossbite (transverse expansion). *See* Transverse occlusal plane correction.
 for incisor intrusion. *See* Anterior open bite; Anterior retraction, and intrusion.
 intrusive component of, 93, 94f, 149-150, 150f
 less-than-ideal, alternatives and solutions, 161-162, 161f, 162f
 line of force in, 93, 118, 119f, 146
 magnitude of forces in, 148, 160, 160f
 moderate force in, 93
 for molar distalization. *See* Molar distalization.

Force system(s)—cont'd
  for molar extrusion. *See* Molar extrusion (uprighting).
  for molar intrusion. *See* Molar intrusion.
  for occlusal plane correction. *See* Occlusal plane correction.
  one-couple and two-couple, 158-160. *See also* Cantilever system.
  of Open Bite Appliance, 346, 348, 348f
  orthopedic, 148
  for pure translation, 134, 134f. *See also* Translation.
  references on, 162-163
  for root movement, 134-135, 135f. *See also* Root movement.
  for root movement and translation, 135, 135f
  in sliding mechanics and loop mechanics, 116, 116f, 117f, 118, 118f, 156-157
  for space closure. *See* Anterior-posterior movement; Missing teeth.
Forced eruption, 282
  of canine, case report, 282f-283f
  as indication for skeletal anchorage, 317, 319, 320t
Fracture, of temporary tooth, 307
Fractured miniscrew, 105, 108, 291
Frenectomy, incisional, 105, 106f
Frenulum, inflammation of, 105, 105f, 154
Friadent system implant, 380, 381f. *See also* Straumann palatal implants.
  dimensions of, 375
  surgical placement of, 376, 378f-379f

G

Gable bends, 116, 116f
Gingiva. *See* Soft tissue.
Gingiva former, 376, 379f, 380
Grafts. *See* Bone grafts.
Guide drill(s), short and long, 97, 98f

H

Healing process. *See also* Complications.
  around titanium implants, 10-11, 10f, 15t, 16
  in osseointegration, 15-16, 15t
  and stability after osseointegration, 16. *See also* Primary stability.
Historical development, of temporary anchorage devices, 3, 4-6, 14-15
Hook screw, LOMAS, 169, 170f
Horton, Tom, 4
Hydroxyapatite coated disk, 14, 73
Hypodontia, 223
Hyrax expansion device, 214, 216f, 217f, 225, 225f
  in counteracting forces of molar intrusion., 149

I

i-CAT, 25
i-CAT software, 25
i-DENT software, 25

I-plate(s), 317, 320f
  fixation of, 320
  in maxillary molar protraction, 324, 325f
i-VIEW software, 25
Ilizarov, Gravial, 252
Immediate loading, of implanted anchorage devices, 15
Impacted molar, uprighting of, 129, 131f
  case report, 132f-133f
Implant(s), 238-239
  definition of, 239
Implant carrier, safe removal of, 379, 380f
Implant modeling, 26, 27f, 28t. *See also* Animal studies; Finite element modeling (FEM) analysis.
Implant supported prostheses (ISPs), 3. *See also* Prosthodontic restoration.
Incision. *See* Insertion.
Incisive canal perforation, in palate, 374
Incisor retraction, and intrusion
  alveolar osseous reaction in, 174, 175f, 176f
  appliance design for, 108-120, 120f, 145, 148-149, 154, 155f. *See also* Anterior retraction.
  lower. *See* Mandibular arch.
Indirect anchorage, 146, 151-159, 198-199. *See also* specific orthodontic process or appliance.
Infection
  after miniplate implantation, 326, 331, 331f
  as complication in predrilling, 88
Inflammation, soft tissue, 15-16, 15t, 49, 150, 151f, 291. *See also* Biological response.
  of labial frenulum, 105, 105f, 154
  in surgical placement of Multipurpose Implant, 344
Infrazygomatic crest. *See* Maxillary infrazygomatic crest.
Insertion, of miniscrew(s), 100, 168-169, 168f, 261-262. *See also* Site assessment.
  in alveolar bone, 100, 103f, 261, 262f
  anesthesia preceding, 261-262, 261f
  angle of, 101, 101f
  based on bone hardness, 169-172, 170t, 171f, 261
  biological response to, 15t, 16. *See also* Biological response; Inflammation.
  bone vasculature, 6-7
  healing, 8, 10-11
  complications of, 105-108, 291
  equipment used in, 97, 98f, 99. *See also* specific implant or anchorage system.
  failure studies of, 78, 84-88
  incision for, 261, 262f
  mesiodistal path of, 101-102, 102f
  in non–tooth-bearing sites, 168-169, 168f
  occlusogingival angle of, 100, 101f
  path of, 101-102, 102f
  postoperative care in, 105-108, 172, 173f
  predrilling in, 261-262, 263f
  procedure for, 261-262

Insertion, of miniscrew(s)—cont'd
   with Aarhus mini-implant, 85-86, 86f
   with Dual Top Anchor microscrew, 289, 289f
   with K-1 System, 58, 61f
   with LOMAS, 169-172, 172f, 173f
   with Orlus miniscrew system, 99-102, 103f-104f
   soft tissue management during, 102
   soft tissue penetration in, 101, 261, 261f
   with tissue punch, 7-8, 8f, 169, 171f
   success of, clinical evaluation, 172-173, 193, 195
Insertion/implantation procedure, for miniplates, 325-326, 327f, 328f
Insufficient anchorage. *See* Bone density; Edentulous space closure; Missing teeth.
Interocclusal clearance, 303, 303f
Interradicular implantation, 289-290, 291f, 393
Interradicular space determination, axial CT scan, 99, 99f
Intrusion, 93, 94f
   in anterior open bite, relapse of, 176f, 193, 195
   of buccal segment or occlusal plane, 151-154. *See also* Buccal segment intrusion; Occlusal plane correction.
   of incisors and molars, 145, 148-149. *See also* Anterior open bite; Anterior retraction; Molar intrusion.
Intrusive component, of force, 93, 94f
IZ crest. *See* Maxillary infrazygomatic crest.

J

Jasper Jumpers, 366, 369f-370f

K

K-1 System, 4, 49-50, 72
K-1 System orthodontics
   in dentoalveolar dysplasia, case report, 58f-72f
     assessment, 58, 59f-60f
     implant insertion surgery, 58, 61f
     orthodontic treatment prior to second surgery, 58, 60, 62f
     posttreatment, 62, 67f, 68f-69f
     removal of implants, 63-64, 70f
     second surgical procedure, 60, 62, 63f
     surgical stent preparation, 58, 61f
     treatment progression after second surgery, 60, 62, 64f, 65f, 66f
     two-year posttreatment, 64, 71f, 72f
   in temporomandibular disorder, case report, 50f-58f
     assessment, 50, 51f, 52f
     CT evaluation before second surgery, 50, 54f
     implant osseointegration, 50, 53f
     posttreatment analysis, 55-58, 57f, 58f
     surgical stent preparation, 50, 53f
     symptom alleviation with splint therapy, 50
     treatment progression and alignment, 50, 54, 55f
     vertical traction application, 50, 54, 55f
Kanomi, Ryuzo, 4, 14-15

L

L-plate(s), 317
   fixation of, 320
     in mandibular molar distalization, 322, 322f
     in mandibular molar intrusion, 323-324, 324f
     in mandibular molar protraction, 325, 326f
Leone miniscrew, stress analysis of, 76
Lever arm, miniscrew combination with, 134, 134f
Lever arms, intruding/extruding, 177
LH. *See* Long head (LH) microimplant.
Ligature placement, correct and incorrect, 86, 87f, 88
Limited skeletal anchorage. *See* Bone density; Edentulous space closure; Missing teeth; Site assessment.
Line of force, 93, 94f, 146
   adjustment and limitations of, 118-119, 119f
Lingual anchorage, on bands, 307, 308-309, 308f
Lingual arch, 199-200, 262, 263f
   and extended arms, 199-200, 200f
Linkow, Leonard, 6
Loading anchorage implants, 307. *See also specific implant.*
   and implant migration, 167-168
   protocols for, 17, 18t, 289, 290f
   stress modeling of, 28f
Local anesthesia, 99, 172, 261, 261f, 289, 289f
   with intravenous sedation, 325
LOMAS (Lin/Liou Orthodontic Mini Anchor System), 169
   appliance mechanics of, 174, 177, 184f-188f, 184t
   bone hardness and insertion procedure for, 169-170, 170t, 171f
   insertion of miniscrew in, 169-172, 171f, 173f
   postoperative care, 172, 173f
   orthodontics using, 177, 188, 190-191
     in Class I anterior open bite, with dentoalveolar protrusion, 190-191, 192f-193f
     in Class I bimaxillary dentoalveolar protrusion, 177, 178f-179f
     in Class II anterior open bite, with high mandibular plane angle, 188, 190, 191f
     in Class II bimaxillary dentoalveolar protrusion, 177, 180f-181f
     in Class III anterior open bite, with mandibular dentoalveolar protrusion, 177, 188, 189f-190f
     in Class III mandibular dentoalveolar protrusion, 177, 182f-183f
     in mandibular micrognathia, 191, 193, 194f-195f
   references on, 195-197
   success of, 173, 193, 195
LOMAS hook screw, 169, 170f, 184t
LOMAS Quattro screw, 169, 170f, 184t
Long-collared miniscrew, 97, 97f
Long head (LH) microimplant, 260, 261f
Long-headed miniscrew, 240f

Loop mechanics, 116, 116f
Loosening, of miniscrew, 88, 103, 104

M

Magnet, for opposing force, 310, 312, 312f
Malocclusion(s)
  Class I
    with dentoalveolar protrusion, case report, 265f-269f
    with high mandibular plane angle, case report, 270f-274f
    with missing incisors, case report, 230f-232f
  Class II
    case report, 202f-205f
    with dentoalveolar protrusion, case report, 233f-236f
    Division I, case report (miniplate anchorage), 361f-365f, 367f-372f
    with retrognathia, 365-367
  Class III
    case report, 205f-208f
    complicated by diabetes and end-stage renal disease, 4f
    Class III tendency and open bite, case report, 208f-211f
  as indication for skeletal anchorage in orthodontic treatment, 317, 319
  orthodontic treatment of, 167, 199-200, 200f. *See also* Anterior open bite; Deep bite; Dentoalveolar dysplasia; Occlusal plane correction.
  using miniplates, 317-341. *See also* Miniplate(s).
Mandible
  anteriorly directed force on, 365-367. *See also* Mandibular retrognathia.
  implantation sites in, 290-291
  miniplate implantation in
    procedure for, 325-326, 328f, 366-367
    sites for, 320, 366, 366f
  miniplate removal in, 326, 330f
  posteriorly directed force on, 367f, 369f-370f
  vascular supply of, 6, 8f
  whole arch movement/rotation of, 226, 226f
    case report, 269f-274f
Mandibular arch. *See also* Mandibular oblique ridge.
  anterior retraction and intrusion in, appliance design, 119, 120f, 177, 182f-183f, 188, 189f-190f, 263, 264f
  boundaries of tooth movement in, 173-174
  distractive lengthening of, 252
  molar distalization in, using miniplates, 321-322, 322f
  molar extrusion in, in vertical occlusal plane correction, 211-212
  molar intrusion in
    using miniplates, 323-324, 324f
    in vertical occlusal plane correction, 212-213

Mandibular arch—cont'd
  molar mesialization in, 224, 225f
  molar protraction in, using miniplates, 324-325, 326f
  sagittal occlusal plane correction in, 199-200, 200f
Mandibular micrognathia, Class II, LOMAS orthodontics in, 191, 193, 194f-195f
Mandibular oblique ridge, 168
  bone hardness in, 169-170, 170t, 171f
  as insertion site, 168, 169
  LOMAS miniscrew insertion procedure in, 169-173, 172f, 173f
Mandibular retrognathia, in Class II malocclusion, 365
  miniplate implantation in, 366, 366f
  treatment progression for, 366, 367f
Manual guide drill(s), short and long, 97, 98f
Manual predrilling, 97, 98f, 102, 289, 289f
MAPS. *See* Miniscrew-assisted push spring.
MARS. *See* Miniscrew-assisted root spring.
MAUS. *See* Miniscrew-assisted uprighting spring.
Maxilla
  implantation sites in, 289-290, 290f. *See also* Maxillary infrazygomatic crest; Zygomatic buttress.
  miniplate implantation sites in, 320, 325-326, 327f
  miniplate removal in, 326, 329f
  whole arch movement in, 225-226, 225f, 226f
Maxillary arch
  anterior retraction and intrusion in, with sliding mechanics, 262-263, 264f
  boundaries of tooth movement in, 173-174
  implantation sites in, 289-290, 290f. *See also* Maxillary infrazygomatic crest.
  molar distalization in, using miniplates, 320-321, 321f
  molar extrusion in, vertical occlusal plane correction, 211-212
  molar intrusion in
    using miniplates, 322-323, 323f
    vertical occlusal plane correction, 213-214
  molar mesialization in, 223-224, 224f
  molar protraction in, using miniplates, 324, 325f
Maxillary infrazygomatic crest, 168-169
  bone hardness of, 169-170, 170t, 171f
  as insertion site, 168-169, 393
  LOMAS miniscrew insertion procedure in, 169-172, 172f, 173f
  migration of implant in, 167-168
Maxillary sinus bone graft procedure, 5
Mechanical strength, determination of, 76. *See also* Finite element modeling (FEM) analysis.
Mechanically retained anchorage devices, 15, 73, 74b
  biological response to, 15t, 16
    bone vasculature, 6-7
    healing, 8, 10-11
  excessive loading of, 16

Mechanically retained anchorage devices—cont'd
  loading protocols for, 17, 18t
  and osseointegrated anchorage devices, distinction between, 16-17
  osseointegration of, studies of, 17
  site assessment for, 7-8, 16
  stability of, 11, 11f, 16
Mesial molar impaction, appliance mechanics in, 128-130. See also Molar extrusion (uprighting).
Mesialization, 156, 223
Mesioangulation. See Mesialization; Molar extrusion; Tipping.
Mesiodistal insertion path, of miniscrew, 101-102
Micro (prefix), definition of, 239
Micro-anchor implant, 238
Micro-anchorage system, 238
Micrognathia, Class II mandibular, LOMAS orthodontics in, 191, 193, 194f-195f
Microimplant(s), 238. See also **Miniscrew(s)/ microscrew(s)**.
  bracket head, for tooth movement in edentulous spaces, 243, 249
    case reports, 243f-245f, 246f-249f
  characteristic features and parts of, 238, 239f, 240f, 260-261, 261f
  definition of term, 239
  Dentos, 260-286. See also Absoanchor microscrew(s).
    with new screwdriver, 252, 253f, 254f
  diameter of, and implant stability, 76, 84f, 169. See also Diameter.
  with noninvasive miniplates, 249, 252
    case report, 250f-252f, 252
  orthodontic treatment using. See **Miniscrew(s)/ microscrew(s)**.
  references on, 258-259, 286
  resorbable, 239-243
  surgical implantation of, 261-262
Microimplant anchorage (MIA) sliding mechanics, 262
  with extraction treatment, 262-263, 262b, 264f
    case report, 265f-269f
  with nonextraction treatment, 269, 269b
    case report, 270f-274f
Micromotion, and postoperative bone remodeling, 11, 11f
Microscrew(s). See **Miniscrew(s)/microscrew(s)**.
Migration of miniscrew, 105, 107f
  avoiding root injury in, 168-169, 168f
  location of mini-implant and, 167-172
  under orthodontic loading, 167-168
Mini-dental implant, 238
Mini-dental screw, 238
Mini-implant(s), 3, 15f, 73, 74b, 238, 241
Mini-implant screw, 238
Mini-Screw Anchorage System (MAS), stress analysis of, 76

Miniplate(s), 73, 74b, 238, 343
  clinical trials of, and case reports, 74t
  Dentos, 252, 252f
    and corresponding microimplant, 252, 253f, 254f
  designs or types of, 252, 252f, 317, 320f
  with fixation screws, 15f, 249-252, 317, 320f
  Multipurpose Implant, 342-346. See also Multipurpose Implant.
  noninvasive, 249, 252, 252f
    in buccal segment intrusion, 151, 153, 153f, 154f
    locking mechanism on, for wire attachment, 152f, 159-160
    magnitude of force generation with, 148
    in molar distalization, 154-155, 155f
    in molar intrusion, 150
    in transverse occlusal plane correction, 250f-252f
  parts of, 317, 320f
  skeletal anchorage using, 342-343, 372. See also Multipurpose Implant; Zygoma implant (Surgi-Tech).
    implantation (fixation) procedure for, 325-326, 327f, 328f
    complications of, 326, 331
    indications for treatment with, 317, 319, 321, 322, 323
    in mandible, 365-367
    in molar distalization, 319, 320-322, 321f, 322f
    in molar intrusion, 322-324, 323f, 324f
    in molar protraction, 324-325, 325f, 326f
    references on, 372-373
    removal procedure for, 326, 329f, 330f
Miniscrew(s)/microscrew(s), 3-15, 73, 74b, 86-88, 238, 260-261, 342, 343. See also **Microimplant(s)**.
  Aarhus, 73-89. See also Aarhus Anchorage System.
  Absoanchor, 260-286. See also Absoanchor microscrew(s).
  animal studies of, 26, 28, 31f, 32. See also Animal studies.
  appliance design using, 74t. See also Appliance mechanics.
    in anterior retraction, 108-120, 154, 155f, 156-157, 157f. See also Anterior retraction, and intrusion.
    in buccal segment intrusion, 151-154. See also Buccal segment intrusion.
  clinical questions about, 6
  clinical trials of, and case reports, 74t. See also specific implant or orthodontic process.
    in edentulous space closure, 223-237. See also Edentulous space closure; Molar protraction.
    in molar distalization, 126-128, 154-156. See also Molar distalization.
    in molar extrusion (uprighting), 128-130
    in molar intrusion, 121-126, 149-151, 150f, 151f. See also Molar intrusion.
    in molar uprighting. See Molar extrusion.

Miniscrew(s)/microscrew(s)—cont'd
    in occlusal plane correction, 198-222. *See also* Occlusal plane correction.
    in rapid canine distalization, 252-256
  biological response to, 6-11, 15t, 16. *See also* Biological response.
  characteristics and design of, 10, 238, 239f, 240f
    Absoanchor, 260, 261f
    Orlus system, 94-95, 97, 97f
  Dentos, 260-286. *See also* Absoanchor microscrew(s).
    with new screw driver, 252, 253f, 254f
  development of, 3, 4-6, 14-15, 239
  diameter of, 95, 96f, 260, 288, 289t
    and implant stability, 76, 84f, 169
      modeling, 26, 28f, 29f, 30f, 31t
    and length, 95, 95f
  Dual Top Anchor, 287-294. *See also* Dual Top Anchor microscrew(s).
  failure of, 10, 104, 173, 193, 195, 286-288. *See also* Failure.
  forces applied with, 93-94, 94f. *See also* Appliance mechanics; Force system(s).
  healing and integration of, 8, 10-11. *See also* Biological response; Complications; Healing process.
  insertion of, 168-170, 168f. *See also* Insertion, of miniscrew(s).
  K-1 System, 49-72. *See also* K-1 System.
  laboratory testing of, 3-4
  LOMAS, 167-197. *See also* LOMAS (Lin/Liou Orthodontic Mini Anchor System).
  manufacturing improvements of, 4, 10. *See also* Titanium implants.
  mechanical features of, 95, 97, 97f, 238, 239f, 240f
  mechanics of, 25-32, 94f. *See also* Appliance mechanics; Finite element modeling (FEM) analysis.
  migration of, under orthodontic loading, 167-168. *See also* Migration of miniscrew.
  moderate force on, 93
  Orlus, 93-144. *See also* Orlus miniscrew system.
  Orlus system, 93-144
  osseointegrated, 4, 49-72. *See also* Osseointegrated anchorage devices.
  references on, 11-13, 47-48, 143-144, 195-197, 258-259, 294
  removal of, 102, 104. *See also specific implant.*
  removal torques for, 17, 17f, 160
  resorbable, 239-243. *See also* Resorbable microimplants.
  self-drilling and self-tapping, 10, 15. *See also* Self-drilling miniscrews.
  site assessment for, 7-8, 16, 25. *See also* Site assessment, and selection.
    in brachyfacial patient, 43-47
    in dolicofacial patient, 32-43

Miniscrew(s)/microscrew(s)—cont'd
  stability of, 4, 11, 11f, 16, 76, 169. *See also* Finite element modeling (FEM) analysis; Stability; Titanium implants.
  taper of, 10, 95, 96f, 238
  types of, and functions, 3, 4f, 10, 95, 97, 97f
Miniscrew assembly, 98f
Miniscrew-assisted push spring (MAPS), 128-129, 130f
Miniscrew-assisted root spring (MARS), 135, 135f
Miniscrew-assisted uprighting spring (MAUS), 129, 131f, 134-135, 135f
Miniscrew capsule, 98f
Missing teeth, 223. *See also* Edentulous space closure.
  acquired, 223
  appliance mechanics in patient(s) with, 223-237
    using bracket-head microimplants, case report, 243f-245f
    large overjet, 76, 77f-78f
    mandibular anterior retraction, case report, 246f-249f
    missing lateral incisors, case report, 229, 230f-232f
    missing mandibular bicuspids and deep bite, case report, 226-227, 227f-229f
    missing maxillary bicuspid, 233, 233f-236f
    molar mesialization, 223-224
    molar protraction, 134-135
    using noninvasive miniplates, 249, 250f-252f, 252
    using palatal implant, case report, 400f-403f
    references on, 236-237
    using resorbable screws, case report, 242f-243f
    whole arch movement, 224-226
  congenital, 223, 226
  and degenerated dentition
    appliance mechanics, 75, 75f-76f, 400f-403f
    as indication for skeletal anchorage, 319
Modeling, implant, 26, 27f, 28t. *See also* Animal studies; Finite element modeling (FEM) analysis.
Molar distalization, 126-128, 145, 154, 177
  appliance mechanics in, 126-128, 154-156
    using Absoanchor microimplants, 269, 269b, 270f-274f, 281f
    buccal miniscrew anchorage in, 126-128, 130f, 155
    direct and indirect anchorage in, 154, 184t
    using LOMAS, 184t, 185f
    using miniplate skeletal anchorage, 320-322, 321f, 322f, 356-359
    using Multipurpose Implant miniplate, 356, 357f, 358f-360f
    using noninvasive miniplates, 154-155, 155f
    using Orlus miniscrew system, 126-128
    using palatal implants, 154, 356, 380, 383f-384f
      case report, 385f-389f

Molar distalization—cont'd
    in sagittal occlusal plane correction, 199-201
        unilateral and bilateral, 127, 127f
    and extrusion, in vertical occlusal plane correction, 211-212, 212f
    in mixed dentition, appliance mechanics, 126-127
    in permanent dentition, appliance mechanics, 128, 128f, 129f
    rotational tendency in, preventing, 155-156
Molar extrusion (uprighting), 128-130, 274, 276
    using Absoanchor microimplants, case reports, 274f-276f
    eruptive, as indication for use of skeletal anchorage, 317, 319, 320f
    of impacted molar, 129, 131f
        case report, 132f-133f
    using joined microimplants, 276, 276f
    in mild mesial tipping, 128, 130f
    in moderate tipping, 128, 131f
    with one retromolar implant, 274, 274f-275f
    using Orlus miniscrew system, 128-130, 132f-133f
    per Y.C. Park, 211, 211f
    preprosthetic, 78f-79f
    in severe tipping, 128, 131f
    in vertical occlusal plane correction, 211-212, 211f, 212f
Molar intrusion, 149-151, 177
    appliance mechanics in, 121-126, 149-151, 150f, 184t
        using Absoanchor microimplants, case reports, 277f-280f
        of adjacent molars, 121, 124f
        on both sides of arch, 126, 126f
        using bracket head implant, 278, 278f-279f
        with buccal and palatal anchorage, 121, 122f, 126, 126f, 277, 277f-278f
        direct and indirect anchorage, 121, 123f, 149-150, 150f, 151f, 279
        using LOMAS, 184f, 184t
        using miniplates, 322-324, 323f, 324f
        using Orlus miniscrew system, 121-126
            case report, 124f-126f
        using palatal implant, 121, 122f, 150, 151f
        in patients with partial edentulism, 297
        of single molar, 121, 122f, 123f
    bone remodeling in, 174
    force magnitude necessary for, 148
    intrusive force control in, 149-150, 150f
    miniscrew insertion for, 149-150
    miniscrew(s) and insertion sites for, 121, 123f
    in vertical occlusal plane correction, 212-214
Molar mesialization, 156, 223
    buccal segment, using miniscrew implants, 201-202, 202f
    using coil springs and mini-implant, 78f-79f, 80f
    direct and indirect anchorage in, 156
    in mandible, 224, 225f

Molar mesialization—cont'd
    in maxilla, 223-224, 224f
    midline deviation in, 224
    using palatal implant, 380, 384f
Molar protraction, 134-135, 134f, 135f, 146, 147f, 148
    in limited anchorage, 135, 135f, 297, 308
    using miniplates, 324-325, 325f, 326f
Molar uprighting. *See* Molar extrusion (uprighting).
Moment/force (M/F) ratio, 118, 119f-120f
Monocortical fixation screws, 317, 320f
Movement
    of whole segments. *See* Anterior retraction, and intrusion; Buccal segment intrusion; Whole arch movement/rotation.
Mucoperiosteum, best method of opening, 7-8, 8f
Multipurpose Implant (MPI), 343, 343f
    molar distalization using, 356-359
        appliance construction, 357, 357f
        case report, 358f-360f
        treatment progress, 357
    placement sites for, on zygomatic buttress, 343, 343f, 344f
    removal of, 344, 346f
    surgical implantation of, 343-344, 345f
        complications of, 344
    use of, with Open Bite Appliance, 346-349
        case reports, 349f-354f, 355f-356f
Myofunctional therapy, 214

N

Nance button, 238, 374, 392
    miniscrew reinforced, in molar distalization, 127, 127f
Natural chewing gum, 348, 349f
NewTom 3G, 25
Nickel-titanium coil spring (wire), 153, 170f, 177, 264f
    in anterior retraction, 267f
    attached to hook screw or Quattro screw, 170f
    attached to Open Bite Appliance, 346, 347f
    compressed, in molar distalization using Multipurpose Implant, 357, 357f
    linear force applied by, 93, 94f
    in maxillary arch, in whole arch movement, 270, 272f
    in push-open coil spring-arm, 225-226, 226f
No head (NH) microimplant, 260, 261f
Nonintegrated miniscrews, 6. *See also* Mechanically retained anchorage devices.
Noninvasive miniplates, 249, 252, 252f
Nonosseointegrated implants, 342. *See also* Mechanically retained anchorage devices.

O

Oblique ridge, of mandible. *See* Mandibular oblique ridge.

Occlusal plane analysis
　dimensions in, 198
　for implant placement, 301, 303-304, 303f
Occlusal plane correction, 198-222. *See also* Malocclusion(s).
　anterior intrusion in, 154, 155f
　appliance mechanics in, 198-199, 199f
　canted, 211-215, 285f
　Class II, case report, 202f-205f
　Class III, case report, 205f-208f
　Class III tendency/open bite, case report, 208f-211f
　dimensions involved in, 198
　in edentulous patient, 296-297
　molar distalization in, 199-201
　molar extrusion in, 211-212
　molar intrusion in, 149-151, 212-214
　references on, 222
　in sagittal plane, appliance mechanics, 118, 199-202
　three dimensional, in treatment of anterior open bite, 218f-221f
　in transverse plane, appliance mechanics, 118, 118f, 214-217
　in vertical plane, appliance mechanics, 116, 116f, 117f, 118, 211-214
Occlusogingival insertion angle, 101, 101f
Occlusogram, 298, 300f, 301
Oligodontia, 223, 246f. *See also* Edentulous space closure; Missing teeth.
One-couple force system, 158-160. *See also* Cantilever.
Onplant(s), 73, 74b, 238, 343, 393
　case report, 74t
Open Bite Appliance, 346-349
　fabrication and application of, 346, 347f, 348
　retention methods after treatment with, 348, 349f
　treatment progress using, 348, 348f
Open bite correction. *See* Anterior open bite.
Orlus miniscrew(s), 95, 97, 97f
　characteristics of, 95, 96f, 97f
　diameter of, 95, 96f
　long-collared, 97, 97f
　standard (universal type) of, 95, 97f
　taper of, 95, 96f
　wide-collared, 95, 97f
Orlus miniscrew system, 93-94
　appliance design using, 93-94, 94f
　compared to conventional orthodontic mechanics, 116-118
　complications after insertion of, 105-108
　equipment required in (armamentarium), 97, 98f-99f, 99
　failure of, 104, 104f
　finite element analysis of, 94-95, 95f, 96f
　insertion procedure for, 99-102, 103f-104f
　　angle of insertion, 101, 101f
　　cortical bone penetration, 102
　　engine-driven hand piece, 102

Orlus miniscrew system—cont'd
　　in frenum area, 105, 106f
　　local anesthesia, 99
　　manual predrilling, 102
　　path of insertion, 101, 102f
　　site assessment and selection, 99-100, 99f, 100f
　　soft tissue management, 102
　　soft tissue penetration, 101
　mechanics of, 93, 94f, 118-120
　　in anterior retraction, and intrusion, 108-120
　　in molar distalization, 126-128
　　in molar extrusion (uprighting), 128-130
　　in molar intrusion, 121-126
　　in molar protraction, 134-135
　　in occlusal plane rotation, 116-118
　　in whole arch movement, 136, 136f-143f
　orthodontic treatment with, case reports, 110-143
　　for anterior open bite (whole arch movement), 136f-143f
　　Class II, Division 2 malocclusion, 110f-115f
　　for extruded molars (molar intrusion), 121-123, 124f-126f
　　for impacted lower molar, 129, 130f, 132f-133f
　predictable tooth movement using, 118-120
　removal procedure in, 102
　stability of, 104
　success rate, and failure of, 104
Ortho-anchor pin, 239
Ortho-anchor screw, 238
Orthodontic implants, 74b
Orthodontic-prosthetic implant anchorage (OPIA), 392. *See also* Straumann palatal implants.
　advantages and permanence of, 393
　indications for, 392-393
　limitations of, 393
Orthognathic-like tooth movement, 76, 84f, 167-169, 174, 177, 184t. *See also* Osseointegrated anchorage devices.
　appliance/system selection for, 148-162, 169, 317. *See also* Appliance mechanics; Miniplate(s); Miniscrew(s)/microscrew(s).
　factors considered in, 148-149
　boundaries of, 167, 173-174, 176f
　implant movement and, 167-168
　indications for, 76, 83f, 167, 174, 177, 317, 319
　non–tooth-bearing insertion sites in, 168-169, 168f
　predictable, 118-120
　rate of, and enhancement, 252-253
Orthopedic implants, 241. *See also* Prosthodontic restoration.
Orthoscrew, 239
Orthosystem palatal implant, 146, 146f, 287, 287f, 393-394. *See also* Straumann palatal implants.
　dimensions of, 375, 394t
Osseointegrated anchorage devices, 3, 6, 15-16, 15t, 73, 74b, 295, 342, 374. *See also specific anchorage system or implant.*

Osseointegrated anchorage devices—cont'd
  importance of, 6
  loading
    early, studies of, 17
      migration of device after, 167-168
      protocols for, 17, 18t
  and mechanically retained devices, distinction between, 16-17
  stability of, 16-17, 287
Osseointegration, 10-11, 15-16, 15t, 288f, 342, 393
  partial, 342
Osteoblast interface, with titanium surface, 15t, 16
Osteocyte response, to implant, 15, 15t
Osteogenesis. *See also* Bone remodeling.
  controlled, 304-305
  distraction, 252-253
    against submucosal screw, 84f
Osteonecrosis of jaw, bisphosphonate implication in, 18-19, 19f

P

Pacific (San Francisco), University of, 3-4
Pain, management of, 108
  after palatal implant surgery, 376
Palatal bars, of Open Bite Appliance, 347f, 348
Palatal implant(s), 3, 14, 15f, 73, 74b, 238, 343, 393-394. *See also* Friadent system implant; *Hyrax entries*; Orthosystem palatal implant; Straumann palatal implants; Transpalatal arch; Transpalatal bar; Transpalatal bar with hooks.
  appliance construction for, 380, 381f-382f, 394, 395f, 396
  appliance mechanics of, 380, 394, 395f, 396
    in anterior retraction, and intrusion, in limited anchorage, 398f-400f
    for en masse anterior retraction, 120f, 383f, 395f
      in Class II malocclusion, case report, 403f-406f
    in growing patients, 126-128, 375, 396
    indirect anchorage in, 146, 154, 393
    in molar distalization, 126-128, 154, 356, 383f-384f, 395f
      case report, 385f-389f
    in molar extrusion, 128-130
    in molar intrusion, 121, 122f, 126f, 150, 151f, 395f
    in molar mesialization, 384f, 395f
    in whole arch movement/rotation, case reports, 136f, 139f, 406f-411f
  histologic section of, after removal, 398f
  indications for, 394, 395f
  mucosal shaping for, 376, 379f
  open versus closed surgery for, 389-390
  for orthodontic treatment in hypodontia and apical root resorption, case report, 400f-403f
  osseointegration period for, 376, 394
  pendulum appliance on, 127, 127f, 395f, 398f
  placement of, 168, 289, 290f, 374, 394

Palatal implant(s)—cont'd
  evaluation of, 376-377, 379, 379f, 396f
  guidelines for, 375b
  median or paramedian, 375
  precautions for, 374-375
  radiography in determining, 374, 375, 376f
  references on, 390-391, 411-412
  removal of, 379, 380f, 389, 389f
  success rate of, 389-390
  surgical insertion of Friadent, 376, 378f-379f, 389-390
    safe removal of implant carrier after, 379, 380f
  surgical insertion of Straumann, 394, 397f
  template construction for surgical placement of, 375-376, 376f, 377f
Palatal/lingual root torque, 177
Palate
  bone height evaluation of, 374, 375, 375b
  hard, bone thickness in, 374
  implant placement in, 168, 289, 290f, 374, 393. *See also* Palatal implant(s).
    guidelines for, 375b
    median or paramedian, 375, 393
    precautions for, 374-375
Panoramic radiographs, for site assessment, 7, 8f-9f, 25, 26f. *See also specific implant and case report.*
Partial osseointegration, 342
Passive extrusion, 276f
Pearl, 213f, 214
Pediatric craniofacial surgery, in development of anchorage devices, 239
Pendulum appliance, fixed palatal, 395f, 396, 398f
  in molar distalization, 127, 127f
Peptides, injection of biologically active, 253
Periapical radiographs, accuracy of, for site assessment, 7-8
Periodontal dressing, 172, 173f
Periodontal probe, 97, 99, 99f
Periodontally compromised teeth, anchorage in patient with, 284f
Periosteum, disruption of, and compromise of venous return, 6-7, 8f
Periotest, 97, 99
Pilot drilling. *See* Predrilling.
Pin(s), 238, 239
Piriform rim, miniplate fixation in, 320
Placement, of anchorage device. *See* Site assessment, and selection.
PLGA 75/25, 242
Polyglycolic acid (PGA), and polylactic acid (PLA), 239-241
  biodegradation of, 241-242
  copolymers of, 242
Posterior intrusion. *See* Molar intrusion.
Posterior intrusion and distalization. *See* Molar distalization.
Posterior open bite, 116, 116f, 117f, 118f

Power arm. *See* Extended arm(s).
Predrilling
   and bone hardness, 169-170, 170t, 171f, 172
   infection problems in, 88
   manual, 97, 98f, 102, 289, 289f
   procedure for, 261-262, 263f, 289
Primary stability, 16
   and failure of implant, 76, 78, 86
   studies of, 76, 78
Prosthetic implants, 3. *See also* Prosthodontic restoration.
Prosthodontic restoration, 295-313
   alveolar bone augmentation in, 304-306
   alveolar bone ridge analysis in, 304
   anterior spacing as indication for, 295, 296f
   financial considerations in, 295-296
   fixed bridges or implant use in, 296-297
   loading implants in, 307
   mechanics of, 307-312
   occlusal plane analysis for implant placement in, 301, 303-304
   occlusion improvement in, 295-296, 310, 312
   placement planning in, 298, 299f
   space restoration in, 310, 312, 312f
   temporary anchorage or dental implant use in, 297
   three-dimensional visualization of, 298, 300f, 301, 301f-302f
   treatment planning in, 297-298
Protraction headgear, using noninvasive miniplates, 148
Protraction of molars, anchorage devices for, 145. *See also* Molar protraction.
Pseudoperiodontium, 5, 6, 49
Push-open coil spring-arm, 224, 225-226, 225f, 226f

Q

Quad Helix screw, 214
Quattro screw, LOMAS, 169, 170f

R

Radiographic analysis software, 25
Radiography. *See also* Cone-beam computed tomography, *or specific case reports.*
   lateral cephalogram, 375, 376f
   panoramic, 7
   periapical, 7
Rapid canine retraction, procedures for, 253
Rapid maxillary expansion, with palatal implant appliance, 136f, 139f, 395f, 396
Reactive forces. *See* Adverse reactive forces; Tipping.
Regional acceleratory phenomenon (RAP), 10-11, 10f
   in bone scintillation scans, 11
Relapse
   of deep bite, in brachycephalic woman, 5f
   of intrusion, in anterior open bite orthodontics, 176f, 193, 195

Removal, of miniscrew(s), 102, 104, 239, 289. *See also specific implant.*
   torques in, 17, 17f, 160
Resorbable microimplants, 239-241, 243
   biocompatibility of, 241-242
   case reports of orthodontics using, 242f-243f
Retraction, 149. *See also* Anterior retraction.
   in mandible and maxilla, boundaries of tooth movement, 173-174
Retrognathia. *See* Mandibular retrognathia.
Retromolar implants, 3, 15f, 73, 74b, 238, 343, 393
   indications for, 75
Ricketts' chart, for force magnitude calculation, 348, 348t
Ricketts-Grummons analysis, 214
Rigid fixation, problems associated with, 239
Root injury
   location of implant and, 167-173
   noninvasive miniplates in avoiding, 151, 153f
   during orthodontic treatment, 105, 107f, 291
      avoiding, 168-169, 168f
   in palatal implantation, 374-375
Root movement, 149
   of incisors, 118-119, 119f
   in limited anchorage, 310, 311f
   of molars, 134-135, 134f, 135f
   and translation, 135, 135f
Root surface area(s), comparisons of, 108, 108f

S

Sagittal occlusal plane correction, 118, 199
   in mandible, 199-200
   in maxilla, 200-202
   using miniscrew implant, case reports, 202-211
Sam II articulator, 198
Screwdriver assembly(ies), 98f, 99f
Screwdriver positioning, correct and incorrect, 87f, 88
Screwdriver tip(s), short and long, 97, 98f
Segmented arch technique, 118
Self-drilling miniscrews, 10, 15, 169, 261. *See also* Aarhus Anchorage System; Dual Top Anchor microscrew(s); K-1 System; LOMAS; Orlus miniscrew system.
   excessive pressure on, results of, 86
   procedure for, 261-262, 262f
Self-reinforcing technique, of Rokkanen and Törmälä, 241
Self-tapping miniscrews, 8, 10, 15, 261, 288f
Sentalloy coil spring, on Aarhus mini-implant, 85f
   asymmetric tooth movement using, 81f-82f
   molar mesialization using, 78f-79f, 80f
SH. *See* Small head (SH) microimplant.
SimPlant software, 25
Site assessment, and selection, 7-8, 10, 16, 25, 88, 148, 289, 393. *See also specific implant or orthodontic process.*
   in brachyfacial patient, 43, 44f-47f

Site assessment, and selection—cont'd
  depending on anchorage types, 108, 109f-110f, 110
  in dolicofacial patient, 32, 33f-43f, 34
  for miniscrew insertion, 99-101. See also Insertion, of miniscrew.
  for orthodontic/prosthodontic treatment, 298
  radiography and computed tomography in, 7-8
Skeletal anchorage
  using miniplates, 73, 74b, 238, 317-341
    clinical trials, and case reports, 74t
    designs or types of, 317, 320f
    implantation (fixation) procedure for, 325-326, 327f, 328f
      complications of, 326, 331
    implantation sites for, 317, 320, 320f
    indications for treatment with, 317, 319, 321, 322, 323
    in molar distalization, 319, 320-322, 321f, 322f
    in molar intrusion, 322-324, 323f, 324f
    in molar protraction, 324-325, 325f, 326f
    removal procedure for, 326, 329f, 330f
  using miniscrews, 3-15, 73, 74b, 86-88, 238, 260-261, 342, 343. See also Miniscrew(s)/microscrew(s).
  using Multipurpose Implant (MPI), 342-360
    in molar distalization, 356-359
      appliance construction, 357, 357f
      case report, 358f-360f
      clinical treatment progress, 357
    with Open Bite Appliance, 346-349
      case reports, 349f-354f, 355f-356f
    placement sites for, on zygomatic buttress, 343, 343f, 344f
    removal of, 344, 346f
    surgical implantation of, 343-344, 345f
      complications of, 344
    palatal, 374-391, 392-412. See also Palatal implant(s).
  using zygoma implant (Surgi-Tech), 361-365
Skeletal deficiencies. See Alveolar bone.
Skeletal open bite, 345
SLA surface, 394
  bioactive, 307
Sliding mechanics
  with extraction treatment, 262-264
  versus loop mechanics, 116-118, 116f, 117f, 156-157
  with miniscrews, 116, 117f
  with nonextraction treatment, 269
Small head (SH) microimplant, 260, 261f
Soft tissue
  coverage of implant by
    miniplates, 326, 331
    miniscrews, 86, 87f, 102, 105, 105f, 172
    Multipurpose Implant, 344
  inflammation of, 105, 105f, 150, 151f

Soft tissue—cont'd
  management of, during insertion of miniscrew, 102, 172
  penetration of, 102
    with tissue punch, 7-8, 8f, 169-170, 171f
    periodontal dressing of, to prevent embedding, 172, 173f
Space closure. See Edentulous space closure.
Springs. See Coil spring(s).
Stability, implant, 4, 11, 11f, 16, 76, 78, 99. See also Failure, of implant anchorage; Finite element modeling (FEM) analysis.
  of Aarhus Anchorage System, 76, 84f
  after osseointegration, 16
  and diameter of miniscrew, 76, 84f, 95, 96f, 169
    modeling, 26, 28f, 29f, 30f, 31t
  factors critical in, 99, 104
  in mechanical retention, 11, 11f, 16
  primary, 76, 78, 86
  studies of, 76, 78, 84-88, 287-288, 374
  titanium and, 11, 16, 76, 169. See also Titanium implants.
Stainless steel. See Surgical steel screws.
Standard miniscrew, 95, 97f
Stationary anchorage, 374
Stent preparation. See Surgical guide (stent) preparation.
Straumann, implant surface developed by, 307
Straumann palatal implants, 146, 146f, 287, 287f, 393-394
  appliance construction for, 394, 395f, 396, 398f
  appliance mechanics using, 394, 395f, 396
    for anterior retraction, and intrusion, in limited anchorage, case report, 398f-400f
    for en masse anterior retraction in Class II malocclusion, case report, 403f-406f
  indirect anchorage in, 146, 154, 393
  in molar distalization, 154, 395f
  in molar intrusion, 150, 151f, 395f
    for orthodontic treatment in hypodontia and apical root resorption, case report, 400f-403f
    for whole arch movement/rotation, case report, 406f-411f
  dimensions of, 375, 394t
  osseointegration period for, 394
  placement of, 394, 396f
  removal procedure for, 394, 398f
  surgical insertion procedure for, 394, 397f
Stress analysis. See Finite element modeling (FEM) analysis.
Superelastic open coil, 292f
Surgical guide (stent) preparation, 25, 304
  for K-1 system implantation, 50, 53f, 58, 61f
  for palatal implant, 375-376, 376f, 377, 377f, 379
Surgical placement, of mini/microimplant. See Insertion, of miniscrew(s); Miniplate(s); Palatal implant(s).

Surgical steel screws, 76
  compared to titanium screws, stress analysis, 76
  and plates, 238, 342

T

T-plate(s), 317, 320f
  orthodontic fixation of, 320
TADs. *See* Temporary anchorage devices.
Taper, of miniscrews, 10, 95, 96f, 238, 241f
Tatum, Hilt, 4, 5
Template construction. *See also* Diagnostic wax-up; Surgical guide (stent) preparation.
  for palatal implant, 375-376, 376f, 377f, 378f
Temporary anchorage devices (TADs), 3, 14, 25, 49, 73, 93, 238, 287, 392
  appliances included in, 3
  biological response to, 6-10, 14-21. *See also* Biological response; Healing process.
  classification of, 15-16, 15f, 15t, 73, 73b, 74b
  clinical studies/case reports on, 73, 74t. *See also specific implant or system.*
  contraindication to, in patients taking bisphosphonates, 19, 19f
  definition of, 3
  direct or indirect anchorage of, 146, 151-159, 198-199, 199f, 393. *See also specific orthodontic process or appliance.*
  distinction between osseointegrated and mechanically retained, 16-17
  drugs affecting implantation of, 18-19
  evaluation and planning in use of, 25-48, 74-75, 145-146, 297. *See also* Brachyfacial patient; Dolicofacial patient; Site assessment.
  failure of, 10, 11, 16, 76, 78. *See also* Failure.
  historical development of, 3, 4-6, 14-15, 295, 342, 392
  indications for, 73, 76, 83f, 167, 174, 177, 319
    alternative to surgery, 76, 83f, 167, 174, 177
    asymmetric tooth movement, 76, 81f-82f
    avoiding adverse reactive forces, 76, 78f-79f, 80f
    bone generation for dental implant, 76, 84f
    insufficient teeth for conventional anchorage, 76, 77f-78f
  loading protocols for, 17, 18t
  mechanically retained, 3-13, 15t, 16. *See also* Mechanically retained anchorage devices.
  mechanics of, 93-144, 145-163, 177, 184t. *See also* Appliance mechanics.
    modeling, 25-32. *See also* Animal studies; Finite element modeling (FEM) analysis.
  nomenclature of, 238-239
  orthodontic treatment strategies using. *See specific clinical condition.*
  osseointegrated, 3, 6, 15-16, 15t, 73, 74b. *See also* Osseointegrated anchorage devices.
  site assessment for, 7-8, 16, 25, 32-48. *See also* Site assessment.

Temporary anchorage devices (TADs)—cont'd
  stability of, 11, 11f, 16, 76, 78. *See also* Stability.
  systems using
    Aarhus mini-implant, 73-89. *See also* Aarhus Anchorage System.
    Absoanchor, 260-286. *See also* Absoanchor microscrew(s).
    K-1 System, 49-72. *See also* K-1 System.
    LOMAS, 167-197. *See also* LOMAS (Lin/Liou Orthodontic Mini Anchor System).
    Orlus miniscrew system, 93-144. *See also* Orlus miniscrew system.
    Orthosystem, 287-294. *See also* Orthosystem.
  treatment strategies using. *See also* Appliance mechanics, *or specific orthodontic condition.*
    in edentulous patients, 295-313. *See also* Prosthodontic restoration.
    for orthognathic-like results, 49-72, 167-197, 198-222. *See also* Dentoalveolar dysplasia; Dentoalveolar protrusion; Malocclusion(s); Occlusal plane correction; Temporomandibular disorder; Whole arch movement/rotation.
    in patients with missing teeth, 223-237. *See also* Edentulous patients; Edentulous space closure; Missing teeth.
Temporary crown, 307
Titanium-Molybdenum Archwire (TMA), 276f, 290f
Temporary orthodontic attachments, 3
Temporomandibular disorder
  K-1 System in orthodontic treatment of, case report, 50, 54, 54f
    assessment, 50, 51f, 52f
    cone-beam CT imaging before second surgery, 50, 54f
    osseointegration of implant, 50, 53f
    posttreatment analyses, 55-58, 57f
    pretreatment evaluation, 51f, 52f
    stent preparation for surgery, 50, 53f
    symptom alleviation with splint therapy, 50
    treatment progression, 50, 54, 55f
    vertical traction application, 50, 54, 55f
  miniplate-based orthodontic treatment of, case report, 331f-341f
    assessment, and treatment goals, 331f, 334f-335f
    posttreatment analyses, 338f-341f
    pretreatment analyses, 332f-334f
    treatment progression, 335f, 336f-337f
TFO (trauma from occlusion), 276f
Three-dimensional computed tomography. *See* Cone-beam computed tomography.
Three-dimensional treatment planning, 298, 300f, 301, 301f-302f
Tip moments, 16
Tipping, 149
  during buccal segment intrusion, prevention of, 153, 154f, 213, 213f

Tipping—cont'd
  controlled, 118, 119f, 149
  lingual, prevention of, 263, 264f
  molar, orthodontic correction of, 126-130, 276f. See also Molar extrusion.
  uncontrolled, 149
Tissue punch, use of, 7-8, 8f, 169, 171f
Titanium alloy(s), 3, 4, 288. See also Nickel-titanium coil spring; Sentalloy.
Titanium implants, 3, 14, 169, 239, 249, 295
  manufacture of, 4, 10
  palatal, 393-394
  stability and failure rate of, 11, 11f, 16, 76, 169
Toe-in bends, necessity of, 116
Torque gauge, 97
Torque spring, conventional, side effects of, 118, 119f
TPA. See Transpalatal arch.
Transitional implant, 239
Translation (translatory movement), 108, 148, 148f
  in buccal segment intrusion, force systems for, 151, 153f
  incisor, force systems for, 119, 119f, 120f
  molar, force systems for, 135, 135f
Transpalatal arch (TPA), 149-150, 177
  attached to temporary implant, in prosthodontics, 307, 308f, 309, 310f
  with bar and hooks, in occlusal plane correction, 198-199, 199f. See also Transpalatal bar with hooks.
  construction of, for palatal implant
    Friadent, 380, 381f-382f
    Straumann palatal implant, 394, 395f, 396
  in limited anchorage
    mesial forces applied with, 309-310, 310f, 311f
    retractive and intrusive forces applied with, 308f, 309, 310f
  in molar distalization, appliance designs, 127, 128f, 129f
  in molar intrusion, appliance designs, 126, 126f, 149-150, 150f
  in tipping prevention during buccal segment intrusion, 153, 154f
  in unilateral expansion, appliance design, 157, 158f
Transpalatal bar, 146, 146f
  for maintaining archform, in anterior retraction, 262-263, 264f, 267f
  modification of
    for mesialization of maxillary molars, 223-224, 224f
    for molar distalization, 281, 281f
    for whole arch movement/rotation, 225-226, 225f, 226f
Transpalatal bar with hooks, 200-201
  conversion to extended arm device, 201f
  with midpalatal miniscrew, 201f
  miniscrew connection to, 201f
  miniscrew placement with, 201f

Transpalatal bar with hooks—cont'd
  modifications of, for molar extrusion in maxilla, 211-212, 212f
  molar distalization using, 200-201
  molar extrusion and distalization using, 212f
  one-sided molar extrusion using, 212f
Transverse expansion. See Transverse occlusal plane correction.
Transverse occlusal plane correction, 118, 118f, 145, 157, 214
  bilateral expansion in, 214, 216f
  direct and indirect anchorage in, 157, 157f, 158f
  in limited skeletal anchorage, case report, 250f-252f
  unilateral expansion in, 214, 217f
Trauma from occlusion (TFO), 276f
Traumatic dental injury, 223
Treatment strategies. See also Appliance mechanics, or specific orthodontic condition..
  in edentulous patients, 295-313. See also Prosthodontic restoration.
  for orthognathic-like results, 49-72, 167-197, 198-222. See also Dentoalveolar dysplasia; Dentoalveolar protrusion; Malocclusion(s); Occlusal plane correction; Temporomandibular disorder; Whole arch movement/rotation.
  in patients with missing teeth, 223-237. See also Edentulous patients; Edentulous space closure; Missing teeth.

U

Ulceration, of buccal mucosa, 105, 105f
Unilateral expansion appliances, 214, 217f
Universal miniscrew, 95, 97f
Uprighting. See Molar extrusion.

V

Vertical dimension of occlusion (VDO), increasing, 6, 7f
Vertical occlusal plane correction, 116, 116f, 117f, 118, 211-215
  mandibular molar extrusion in, 211, 211f
  mandibular molar intrusion in, 212-213
  maxillary molar extrusion in, 211-212, 212f
  maxillary molar intrusion in, 213-214
  myofunctional therapy in, 214
Visualized treatment objective (VTO), 298, 301f
  importance of, in predicting occlusal plane changes, 303-304
Vitallium. See Cobalt-chromium alloy.
Vitreous screws, 238

W

Wax-up, diagnostic, 298, 300f, 301, 301f-302f
Whole arch movement/rotation, 224. See also Anterior retraction, and intrusion.
  in closing edentulous spaces, 224-226
  in mandible, 226, 226f

Whole arch movement/rotation—cont'd
　　in maxilla, 225-226, 225f, 226f
　　in maxilla and mandible, case report, 269f-274f
　　　　placement of microimplants and arches, 272f
　　in occlusal plane correction, 198-222. *See also*
　　　　Malocclusion(s); Occlusal plane correction.
　　using Orlus miniscrew system, case report,
　　　　136f-143f
　　using Straumann palatal implant, case report,
　　　　406f-411f
Wide-collared miniscrew, 95, 97f
Wire-receiving attachment, on Aarhus mini-implant,
　　85f

Y

Y-plate(s), 317, 320f
　　fixation of, 320
　　　　in maxillary molar distalization, 321, 321f
　　　　in maxillary molar intrusion, 323, 323f

Z

Zygoma implant (Surgi-Tech), 361, 361f
　　case report of treatment with, 362f-365f
　　mechanics of, 361, 361f
Zygoma ligatures, for anterior retraction and intrusion,
　　75, 75f-76f
Zygomatic buttress, 343f
　　implant anchorage in. *See also* Multipurpose
　　　　Implant; Zygoma implant (Surgi-Tech).
　　implantation (fixation) procedure for, 325-326,
　　　　327f, 328f
　　complications of, 326, 331
　　indications for, 317, 319, 321, 322, 323
　　in molar distalization, 319, 320-322, 321f, 322f
　　in molar intrusion, 322-324, 323f, 324f
　　in molar protraction, 324-325, 325f, 326f
　　removal procedure for, 326, 329f, 330f
　　miniplate fixation sites in, 320, 321f, 325-326, 327f
Zygomatic wires, 238, 343